ACLS
STUDY GUIDE

Third Edition

ACLS
STUDY GUIDE

Third Edition

Barbara Aehlert, RN, BSPA
Southwest EMS Education, Inc.
Phoenix, Arizona/Pursley, Texas

MOSBY JEMS

ELSEVIER

MOSBY JEMS
ELSEVIER

11830 Westline Industrial Drive
St. Louis, Missouri 63146

Notice

Knowledge and best practice in this field are constantly changing. As new research and experience broaden our knowledge, changes in practice, treatment and drug therapy may become necessary or appropriate. Readers are advised to check the most current information provided (i) on procedures featured or (ii) by the manufacturer of each product to be administered, to verify the recommended dose or formula, the method and duration of administration, and contraindications. It is the responsibility of the practitioner, relying on their own experience and knowledge of the patient, to make diagnoses, to determine dosages and the best treatment for each individual patient, and to take all appropriate safety precautions. To the fullest extent of the law, neither the Publisher nor the Author assumes any liability for any injury and/or damage to persons or property arising out or related to any use of the material contained in this book.

The Publisher

ISBN-13: 978-0-323-04695-4
ISBN-10: 0-323-04695-9

Executive Editor: Linda Honeycutt
Developmental Editor: Katherine Tomber
Publishing Services Manager: Julie Eddy
Project Manager: Gail Michaels
Text Designer: Jyotika Shroff

Printed in Canada

Last digit is the print number: 9 8 7 6 5 4 3 2

DEDICATED

to
my father, Bobby R. Mahoney,
for your inspiration, guidance, love, and support

and
in loving memory of
my grandfather, John Dallas Mahoney,

and uncles,
William Jarrell Mahoney and Donald C. Mahoney

Preface to Third Edition

The *ACLS Study Guide* is designed for use by paramedic, nursing, and medical students, ECG monitor technicians, nurses, and other allied health personnel working in emergency departments, critical care units, post-anesthesia care units, operating rooms, and telemetry units preparing for an Advanced Cardiac Life Support provider course.

The third edition of this book is based on the following science, treatment recommendations, and guidelines:

- 2005 International Consensus Conference on Cardiopulmonary Resuscitation and Emergency Cardiovascular Care Science with Treatment Recommendations hosted by the American Heart Association in Dallas, Texas, January 23–30, 2005, *Circulation* 112: III-5-III-16, 2005, and *Resuscitation* 67(supp 1): S1-S190, December 2005. © 2005 International Liaison Committee on Resuscitation, American Heart Association, Inc. and European Resuscitation Council.

- 2005 American Heart Association Guidelines for Cardiopulmonary Resuscitation and Emergency Cardiovascular Care, *Circulation* 112:IV-1-211, 2005. © 2005 American Heart Association, Inc.

- Other evidence-based treatment recommendations or sources are cited in the reference section of relevant chapters.

This book is designed for use with the American Safety and Health Institute (ASHI) Advanced Cardiac Life Support provider course. ASHI is a collaborating organization of the National First Aid Science Advisory Board cofounded by the American Red Cross and American Heart Association, Inc., and a participant in the International Committee on Resuscitation (ILCOR) 2005 International Conference on Cardiopulmonary Resuscitation and Emergency Cardiovascular Care Science with Treatment Recommendations, hosted by the American Heart Association, Inc. This book may be used as supplemental material by participants of ACLS courses offered by other organizations.

This book consists of two primary sections. The first section of this book, Chapters 1 through 8, provides the "why," "when," and "how" for the case studies in the second section. Each chapter contains instructional objectives, quick review questions throughout the chapter, and a chapter quiz. Answers and rationales are provided for all multiple-choice questions in this text, including those in the 50-question pretest and posttest.

It has been proven that in order to learn how to do something, you must actually *do* it. The opportunity to "do" the skills taught in an ACLS course and make decisions regarding patient care is provided by 10 "core" case studies in an ACLS provider course. A sample case study has been provided for each of the standard "core" cases presented in an ACLS course. The case studies are not intended to cover every possible dysrhythmia that may be presented in an actual ACLS course. Rather, they are provided as examples to help you understand the information presented in the preparatory section of the text. To help you prepare for the ACLS course, each case study includes a scenario sheet that represents dialogue between an ACLS "coach" and team leader. This has been done to simulate the interaction between an ACLS instructor and student (team leader) in an ACLS course. After you have read each of the case studies, ask another person to assist you by assuming the role of the "coach."

Every attempt has been made to provide information that is consistent with current literature, including current resuscitation guidelines. However, medicine is a dynamic field. Resuscitation guidelines change, new medications and technology are being developed, and medical research is ongoing. As a result, be sure to learn and follow local protocols as defined by your medical advisors. The author and publisher assume no responsibility or liability for loss or damage resulting from the use of information contained within.

I hope you find this text helpful. If you have comments or suggestions about how I could improve this text, please visit my web site (http://www.swemsed.com) and drop me a line. I would like to hear from you.

Best regards,

Barbara Aehlert

Acknowledgments

I took my first ACLS class many years ago. I was terrified (and lost) throughout the entire course. Although I spent weeks studying before the course, the information I read seemed to me to be written in a foreign language. I could find no resources to "translate" the information into something that was useful to me. The course consisted of very long lectures by instructors who read slides and offered little useful insight. The most memorable part of the course was the "patient management" station in which each course participant was evaluated one-on-one by an instructor. (For those of you who have been around a while, you are probably having flashbacks of those days). I will *never* forget that experience.

Despite the time spent studying, as soon as the door closed behind me I was a mental wreck. The instructor proceeded to methodically strip away any self-confidence I might have had in treating a patient who had a cardiac-related emergency. I was able to answer the questions asked of me until I was presented with a patient who had asymptomatic bradycardia. Atropine had not worked (transcutaneous pacing was not a readily available option that many years ago), and the next drug that was recommended at that time was isoproterenol. I knew that. What I could not recall was whether isoproterenol was given in mcg/min (correct) or mg/min. I took a "50/50" guess and said mg/min. Since that was the wrong decision, I was told I had failed the course and would need to schedule myself to attend another 2-day class.

Before driving home, I sat outside for a few minutes contemplating what had happened and what I could have done to change the outcome. On that day, I made a promise to myself that I would become an ACLS instructor someday and find a way to teach the information in a more user-friendly atmosphere. I promised myself that I would be a part of teaching courses that were useful to practicing healthcare professionals and delivered in an environment in which the participants looked forward to the class—instead of dreading it. Although I was an instructor and regional faculty for another organization for many years, I found my "home" with the American Safety and Health Institute.

My sincerest thanks to Andrew Allen, Linda Honeycutt, Laura Bayless, and Katherine Tomber for their advice, encouragement, and the resources necessary to complete this project. Thanks to the manuscript reviewers who provided insightful comments and suggestions.

A special thanks to these instructors who share the same philosophy about teaching ACLS as I do: Andrew Baird, CEP; Eileen Blackstone, CEP; Lynn Browne-Wagner, RN; Ken Bruck, CEP; Randy Budd, CEP; Thomas Cole, CEP; Mike Connor, CEP; Bob Dotterer, CEP; David Farrow, CEP; Cathy Griggs, RN: Paul Honeywell, CEP; Willadine Hughes, RN: Bill Loughran, RN; Sean Newton, CEP; Jason Payne, CEP; Jeff Pennington, CEP; Greg Ruiz, CEP; Jeanne Shepard, CEP; Gary Smith, MD; David Stockton, CEP; Ed Tirone, CEP; Nicky Treece, RN: and Maryalice Witzel, RN.

Publisher Acknowledgments

The editors wish to acknowledge and thank the many reviewers of this book, who devoted countless hours to intensive review. Their comments were invaluable in helping develop and fine-tune the manuscript.

Tom Bausman, BS, NREMT-P, I/C, T, W
USAF Pararescueman, Retired
Tier One EMT, Inc.
Twin Falls, Idaho

Jeffrey K. Benes, BS, NREMT-P
Owner/Consultant/Educator
Jeff Benes Company
Antioch, Illinois

Kristen D. Borchelt, NREMT-P
Paramedic
Cincinnati Children's Hospital
Cincinnati, Ohio

Robert Joseph Carter, EMT-P
Law Enforcement Instructor
Emergency Services Section – United States Secret Service
Washington, DC

Thomas P. Fogarty III
Training Center Coordinator
George Washington University
Department of Emergency Medicine
Washington, DC

Fidel O. Garcia, EMT-P
EMS Education Coordinator
St. Mary's Hospital
Grand Junction, Colorado

J. Hudson Garrett Jr., MSN, MPH, CCRN
President and CEO
Community Health Associates, LLC
Atlanta, Georgia

Karen F. Marlowe, PharmD, BCPS
Associate Professor
Auburn University, Harrison School of Pharmacy
Auburn, Alabama

Joanne McCall, RN, BS, MA, CEN, SANE-A
Emergency Department Nurse Educator
Providence Park Hospital
Novi, Michigan

Christine C. McEachin, RN, BSN, CEN, Paramedic/IC
Clinical Nurse Specialist – Emergency Services
William Beaumont Hospital, Troy
Troy, Michigan

Lynn Pierzchalski-Goldstein, RPh, BS Pharm, PharmD
Emergency Medicine Specialist
William Beaumont Hospital
Royal Oak, Michigan

Sandie L. Sanders, RN
Emergency Department
The Toledo Hospital
Toledo, Ohio

Howard A. Werman, MD, FACEP
Professor of Clinical Emergency Medicine
The Ohio State University
Columbus, Ohio
Medical Director
MedFlight of Ohio
Columbus, Ohio

About the Author

Barbara Aehlert, RN, BSPA, is the President of Southwest EMS Education, Inc. in Phoenix, Arizona and Pursley, Texas. She has been a registered nurse for more than 30 years with clinical experience in medical/surgical and critical care nursing and, for the past 20 years, in prehospital education. Barbara is an active CPR, First Aid, Paramedic, ACLS, and PALS instructor and takes a special interest in teaching basic dysrhythmia recognition and ACLS to nurses and paramedics. She is a consultant with the Southwest Ambulance, Mesa, Arizona paramedic program and an active member of the Pursley, Texas Volunteer Fire Department.

Contents

Pretest

1. The drug of choice for most forms of narrow-QRS tachycardia is:
   a. Amiodarone
   b. Atropine
   c. Adenosine
   d. Epinephrine

2. Vasopressin may be used in the management of:
   a. Symptomatic first-degree atrioventricular block
   b. Ventricular fibrillation
   c. Narrow-QRS tachycardia
   d. Atrial fibrillation with a rapid ventricular response

3. Which of the following could be administered endotracheally if necessary?
   a. Amiodarone, dopamine, procainamide, naloxone, and adenosine
   b. Naloxone, atropine, vasopressin, epinephrine, and lidocaine
   c. Lidocaine, amiodarone, procainamide, vasopressin, and naloxone
   d. Procainamide, epinephrine, lidocaine, adenosine, and dopamine

4. The most common side effects of giving amiodarone are:
   a. Nausea and asystole
   b. Bradycardia and hypotension
   c. AV block and hypertension
   d. Blurred vision and abdominal pain

5. A 75-year-old man has suffered a cardiac arrest. The arrest was not witnessed. CPR is in progress. The cardiac monitor reveals ventricular fibrillation. A monophasic waveform defibrillator is available to you. Your next action will be to:
   a. Deliver three stacked shocks using 200, 300, and 360 joules after 5 cycles (about 2 minutes) of CPR
   b. Give a 2.5- to 5-mg IV bolus of verapamil over 3 minutes
   c. Deliver a single shock using 360 joules after 5 cycles of CPR and then immediately resume CPR
   d. Give magnesium sulfate 1 to 2 g IV over 10 minutes

6. Which of the following approaches is recommended during an <u>initial</u> patient evaluation?
   a. Oxygen, IV, monitor
   b. Level of responsiveness, airway, breathing, circulation, defibrillation if necessary
   c. Temperature, pulse, respirations, blood pressure
   d. Oxygen, IV fluid challenge, vital signs, level of responsiveness

7. A 37-year-old woman is complaining of shortness of breath and palpitations. You have placed the patient on oxygen and an IV has been established. Her mental status is rapidly decreasing and she is very pale. Her initial blood pressure was 148/70. It is now 62/38. Breathing is shallow at 8 to 12 breaths/minute. The cardiac monitor shows the following rhythm:

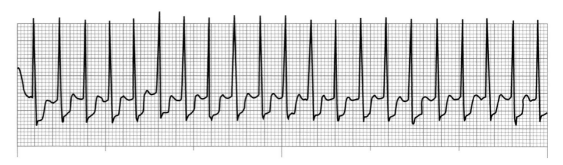

Your best course of action will be to:
   a. Perform synchronized cardioversion starting with 50 joules
   b. Give sublingual nitroglycerin
   c. Perform CPR for 2 minutes, then defibrillate with 200 joules
   d. Perform CPR and give epinephrine 1 mg IV push

8. At doses recommended for use in cardiac arrest, epinephrine and vasopressin:
   a. Cause significant peripheral vasoconstriction
   b. Neutralize acid accumulated during cardiac arrest
   c. Slow conduction through the atrioventricular node
   d. Cause profound peripheral vasodilation

9. The first antiarrhythmic administered in the management of the patient in pulseless ventricular tachycardia or ventricular fibrillation is:
   a. Epinephrine or vasopressin
   b. Amiodarone or lidocaine
   c. Vasopressin or amiodarone
   d. Epinephrine or lidocaine

10. During cardiac arrest:
   a. Chest compressions should be interrupted for 2 to 3 minutes to start an IV and insert an advanced airway
   b. Chest compressions should never be interrupted
   c. Interruptions in chest compressions to analyze the ECG, charge the defibrillator, place an advanced airway, check a pulse, or other procedures must be kept to a minimum
   d. Chest compressions and ventilations should be interrupted every 3 to 5 minutes to permit the members of the resuscitation team to change positions

11. A 56-year-old woman is complaining of palpitations. When questioned, she denies chest discomfort or shortness of breath. Her blood pressure is 134/82, pulse 180, respirations 18. The cardiac monitor shows a narrow-QRS tachycardia without visible P waves. Recommended treatment for this patient includes:
   a. Airway, breathing, circulation (ABCs); O_2; IV; sedation; and synchronized cardioversion with 200 joules
   b. ABCs, O_2, IV, vagal maneuvers, and lidocaine 1- to 1.5-mg/kg IV bolus
   c. ABCs, O_2, IV, and atropine 1-mg IV every 3 to 5 minutes to a maximum of 3 mg
   d. ABCs, O_2, IV, vagal maneuvers, and adenosine 6-mg rapid IV bolus

Questions 12 through 16 pertain to the following scenario.

A 78-year-old woman is found unresponsive.

12. From across the room, your first impression of the patient is that she is not moving, you can see no rise and fall of her chest or abdomen, and her skin color is pale. When you arrive at the patient's side, you confirm that she is unresponsive. As you shout for help, your next action in this situation should be to:
    a. Apply the automated external defibrillator
    b. Open her airway and check breathing
    c. Begin chest compressions
    d. Prepare the necessary equipment to insert an advanced airway

13. If no head or neck trauma is suspected, which of the following techniques should healthcare professionals use to open the airway?
    a. Jaw-thrust without head tilt
    b. Head tilt–neck lift
    c. Head tilt–chin lift
    d. Tongue–jaw lift

14. The primary survey reveals that the patient is unresponsive and not breathing. A weak pulse is present at a rate of about 70. Your best course of action will be to:
    a. Begin mouth-to-mouth breathing
    b. Begin ventilating with a bag-mask
    c. Begin chest compressions
    d. Insert an endotracheal tube, Combitube, or laryngeal mask airway

15. An oral airway:
    a. May help in the delivery of adequate ventilation with a bag-mask device by preventing the tongue from blocking the airway
    b. Is of proper size if it extends from the tip of the nose to the tip of the ear
    c. Is usually well tolerated in responsive or semi-responsive patients
    d. Can only be used in spontaneously breathing patients

16. An oral airway is in place. In this situation, the proper rate for bag-mask ventilation is:
    a. 8 to 10 ventilations per minute; each ventilation delivered over 1 second
    b. 10 to 12 ventilations per minute; each ventilation delivered over 1 second
    c. 12 to 20 ventilations per minute; each ventilation delivered over 1½ to 2 seconds
    d. 20 to 24 ventilations per minute; each ventilation delivered over 1½ to 2 seconds

17. Which of the following reflects correct operation of a transcutaneous pacemaker for a patient experiencing a symptomatic bradycardia?
    a. The rate should be set between 20 and 60; the current (milliamps) should be increased slowly to maximum output.
    b. The rate should be set between 40 and 100; the current should be increased rapidly to a maximum of 160 milliamps.
    c. The rate should be set between 60 and 80; the current should be increased slowly until capture is achieved.
    d. The rate should be set between 80 and 100; the current should be increased rapidly to maximum output.

18. A patient who presents with a possible (or definite) acute coronary syndrome should receive a targeted history and physical exam and initial 12-lead ECG within _____ of patient contact (prehospital) or arrival in the emergency department.
    a. 5 minutes
    b. 10 minutes
    c. 30 minutes
    d. 60 minutes

19. The approximate percentage of oxygen delivered by a simple face mask at 8 to 10 L/min is:
   a. 20% to 40%
   b. 40% to 60%
   c. 60% to 80%
   d. 80% to 100%

20. Most myocardial infarctions occur because of:
   a. Coronary thrombosis
   b. Acute respiratory failure
   c. Coronary artery spasm
   d. Acute volume overload

Questions 21 through 25 pertain to the following scenario.

A 65-year-old woman is found unresponsive and not breathing. You are unable to feel a pulse.

21. The cardiac monitor reveals the following rhythm.

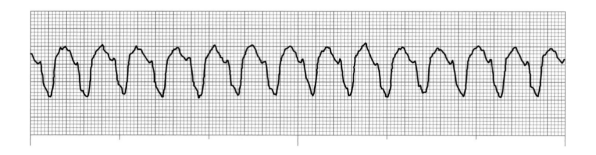

Which of the following statements is true about this rhythm?
   a. This rhythm is ventricular fibrillation, a "shockable" rhythm
   b. This rhythm is a narrow-QRS tachycardia, a "nonshockable" rhythm
   c. This rhythm is monomorphic ventricular tachycardia, a "shockable" rhythm
   d. This rhythm is a wide-QRS tachycardia, a "nonshockable" rhythm

22. When a shockable rhythm is present during cardiac arrest and a biphasic manual defibrillator is available, the initial energy level selected should be:
   a. 120 joules
   b. 200 joules
   c. 360 joules
   d. The dose recommended by the manufacturer for terminating the rhythm

23. An IV is not in place. The preferred site for initial placement of a large IV catheter is the:
   a. Saphenous vein
   b. Antecubital vein
   c. Subclavian vein
   d. Internal jugular vein

24. Drugs given during cardiac arrest should be given:
   a. By the endotracheal route whenever possible
   b. By continuous IV infusion
   c. By IV bolus and followed with a 20-mL flush of IV fluid
   d. By IV bolus over 2 to 3 minutes and then followed with a 10-mL flush of IV fluid

25. Attempts to establish a peripheral IV have been unsuccessful. Your best course of action at this time will be to:
    a. Attempt intraosseous access
    b. Insert a central line
    c. Continue peripheral IV attempts until successful
    d. Discontinue resuscitation efforts

26. Amiodarone:
    a. Is given as an initial IV dose of 300 mg and one repeat dose of 150 mg in cardiac arrest due to pulseless ventricular tachycardia or ventricular fibrillation
    b. Should be given IV or endotracheally in cardiac arrest due to pulseless electrical activity
    c. Is given as a loading dose of 150-mg IV bolus over 10 minutes in cardiac arrest
    d. Should be given only if there is a return of spontaneous circulation after cardiac arrest

27. Rapid heart rates may produce serious signs and symptoms. The physiologic reason for this is that increases in heart rate result in _____ ventricular filling time, which frequently results in _____ stroke volume.
    a. Decreased, decreased
    b. Decreased, increased
    c. Increased, decreased
    d. Increased, increased

28. Dobutamine:
    a. Stimulates alpha, beta-1, and beta-2 receptors
    b. Is the drug of choice in the treatment of symptomatic narrow-QRS bradycardia
    c. May result in asystole when given in high doses
    d. Is given as a 2- to 20-mcg/kg IV bolus

29. A 56-year-old woman presents with a sudden onset of chest discomfort that has been present for about 1 hour. The patient describes her discomfort as a "squeezing" sensation in the middle of her chest. She rates her discomfort an 8 on a 0 to 10 scale. Her blood pressure is 126/72, respirations 14. Oxygen has been applied, an IV has been started, and the cardiac monitor reveals the rhythm below.

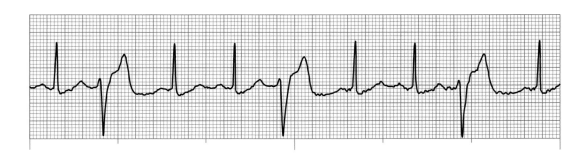

Immediate management of this patient should include:
    a. Vagal maneuvers and adenosine rapid IV push
    b. Nitroglycerin, morphine, lidocaine or amiodarone, and aspirin
    c. Aspirin, nitroglycerin, and morphine
    d. Vagal maneuvers and an amiodarone IV infusion

30. Atropine:
    a. Is used to slow the ventricular rate in narrow-QRS tachycardias
    b. Is given in doses of 1 mg to a maximum of 3 mg in asystole or slow pulseless electrical activity
    c. Is most effective for atrioventricular (AV) blocks below the level of the AV node
    d. Is given in doses of 1 to 1.5 mg/kg for symptomatic bradycardia

31. Which of the following statements is true about ventilation with a bag-mask?
    a. A bag-mask device should be equipped with a pop-off (pressure release) valve to overcome increased air resistance in cardiac arrest patients
    b. When an advanced airway is in place, ventilations with a bag-mask must be synchronized with compressions during cardiac arrest
    c. Bag-mask ventilation can produce gastric distention that can lead to vomiting and subsequent aspiration
    d. Bag-mask ventilation can be used only for patients who are not breathing

32. Which of the following statements is true of right ventricular infarction (RVI)?
    a. Nitrates, diuretics, and other vasodilators should be avoided in RVI because severe hypotension may result
    b. Typical signs and symptoms of RVI include hypertension, jugular venous distention, and bilateral rales/crackles
    c. RV infarction or ischemia usually occurs in patients with an anterior wall infarction
    d. Caution should be used when administering IV fluids because the development of pulmonary edema is increased in patients with RVI

33. Defibrillation is indicated in the management of:
    a. Asystole and pulseless electrical activity
    b. Pulseless ventricular tachycardia and ventricular fibrillation
    c. Ventricular fibrillation and asystole
    d. Pulseless ventricular tachycardia and pulseless electrical activity

34. Verapamil:
    a. Should be given <u>only</u> to patients with narrow-QRS tachycardia or dysrhythmias known with certainty to be of supraventricular origin
    b. Is given rapidly as a 2.5- to 5-mg IV bolus (over 1 to 3 seconds)
    c. Can be safely given to patients with impaired ventricular function or heart failure
    d. Is the drug of choice for patients with atrial fibrillation or atrial flutter associated with known preexcitation (Wolff-Parkinson-White [WPW]) syndrome

35. Lidocaine may be <u>lethal</u> if administered for which of the following rhythms?
    a. Monomorphic ventricular tachycardia
    b. Idioventricular (ventricular escape) rhythm
    c. Polymorphic ventricular tachycardia
    d. Sinus tachycardia

36. True or False: Side effects associated with transcutaneous pacing are most often related to muscle contraction, pain, and patient intolerance of the pacing stimulus.

37. A 58-year-old man is complaining of chest pain. Select the question that best evaluates the <u>quality</u> of the patient's pain.
    a. "When did the pain begin?"
    b. "How would you describe your pain?"
    c. "Does anything make the pain better or worse?"
    d. "Where is your discomfort?"

38. Angiotensin-converting-enzyme (ACE) inhibitors:
    a. Increase blood pressure
    b. Increase myocardial workload
    c. May be used in the management of ST-segment elevation myocardial infarction
    d. Include medications such as metoprolol, atenolol, and propranolol

39. A 72-year-old man presents with severe substernal chest pain. His level of consciousness suddenly decreased as an alarm sounded on the monitor. A quick glance at the cardiac monitor reveals the rhythm below. He now responds by moaning when his name is spoken. His skin is pale and clammy. BP 68/40, R 12. His pulse is weak and fast.

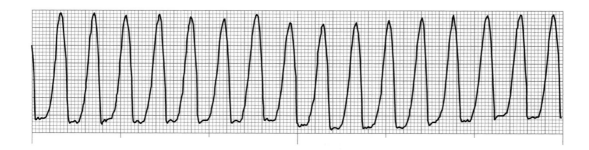

Your best course of action in this situation will be to:
    a. Consider sedation and perform synchronized cardioversion with 100 joules
    b. Start an IV and give a 300-mg dose of amiodarone
    c. Ask the patient to bear down; if unsuccessful, give adenosine IV
    d. Begin CPR and then defibrillate with 360 joules as soon as a defibrillator is available

40. The most common cause of a stroke is:
    a. A clot (thrombus)
    b. An arteriovenous malformation
    c. A ruptured blood vessel
    d. Spasm of a cerebral artery

41. True or False: Simultaneous, bilateral carotid massage should be attempted to try to slow the heart rate of a stable patient with a narrow-QRS tachycardia before medication administration.

42. A 46-year-old woman is found unresponsive, not breathing, and pulseless. The patient's sister states that 15 minutes ago, the patient said she couldn't breathe and then lost consciousness. The patient has a history of congestive heart failure and asthma. CPR is in progress. The cardiac monitor displays asystole. Examination of the patient reveals no signs of trauma. How should this patient be managed?
    a. Defibrillate once as soon as possible, resume CPR, start an IV, and give epinephrine
    b. Continue CPR, start an IV, intubate using the largest endotracheal tube available, and give epinephrine and atropine
    c. Stop CPR and attempt transcutaneous pacing, then start an IV and begin a dopamine infusion
    d. Attempt synchronized cardioversion using 100 joules; if the rhythm is unchanged, start an IV, and intubate using the largest endotracheal tube available

43. True or False: Rapid, wide-QRS rhythms associated with pulselessness, shock, or congestive heart failure should be presumed to be ventricular tachycardia.

44. The maximum length of time for a suctioning attempt is:
   a. 10 to 15 seconds
   b. 15 to 20 seconds
   c. 20 to 25 seconds
   d. 25 to 30 seconds

45. Which of the following factors reduces transthoracic resistance and enhances the chance for successful defibrillation in cardiac arrest?
   a. Phase of patient's respiration
   b. The use of lower energy levels (10 to 25 joules)
   c. Giving calcium chloride before each defibrillation attempt
   d. The delivery of shocks in sets of three when a shock is indicated

46. Successful placement of an endotracheal tube in an adult usually results in the depth marking on the side of the tube lying between the _____ mark at the front teeth.
   a. 15 and 20 cm
   b. 16 and 22 cm
   c. 19 and 23 cm
   d. 20 and 25 cm

47. What is the most common complication in the first few hours of an acute myocardial infarction?
   a. Pulmonary embolism
   b. Hypertension
   c. Ventricular aneurysm
   d. Dysrhythmias

48. Select the <u>incorrect</u> statement regarding the automated external defibrillator (AED).
   a. Some AEDs are programmed to detect spontaneous movement by the patient or others
   b. If a fully automated AED is used and a shockable rhythm is detected, the AED will instruct the AED operator to press the shock control to deliver a shock
   c. Some AEDs have adapters available for many popular manual defibrillators, enabling the AED pads to remain on the patient when patient care is transferred
   d. AEDs will recommend a shock for monomorphic ventricular tachycardia, polymorphic ventricular tachycardia, and ventricular fibrillation

49. Which of the following may be used for rhythm control of atrial fibrillation ≤48 hours in duration?
   a. Calcium chloride
   b. Sodium bicarbonate
   c. Lidocaine
   d. Magnesium sulfate

50. Paramedics arrive in the emergency department with a 40-year-old man. When they arrived at the patient's home, the patient was complaining of a severe chest pain. While taking the patient's history and vital signs, he experienced a cardiac arrest. The cardiac monitor showed VF. The paramedics defibrillated immediately with successful conversion to a sinus rhythm. The patient responds to a painful stimulus, but does not respond to verbal stimuli. His blood pressure is 104/70, respirations 12/min. Which of the following should be done at this time?
   a. The patient's baseline temperature should be obtained and warming measures should be started until the patient's temperature reaches 101° F
   b. The patient should be cooled to 89.6° F to 93.2° F (32° C to 34° C) for 12 to 24 hours
   c. Heat packs should be applied to the patient's axilla, neck, and groin to prevent hypothermia
   d. Give 50% dextrose in water IV push to make sure sufficient glucose is available for adequate brain function

PRETEST ANSWERS

1. c. Adenosine is the first drug used for most forms of narrow-QRS tachycardia. Narrow-QRS tachycardia includes atrioventricular nodal reentrant tachycardia (AVNRT) and AV reentrant tachycardia (AVRT). In AVNRT, fast and slow pathways in the AV node form an electrical circuit or loop. The impulse spins around the AV nodal (junctional) area. In AVRT, the impulse begins above the ventricles but travels via a pathway other than the AV node and bundle of His. Adenosine slows conduction time through AV node and can interrupt reentry pathways through AV node.

2. b. Vasopressin may be used in place of the first or second dose of epinephrine in pulseless arrest due to ventricular fibrillation, ventricular tachycardia, asystole, and (possibly) pulseless electrical activity (PEA). There is insufficient evidence to recommend for or against vasopressin use in PEA.

3. b. Although IV or intraosseous (IO) administration of drugs is preferred, some drugs can be given endotracheally if vascular access is delayed or cannot be achieved. Drugs that can be given via the endotracheal route during an adult cardiac arrest can be remembered by using the memory aid "NAVEL"— *N*aloxone, *A*tropine, *V*asopressin, *E*pinephrine, and *L*idocaine.

4. b. Hypotension and bradycardia are most common side effects of amiodarone administration. Slow the infusion rate or discontinue if seen.

5. c. After 5 cycles of CPR, deliver a single shock using 360 joules and then immediately resume CPR, starting with chest compressions. In cardiac arrest, magnesium sulfate is used to treat torsades de pointes (not ventricular fibrillation). Verapamil is not indicated in cardiac arrest.

6. b. The initial patient evaluation should consist of evaluation of the patient's level of responsiveness, airway, breathing, circulation, and the need for defibrillation.

7. a. This patient is clearly unstable (acute altered mental status, hypotension, and shortness of breath). Consider sedation and perform synchronized cardioversion starting with 50 joules or equivalent biphasic energy. Since the patient has a pulse, CPR is not indicated. Epinephrine causes vasoconstriction and increases heart rate. Since the patient is already tachycardic, epinephrine is contraindicated. Nitroglycerin is not indicated because the patient has no complaint of chest discomfort and is severely hypotensive.

8. a. Epinephrine and vasopressin are potent vasoconstrictors. Drugs given during cardiac arrest that constrict blood vessels (vasopressors) may improve coronary perfusion pressure.

9. b. The first *antiarrhythmic* administered in the management of the patient in pulseless ventricular tachycardia (VT) or ventricular fibrillation (VF) is amiodarone (or lidocaine if amiodarone is unavailable). Epinephrine and vasopressin are vasopressors, not antiarrhythmics.

10. c. During cardiac arrest, coronary perfusion declines rapidly if chest compressions are stopped for even a few seconds. When caring for a patient in cardiac arrest, it is *essential* that interruptions to analyze the ECG, charge the defibrillator, place an advanced airway, check a pulse, or other procedures be kept to a minimum.

11. d. From the information provided, this patient appears stable. Initial treatment should include ABCs, oxygen, IV, and vagal maneuvers. If vagal maneuvers are ineffective, give 6 mg of adenosine rapid IV push and reassess. Atropine is used to increase heart rate. Since this patient is tachycardic, atropine is not indicated in the treatment of this pa-

tient. Lidocaine is an antiarrhythmic used to treat ventricular (not supraventricular) dysrhythmias. Therefore, lidocaine is not indicated in this situation.

12. b. After forming a first impression, you should perform a primary survey using the ABCD approach—*A*irway, *B*reathing, *C*irculation, and *D*efibrillation (if necessary).

13. c. If no head or neck trauma is suspected, use the head tilt-chin lift maneuver to open the airway. If trauma is suspected, the jaw thrust without head tilt maneuver should be used.

14. b. The patient has experienced a respiratory arrest. Chest compressions are not indicated since the patient has a pulse. Begin ventilating with a bag-mask. Although insertion of an advanced airway is appropriate, it must be preceded by another form of ventilation (such as bag-mask ventilation) while preparations are made to insert the airway.

15. a. When properly positioned, an oral airway positions the tongue forward and away from the back of the throat. It may be used to help maintain an open airway in an unresponsive patient who is not intubated, to help maintain an open airway in an unresponsive patient with no gag reflex who is being ventilated with a bag-mask or other positive-pressure device, and as a bite block after insertion of an endotracheal tube or orogastric tube. An oral airway may produce vomiting if used in a responsive or semiresponsive patient with a gag reflex. Correct size is determined by selecting an oral airway that extends from the corner of the mouth to the tip of the earlobe or the angle of the jaw.

16. b. The proper rate for bag-mask ventilation in this situation is 10 to 12 ventilations per minute with each ventilation delivered over 1 second.

17. c. When transcutaneous pacing is used to treat a symptomatic bradycardia, the rate is set at a nonbradycardic rate, generally between 60 and 80 pulses per minute (ppm). After the rate has been regulated, set the stimulating current. Increase the current slowly but steadily until capture is achieved. Sedation and/or analgesia may be needed to minimize the discomfort associated with this procedure (common with currents of 50 mA or more).

18. b. If patient findings are consistent with a possible or definite acute coronary syndrome, a targeted history and a physical exam and initial 12-lead ECG should be performed within 10 minutes of patient contact (prehospital) or arrival in the emergency department.

19. b. At 6 to 10 L/min, a simple face mask can provide an inspired oxygen concentration of approximately 40%-60%. The recommended flow rate is 8 to 10 L/min. The patient's actual inspired oxygen concentration will vary because the amount of air that mixes with supplemental oxygen is dependent on the patient's inspiratory flow rate. When a simple face mask is used, the oxygen flow rate must be higher than 5 L/min to flush the buildup of the patient's exhaled carbon dioxide from the mask.

20. a. Acute coronary syndromes (ACS) include unstable angina, non-ST-segment elevation myocardial infarction (NSTEMI), and ST-segment elevation MI (STEMI). ACS are conditions caused by a similar sequence of pathologic events—a temporary or permanent blockage of a coronary artery, most often due to rupture of an atherosclerotic plaque. This sequence of events results in conditions ranging from myocardial ischemia or injury to death (necrosis) of heart muscle.

21. c. The rhythm shown is monomorphic VT. Monomorphic VT and VF are shockable cardiac arrest rhythms.

22. d. When using a biphasic waveform defibrillator to treat pulseless VT/VF, use the energy levels recommended by the manufacturer for the initial and subsequent shocks. If you do not know what the recommended energy levels are, it is reasonable to use 200 joules for the first shock. Use either an equal or higher dose for the second or subsequent shocks, depending on the capabilities of the device.

23. b. During circulatory collapse or cardiac arrest, the preferred vascular access site is the largest, most accessible vein that does not require the interruption of resuscitation efforts. If no IV is in place before the arrest, establish IV access using a peripheral vein—preferably the antecubital or external jugular vein.

24. c. During cardiac arrest, give IV drugs rapidly by bolus injection. Follow each drug with a 20-mL bolus of IV fluid and raise the extremity for 10 to 20 seconds to aid delivery of the drug(s) to the central circulation.

25. a. If peripheral IV access is unsuccessful during cardiac arrest, consider an IO infusion before considering placement of a central line.

26. a. Amiodarone is given as an initial IV dose of 300 mg and one repeat dose of 150 mg in cardiac arrest due to pulseless VT or VF.

27. a. Rapid heart rates may produce serious signs and symptoms. The physiologic reason for this is that increases in heart rate result in <u>decreased</u> ventricular filling time, which frequently results in <u>decreased</u> stroke volume.

28. a. Dobutamine stimulates alpha, beta-1, and beta-2 receptors and is used for the short-term management of patients with cardiac decompensation due to depressed contractility (e.g., CHF, pulmonary congestion) with a systolic BP of 70 to 100 mm Hg <u>and no signs of shock</u>. Hypovolemia must be corrected before treatment with dobutamine. Dobutamine is given as a continuous IV infusion at a rate of 2 to 20 mcg/kg/min, and may result in tachycardia when administered in high doses.

29. c. Antiarrhythmics such as lidocaine and amiodarone should not be used to treat the ventricular ectopy seen on the patient's cardiac monitor. Treat the <u>cause</u> of the premature ventricular complexes. Give 160 to 325 mg of nonenteric aspirin as soon as possible after symptom onset, if there are no contraindications. Nitroglycerin relaxes vascular smooth muscle, including dilation of the coronary arteries (particularly in the area of plaque disruption). It also decreases myocardial oxygen consumption. Before giving nitroglycerin, make sure an IV is in place, the patient's systolic BP is >90 mm Hg, the patient's heart rate is >50 and <100 bpm, there are no signs of right ventricular infarction, and the patient has not used Viagra, Cialis, or similar medication in the previous 24 to 48 hours. Morphine is the drug of choice to relieve pain associated with ACS. It decreases anxiety, pain, and myocardial oxygen requirements. Vagal maneuvers are used to slow the heart rate in a patient who has a narrow-QRS tachycardia. They are not indicated in this situation.

30. b. Atropine is a first-line drug for symptomatic narrow-QRS bradycardia. It is also indicated in the treatment of asystole (after epinephrine) and slow pulseless electrical activity (PEA) (after epinephrine). When given for a symptomatic bradycardia, the dose of atropine is 0.5 mg IV push every 3 to 5 min to a total dose of 3.0 mg. In asystole or slow PEA, the IV/IO dose of atropine is 1.0 mg every 3 to 5 minutes to a total dose of 3 mg. Atropine is useful for treating AV blocks at the level of the AV node. Use transcutaneous pacing without delay for symptomatic wide-QRS bradycardias.

31. c. Bag-mask ventilation can be used with the spontaneously breathing patient as well as the nonbreathing patient. A bag-mask used during a cardiac arrest should have either no pop-off valve (pressure-release valve) or a pop-off valve that can be disabled

during resuscitation. During cardiac arrest, if the patient does not have an advanced airway in place, deliver cycles of 30 compressions and 2 breaths. Deliver the breaths during pauses in compressions. Deliver each breath over 1 second with just enough force to cause gentle chest rise. Delivering breaths that are too large or too forceful is unnecessary and may cause gastric distention that can lead to vomiting and subsequent aspiration. Once an advanced airway (endotracheal tube, Combitube, or laryngeal mask airway) is in place during 2-person CPR, ventilate at a rate of 8 to 10 breaths per minute without pausing chest compressions for delivery of ventilations.

32. a. Suspect a right ventricular infarction (RVI) when ECG changes suggesting an <u>inferior</u> infarction (ST-segment elevation in leads II, III, and/or aVF) are seen. About 50% of patients with inferior infarction have some involvement of the right ventricle. RVI can result in hypotension (of varying degrees), jugular venous distention, and absence of pulmonary edema (clear lung sounds). These signs are considered the clinical triad of RVI. This triad is present in only about 10% to 15% of patients with RVI. Vasodilators reduce preload. This reduction in preload, while usually beneficial, can be undesirable in the setting of RVI and may cause profound hypotension. Caution must be exercised when giving nitroglycerin and morphine to patients experiencing RVI. If hypotension does occur, it will bring with it the serious consequence of a decrease in coronary artery perfusion. If the decision is made to give vasodilators, establish an IV before giving a vasodilator. This should be routinely done for all patients; however, it is particularly important in RVI. If the patient's breath sounds are clear, give an IV fluid challenge of 250 to 500 mL (usually with normal saline) and reassess the patient's response. This approach attempts to increase preload and offset the anticipated decrease in preload. In the setting of RVI, blood does not back up from the left ventricle into the lungs, so pulmonary edema is not expected.

33. b. Defibrillation is indicated in the management of pulseless VT and VF.

34. a. Verapamil is indicated in the management of stable narrow-QRS tachycardia due to reentry if the rhythm persists despite vagal maneuvers or adenosine, the management of stable narrow-QRS tachycardia due to automaticity (junctional, ectopic atrial, multifocal atrial tachycardia) if the rhythm persists despite vagal maneuvers or adenosine, and control of the ventricular rate in patients with atrial fibrillation or atrial flutter. It should <u>not</u> be given to patients with atrial fibrillation or atrial flutter associated with known preexcitation (WPW) syndrome. The initial dose of verapamil is 2.5 to 5.0 mg given slow IV push over 2 minutes (give over 3 to 4 minutes in the elderly or when BP is within the lower range of normal). Because verapamil decreases myocardial contractility, it is contraindicated in patients who have severe heart failure.

35. b. Lidocaine may be lethal if administered for a bradycardia with a ventricular escape rhythm (e.g., idioventricular rhythm, second-degree AV block type II, third-degree AV block).

36. True. Side effects associated with transcutaneous pacing are most often related to muscle contraction, pain, and patient intolerance of the pacing stimulus.

37. b. The quality of the patient's pain may be assessed by asking, "How would you describe your discomfort?" (Pressure, pain, crushing, dull, burning, tearing, throbbing, squeezing, stabbing, vise-like). "When did the pain begin?" determines the onset of the patient's symptoms. "Does anything make the pain better or worse?" is asked to determine what provokes the patient's symptoms. "Where is your discomfort?" pinpoints the region/radiation of the patient's symptoms.

38. c. ACE inhibitors prevent the conversion of angiotensin I to angiotensin II. As a result, blood vessels relax, reducing the pressure the heart must pump against and decreasing

myocardial workload. ACE inhibitors are recommended within the first 24 hours after on-set of symptoms in STEMI patients with pulmonary congestion or left ventricular ejection fraction <40%, in the absence of hypotension (systolic BP <100 mm Hg or more than 30 mm Hg below baseline). Metoprolol, atenolol, and propranolol are beta-blockers.

39. a. The rhythm shown is monomorphic VT. The patient is clearly unstable as evidenced by his acute altered mental status and severe hypotension. Consider sedation and per-form synchronized cardioversion with 100 joules or equivalent biphasic energy.

40. a. A clot (thrombus) is the most common cause of stroke. In a thrombotic stroke, ath-erosclerosis of large vessels in the brain causes progressive narrowing and platelet clumping. Platelet clumping results in the development of blood clots within the brain artery itself (cerebral thrombosis). When the blood clots are of sufficient size to block blood flow through the artery, the area previously supplied by that artery becomes isch-emic. Ischemia occurs because the tissue supplied by the blocked artery does not re-ceive oxygen and the essential nutrients needed for normal brain function. The patient's signs and symptoms depend on the location of the artery affected and the areas of brain ischemia.

41. False. Carotid sinus pressure is a type of vagal maneuver. Vagal maneuvers are used to slow the heart rate of stable patients with a narrow-QRS tachycardia (assuming there are no contraindications to the procedure). Carotid sinus pressure is performed with the patient's neck extended. Firm pressure is applied just underneath the angle of the jaw for up to 5 seconds. Carotid pressure should be avoided in older patients and in pa-tients with carotid artery bruits. Simultaneous, bilateral carotid pressure should *never* be performed.

42. b. Confirm asystole in a second lead. If the rhythm is asystole, continue CPR, start an IV, intubate using the largest endotracheal tube available, and give epinephrine and atropine. Based on the patient's medical history, additional drugs that may be ordered include albuterol, ipratropium bromide, and nebulized magnesium sulfate among oth-ers.

43. True. Most wide-QRS tachycardias are VT. Any rapid, wide-QRS rhythm associated with pulselessness, shock, or congestive heart failure should be presumed to be VT until proven otherwise.

44. a. The maximum length of time for a suctioning attempt is 10 to 15 seconds.

45. a. Factors known to affect transthoracic resistance include paddle/electrode size, paddle/electrode position, use of conductive material (when using hand-held paddles), phase of patient's respiration, paddle pressure (when using hand-held paddles), and selected energy. Because frequent or long interruptions of chest compressions are detrimental, a single shock is recommended during cardiac arrest associated with a "shockable" rhythm. After the shock is delivered, immediately resume CPR, starting with chest compressions.

46. c. Successful placement of an endotracheal tube in an adult usually results in the depth marking on the side of the tube lying between the 19- and 23-cm mark at the front teeth.

47. d. Dysrhythmias are the most common complication in the first few hours following MI. Cardiac dysrhythmias are the primary <u>electrical</u> complication of acute MI. The primary <u>mechanical</u> complications of acute MI are heart failure and cardiogenic shock.

48. b. If a fully automated AED is used and a shockable rhythm is detected, the AED will signal everyone to stand clear of the patient and then deliver a shock by means of the adhesive pads that were applied to the patient's chest. If the machine is a semi-automated AED and a shockable rhythm is detected, it will instruct the AED operator (by means of voice prompts and visual signals) to press the shock control to deliver a shock.

49. d. Magnesium sulfate may be used for rhythm control of atrial fibrillation (≤48 hours in duration). Give 1 to 2 g IV in 50 to 100 mL D5W over 5 to 60 min. Give the infusion slowly if the patient is stable and more rapidly if the patient is unstable.

50. b. After prehospital cardiac arrest, unresponsive adults who have a return of spontaneous circulation should be cooled to 89.6° F to 93.2° F (32° C to 34° C) for 12 to 24 hours when the initial rhythm was VF. Similar therapy may be beneficial for prehospital patients with cardiac arrest due to other rhythms or for in-hospital arrest. Fever can impair brain recovery by creating an imbalance between oxygen supply and demand; avoid hyperthermia. Studies have documented poor neurologic outcomes in patients who have high blood glucose levels after resuscitation from cardiac arrest. Monitor serum glucose levels closely.

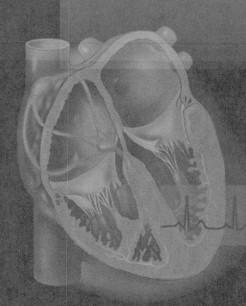

PART

I

PREPARATORY

The ABCDs of Emergency Cardiac Care

OBJECTIVES

Upon completion of this chapter, you will be able to:

1. Identify the risk factors for coronary artery disease.
2. Define "cardiac arrest" and "sudden cardiac death."
3. Identify and describe the links in the Chain of Survival.
4. Name four heart rhythms associated with cardiac arrest.
5. Differentiate "shockable" cardiac arrest rhythms from "nonshockable" cardiac arrest rhythms.
6. Identify the components of advanced cardiac life support.
7. Describe the phases of cardiopulmonary resuscitation.
8. List the purpose and components of the primary and secondary surveys.
9. Explain advance directives and do not resuscitate (DNR) orders.

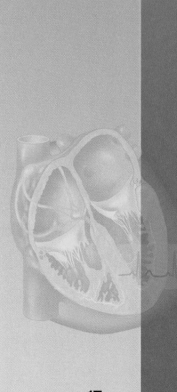

INTRODUCTION

Heart disease is the leading cause of death in the United States. According to the National Center for Chronic Disease Prevention and Health Promotion[1]:

■ About 950,000 Americans die of cardiovascular disease each year. This amounts to about one death every 33 seconds; 400,000 to 460,000 Americans die of heart disease in an emergency department or before reaching a hospital each year.[2]

■ Almost one fourth of the American population has some form of cardiovascular disease.

■ Coronary heart disease is a leading cause of premature, permanent disability among working adults.

As you can see from these statistics, the likelihood of encountering a patient who needs basic life support (BLS) or advanced cardiac life support (ACLS) care is high. In this chapter, you'll read about the essentials of ACLS. Just as BLS is a systematic way of providing care to a choking victim or one who needs cardiopulmonary resuscitation (CPR), ACLS is an orderly approach to providing advanced emergency care to a patient experiencing a cardiac-related problem.

This chapter discusses risk factors for coronary artery disease (CAD), sudden cardiac death, the Chain of Survival, the phases of CPR, a systematic approach to patient assessment, advance directives, and the 2005 resuscitation guidelines classification of treatment recommendations.

RISK FACTORS FOR CORONARY ARTERY DISEASE

Cardiovascular disorders are a collection of diseases and conditions that involve the heart (cardio) and blood vessels (vascular). **Heart disease** is a broad term that refers to conditions affecting the heart. **Coronary heart disease (CHD)** refers to disease of the coronary arteries and their resulting complications, such as angina pectoris or acute myocardial infarction. **Coronary artery disease** affects the arteries that supply the heart muscle with blood.

Prevention of cardiovascular disease requires managing risk factors. **Risk factors** are traits and lifestyle habits that may increase a person's chance of developing a disease. More than 300 risk factors have been associated with coronary heart disease and stroke. Major risk factors meet three criteria[3]:

1. High frequency in many populations
2. Significant independent impact on the risk of coronary heart disease or stroke
3. Treatment and control of the risk factor results in reduced risk

Some risk factors can be modified. Risk factors that cannot be modified are called nonmodifiable or fixed risk factors. Modifiable risk factors can be changed or treated. Contributing risk factors are thought to lead to an increased risk of heart disease, but their exact role has not been defined (Table 1-1).

TABLE 1-1	Cardiovascular Disease Risk Factors		
Nonmodifiable (Fixed) Factors	**Modifiable Factors**	**Contributing Factors**
• Heredity • Race • Gender • Age	• High blood pressure • Elevated serum cholesterol levels • Tobacco use • Diabetes • Physical inactivity • Obesity • Metabolic syndrome	• Stress • Inflammatory markers • Psychosocial factors • Alcohol intake

NONMODIFIABLE (FIXED) FACTORS

■ *Heredity.* A positive family history plays an important part in the development of cardiovascular disease and affects some of the modifiable risk factors. The younger the onset in a first-degree relative (age of 55 years for a male relative or 65 years for a female relative), the greater the risk of cardiovascular disease. Examples of first-degree relatives include parents, children, and siblings.

■ *Race/ethnicity.* Heart disease is the leading cause of death for American Indians and Alaska Natives, blacks, Hispanics, and whites.[4]

■ *Gender.* The incidence of CAD in men is about the same as that in women 10 years older.[5]

■ *Age.* The incidence of cardiovascular disease increases sharply with age.

MODIFIABLE FACTORS

■ *High blood pressure.* High blood pressure is a major risk factor for heart disease, stroke, and end-stage renal disease.

  ▶ According to the National Heart, Lung, and Blood Institute (NHLBI), an adult's normal blood pressure is considered to be a systolic blood pressure less than 120 mm Hg and a diastolic blood pressure less than 80 mm Hg (Table 1-2).

  ▶ A person who has a systolic blood pressure of 120–139 mm Hg or diastolic blood pressure of 80–89 mm Hg is considered to have "prehypertension."

  ▶ A person who has diabetes or chronic kidney disease has high blood pressure if his or her blood pressure is 130/80 or higher.

According to the World Health Organization, the risk of cardiovascular disease doubles for every 10-point increase in diastolic blood pressure or every 20-point increase in systolic blood pressure.[3]

■ *Elevated serum cholesterol levels.* Increased serum cholesterol and triglyceride levels are associated with an increased risk of coronary heart disease.

  ▶ Low-density lipoproteins (LDLs), or "bad cholesterol," transport cholesterol from the liver to other parts of the body where it can be used. LDLs carry most of the cholesterol in the blood. If these lipoproteins are not removed from the blood, cholesterol and fat can build up in arteries and contribute to atherosclerosis. For patients with familial hypercholesterolemia, heredity affects how quickly LDLs are made and removed from the blood. Lowering total cholesterol and LDL levels significantly reduces the risk of CHD.

TABLE 1-2	Blood Pressure Values in Adults*	
Category	Systolic Blood Pressure (in mm Hg)	Diastolic Blood Pressure (in mm Hg)
Normal	<120	<80
Prehypertension	120-139	80-89
Stage 1 high blood pressure	140-159	90-99
Stage 2 high blood pressure	≥160	≥100

* For adults 18 and older who:
   Are not on medicine for high blood pressure
   Are not having a short-term serious illness
   Do not have other conditions such as diabetes and kidney disease

From National Heart, Lung, and Blood Institute. *High blood pressure:* www.nhlbi.nih.gov/health/dci/Diseases/Hbp/HBP_WhatIs.html. Accessed 5/15/2005.

▶ High-density lipoproteins (HDLs) or "good cholesterol," help remove cholesterol from the blood, preventing buildup of cholesterol in the arterial walls. Increasing physical activity, regular exercise, and losing weight have been shown to increase the concentration of HDL in the blood.

■ *Tobacco use.* Smoking greatly increases the risk of heart disease and peripheral vascular disease (disease in the vessels that supply blood to the arms and legs). The likelihood of a heart attack is increased sixfold in women and threefold in men who smoke at least 20 cigarettes per day compared with persons who have never smoked.[6]

▶ Research has shown that smoking damages the inner lining of blood vessels and speeds up the process of atherosclerosis. The chemicals in cigarettes affect levels of fibrinogen, increasing clotting. Nicotine increases heart rate and blood pressure. Smoking also promotes coronary artery spasm.[3]

Quitting smoking reduces the risk of heart disease by 50 percent after only 1 year. Within 2 to 6 years, the risk of developing coronary heart disease is similar to that of a nonsmoker.

■ *Diabetes.* Diabetes increases the risks of coronary heart disease, cerebrovascular disease, peripheral vascular disease, and congestive heart failure (CHF). CHD occurs more often in diabetic patients than in the general population, affecting approximately 55% of patients.[7] Adult-onset or Type II diabetes (also known as non–insulin-dependent diabetes) is largely preventable because it is related to physical inactivity, excess calorie intake, and obesity. Persons with Type II diabetes have a 2- to 4-fold increased risk of CHD and a 4-fold increase in death from CHD.[8]

■ *Physical inactivity.* Sedentary Death Syndrome (SeDS) is a term used by researchers to represent the growing number of health conditions caused or worsened by a lack of adequate physical activity (Table 1-3). People who are not active have a greater risk of cardiovascular disease than do people who exercise regularly. Physical activity reduces the risk of CHD, diabetes, high blood pressure, and obesity. It can also help reduce stress.

According to the World Health Organization, doing more than 150 minutes of moderate physical activity or 60 minutes of vigorous physical activity a week can reduce the risk of coronary heart disease by about 30%.[3]

TABLE 1-3	Conditions That Are Caused or Worsened by Sedentary Lifestyle	
Sedentary Living Increases the Risk of These Conditions:		**Sedentary Living Increases the Progression of These Conditions:**
• Angina, heart attack, coronary artery disease	• Osteoporosis	• Chemotherapy
• Breast cancer	• Pancreatic cancer	• Chronic back pain
• Colon cancer	• Peripheral vascular disease	• Debilitating illness
• Congestive heart failure	• Physical frailty	• Disease cachexia
• Depression	• Premature mortality	• Falls resulting in broken hips
• Gallstone disease	• Prostate cancer	• Physical frailty
• High blood cholesterol	• Sleep apnea	• Spinal cord injury
• High blood triglycerides	• Stiff joints	• Stroke
• Hypertension	• Stroke	• Vertebral/femoral fractures
• Less cognitive function	• Type II diabetes	
• Low blood HDL		
• Lower quality of life		
• Obesity (more difficult time with weight control)		

From US President's Council on Physical Fitness and Sports: *Research Digest,* Series 3, No. 16, March 2002: www.fitness.gov/researchdigestmarch2002.pdf. Accessed 5/16/2005.

■ *Obesity and body fat distribution.* Obesity is associated with an increased risk of heart disease. It also increases the likelihood of developing other coronary heart disease risk factors, including high blood pressure, diabetes, and high cholesterol. Body mass index (BMI) is a calculation used to assess body weight in relation to body height. Calculation: (Weight in pounds) divided by (height in inches^2) $\times$ 704.5 = BMI. This formula, used for adult men and women, has been shown to be an effective predictor of body fat (Table 1-4).

Studies have shown that even a 10% reduction in body weight can help reduce the risks associated with obesity.

▶ Body fat distribution appears to be an important factor in determining the risk of CHD. Persons who have abdominal (central) obesity are referred to as "apple-shaped." In "apple-type" obesity, fat is distributed more on the upper body than around the hips. This type of fat distribution is more common in men. In "pear-shaped" or "pear-type" obesity, fat distribution is more around the hips. This type of distribution is more common in women. Individuals who have abdominal obesity are at greatest risk of coronary heart disease. An increased waist circumference (>40 inches in men and >35 inches in women) is a stronger predictor of cardiovascular risk in both genders than BMI.[7]

■ *Metabolic syndrome.* Metabolic syndrome (sometimes called syndrome X, the deadly quartet, or insulin resistance syndrome) is a group of disorders related to body metabolism. The disorders include high blood pressure, elevated insulin levels, excess body weight (particularly around the abdomen), and one or more abnormal cholesterol levels. It is estimated that 1 in 4 adults in the United States meets the criteria for metabolic syndrome.[9] In the United States, the frequency with which this syndrome occurs appears to be increasing, as the incidence of obesity and sedentary lifestyle is increasing.

▶ One of the main features of this syndrome is insulin resistance. **Insulin resistance** is a condition in which the normal amount of insulin secreted by the pancreas isn't enough to cause an effect in body cells. The pancreas responds by secreting even more insulin in order for insulin to have an effect on body cells. As a result, insulin levels rise. Blood glucose levels also begin to rise when the pancreas is no longer able to produce enough insulin.

▶ Insulin resistance is aggravated by obesity and physical inactivity. Some patients eventually develop Type II diabetes, further increasing their risk of cardiovascular disease. In many cases, metabolic syndrome can be prevented with weight loss and increased physical activity.

TABLE 1-4	Body Mass Index
BMI Category	**Value**
Underweight	<18.5
Normal weight	18.5 to 24.9
Overweight	25 to 29.9
Obese	≥30
Morbidly obese	≥40

(Weight in pounds) ÷ (height in inches^2) $\times$ 704.5 = BMI

CONTRIBUTING RISK FACTORS

■ *Stress*. Because we all deal with stress differently, researchers aren't sure how stress increases the risk of heart disease. We do know that hormones such as epinephrine are released during times of stress. The release of epinephrine results in an increase in heart rate, blood pressure, and the body's need for oxygen. Chronic stress exposes the body to persistent levels of epinephrine.

» Stress has been shown to increase the amount of clotting factors in the blood. This increases the risk of a clot lodging in an artery, which increases the risk of a heart attack. The body's response to stress can worsen other risk factors. For example, a person who is stressed may exercise less, overeat, start smoking, or smoke more than usual.

■ *Inflammatory markers*. **C-reactive protein** (CRP) is a protein produced by the liver and released into the bloodstream when there is active inflammation in the body. Atherosclerosis is an inflammatory disease. An elevated level of CRP in the bloodstream suggests that persistent inflammation is present. Studies have shown that inflammation markers such as CRP predict future CHD complications better than LDL cholesterol.[10] High blood levels of CRP can be used to predict serious events such as heart attack, stroke, peripheral vascular disease, and sudden cardiac death. High-sensitivity C-reactive protein (hsCRP) levels of less than 1, 1 to 3, and greater than 3 mg/L are associated with lower, moderate, and higher cardiovascular risks, respectively.[11] CRP levels are elevated with other conditions such as hypertension, cancer, gum disease, obesity, cigarette smoking, metabolic syndrome, diabetes, sepsis, postmenopausal hormone use, chronic infections, and chronic inflammation. CRP levels are decreased with moderate alcohol consumption, aspirin use, physical activity, and weight loss.

» **Fibrinogen** is a protein produced by the liver and necessary for normal blood clotting. High blood levels of fibrinogen increase the thickness (viscosity) of the blood and may play a direct role in the clumping (aggregation) of platelets. Several studies have shown that fibrinogen levels can be used to predict the future risk of heart attack and stroke. Fibrinogen levels increase with age, smoking, obesity, diabetes, and oral contraceptive use. Physical activity decreases fibrinogen levels.

■ *Psychosocial factors*. People with depression are at greater risk for developing heart disease than those who are otherwise healthy.[12] Depression is common in people with coronary heart disease and is predictive of a poor prognosis for patients after a heart attack.[13,14]

» Factors such as education, family income, and employment affect risk factors for heart disease and stroke.[15] Poor social support and poverty are associated with an increased risk of CHD. People from lower socioeconomic groups may not have easy access to healthcare, are more likely to smoke, and less likely to eat a healthy diet. For those who do have access to healthcare, they may be less likely to report warning signs of CHD such as chest discomfort to their doctor.

■ *Alcohol intake*. Heavy alcohol intake (three or more drinks per day) is associated with an increased risk of death from several causes, including stroke, several kinds of cancer, cirrhosis, and pancreatitis, as well as accidents, suicide, and homicide.[16,17]

» However, several studies have shown that light to moderate alcohol intake (one drink per day for women and two drinks for men) has a protective effect for coronary disease in both men and women. Alcohol intake increases HDL levels and may protect against coronary heart disease through an antiinflammatory mechanism.[18]

» Alcohol may also reduce fibrinogen and inhibit platelet clumping.

QUICK REVIEW 1-1

1. Can you name four nonmodifiable risk factors for coronary artery disease?
2. Can you name four modifiable risk factors?
3. Can you name three contributing risk factors?
Answers can be found at the end of this chapter.

SUDDEN CARDIAC DEATH

■ **Cardiopulmonary (cardiac) arrest** is the absence of cardiac mechanical activity, confirmed by the absence of a detectable pulse, unresponsiveness, and apnea or agonal, gasping respiration. The term "cardiac arrest" is more commonly used than "cardiopulmonary arrest" when referring to a patient who is not breathing and has no pulse. Possible causes of cardiac arrest are shown in Table 1-5.

TABLE 1-5	Possible Causes of Cardiac Arrest
Cardiac Causes	**Noncardiac Causes (partial list)**
• Coronary artery disease (most common cause) • Cardiac dysrhythmias • Acute myocardial infarction • Valvular heart disease • Cardiomyopathy or myocarditis • Prolonged QT interval • Congenital heart disease • Intracardiac tumor • Wolff-Parkinson-White syndrome • Pericardial tamponade	• Pulmonary embolism • Choking and asphyxia • Drug ingestion (prescribed or nonprescribed) • Substance abuse • Stroke • Hypoxia • Hypoglycemia • Alcoholism • Allergic reactions • Electrical shock

■ **Sudden cardiac death** (SCD) is an unexpected death due to a cardiac cause that occurs either immediately or within one hour of the onset of symptoms.
  ▶ Studies have shown that there is an increased risk of SCD during the morning hours, on Mondays, and during the winter months.[19]
  ▶ Some victims of SCD have no warning signs of the impending event. For others, warning signs may be present up to 1 hour before the actual arrest (Figure 1-1).
  ▶ Because of irreversible brain damage and dependence upon life support, some patients may live days to weeks after the cardiac arrest before biological death occurs. These factors influence interpretation of the 1-hour definition of SCD.[20]

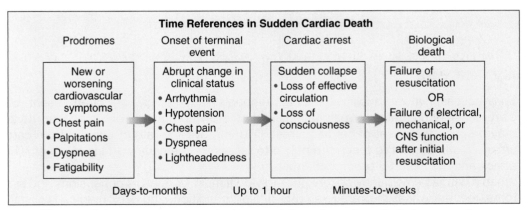

Figure 1-1 • Sudden cardiac death viewed from four chronological perspectives: (1) warning signs (prodromes), (2) onset of the terminal event, (3) cardiac arrest, and (4) progression to biological death. *CNS*, Central nervous system.

CHAIN OF SURVIVAL

The **Chain of Survival** represents the ideal series of events that should take place immediately following the recognition of onset of sudden illness. The chain consists of four key steps that are interrelated (Figure 1-2). Following these steps gives the victim the best chance of surviving a heart attack or sudden cardiac arrest. The links in the chain of survival for adults (and children over 12 to 14 years of age) include early access, early CPR, early defibrillation, and ACLS.

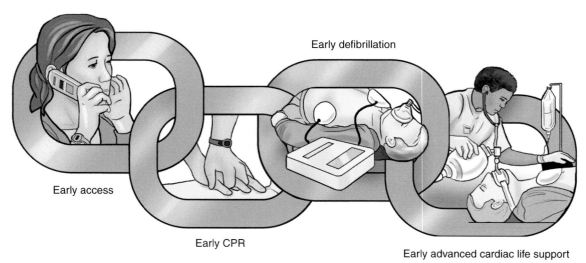

Figure 1-2 • The Chain of Survival.

KEEPING IT SIMPLE

Links in the Chain of Survival
- Early access
- Early CPR
- Early defibrillation
- Early ACLS

Early Access

■ Early access involves public education. Although warning signs are often absent, chest pain, difficulty breathing, or palpitations and other symptoms of abnormal heart rhythms may precede the onset of cardiac arrest.[20] To improve the rate of survival from cardiac arrest, it is important to teach the public to recognize the early warning signs of a heart attack and the need for prompt attention.

■ When a cardiac emergency occurs, the individual must identify his or her signs and symptoms, recognize that they are related to a heart condition, and seek medical assistance. Time delays occur from the call for assistance to arrival of assistance and from arrival of assistance to arrival at the hospital. Studies have found that about one third to one half of patients delay for more than 4 hours before calling for help and greater delays in seeking help occur in female patients, older patients, nonwhite patients, and those who had a history of angina, congestive heart failure (CHF), diabetes, and hypertension.[21]

■ Public education must also include early recognition of patient collapse and how to gain rapid access to the emergency medical services (EMS) system (usually by telephone) via EMS dispatchers. When a call is placed to 9-1-1 (or similar emergency number), rapid recognition by EMS dispatchers of the bystander's description of a potential heart attack or cardiac arrest is important. Dispatchers quickly send appropriately trained and equipped EMS personnel to the scene (Figure 1-3). With appropriate training, EMS dispatchers provide telephone instructions to bystanders. They can ask bystanders to find out if the patient is unresponsive and if normal breathing is present. They can also provide telephone CPR instructions when needed until EMS personnel arrive.

■ Patients who experience a cardiac arrest in the hospital often show signs of deterioration several hours before the arrest.[22] Early recognition of the critically ill patient and activation of a **Medical Emergency Team** (MET) (also known as a Rapid Response Team) may prevent the development of cardiac arrest and improve patient outcome. A MET typically consists of a physician and nurse with critical care training who are available at all times. They are summoned by other hospital staff based on well-defined criteria for activation of the team.

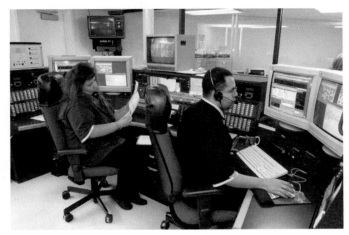

Figure 1-3 • 9-1-1 dispatch center.

Early CPR

■ Cardiopulmonary resuscitation is a part of basic life support (BLS). The components of BLS are shown in Box 1-1.

BOX 1-1

Components of Basic Life Support

- Recognition of signs of:
  - Cardiac arrest
  - Heart attack
  - Stroke
  - Foreign-body airway obstruction (FBAO)
- Relief of FBAO
- CPR
- Defibrillation with an automated external defibrillator

■ Bystander CPR affects survival and is the best treatment a cardiac arrest victim can receive until arrival of a defibrillator and ACLS. CPR training teaches citizens how to contact the EMS system, decreasing the time to defibrillation. It has been shown that victims of cardiac arrest are more likely to receive CPR when the event is witnessed by bystanders unknown to the victim than if the arrest is witnessed by friends or family.[23]

■ After recognizing that an emergency exists, assess the scene to ensure that it is safe. If the scene is safe, quickly assess the patient for life-threatening conditions and determine the nature of the emergency. Alert EMS for medical assistance if not already done. Provide necessary care until advanced medical help arrives and assumes responsibility for the patient's care. Necessary care may include:

▶ Patient positioning
▶ Rescue breathing for victims of respiratory arrest
▶ Recognition and relief of foreign body airway obstruction (FBAO)
▶ Chest compressions and rescue breathing for victims of cardiopulmonary arrest
▶ Defibrillation with an automated external defibrillator (AED) (see Chapter 4)

 Three of the four links of the Chain of Survival can be performed by bystanders.

■ Until recently, resuscitation guidelines for an infant referred to a child less than 1 year of age. A child was considered 1 to 8 years of age, and adult resuscitation guidelines applied to individuals more than 8 years of age. The 2005 resuscitation guidelines redefined the age of a child for healthcare professionals. Child resuscitation guidelines apply to victims from 1 year of age to the onset of puberty (about 12 to 14 years of age). A summary of the treatment for adult, child, and infant choking and CPR can be found in Table 1-6.

Early Defibrillation

■ Heart rhythms that may be observed in a cardiac arrest include the following:

▶ Pulseless ventricular tachycardia (VT), in which the electrocardiogram (ECG) displays a wide QRS complex at a rate faster than 120 bpm
▶ Ventricular fibrillation (VF), in which irregular chaotic deflections that vary in shape and height are observed on the ECG but there is no coordinated ventricular contraction
▶ Asystole, in which no cardiac electrical activity is present
▶ Pulseless electrical activity (PEA), in which electrical activity is visible on the ECG but central pulses are absent

---

KEEPING IT SIMPLE

Cardiac Arrest Rhythms

Shockable rhythms
• Ventricular tachycardia
• Ventricular fibrillation

Nonshockable rhythms
• Asystole
• Pulseless electrical activity

■ VT and VF are "shockable" rhythms. This means that delivering a shock to the heart by means of a defibrillator may result in termination of the rhythm. Asystole and PEA are nonshockable rhythms.

■ When a cardiac arrest is witnessed and the patient's heart rhythm is VF, the patient's survival rate decreases 7% to 10% for every minute that passes between collapse and defibrillation if no CPR is provided.[24] The decrease in survival rates is less rapid (averaging 3% to 4% per minute from collapse to defibrillation) when bystander CPR is provided.[25]

■ An **automated external defibrillator** is a machine with a sophisticated computer system that analyzes the patient's heart rhythm (Figure 1-4). The AED uses an algorithm to distinguish shockable rhythms from non-shockable rhythms. If the AED detects a shockable rhythm, it directs the rescuer to deliver an electrical shock. Defibrillation performed by citizens at the scene is called **public access defibrillation**. The deployment of AEDs in our communities can contribute to better patient outcomes from cardiac arrest (Figure 1-5).

TABLE 1-6	Summary of Treatment for Adult, Child, and Infant Choking and CPR		
CPR/Rescue Breathing	**Infant**	**Child**	**Adult/Older Child**
Age	<1 year	1 to about 12 to 14 years	>12 to 14 years
Level of responsiveness	Establish unresponsiveness	Establish unresponsiveness	Establish unresponsiveness
A = Airway	Open airway with head tilt-chin lift. If trauma is present, use jaw-thrust without head tilt maneuver.	Open airway with head tilt-chin lift. If trauma is present, use jaw-thrust without head tilt maneuver.	Open airway with head tilt-chin lift. If trauma is present, use jaw-thrust without head tilt maneuver.
B = Breathing (assess up to 10 sec)	Look, listen, feel. If breathing adequate, place in recovery position. If no breathing, give 2 breaths.	Look, listen, feel. If breathing adequate, place in recovery position. If no breathing, give 2 breaths.	Look, listen, feel. If breathing adequate, place in recovery position. If no breathing, give 2 breaths.
Initial breaths	2 breaths, each breath lasting 1 sec	2 breaths, each breath lasting 1 sec	2 breaths, each breath lasting 1 sec
Breaths/minute	About 12-20 breaths/min 1 breath every 3-5 sec	About 12-20 breaths/min 1 breath every 3-5 sec	About 10-12 breaths/min 1 breath every 5-6 sec
If airway obstruction present:			
Conscious victim	Give 5 back blows, then 5 chest thrusts if object is not expelled.	Give abdominal thrusts until object is expelled.	Give abdominal thrusts until object is expelled.
Unconscious victim	Try to ventilate. If no chest rise, reposition, try again. If no chest rise, begin CPR.	Try to ventilate. If no chest rise, reposition, try again. If no chest rise, begin CPR.	Try to ventilate. If no chest rise, reposition, try again. If no chest rise, begin CPR.
C = Circulation Check pulse	Brachial or femoral If pulse present, support airway and breathing. If no pulse, start compressions.	Carotid If pulse present, support airway and breathing. If no pulse, start compressions, call for AED.	Carotid If pulse present, support airway and breathing. If no pulse, start compressions, call for AED.
Chest landmarks	Lower half of sternum, 1 finger-width below nipple line	Lower half of sternum	Lower half of sternum
Compress chest with	2 fingers (1 rescuer) or 2 thumbs encircling chest (2 rescuers)	Heel of 1 hand or as for adult	Heel of 1 hand, other hand on top
Compression depth	½ to 1 inch About ⅓ to ½ depth of chest	1 to 1½ inches About ⅓ to ½ depth of chest	1½ to 2 inches About 100/min
Compression rate	About 100/min	About 100/min	1 or 2 rescuers = 30:2
Compression/ventilation ratio	1 rescuer = 30:2 2 rescuers = 15:2	1 rescuer = 30:2 2 rescuers = 15:2	
D = Defibrillation, if necessary	CPR for 5 cycles, recheck pulse. If no pulse, continue CPR. Recheck pulse every 5 cycles (about every 2 minutes). Although AEDs exist for use in infants, resuscitation guidelines currently make no recommendation for or against AED use in infants.	If witnessed arrest, use AED. Power on AED, apply pads. Analyze rhythm, shock if indicated using pediatric pads/cable system. If unwitnessed arrest, 5 cycles of CPR, then use AED. If shockable rhythm, give 1 shock, resume CPR for 5 cycles, recheck rhythm. If rhythm is not shockable, resume CPR.	If witnessed arrest, use AED. Power on AED, apply pads. Analyze rhythm, shock if indicated. If unwitnessed arrest, 5 cycles of CPR, then use AED. If shockable rhythm, give 1 shock, resume CPR for 5 cycles, recheck rhythm. If rhythm is not shockable, resume CPR.

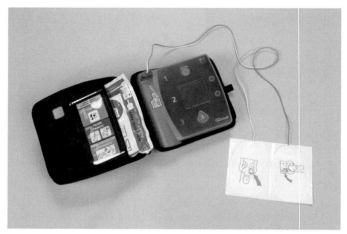

Figure 1-4 • An automated external defibrillator uses an algorithm to distinguish shockable rhythms from nonshockable rhythms.

AED Deployment Strategies				
Deployment	**Examples**	**Rescuers**	**Advantages**	**Limitations**
Emergency vehicles	Police cars Fire engines Ambulances	Trained emergency personnel	Experienced users Broad deployment Objectivity	Deployment time Arrival delays Community variations
Public access sites	Public buildings Stadiums, malls Airports Airliners	Security personnel Designated rescuers Random lay persons	Population density Shorter delays Lay and emergency personnel access	Low event rates Inexperienced users Panic and confusion
Multi-family dwellings	Apartments Condominiums Hotels	Security personnel Designated rescuers Family members	Familiar locations Defined personnel Shorter delays	Infrequent use Low event rates Geographic factors
Single-family dwellings	Private homes Apartments Neighborhood "Heart Watch"	Family members Security personnel Designated rescuers	Immediate access Familiar setting	Acceptance Victim may be alone One-time user; panic

Figure 1-5 • Deployment strategies for automated external defibrillators.

QUICK REVIEW 1-2

Can you name the four cardiac arrest rhythms? Which of these are considered shockable rhythms?

When an individual experiences a cardiac arrest, the likelihood of successful resuscitation is affected by the speed with which CPR and defibrillation are performed. Because time is critical when dealing with a victim of SCD, a weak or missing link in the Chain of Survival can reduce the likelihood of a positive outcome.

Early ACLS

■ In the prehospital setting, early advanced care is provided by paramedics arriving on the scene. Paramedics work quickly to stabilize the patient by providing ventilation support and vascular access and by giving emergency drugs, among other interventions. They then transfer the patient to the Emergency Department (ED) where definitive care can be provided.

■ In the hospital setting, healthcare professionals provide advanced care, including advanced airway management, ventilation support, and possible surgical interventions (Box 1-2).

■ A resuscitation effort requires coordination of four critical tasks: (1) airway management, (2) chest compressions, (3) ECG monitoring and defibrillation, and (4) vascular access and drug administration.

■ Regardless of where a cardiac arrest occurs, the goals of the resuscitation team are to restore spontaneous breathing and circulation and preserve vital organ function throughout the resuscitation effort. **Cerebral resuscitation** is a term used to emphasize the need to preserve the viability of the cardiac arrest victim's brain.

BOX 1-2

Components of Advanced Cardiac Care

- Basic life support
- Advanced airway management
- Ventilation support
- ECG/dysrhythmia recognition
- 12-lead ECG interpretation
- Vascular access and fluid resuscitation
- Electrical therapy including defibrillation, synchronized cardioversion, and pacing
- Giving medications
- Coronary artery bypass, stent insertion, angioplasty

QUICK REVIEW 1-3

1. Can you name the components of the Chain of Survival?

2. What are the goals of the resuscitation team in a cardiac arrest?

3. Can you name the four critical tasks of resuscitation?

THE PHASES OF CPR

Research has shown that cardiac arrest due to VF occurs in a 3-phase, time-dependent manner.[26]

■ Phase 1

▶ The first phase is called the *electrical phase* (Table 1-7). It extends from the time of cardiac arrest to about 5 minutes following the arrest.

▶ Prompt defibrillation is the most important treatment during this phase. If you witness a cardiac arrest (see the patient collapse), assess the patient's airway, breathing, and circulation, and then quickly apply an AED (or check the patient's cardiac rhythm using a manual defibrillator).

▶ Since 70% of cardiac arrests occur in the home, CPR training for families and having an AED in the home can help increase the number of survivors of cardiac arrest due to VF.[27] Even if an AED is present in the home, family members should be taught to call for help as soon as possible to mobilize resources.

Phase	Phase Name	Time from VF Arrest	Important Intervention
	TABLE 1-7 Phases of CPR		
1	Electrical phase	From time of arrest to about the first 5 min after arrest	Electrical therapy
2	Circulatory (hemodynamic) phase	About 5 min to 10 or 15 min after arrest	CPR before electrical therapy
3	Metabolic phase	After about 10 to 15 min	Possible therapeutic hypothermia or other new concept

- **Phase 2**
  - The second phase is called the *circulatory phase* or *hemodynamic phase*. It lasts from about 5 to 10 or 15 minutes after the cardiac arrest. CPR is very important during this phase.
  - Adequate cerebral and coronary perfusion pressure is critical to neurologically normal survival. **Coronary perfusion pressure** (CPP) is the difference between the aortic relaxation (diastolic) pressure and the right atrial relaxation (diastolic) blood pressure during CPR. When performing external chest compressions, systole is the chest compression phase and diastole is the release phase.[28] CPP is related to myocardial blood flow and is a major determinant of success in resuscitation.
  - Factors affecting perfusion pressures during cardiac arrest include the following[28]:
    - CPPs are generated during chest compressions. When performing chest compressions, it takes time to develop cerebral and coronary perfusion pressures. When chest compressions are stopped for even a few seconds to give rescue breaths or perform other interventions (such as inserting an advanced airway), cerebral and coronary perfusion pressures fall quickly.

 During cardiac arrest, coronary perfusion declines rapidly if chest compressions are stopped for even a few seconds. When caring for a patient in cardiac arrest, it is *essential* that interruptions to analyze the ECG, charge the defibrillator, place an advanced airway, check a pulse, or other procedures be kept to a minimum.[29]

    - *Vascular resistance.* Drugs given during cardiac arrest that constrict blood vessels (vasopressors) may improve perfusion pressures. Drugs given that dilate blood vessels (vasodilators) decrease perfusion pressures.
    - *Vascular volume.* An adequate blood volume is necessary for adequate perfusion. An adequate perfusion pressure cannot be obtained and patients cannot be resuscitated if their blood volume is low (such as that due to blood loss or significant venous dilation).
    - *Intrathoracic pressure.* During the release (diastolic) phase of chest compression, intrathoracic pressure is low. This helps increase the return of venous blood into the chest. If intrathoracic pressure is too high during this phase, venous return is inhibited. Hyperventilation is a common cause of excessive intrathoracic pressure during CPR.
  - Studies have shown that if an AED is the first intervention applied during this phase, the patient is less likely to survive. The 2005 resuscitation guidelines recommend that EMS personnel who do not witness a prehospital cardiac arrest may perform 5 cycles of CPR (about 2 minutes) and then analyze the patient's rhythm with an AED.[30] There is insufficient evidence for or against CPR before defibrillation for in-hospital cardiac arrest.[25]

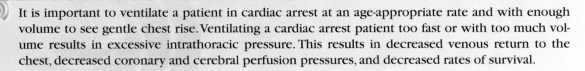

It is important to ventilate a patient in cardiac arrest at an age-appropriate rate and with enough volume to see gentle chest rise. Ventilating a cardiac arrest patient too fast or with too much volume results in excessive intrathoracic pressure. This results in decreased venous return to the chest, decreased coronary and cerebral perfusion pressures, and decreased rates of survival.

- Phase 3
  - The third phase is the *metabolic phase*. It extends beyond about 10 to 15 minutes after cardiac arrest. During this phase, the effectiveness of immediate defibrillation and CPR followed by defibrillation decreases rapidly and survival rates appear to be poor.[26]
  - Studies have shown the benefit of inducing hypothermia (therapeutic hypothermia) within minutes to hours after the return of spontaneous circulation following resuscitation of adults from VF.[31]
    - Although research is ongoing, therapeutic hypothermia appears to provide the following beneficial effects[32]:
      - Suppression of many of the chemical reactions associated with reperfusion injury
      - Possible improvement in oxygen delivery to the brain
      - Decrease in heart rate and an increase in systemic vascular resistance, while stroke volume and arterial blood pressure are maintained
  - The 2005 resuscitation guidelines recommend that unconscious adult patients who have a return of spontaneous circulation after out-of-hospital cardiac arrest should be cooled to between 89.6° F and 93.2° F (32° C to 34° C) for 12 to 24 hours when the patient's initial cardiac rhythm was VF. Similar therapy may be helpful for patients with non-VF arrest out of hospital or for in-hospital arrest.[33]

QUICK REVIEW 1-4

Can you name the three phases of CPR?
1.
2.
3.

PATIENT ASSESSMENT

The interval preceding a cardiac arrest is called the **prearrest period**. The **periarrest period** is considered 1 hour before and 1 hour after a cardiac arrest. Recognizing and promptly treating critical conditions in the "prearrest" or "periarrest" period may prevent a full cardiac arrest. Recognition of critical conditions requires good patient assessment skills.

SCENE SAFETY

Before approaching the patient, make sure that the scene is safe. Note any hazards or potential hazards and any visible mechanism or injury or illness. Always take appropriate body substance isolation precautions.

FIRST IMPRESSION

When you first see a patient, pause for a moment and form a first impression. Does the patient appear to be "sick" or "not sick"? Forming a first impression will help you quickly determine if a life-threatening problem exists that requires immediate care. The "ABCs" have been a part of emergency care for many years. When forming a first impression, the ABCs stand for *Ap-pearance*, (work of) *Breathing*, and *Circulation* (Figure 1-6).

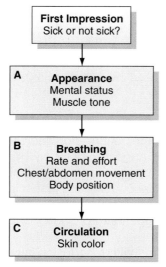

Figure 1-6 • Patient assessment: First impression.

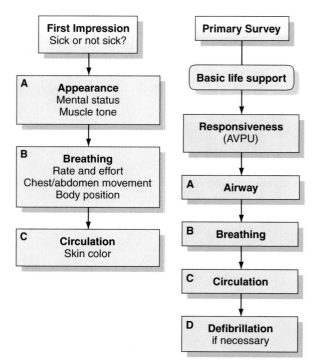

Figure 1-7 • Patient assessment: Primary survey.

- Normal findings
  - ▶ Appearance—Aware of your approach, normal muscle tone, equal movement of all extremities
  - ▶ Breathing—Quiet, unlabored respirations; equal chest rise and fall, respiratory rate within normal range for age
  - ▶ Circulation—Skin color appears normal for patient's ethnic group
- Abnormal findings
  - ▶ Appearance—Decreased responsiveness, limp or rigid muscle tone
  - ▶ Breathing—Abnormal body position (tripod position), retractions, accessory muscle use, noisy breathing, respiratory rate outside normal range
  - ▶ Circulation—Pallor, mottling, cyanosis

If the patient appears sick (abnormal findings are present), move quickly. Proceed *immediately* to the primary survey. If the patient's condition does not appear to be urgent, proceed systematically, starting with the primary survey and then the secondary survey.

Quick Review 1-5

What are the first impression ABCs?
A =
B =
C =

PRIMARY SURVEY

■ Approach the patient and perform a primary survey only after making sure that the scene is safe.
■ The primary survey is a rapid hands-on assessment of the patient that usually requires less than 60 seconds to complete, but may take longer if you must provide emergency care at any point.
■ The purpose of the primary survey is to detect the presence of life-threatening problems and immediately correct them. During this phase of patient assessment, assessment and management occur at the same time—"Treat as you find."
■ The primary survey is performed in the following order (Figure 1-7):
   ▶ Level of responsiveness
   ▶ A = Airway
   ▶ B = Breathing
   ▶ C = Circulation
   ▶ D = Defibrillation, if necessary
■ The primary survey should be periodically repeated, particularly after any major intervention or when a change in the patient's condition is detected.

Assess Responsiveness

■ After determining that the scene is safe, quickly determine the patient's level of responsiveness (Figure 1-8). If trauma to the head or neck is suspected, have someone maintain in-line stabilization of the cervical spine to minimize movement and avoid further injury.
■ Use the AVPU acronym when evaluating level of responsiveness:
   ▶ A = *A*lert
   ▶ V = Responds to *v*erbal stimuli
   ▶ P = Responds to *p*ainful stimuli
   ▶ U = *U*nresponsive
■ A patient oriented to person, place, time, and event is "alert and oriented times four." Alert does not necessarily mean oriented. Alert only means the patient is spontaneously aware of his or her environment.
■ If the patient is responsive, ask the patient questions to determine his or her level of responsiveness and the adequacy of his or her airway and breathing. Momentarily leave the patient to call 9-1-1 and then return as quickly as possible and continue your assessment. If the emergency occurred in a facility with an established medical response system, notify that system instead of calling 9-1-1.

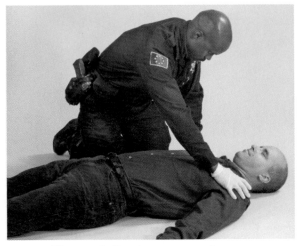

Figure 1-8 • Assess responsiveness.

- If the patient appears unresponsive, questions such as "Are you okay?" or "Can you hear me?" may elicit a response. If there is no response, try rubbing the patient's shoulder or pinching the skin of the patient's earlobe or neck muscles to elicit a response.
  - ▶ If there is no response and you are by yourself in the prehospital setting, activate the EMS system (call 9-1-1), get an AED (if available), and quickly return to the patient to provide CPR and defibrillation if needed.
  - ▶ If another rescuer is present, one rescuer should continue the primary survey while the other activates the EMS system and gets the AED.
  - ▶ If the patient is unresponsive and in a facility with an established medical response system, notify that system instead of activating the EMS system.
- An unresponsive patient should be positioned face up and flat on a firm surface to aid assessment and treatment.

Assess the Airway

- If the patient is responsive and the airway is open, move on and assess the patient's breathing. If the patient is responsive but cannot talk, cry, or cough forcefully, evaluate for possible airway obstruction.
- If the patient is unresponsive, open the airway using a head-tilt/chin-lift (Figure 1-9). If trauma is suspected, use the jaw-thrust without head tilt maneuver to open the airway (see Chapter 2). If the airway is now open, move on and assess the patient's breathing.
  - ▶ Assess for sounds of airway compromise (snoring, gurgling, stridor). Gurgling is an indication for immediate suctioning. Look in the mouth for blood, broken teeth or loose dentures, gastric contents, and foreign objects. If present, position the patient to facilitate drainage and suction the mouth. If solid material is visualized, remove it with a gloved finger covered in gauze.
  - ▶ Insert an airway adjunct (such as an oral or nasal airway) as needed to maintain an open airway.

If dentures are loose or broken, remove them. If they are intact and well fitting, leave them in place to help maintain the contour of the mouth and provide a firm surface when performing mouth-to-mask or bag-valve-mask ventilation.

Assess Breathing

- An open airway does not assure adequate breathing. Take up to 10 seconds to look, listen, and feel for breathing (Figure 1-10). If the patient is breathing, determine if breathing is adequate or inadequate (Table 1-8). If breathing is adequate, move on to assessment of circulation.

■ Look at the chest and abdomen for movement. Evaluate the depth (tidal volume) and symmetry of movement with each breath. Chest expansion should be adequate with sufficient tidal volume to make the chest rise and equal with no excessive use of accessory muscles during inspiration or expiration.

■ Estimate the respiratory rate. The normal respiratory rate for an adult at rest is 12 to 20 breaths/min. A patient who has breathing difficulty often has a respiratory rate outside the normal limits for his or her age. An increase in the respiratory rate is an early sign of respiratory distress.

■ Look for signs of increased work of breathing (respiratory effort)—pursed-lip breathing, use of accessory muscles, leaning forward to inhale, and/or retractions.

■ Listen to the patient's breathing. Note if respirations are quiet, absent, or noisy (stridor, wheezing, snoring, crowing, gurgling). Wheezing may be heard throughout the lungs or, in the case of a foreign body obstruction, may be localized.

■ Feel for air movement from the nose or mouth against your chin, face, or palm of your hand.

■ If the unresponsive patient is breathing adequately and there are no signs of trauma, place the patient in the recovery position. If breathing is difficult and the rate is too slow or too fast, provide supplemental oxygen and, if necessary, **positive-pressure ventilation** (forcing air into the lungs).

■ If breathing is absent, deliver two breaths (Figure 1-11). Each breath should be delivered over 1 second. Make sure the patient's chest rises with each breath. Insert an airway adjunct (oral or nasal airway) if not previously done and provide positive-pressure ventilation (see Chapter 2). Continue the primary survey.

TABLE 1-8	Signs of Adequate and Inadequate Breathing	
	Adequate Breathing	**Inadequate Breathing**
Rate	12 to 20 breaths/min (adult) at rest	Respiratory rate outside normal range for age and situation
Rhythm	Regular	Irregular
Quality	Breath sounds present and equal bilaterally	Breath sounds diminished or absent
	Chest expansion adequate and equal with each breath	Chest expansion unequal or inadequate
	No excessive use of accessory muscles during inspiration or expiration	Increased effort (work) of breathing
		Cannot complete full sentences
Depth (tidal volume)	Adequate	Inadequate/shallow
Skin	Pink, warm, dry	Pale, cyanotic, cool, clammy

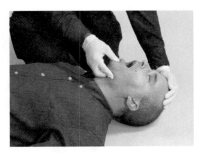

Figure 1-9 • Open the airway.

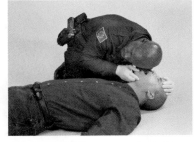

Figure 1-10 • Assess breathing.

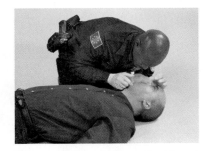

Figure 1-11 • If the patient is not breathing, give rescue breaths.

Assess Circulation

■ Check for the presence of a pulse and other signs of circulation for up to 10 seconds. If the patient is responsive, assess the radial pulse. If the patient is unresponsive, assess the carotid pulse on the side of the patient's neck nearest you (Figure 1-12).

■ If a pulse is present, quickly estimate the rate and determine the quality of the pulse (fast/slow, regular/irregular, weak/strong), then move on to the secondary survey.

■ If there is no pulse, and you witnessed the patient's collapse, perform CPR until an AED (or monitor/defibrillator) is available. For adults, the ratio of chest compressions to ventilations is 30 to 2 for both one-rescuer and two-rescuer CPR. An adult should be given 10 to 12 ventilations/minute (1 ventilation every 5 to 6 seconds). Give compressions at a rate of about 100/minute. If there is no pulse and you did not witness the arrest, perform CPR for about 2 minutes and then analyze the patient's heart rhythm with the AED.

■ If two or more rescuers are present, the rescuer giving chest compressions should switch roles with the rescuer giving ventilations about every 2 minutes (when the patient's rhythm is checked). This change should optimize the rate and quality of chest compressions by preventing compressor fatigue. To minimize the interruption in chest compressions, try to accomplish the switch in less than 5 seconds.

Defibrillation

■ If there is no pulse, turn the power on to the AED. Attach AED pads to the patient's bare chest according to the manufacturer's instructions (Figure 1-13). Analyze the patient's heart rhythm using the AED. Deliver a shock if instructed to do so by the AED. After delivery of the shock, immediately resume CPR, starting with chest compressions.

KEEPING IT SIMPLE

Repeat the primary survey:
• With any sudden change in the patient's condition
• When interventions do not appear to be working
• When vital signs are unstable
• Before any procedures
• When a change in rhythm is observed on the cardiac monitor

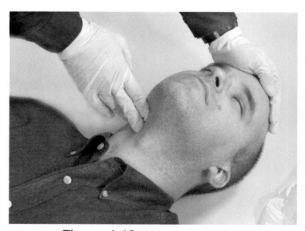

Figure 1-12 • Assess circulation.

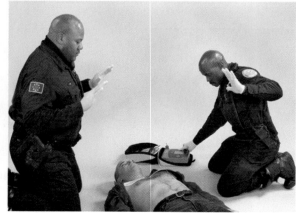

Figure 1-13 • If there is no pulse, attach an AED or conventional monitor/defibrillator when available. Defibrillate if necessary.

QUICK REVIEW 1-6

1. What is the purpose of the primary survey?

2. Can you name the components of the primary survey?

3. During the primary survey, for what length of time should you assess for the presence of a pulse and other signs of circulation?
4. What is the normal respiratory rate for an adult at rest?
5. True or False. An open airway ensures adequate ventilation.

THE SECONDARY SURVEY

KEEPING IT SIMPLE

The Secondary Survey
(Advanced) **A**irway
Breathing
Circulation
Differential **D**iagnosis, diagnostic procedures
Evaluate interventions, pain management
Facilitate family presence for invasive and resuscitative procedures

- The purpose of the physical examination in the secondary survey is to detect potentially life-threatening conditions and provide care for those conditions. The secondary survey focuses on *advanced* life support (ALS) interventions and management.
- Obtain vital signs and attach a pulse oximeter, ECG, and blood pressure monitor (Figure 1-14).
- Obtain a focused history. The history is often obtained while the physical examination is being performed and emergency care is being given. Ask the patient, family, bystanders, or others questions regarding the patient's history. SAMPLE is a memory aid used to organize the information obtained when taking a patient history.
  - *Signs/symptoms*—Assessment findings and history as they relate to the emergency
    - When did it start/occur (time, sudden, gradual)? What was the patient doing when it started/occurred?
    - How long did it last? Does it come and go? Is it still present?
    - Where is the problem? Describe character and severity if painful (use 0 to 10 pain scale).
    - Radiation? Aggravating or alleviating factors?
    - Previous history of same? If yes, what was the diagnosis?
  - *Allergies*—to medications, food, environmental causes (pollen), and products (latex)
  - *Medications*
    - Prescription and over-the-counter medications (including herbal supplements) the patient is currently taking
    - Determine name of medication, dose, route, frequency, and indication for the medication

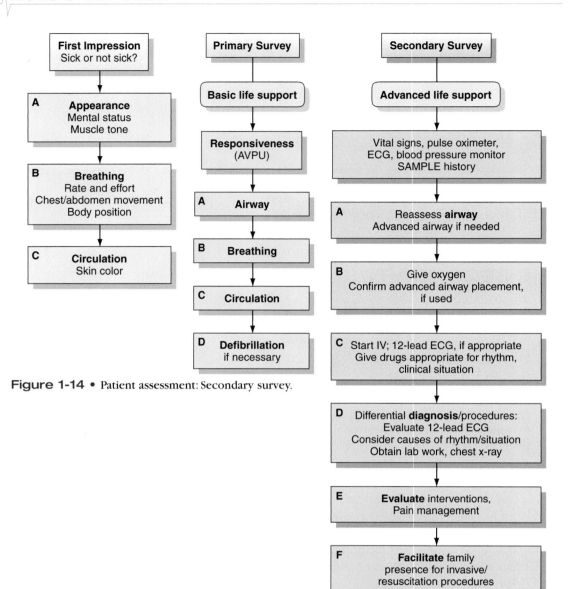

First Impression
Sick or not sick?

A **Appearance**
Mental status
Muscle tone

B **Breathing**
Rate and effort
Chest/abdomen movement
Body position

C **Circulation**
Skin color

Primary Survey

Basic life support

Responsiveness
(AVPU)

A **Airway**

B **Breathing**

C **Circulation**

D **Defibrillation**
if necessary

Secondary Survey

Advanced life support

Vital signs, pulse oximeter,
ECG, blood pressure monitor
SAMPLE history

A Reassess **airway**
Advanced airway if needed

B Give oxygen
Confirm advanced airway placement,
if used

C Start IV; 12-lead ECG, if appropriate
Give drugs appropriate for rhythm,
clinical situation

D Differential **diagnosis**/procedures:
Evaluate 12-lead ECG
Consider causes of rhythm/situation
Obtain lab work, chest x-ray

E **Evaluate** interventions,
Pain management

F **Facilitate** family
presence for invasive/
resuscitation procedures

Figure 1-14 • Patient assessment: Secondary survey.

▶ (Pertinent) *P*ast medical history
  • Is the patient currently under a physician's care?
  • Hospitalizations—age, reason for admission
  • Surgical procedures—age, reason for procedure, complications
  • Trauma/injuries and fractures/ingestions, burns—age, circumstances surrounding event, treatment, complications
▶ *L*ast oral intake
  • Time of most recent meal and fluid intake
  • Changes in eating pattern or fluid intake
▶ *E*vents leading to the illness or injury
  • Onset, duration, and precipitating factors
  • Associated factors such as drugs, alcohol
  • Treatment given by caregiver, bystanders

(Advanced) Airway

■ Reassess the effectiveness of initial airway maneuvers and interventions.

■ If needed, insert an advanced airway (endotracheal tube, Combitube, or laryngeal mask airway [LMA]).

Insertion of advanced airways in cardiac arrest has not been shown to increase survival to hospital discharge.

Reassess Breathing

■ Assess the adequacy of ventilations.

■ If an advanced airway has been inserted, confirm proper placement using at least two methods (see Chapter 2). Provide positive-pressure ventilation with 100% oxygen and assess the effectiveness of ventilations. Make sure the tube is adequately secured.

■ In cardiac arrest, the patient may be ventilated using a bag-valve mask alone or in combination with endotracheal intubation. Remember that it is *essential* to minimize interruption of chest compressions during cardiac arrest.

  ▶ Placement of an advanced airway requires a brief interruption in chest compressions. However, once an advanced airway is in place, ventilation will not require interruption (or even pausing) of chest compressions.

KEEPING IT SIMPLE

The Primary and Secondary Surveys

Time: 9:30 a.m. Your patient is a 69-year-old man complaining of chest pain. The patient is sitting upright in bed.

Patient History (SAMPLE)

• Signs/symptoms—Chest pain earlier today that has returned and radiating to left hand.
• Allergies—None known.
• Medications—The patient has taken one Advil. He takes an unknown medication for high cholesterol once daily.
• Past medical history—High cholesterol.
• Last oral intake—Breakfast at 6 a.m. today.
• Events prior—The patient states he was shopping earlier today when he experienced chest pain. The pain began in the center of his chest and radiated to both shoulders. Upon return home, the patient took one Advil and the pain subsided. Two hours later, the pain has returned and is radiating to his left hand.

Primary Survey

• Level of responsiveness—Awake and talking with you; alert and oriented to person, place, time, and event.
• Airway—Open.
• Breathing—Respiratory rate 14, equal chest rise and fall, good tidal volume.
• Circulation—Carotid and radial pulses present, rate about 80; strong and regular.
• Defibrillation—Not indicated at this time.

Secondary Survey

• Assess vital signs; place patient on pulse oximeter, ECG, and BP monitor.
• Airway—Open; no advanced airway needed.
• Breathing—Give oxygen by nonrebreather mask at 15 L/min; breath sounds clear bilaterally.
• Circulation—Establish IV of normal saline.
• Differential diagnosis—Ask the patient questions to determine if he may be experiencing an acute coronary syndrome (Chapter 6). Give medications appropriate for his cardiac rhythm/clinical situation.
• Evaluation interventions, pain management—Reassess patient's response to care given thus far (reassess vital signs, cardiac rhythm). Assess the patient's discomfort on a 0 to 10 scale. If his BP will tolerate it, give pain medication and reassess response using pain scale.
• Facilitate family presence—Explain what is being done for the patient to family members who are present.

KEEPING IT SIMPLE

PATCH-4-MD

Pulmonary embolism
Acidosis
Tension pneumothorax
Cardiac tamponade
Hypovolemia
Hypoxia
Heat/cold (hypo-/hyperthermia)
Hypo-/hyperkalemia (and other electrolytes)
Myocardial infarction
Drug overdose/accidents

Five H's and Five T's

Hypovolemia	**T**amponade, cardiac
Hypoxia	**T**ension pneumothorax
Hypothermia	**T**hrombosis: lungs (massive pulmonary embolism)
Hypo-/Hyperkalemia	**T**hrombosis: heart (acute coronary syndromes)
Hydrogen ion (acidosis)	**T**ablets/toxins: drug overdose

▶ If an advanced airway is in place, the team member giving the ventilations should give 8 to 10 breaths/minute and should be careful to avoid delivering an excessive number of ventilations.

▶ Members of the resuscitation team may opt to wait to insert an advanced airway until there is a return of spontaneous circulation.

Assess Circulation

■ If the patient has a pulse, check its rate and quality often. If a pulse is present, assess the patient's blood pressure.

■ If not already done, attach ECG electrodes and connect the patient to an ECG monitor to allow continuous recording and reassessment of the cardiac rhythm. Obtain a 12-lead ECG if appropriate.

■ Establish vascular access with normal saline (NS) or lactated Ringer's (LR) solution. Vascular access is usually established via a peripheral IV; however, intraosseous access in cardiac arrest is safe, effective, and appropriate for patients of all ages. During cardiac arrest, establishing vascular access is important, but it should not interfere with CPR and the delivery of shocks. Each drug given in a cardiac arrest should be followed with a 20-mL IV fluid bolus and elevation of the extremity.

■ Give medications appropriate for the cardiac rhythm/clinical situation. During a cardiac arrest, drugs should be given at the time of the rhythm check.

Differential Diagnosis/Diagnostic Procedures

Search for, find, and treat reversible causes of the cardiac arrest, rhythm, or clinical situation. The memory aids "PATCH-4-MD" and "The 5 H's and 5 T's" may be used to recall possible treatable causes of cardiac emergencies.

Evaluate Interventions, Pain Management

Reassess the effectiveness of the care given thus far. Troubleshoot as needed. If the patient is responsive and complaining of discomfort, begin appropriate pain management if his or her blood pressure and other vital signs will tolerate it.

 The safe and effective relief of pain should be a priority in the management of a patient of any age.

QUICK REVIEW 1-7

1. In the primary survey, the focus of care is on _____ _____ _____.
2. In the secondary survey the focus of care is on _____ _____ _____ interventions and management.

Facilitate Family Presence

Witnessed resuscitation is a phrase used to describe the process of active "medical" resuscitation in the presence of family members. Although acceptance of witnessed resuscitation programs is not universal among all groups of healthcare professionals and concerns exist about the ethics of witnessed resuscitation and its medical-legal implications,[34] some institutions have allowed family members to be present in these situations with positive results.

The Emergency Nurses Association has resolved that family presence during invasive procedures and resuscitation is the right of the patient and is beneficial for both patients and family members.

ADVANCE DIRECTIVES

In the United States, the patient's consent to the performance of CPR is presumed under the theory of implied consent. The presence of an advance directive is a recognized exception to this presumption. An **advance directive** is a written document recording an individual's decisions concerning medical treatment that is to be applied (or not applied) in the event of physical or mental inability to communicate these wishes.

TYPES OF ADVANCE DIRECTIVES

Although a patient may have an advance directive, consent for medical treatment must be obtained from the patient as long as he or she remains able to make decisions about his or her healthcare.

■ A **living will** is a type of advance directive in which the patient puts in writing his or her wishes about medical treatment if he or she becomes terminally ill and incapable of making decisions about his or her medical care. A living will directs physicians to withhold or withdraw "death-delaying" treatments (not including nutrition and hydration). Living wills have limitations. For example, they do not apply to patients who do not have a terminal illness but are in a persistent vegetative state.

- The Patient Self-Determination Act (PSDA) went into effect December 1, 1991. This law requires that hospitals and nursing homes ask individuals at the time of admission if they have an advance directive. If the individual does not, the facility must ask if he or she wishes to complete one.
- A **durable power of attorney for healthcare** (DPAHC) is a type of advance directive that overcomes the limitations of a living will. A DPAHC is a written document that identifies a legal guardian to make healthcare decisions for a patient when the patient can no longer make such decisions for himself or herself. It may also be called a "healthcare proxy" or "appointment of a healthcare agent." The person appointed may be called the patient's healthcare agent, surrogate, attorney-in-fact, or proxy. In many states, a durable power of attorney applies to any medical situation in which the patient is unable to make his or her own medical decisions, not just terminal illness. Withdrawal of nutrition and hydration by a feeding tube is permissible.[35]
- Some advance directives are combination documents that combine elements of a living will and DPAHC decisions into one document.
  - The Five Wishes Document developed by Aging with Dignity is an innovative document that addresses the patient's healthcare wishes, as well as his or her personal, emotional, and spiritual needs. As this book goes to press, the Five Wishes Document meets the technical requirements for an advance directive in 37 states.
    - Wish 1. The person I want to make healthcare decisions for me when I can't make them for myself.
    - Wish 2. My wish for the kind of medical treatment I want or don't want.
    - Wish 3. My wish for how comfortable I want to be.
    - Wish 4. My wish for how I want people to treat me.
    - Wish 5. My wish for what I want my loved ones to know.

The Five Wishes Advance Directive document can be ordered by calling Aging with Dignity (888-5-WISHES). It is also available at http://www.agingwithdignity.org/. The Caring Conversations Advance Directive document is available at http://www.midbio.org/mbc-ccorder.htm or from the Midwest Bioethics Center (800-344-3829).

- Caring Conversations, published by the Midwest Bioethics Center, is a short workbook that encourages discussion about end-of-life decisions and advance care planning with family and friends. Examples of questions include, "What are your fears regarding the end of your life?" "If you could plan it today, what would the last day of your life be like?" and "If you wrote your own epitaph or obituary, what would it say?"

- The phrases "do not resuscitate" (DNR), "do not attempt resuscitation" (DNAR), and "no CPR" are often used interchangeably. Some physicians are changing those designations to "AND" which stands for "Allow Natural Death." This designation is more positive and takes away the stigma of withholding care.
- All 50 states and the District of Columbia recognize both the living will and the DPAHC advance directives. However, the laws of each state vary considerably in terminology, the scope of decision making addressed, restrictions, and the formalities required for making an advance directive.

COMPLICATIONS ASSOCIATED WITH ADVANCE DIRECTIVES

- Despite the existence of an advance directive, complications may exist when the healthcare team or facility is not aware of its existence. It is essential that the patient, his or her healthcare agent or guardian, and those close to the patient make sure that everyone who might need a copy of the directive in fact has a copy.
- Another complication may arise when the patient has not expressed his or her wishes clearly in the advance directive. Use of vague language that requests "no heroic mea-

sures" or "no treatment measures that only prolong the process of dying" may result in problems with interpretation of the patient's wishes. These issues can be avoided if the patient and his or her healthcare agent or guardian have previously discussed the patient's wishes. Unfortunately, the healthcare agent or guardian is sometimes unaware of what it is the patient would want done in a given situation.

▪ In the prehospital setting, challenges may arise when a dying patient with an advance directive (or the patient's family) calls 9-1-1. In general, EMS personnel are required to resuscitate and stabilize patients and, when necessary, transport them to an appropriate facility.

  ▶ States have begun to address this situation by developing protocols that allow EMS personnel to refrain from resuscitating patients who possess a legal document or other approved identifier (such as a special bracelet or form) verifying a DNR order (Figure 1-15). The names of these protocols vary, such as "Prehospital Medical Care Directive" and "Comfort Care/Do Not Resuscitate" (CC/DNR) protocols. When in place, these protocols enable EMS professionals to honor DNR orders in the prehospital setting.

  ▶ Confusion may occur when a patient who has a valid DNR order is ill or injured, but not in full cardiac or respiratory arrest.

    • Consider this real-life example. Paramedics respond to a private residence for an elderly man with difficulty breathing. The EMS crew recognizes the bracelet the patient is wearing as a state-approved DNR identifier. The patient's heart rate and breathing are adequate, although the patient states it is harder to breathe than usual. The members of the EMS crew disagree about how to handle the situation. One paramedic believes the patient's DNR does not apply because the patient is obviously breathing and has a pulse. His paramedic partner believes that the presence of a valid DNR means "do not treat." They phone Medical Control for advice and direction. After quickly relaying the circumstances at the scene, the Emergency Department physician angrily states that the patient's family should not have called 9-1-1 in the first place if the patient has a DNR order. The crew is instructed to transport the patient without giving any advanced life support care.

PREHOSPITAL MEDICAL CARE DIRECTIVE
(side one)

IN THE EVENT OF CARDIAC OR RESPIRATORY ARREST, I REFUSE ANY RESUSCITATION MEASURES, INCLUDING CARDIAC COMPRESSION, ENDOTRACHEAL INTUBATION, AND OTHER ADVANCED AIRWAY MANAGEMENT, ARTIFICIAL VENTILATION, DEFIBRILLATION, ADMINISTRATION OF ADVANCED CARDIAC LIFE SUPPORT DRUGS, AND RELATED EMERGENCY MEDICAL PROCEDURES.

Patient:_____ Date:_____

_____
(Signature or mark)

Attach recent photograph here or provide all of the following information below:

Date of Birth_____
Sex_____ Race_____
Eye Color_____
Hair Color_____

PHOTO

Hospice Program (if any)

_____

Name and telephone number of patient's physician___

_____

(side two)

I have explained this form and its consequences to the signer and obtained assurance that the signer understands that death may result from any refused care listed above (on reverse side).

_____ Date:_____
(Licensed health care provider)

I was present when this was signed (or marked). The patient then appeared to be of sound mind and free from duress.

_____ Date:_____
(Witness)

Figure 1-15 • An example of a prehospital medical care directive.

▓ To address these types of situations, some state protocols now spell out the responsibilities of EMS personnel at the scene and/or during transport of patients possessing a valid CC/DNR form (or other identifier). They also permit EMS personnel to provide comfort care (within their scope of practice) for patients who have a valid order. For example, protocols developed by the state of Massachusetts provide the following specific instructions:[36]

> ❱ "**If the patient is *not* in respiratory or cardiac arrest** and the patient's heart beat and breathing are adequate, but there is some other emergency illness or injury, the EMS personnel shall provide full treatment and transport, as appropriate, within the scope of their training and level of certification.

> ❱ **If the patient is in full respiratory or cardiac arrest,** the EMS personnel **shall not resuscitate,** which means:
> - Do not initiate CPR;
> - Do not insert an oropharyngeal airway (OPA);
> - Do not provide ventilatory assistance;
> - Do not artificially ventilate the patient (mouth-to-mouth, bag valve mask, positive pressure, etc.);
> - Do not administer chest compressions;
> - Do not initiate advanced airway measures such as endotracheal intubation;
> - Do not administer cardiac resuscitation drugs; and
> - Do not defibrillate.

> ❱ **If the patient is *not* in full respiratory or cardiac arrest**, but the patient's heart beat or breathing is inadequate, EMS personnel shall not resuscitate but **shall** provide, within the scope of their training and level of certification, full palliative care and transport, as appropriate, including:
> - Emotional support;
> - Suction airway;
> - Administer oxygen;
> - Application of cardiac monitor;
> - Control bleeding;
> - Splint;
> - Position for comfort;
> - Initiate IV line; and
> - Contact Medical Control, if appropriate, for further orders, including necessary medications."

▓ In the absence of such documentation (or other identifier), prehospital personnel will generally begin resuscitation procedures while simultaneously attempting to obtain orders from a physician medical director. This occurs because these situations raise doubts about the validity of the DNR order. EMS professionals should always defer to their local or regional protocols.

CRITERIA FOR NOT STARTING CPR

▓ The 2005 Resuscitation Guidelines recommend that all patients in cardiac arrest receive resuscitation unless:
> ❱ The patient has a valid DNAR order
> ❱ The patient has signs of irreversible death (e.g., rigor mortis, decapitation, decomposition, or dependent lividity)
> ❱ No physiologic benefit can be expected because vital functions have deteriorated despite maximal therapy (e.g., progressive septic or cardiogenic shock)

▓ According to the American Heart Association, prehospital professionals should begin CPR and ACLS if there is reason to believe that:[37]
> ❱ There is reasonable doubt about the validity of a DNAR order or advance directive
> ❱ The patient may have changed his or her mind
> ❱ The best interests of the patient are in question

Rigor mortis and decapitation are obvious signs of death. Dependent lividity is considered an obvious sign of death only when there are extensive areas of reddish-purple discoloration of the skin in dependent areas of an unresponsive, breathless, and pulseless patient. In some areas, both lividity and rigor mortis must be present to be considered signs of obvious death.

■ In some cases, the patient in cardiac arrest will not respond despite appropriate basic and advanced life support care. Most EMS systems have developed obvious death, field termination, death in the field, or similar protocols that allows field termination of resuscitation efforts in specific circumstances.

■ The National Association of EMS Physicians (NAEMSP) has recommended factors that should be considered when establishing prehospital termination of resuscitation protocols.[38] The NAEMSP recommendations include the following:

  ▶ Termination of resuscitation may be considered for any adult patient who suffers SCD that is likely to be medical.

  ▶ Unwitnessed cardiac arrest with delayed initiation of cardiopulmonary resuscitation (CPR) beyond 6 minutes and delayed defibrillation beyond 8 minutes has a poor prognosis.

  ▶ In the absence of DNR or advance directives, a full resuscitative effort including CPR, definitive airway management, medication administration, defibrillation if necessary, and at least 20 minutes of treatment following ACLS guidelines should be performed prior to declaring the patient dead.

  ▶ A patient whose rhythm changes to, or remains in, VF or VT should have continued resuscitative efforts. Patients in asystole or pulseless electrical activity (PEA) should be strongly considered for out-of-hospital termination of resuscitation.

  ▶ Logistic factors should be considered, such as collapse in a public place, family wishes, and safety of the crew and public.

  ▶ Online medical direction should be established prior to termination of resuscitation. The decision to terminate efforts should be a consensus between the on-scene paramedic and the online physician.

  ▶ The on-scene providers and family should have access to resources such as clergy, crisis workers, and social workers.

  ▶ Quality review is necessary to ensure appropriate application of the termination protocol, law enforcement notification, medical examiner or coroner involvement, and family counseling.

■ At the scene, law enforcement personnel may need to communicate with the patient's physician for the death certificate. They may also determine if the event/patient requires assignment to the medical examiner. This may occur if there is any suspicion about the nature of the death or if the patient's physician refuses or hesitates to sign the death certificate. If the patient does not have a personal physician, the patient will be assigned to the medical examiner.

QUICK REVIEW 1-8

1. True or False. A DPAHC is a type of advance directive that identifies a legal guardian to make healthcare decisions for a patient when the patient can no longer make such decisions for him or herself.
2. A written document recording an individual's decisions concerning medical treatment that is to be applied (or not applied) in the event of physical or mental inability to communicate these wishes is called a(n) _____ _____ .
3. Complete the following. In general, patients in cardiac arrest receive resuscitation unless:
   • The patient has a valid DNAR order.
   • The patient has signs of irreversible death:

   _____

   _____

   _____

   • No physiologic benefit can be expected because vital functions have deteriorated despite maximal therapy for such conditions as progressive septic or cardiogenic shock.

CLASSIFICATION OF TREATMENT RECOMMENDATIONS

The 2005 resuscitation guidelines and treatment recommendations have been classified as follows:[39]

■ Class I—Procedure/treatment or diagnostic test/assessment should be performed/administered.

■ Class IIa—It is reasonable to perform procedure/administer treatment or perform diagnostic test/assessment.

■ Class IIb—Procedure/treatment or diagnostic test/assessment may be considered.

■ Class III—Procedure/treatment or diagnostic test/assessment should not be performed/administered. It is not helpful and may be harmful.

■ Indeterminate—Research just getting started; continuing area of research; no recommendations until further research (e.g., cannot recommend for or against).

QUICK REVIEW ANSWERS

Quick Review Number	Answers
1-1	1. Nonmodifiable risk factors for coronary artery disease include heredity, gender, race, and age. 2. Modifiable risk factors include high blood pressure, elevated blood cholesterol levels, tobacco use, physical inactivity, obesity, and metabolic syndrome. 3. Contributing risk factors include stress, inflammatory markers, psychosocial factors, and alcohol intake.
1-2	The four cardiac arrest rhythms are VT, VF, asystole, and PEA. Ventricular tachycardia and ventricular fibrillation are shockable rhythms. Asystole and PEA are nonshockable rhythms.
1-3	1. The steps in the Chain of Survival are (1) early access, (2) early CPR, (3) early defibrillation, and 4) early ACLS. 2. The goals of the resuscitation team are to restore spontaneous breathing and circulation and preserve vital organ function throughout the resuscitation effort. 3. Airway management, chest compressions, ECG monitoring and defibrillation, vascular access, and drug administration.
1-4	The three phases of CPR are the electrical phase, circulatory (hemodynamic) phase, and metabolic phase. The electrical phase lasts from the time of arrest to about the first 5 minutes after the arrest. The circulatory phase lasts about 5 minutes to 10 or 15 minutes after the arrest. The metabolic phase occurs after about 10 to 15 minutes.
1-5	The first impression ABCs are appearance, (work of) breathing, and circulation.
1-6	1. The purpose of the primary survey is to detect the presence of life-threatening problems that require rapid intervention. 2. The components of the primary survey are Airway, Breathing, Circulation, and Defibrillation, if necessary. 3. A pulse and other signs of circulation should be assessed for up to 10 seconds. 4. The normal respiratory rate for an adult at rest is 12 to 20 breaths/minute. 5. False. An open airway does not ensure adequate ventilation.
1-7	1. In the primary survey, the focus of care is on basic life support. 2. In the secondary survey the focus of care is on advanced life support interventions and management.
1-8	1. True 2. Advance directive 3. Rigor mortis, decapitation, dependent lividity (or decomposition)

STOP & REVIEW

Questions 1–18. Match each answer below (a through r) with its corresponding description.

a) Rhythm
b) LDL
c) Abdominal
d) First-degree
e) Syndrome X
f) Appearance
g) Circulatory
h) Acidosis
i) Witnessed
j) AVPU
k) Coronary perfusion
l) Periarrest
m) Cerebral
n) Electrical
o) Team leader
p) Metabolic
q) Risk factors
r) OPQRST

_____ 1. The period 1 hour before and 1 hour after a cardiac arrest

_____ 2. _____ resuscitation is a term used to emphasize the need to preserve the viability of the cardiac arrest victim's brain

_____ 3. "Bad" cholesterol

_____ 4. Second phase of CPR

_____ 5. This drops rapidly if chest compressions are stopped for even a few seconds in cardiac arrest

_____ 6. Memory aid used to assess level of responsiveness

_____ 7. First phase of CPR

_____ 8. The younger the onset in a _____ _____ relative, the greater the risk of cardio-vascular disease

_____ 9. Third phase of CPR

_____10. Drugs given during cardiac arrest should be given during _____ checks

_____11. The "A" assessed when you form a first impression of a patient

_____12. The person in charge of a resuscitation effort

_____13. Persons who have _____ obesity are at greatest risk of coronary heart dis-ease

_____14. Traits and lifestyle habits that may increase a person's chance of developing a disease

_____15. The "A" in PATCH-4-MD

_____16. Memory aid used to assess a complaint of pain or discomfort

_____17. _____ resuscitation refers to the process of active medical resuscitation in the presence of family members

_____18. Another name for metabolic syndrome

19. A person who has a systolic blood pressure of 120–139 mm Hg or diastolic blood pressure of 80–89 mm Hg is considered to have _____.

20. A 78-year-old man is in cardiac arrest. CPR is in progress and an IV line has not yet been established. The preferred sites for IV cannulation while chest compressions are being performed are the:
    a. Antecubital or external jugular veins
    b. Subclavian or antecubital veins
    c. Internal or external jugular veins
    d. Femoral or internal jugular veins

21. In the hospital setting, early recognition of the critically ill patient and activation of a _____ _____ _____ may prevent the development of cardiac arrest and improve patient outcome.

22. Which of the following statements about two-rescuer adult CPR is correct?
    a. The compression to ventilation ratio is 15 to 2.
    b. Pause compressions to give a breath once every 3 to 5 seconds.
    c. The switch of compressor and ventilator roles should occur in 5 seconds or less when possible.
    d. Perform CPR for at least 5 minutes before analyzing the patient's heart rhythm with an AED.

23. Which of the following memory aids may be used when evaluating a patient's level of responsiveness?
    a. ABCD
    b. AVPU
    c. OPQRST
    d. NAVEL

24. Drugs given during cardiac arrest that _____ blood vessels (vasopressors) may improve perfusion pressures.
    a. Constrict
    b. Dilate

25. The "D" in the primary ABCD survey stands for:
    a. Disability
    b. Decision
    c. Defibrillation
    d. Differential diagnosis

26. Establishing vascular access is part of:
    a. "A" in the primary survey
    b. "B" in the secondary survey
    c. "C" in the secondary survey
    d. "D" in the primary survey

27. When an IV line is established during CPR:
    a. 5% dextrose in water is the preferred solution for use during cardiac arrest
    b. It is preferable to give some medications by intramuscular injection rather than IV
    c. IV drugs given by bolus injection should be followed with a 20-mL flush of IV fluid
    d. Attempts should focus on accessing the central venous circulation rather than peripheral veins

28. "Shockable" cardiac arrest rhythms include:
    a. Asystole and pulseless electrical activity
    b. Ventricular tachycardia and asystole
    c. Pulseless electrical activity and ventricular fibrillation
    d. Ventricular fibrillation and ventricular tachycardia

STOP & REVIEW ANSWERS

1. l	10. a
2. m	11. f
3. b	12. o
4. g	13. c
5. k	14. q
6. j	15. h
7. n	16. r
8. d	17. i
9. p	18. e

19. A person who has a systolic blood pressure of 120–139 mm Hg or diastolic blood pressure of 80–89 mm Hg is considered to have <u>prehypertension.</u>

20. a. If no IV line exists at the time of arrest, a large-gauge IV catheter should be inserted into the antecubital vein. An alternate site is the external jugular vein, which is considered a peripheral vein. If IV attempts are unsuccessful, intraosseous access should be attempted before considering cannulating a central vein.

21. Early recognition of the critically ill patient and activation of a <u>medical</u> <u>emergency</u> <u>team</u> (also known as a Rapid Response Team) may prevent the development of cardiac arrest and improve patient outcome.

22. c. When possible, the switch of compressor and ventilator roles should occur in 5 seconds or less to minimize interruption of chest compressions. An adult should be given 10 to 12 ventilations/minute (1 ventilation every 5 to 6 seconds) and compressions at a rate of about 100/minute. If there is no pulse and you did not witness the arrest, perform CPR for about 2 minutes and then analyze the patient's heart rhythm with the AED.

23. b. The AVPU acronym is used to quickly assess a patient's level of responsiveness. AVPU— *A*lert, responds to *v*erbal stimuli, responds to *p*ainful stimuli, *u*nresponsive. ABCD are components of the primary and secondary surveys. OPQRST is an acronym used when evaluating a patient's complaint of pain. NAVEL is an acronym used to recall medications that may be administered via an endotracheal tube (naloxone, atropine, vasopressin, epinephrine, and lidocaine).

24. a. Drugs given during cardiac arrest that *constrict* blood vessels (vasopressors) may improve perfusion pressures. Drugs given that dilate blood vessels (vasodilators) decrease perfusion pressures.

25. c. The "D" in the primary ABCD survey stands for defibrillation. If the primary ABCD survey reveals the patient has no pulse, an AED should be attached to the patient (or a monitor/defibrillator) when available.

26. c. The primary survey focuses on basic life support assessment and intervention. The secondary survey focuses on advanced life support assessment and interventions. Thus, establishing vascular access is part of "C" (Circulation) in the secondary survey.

27. c. IV drugs given by bolus injection in a cardiac arrest should be followed with a 20-mL flush of IV fluid. Because a rapid onset of action is needed for any drug given during cardiac arrest, the intramuscular and subcutaneous routes are not used. If no IV is in place at the start of a cardiac arrest, efforts should focus on establishing a peripheral IV with a large-gauge catheter. Normal saline or lactated Ringer's solution is the preferred IV solution in cardiac arrest. Solutions containing dextrose should not be used unless there is documented evidence of hypoglycemia.

28. d. There are four cardiac arrest rhythms: 1) Ventricular fibrillation, 2) ventricular tachycardia, 3) asystole, and 4) pulseless electrical activity. "Shockable" cardiac arrest rhythms include ventricular fibrillation and ventricular tachycardia. Defibrillation is not indicated for asystole or pulseless electrical activity.

REFERENCES

1. National Center for Chronic Disease Prevention and Health Promotion: Chronic disease prevention, *Preventing Heart Disease and Stroke* (serial online): http://www.cdc.gov/nccdphp/bb_heartdisease/ Accessed 5/18/2005.
2. *Morb Mortal Wkly Rep* 51(6):123-6, 2002.
3. Mackay J, Mensah GA: *Atlas of Heart Disease and Stroke*. World Health Organization, 2004.
4. National Center for Chronic Disease Prevention and Health Promotion: Cardiovascular health, *Heart Disease Fact Sheet* (serial online): http://www.cdc.gov/cvh/library/fs_heart_disease.htm. Accessed 5/14/2005.
5. Castelli WP: Epidemiology of coronary heart disease: the Framingham study, *Am J Med* 1994;76(2A):4-12, 1984.
6. Prescott E, Hippe M, Schnohr P, Hein HO, Vestbo J: Smoking and risk of myocardial infarction in women and men: longitudinal population study, *BMJ* 1998;316(7137):1043.
7. Fodor J, Tzerovska R: Coronary heart disease: is gender important? *J Men's Health Gend* 2004;1(1):32.
8. Haffner SJ, Cassells H: Hyperglycemia as a cardiovascular risk factor, *Am J Med* 2003;115 (suppl 8A):6S-11S (review).
9. Ford ES, Giles WH, Dietz WH: Prevalence of the metabolic syndrome among US adults: findings from the third National Health and Nutrition Examination Survey, *JAMA 2002;*287(3):356-9.
10. Ridker PM: Clinical application of C-reactive protein for cardiovascular disease detection and prevention, *Circulation* 2003;107(3):363-9.
11. Bassuk SS, Rifai N, Ridker PM: High-sensitivity C-reactive protein: clinical importance, *Curr Probl Cardiol* 2004;29(8):439-93 (review).
12. Nemeroff CB, Musselman DL, Evans DL: Depression and cardiac disease, *Depress Anxiety* 1998;8 (suppl 1):71-9 (review).
13. Shimbo D, Davidson KW, Haas DC, Fuster V, Badimon JJ: Negative impact of depression on outcomes in patients with coronary artery disease: mechanisms, treatment considerations, and future directions, *J Thromb Haemost* 2005;3(5):897-908.
14. Rowan PJ, Haas D, Campbell JA, Maclean DR, Davidson KW: Depressive symptoms have an independent, gradient risk for coronary heart disease incidence in a random, population-based sample, *Ann Epidemiol* 2005;15(4):316-20.
15. Centers for Disease Control and Prevention: Racial/ethnic and socioeconomic disparities in multiple risk factors for heart disease and stroke—United States, 2003. *Morb Mortal Wkly Rep* 2005;54(5):113-7.
16. Friedman GD, Klatsky AL: Is alcohol good for your health? *N Engl J Med* 1993;329(25):1882-3 (editorial).
17. Pearson T:. Alcohol and heart disease, *Circulation* 1996;94(11):3023-5.
18. Zairis MN, Ambrose JA, Lyras AG, Thoma MA, Psarogianni PK, Psaltiras PG, Kardoulas AD, Bibis GP, Pissimissis EG, Batika PC, DeVoe MC, Prekates AA, Foussas SG, GENERATION Study Group: C Reactive protein, moderate alcohol consumption, and long term prognosis after successful coronary stenting: four year results from the GENERATION study, *Heart* 2004;90(4):419-24.

19. Arntz HR, Willich SN, Schreiber C, Bruggemann T, Stern R, Schultheiss HP: Diurnal, weekly and seasonal variation of sudden death. Population-based analysis of 24,061 consecutive cases, *Eur Heart J* 2000;21(4):315-20.

20. Myerburg RJ, Castellanos A: Cardiac arrest and sudden cardiac death. In Zipes DP, Libby P, Bonow RO, Braunwald EB, editors: *Braunwald's heart disease: A textbook of cardiovascular medicine,* 7th ed, 2005, Saunders. pp. 865-908.

21. Hankins DG, Luke A: Emergency medical service aspects of emergency cardiac care, *Emerg Med Clin North Am* 2005;23(4):1219-31.

22. International Liaison Committee on Resuscitation: Advanced life support. *Resuscitation* 2005;67 (suppl 1): 213.

23. Casper K, Murphy G, Weinstein C, Brinsfield K: A comparison of cardiopulmonary resuscitation rates of strangers versus known bystanders, *Prehosp Emerg Care* 2003;7(3):299-302.

24. Larsen MP, Eisenberg MS, Cummins RO, Hallstrom AP: Predicting survival from out-of-hospital cardiac arrest: a graphic model, *Ann Emerg Med* 1993;22(11):1652-8.

25. 2005 American Heart Association guidelines for cardiopulmonary resuscitation and emergency cardiovascular care, part 5. Electrical therapies: automated external defibrillators, defibrillation, cardioversion, and pacing, *Circulation* 2005;112 (suppl IV):IV-36.

26. Weisfeldt ML, Becker LB: Resuscitation after cardiac arrest: a 3-phase time-sensitive model, *JAMA* 2002;288(23):3035-8.

27. Weisfeldt ML: Public access defibrillation: good or great? *BMJ* 328(7438):E271-2, 2004.

28. Ewy GA: Cardiocerebral resuscitation: the new cardiopulmonary resuscitation, *Circulation* 2005;111(16):2134-42.

29. Eftestol T, Wik L, Sunde K, Steen PA: Effects of cardiopulmonary resuscitation on predictors of ventricular fibrillation defibrillation success during out-of-hospital cardiac arrest, *Circulation* 2004;110(1):10-5.

30. 2005 American Heart Association guidelines for cardiopulmonary resuscitation and emergency cardiovascular care, Part 7. Advanced cardiovascular life support, *Circulation* 2005;112(suppl IV): IV-58.

31. Bernard SA, Gray TW, Buist MD, Jones BM, Silvester W, Gutteridge G, Smith K: Treatment of comatose survivors of out-of-hospital cardiac arrest with induced hypothermia, *N Engl J Med* 2002;346(8):557-63.

32. Bernard S: Therapeutic hypothermia after cardiac arrest, *Neurol Clin* 24(1):61-71, 2006.

33. 2005 American Heart Association guidelines for cardiopulmonary resuscitation and emergency cardiovascular care, Part 7. Advanced cardiovascular life support. *Circulation* 2005;112(suppl IV): IV-85.

34. Boyd R: Witnessed resuscitation by relatives, *Resuscitation* 2000;43(3):171-6.

35. Kirschner KL: When written advance directives are not enough, *Clin Geriatr Med* 2005;21(1): 193-209.

36. Office of Emergency Medical Services, Department of Health, Commonwealth of Massachusetts. *Comfort Care/DNR Order Verification Protocol* (serial online), http://www.mass.gov/dph/oems/comfort/ccprot2a.htm. Accessed January 6, 2006.

37. 2005 American Heart Association guidelines for cardiopulmonary resuscitation and emergency cardiovascular care, Part 2. Ethical issues. *Circulation* 2005;112(suppl IV):IV-8.

38. Bailey ED, Wydro GC, Cone DC: Termination of resuscitation in the prehospital setting for adult patients suffering nontraumatic cardiac arrest. National Association of EMS Physicians Standards and Clinical Practice Committee, *Prehosp Emerg Care* 2000;4(2):190-5 (review).

39. 2005 American Heart Association guidelines for cardiopulmonary resuscitation and emergency cardiovascular care, Part 1. Introduction. *Circulation* 2005;112(suppl IV):IV-2.

Airway Management: Oxygenation and Ventilation

OBJECTIVES

Upon completion of this chapter, you will be able to:

1. Name the major structures of the respiratory system.
2. Describe the oxygen liter flow per minute and estimated oxygen percentage delivered for each of the following devices:
   - Nasal cannula
   - Simple face mask
   - Partial nonrebreather mask
   - Nonrebreather mask
   - Venturi mask
3. Describe the steps in performing the head-tilt/chin-lift and jaw thrust without head-tilt maneuvers for opening the airway.
4. Relate mechanism of injury to opening the airway.
5. Describe correct suctioning technique and complications associated with this procedure.
6. Describe how to correctly size and insert an oral airway and a nasal airway.
7. Describe indications for positive-pressure ventilation.
8. Describe the oxygen liter flow per minute and estimated inspired oxygen concentration delivered for a pocket mask and bag-mask device.
9. Describe how to ventilate a patient with a bag-mask using one and two rescuers.
10. Describe the signs of adequate and inadequate bag-mask ventilation.
11. Describe advantages and disadvantages associated with the use of an automatic transport ventilator (ATV) and a flow-restricted, oxygen-powered ventilation device.
12. Describe the indications, advantages, and technique for advanced airways including the Combitube, laryngeal mask airway (LMA), and endotracheal (ET) tube.

ANATOMY OF THE RESPIRATORY SYSTEM

DIVISIONS OF THE AIRWAY

- Upper airway
  - ▶ Consists of structures located outside the chest cavity including the nose and nasal cavities, pharynx, and larynx.
  - ▶ Function—filter, warm, and humidify the air, protecting the surfaces of the lower respiratory tract.
- Lower airway
  - ▶ Contains the organs located in the chest cavity including the trachea, bronchi, bronchioles, alveoli, and lungs (Figure 2-1).
  - ▶ Functions in the exchange of oxygen and carbon dioxide.

 For the purposes of this text, airway structures located above the glottis are considered upper airway structures. Structures located below the glottis are considered lower airway structures.

Upper Airway

- The nasal cavity and the mouth meet at the pharynx (throat).
- The pharynx extends from the nasal cavities to the larynx and includes three parts: the nasopharynx, oropharynx, and laryngopharynx (or hypopharynx) (Figure 2-2). The pharynx is a passageway common to both the respiratory and digestive systems.
- Nasopharynx
  - ▶ Functions in respiration; the portion of the pharynx immediately behind the nasal cavities and above the soft palate.
  - ▶ The mucous lining of the nasopharynx filters, warms, and moistens the air.
  - ▶ The nasopharynx contains adenoid tissue and eustachian tube openings.
  - ▶ Tissues of the nasopharynx are extremely delicate and vascular. Improper or overly aggressive placement of tubes or airways may result in significant bleeding.

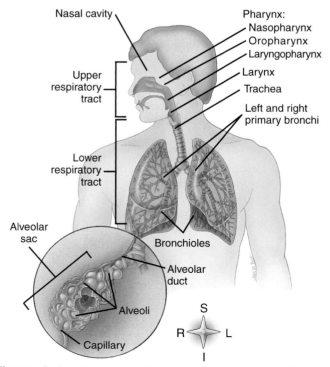

Figure 2-1 • Structures of the upper and lower respiratory tract.

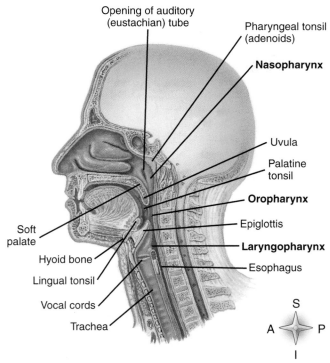

Figure 2-2 • Pharynx. Midsagittal section illustrating the three divisions of the pharynx—nasopharynx, oropharynx, and laryngopharynx.

■ Oropharynx
  ▶ Functioning in respiration and digestion, the oropharynx is the portion of the pharynx that is visible via the mouth.
  ▶ The oropharynx includes the teeth, tongue, palate, adenoids, epiglottis, and **vallecula** and extends from the soft palate superiorly to the vallecula inferiorly.
    • "Vallecula" means "little valley" and is the space (or "pocket") between the base of the tongue and the epiglottis.
  ▶ **Soft palate**—the back part of the roof of the mouth that is made up of mucous membrane, muscular fibers, and mucous glands.
  ▶ **Uvula**—fleshy tissue resembling a grape that hangs down from the soft palate.
  ▶ **Hard palate**—bony portion of the roof of the mouth that forms the floor of the nasal cavity (Figure 2-3).

The vallecula is an important landmark when performing orotracheal intubation with a curved laryngoscope blade.

■ Laryngopharynx (hypopharynx)
  ▶ The portion of the throat below the epiglottis, the laryngopharynx (hypopharynx) connects to the esophagus.
  ▶ The laryngopharynx functions in respiration and digestion.
  ▶ Larynx (voice box)
    • Connects the pharynx and trachea at the level of the cervical vertebrae.
    • Tubular structure made up of cartilage, muscles, and ligaments.
    • Conducts air between the pharynx and the lungs, prevents food and foreign substances from entering the trachea and houses the vocal cords (involved in speech production).
    • Most of the larynx is innervated with nerve endings from the vagus nerve.
      • Bradycardia can result from stimulation of the larynx by a laryngoscope blade or tracheal tube.

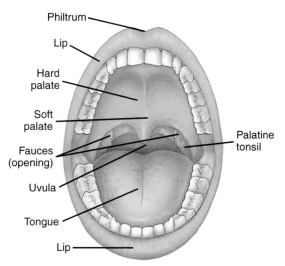

Figure 2-3 • The oral cavity illustrating the hard and soft palate.

- Consists of connective tissue that contains nine cartilages. The three largest cartilages are the thyroid cartilage, the epiglottis, and the cricoid cartilage.
- Thyroid cartilage (Adam's apple)
  - Largest and most superior cartilage.
  - Shaped like a shield (Figure 2-4).
  - More pronounced in adult males than adult females.
  - The true vocal cords and the space between them make up the **glottis.** The glottic opening is located directly behind the thyroid cartilage and is the narrowest part of the adult larynx (Figure 2-5).
- Cricoid cartilage
  - Shaped liked a signet ring.
  - Most inferior of the nine laryngeal cartilages.
    — First tracheal ring and the only completely cartilaginous ring in the larynx.
    — Narrowest diameter of the airway in infants and children younger than 10 years of age is at the cricoid cartilage.
    — During positive-pressure ventilation, compression of the cricoid cartilage occludes the esophagus, reducing the risk of aspiration. This technique is called cricoid pressure or the **Sellick maneuver.**

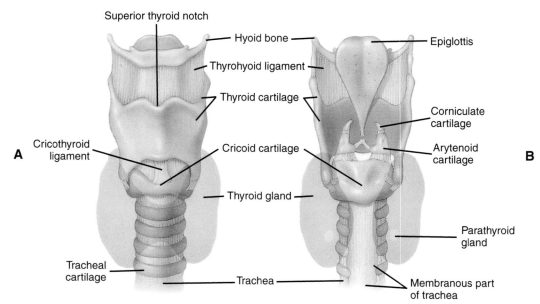

Figure 2-4 • Anatomy of the larynx. **A,** Anterior view. **B,** Posterior view.

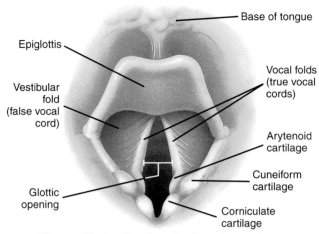

Figure 2-5 • Vocal cords viewed from above.

- **Cricothyroid membrane**—a fibrous membrane located between the cricoid and thyroid cartilages. This site may be used for surgical and alternative airway placement.
- **Epiglottis**—a small, leaf-shaped cartilage located at the top of the larynx that prevents food from entering the respiratory tract during swallowing.

Lower Airway

■ Consists of the trachea, the bronchial tree (primary bronchi, secondary bronchi, and bronchioles), alveoli, and the lungs.

■ Functions in the exchange of oxygen and carbon dioxide.

■ Trachea
  ▶ A rigid tube approximately 4 to 5 inches long and about 1 inch in diameter.
  ▶ Conducts air to and from the lungs.
  ▶ Extends from the larynx in the neck to the primary bronchi in the thoracic cavity, where it divides (bifurcates) into the right and left bronchi (Figure 2-6).
    • The point where the trachea divides into the right and left mainstem bronchi is called the **carina** (about the level of the 5th or 6th thoracic vertebra).
  ▶ The walls of the trachea are supported and held open by a series of C-shaped rings of cartilage that are open (incomplete) on the posterior surface. These rings are open to permit the esophagus, which lies behind the trachea, to bulge forward as food moves from the esophagus to the stomach.
  ▶ The area between the tracheal cartilages is made up of connective tissue and smooth muscle. Tracheal smooth muscle is innervated by the parasympathetic division of the autonomic nervous system.
  ▶ The trachea is lined with mucus-producing cells and cilia that filter the air before it enters the bronchi.

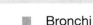

Obstruction of the trachea will result in death if not corrected within minutes.

■ Bronchi
  ▶ The trachea divides at the carina into the right and left mainstem bronchi, which have the same structure as the trachea.
  ▶ Primary (mainstem) bronchi branch into narrowing secondary and tertiary bronchi that branch into bronchioles.

■ Bronchioles
  ▶ Composed entirely of smooth muscle supported by connective tissue.
  ▶ Responsible for regulating the flow of air to the alveoli. The bronchioles subdivide into terminal bronchioles, which extend into the alveoli.
  ▶ Right mainstem bronchus is shorter, wider, and straighter than the left.

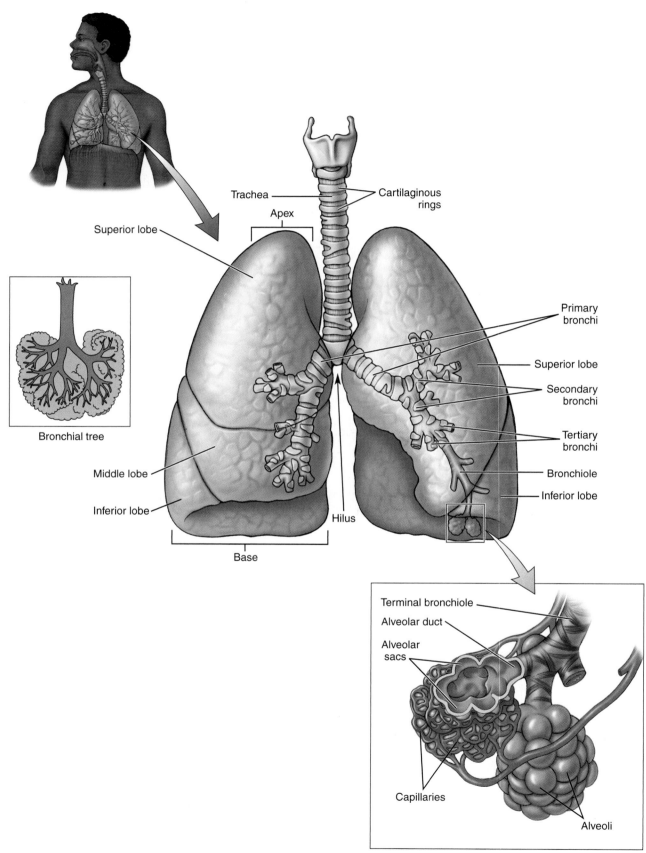

Figure 2-6 • Trachea, bronchi, bronchioles, and alveoli.

- A tracheal tube that is inserted too far or foreign material that is aspirated is more likely to enter the right mainstem bronchus than the left.
- Stimulation of beta-2 receptor sites in the bronchioles results in relaxation of bronchial smooth muscle.

■ Alveoli
  ▶ Bronchioles subdivide into tiny tubes called alveolar ducts. These ducts end in alveoli, which are tiny, hollow air sacs.
  ▶ Each alveolus is surrounded by a pulmonary capillary. Oxygen passes through the thin walls of the alveoli to capillaries, and carbon dioxide passes from the capillaries to the alveoli.
  ▶ Each lung of an average adult contains about 300 million alveoli.

LUNG VOLUMES

■ **Tidal volume**—the volume of air moved into or out of the lungs during a normal breath
  ▶ Average tidal volume for an adult male at rest is about 500 mL (5-7 mL/kg) (Figure 2-7).
  ▶ Because tidal volume equals lung inflation (and oxygenation), it can be indirectly evaluated by observing the rise and fall of a patient's chest.
■ **Minute volume**—the amount of air moved in and out of the lungs in 1 minute
  ▶ Determined by multiplying the tidal volume by the respiratory rate.
  ▶ A change in either the tidal volume *or* respiratory rate will affect minute volume.

Evaluation of a patient's breathing should include assessment of the patient's tidal volume (depth of respiration) and respiratory rate.

Personal protective equipment (PPE) must be worn when an exposure to blood or other potentially infectious material can be reasonably anticipated. PPE includes eye protection, protective gloves, gowns, and masks.

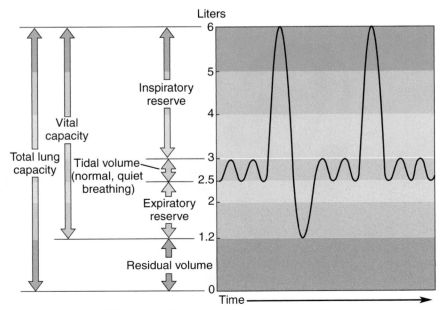

Figure 2-7 • Lung volumes and capacities.

OXYGEN DELIVERY DEVICES

 Oxygen therapy is referred to as the fraction of inspired gas that is oxygen (FIO_2).

NASAL CANNULA

- A **nasal cannula** (also called nasal prongs) is a piece of plastic tubing with two soft prongs that project from the tubing. The prongs are inserted into the patient's nostrils. The tubing is then secured to the patient's face (Figure 2-8). Oxygen flows from the cannula into the patient's nasopharynx, which acts as an anatomic reservoir.
- Although the actual inspired oxygen concentration depends on the patient's respiratory rate and depth, a nasal cannula can deliver oxygen concentrations of about 25% to 45% at 1 to 6 L/min flow. Flow rates of 6 L/min and more dry the mucous membranes of the nasal cavity and often cause discomfort, such as headaches.
- In an adult, oxygen delivery by means of a nasal cannula does not need to be humidified if the flow rate is ≤4 L/min.
- Advantages and disadvantages of using a nasal cannula are shown in Table 2-1.

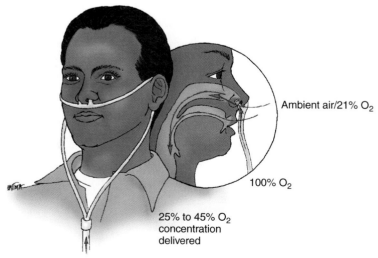

Figure 2-8 • At flow rates of 1 to 6 L/min, a nasal cannula can deliver an oxygen concentration of 25% to 45%.

KEEPING IT SIMPLE

Nasal Cannula

Formula = (4 × the oxygen flow rate in L/min) + 21% (room air)
- 1 L/min = 25%
- 2 L/min = 29%
- 3 L/min = 33%
- 4 L/min = 37%
- 5 L/min = 41%
- 6 L/min = 45%

TABLE 2-1	Nasal Cannula—Advantages and Disadvantages
Advantages	**Disadvantages**
• Comfortable, well tolerated by most patients • Does not interfere with patient assessment or impede patient communication with healthcare personnel • Allows for talking and eating • No rebreathing of expired air • Can be used with mouth breathers • Useful in patients predisposed to carbon dioxide retention • Can be used for patients who require oxygen but cannot tolerate a nonrebreather mask	• Can only be used in a spontaneously breathing patient • Easily displaced • Nasal passages must be open • Drying of mucosa • May cause sinus pain

SIMPLE FACE MASK (STANDARD MASK)

■ A **simple face mask** is a plastic reservoir designed to fit over the patient's nose and mouth. The mask is secured around the patient's head by means of an elastic strap. The internal capacity of the mask produces a reservoir effect. Small holes on each side of the mask allow the passage of inspired and expired air. Supplemental oxygen is delivered through a small-diameter tube connected to the base of the mask (Figure 2-9).

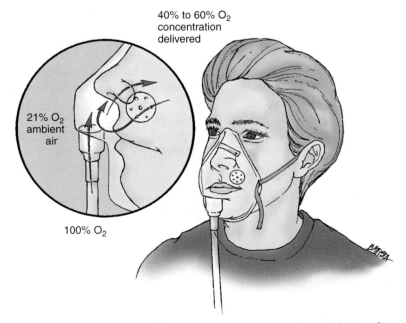

40% to 60% O_2 concentration delivered

21% O_2 ambient air

100% O_2

Figure 2-9 • The simple face mask can deliver an oxygen concentration of 40% to 60% with an oxygen flow rate of 6 to 10 L/min. (recommended flow rate is 8 to 10 L/min).

- At 6 to 10 L/min, the simple face mask can provide an inspired oxygen concentration of about 40% to 60%. The recommended flow rate 8 to 10 L/min. The patient's actual inspired oxygen concentration will vary, because the amount of air that mixes with supplemental oxygen depends on the patient's inspiratory flow rate.
- Advantages and disadvantages of using a simple face mask are shown in Table 2-2.

 When using a simple face mask, the oxygen flow rate must be higher than 5 L/min to flush the buildup of the patient's exhaled CO_2 from the mask.

TABLE 2-2	Simple Face Mask—Advantages and Disadvantages	
Advantages	**Disadvantages**	
• Delivers higher oxygen concentration than by nasal cannula	• Can only be used in a spontaneously breathing patient • Not tolerated well in severely dyspneic patients • Can be uncomfortable • Difficult to hear the patient speaking when the device is in place • Must be removed at meals • Requires a tight face seal to prevent leakage of oxygen • Oxygen flow rates of more than 10 L/min do not enhance delivered oxygen concentration	

 Pulse oximetry is a noninvasive method of measuring the percentage of oxygen saturated in the blood (SpO_2). Because it can provide a continuous measurement of oxygenation, use of pulse oximetry provides healthcare professionals with an early warning of decreased oxygenation. An SpO_2 reading between 96% and 100% generally indicates adequate oxygenation. A reading between 91% and 95% suggests mild hypoxia. An SpO_2 reading less than 91% generally represents severe hypoxia.

Pulse oximetry may be inaccurate in situations involving poor capillary blood flow, an abnormal hemoglobin concentration, or an abnormal shape of the hemoglobin molecule. For example, pulse oximetry may give misleading results in cardiac arrest, shock, hypothermia, carbon monoxide poisoning, and sickle cell disease. Results may also be inaccurate if the patient is wearing dark or metallic nail polish or if there is patient movement, such as that due to shivering.

PARTIAL REBREATHER (REBREATHING) MASK

- A partial rebreather mask is similar to a simple face mask but has an attached oxygen-collecting device (reservoir) at the base of the mask that is filled before patient use. Pure oxygen is delivered through oxygen tubing to the reservoir bag. The reservoir collects the oxygen and allows some of the patient's exhaled air (approximately equal to the volume of the patient's anatomic dead space) to enter the reservoir bag and be reused (Figure 2-10).
- The oxygen concentration of the patient's exhaled air, combined with the supply of 100% oxygen, allows the use of oxygen flow rates lower than those necessary for a nonrebreather mask.
- Depending on the patient's respiratory pattern, oxygen concentrations of 35% to 60% can be delivered when using an oxygen flow rate (typically 6-10 L/min) that prevents the reservoir bag from collapsing completely on inspiration.
- Advantages and disadvantages of using a partial rebreather mask are shown in Table 2-3.

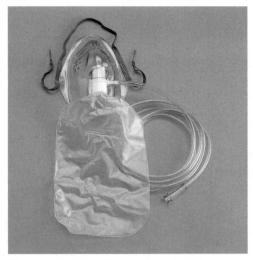

Figure 2-10 • The partial rebreather mask has an attached oxygen-collecting device (reservoir) at the base of the mask. The reservoir collects oxygen and allows some of the patient's exhaled air to enter the reservoir bag and be reused.

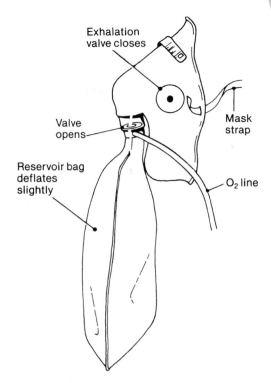

Inhalation

Figure 2-11 • In the nonrebreather mask, oxygen collects in the reservoir (bag) below the mask before inhalation. A one-way valve separates the reservoir from the mask. Exhaled air leaves the mask through the side ports on the mask.

TABLE 2-3	**Partial Rebreather Mask—Advantages and Disadvantages**
Advantages	**Disadvantages**
• Delivers higher oxygen concentration than by nasal cannula • Inspired oxygen not mixed with room air	• Can only be used in a spontaneously breathing patient • Not tolerated well in severely dyspneic patients • Can be uncomfortable • Difficult to hear the patient speaking when the device is in place • Must be removed at meals • Requires a tight face seal to prevent leakage of oxygen • Oxygen flow rates of more than 10 L/min do not enhance delivered oxygen concentration

NONREBREATHER (NONREBREATHING) MASK

■ A nonrebreather mask is similar to a partial rebreather mask but does not permit mixing of the patient's exhaled air with 100% oxygen. Rubber flaps cover the side ports on the mask, preventing inhalation of room air. When the patient breathes in, oxygen is drawn into the mask from the reservoir (bag) through a one-way valve that separates the bag from the mask. When the patient breathes out, the exhaled air exits through the side ports on the mask. The one-way valve prevents the patient's exhaled air from returning to the reservoir bag (thus the name "nonrebreather"). This ensures a supply of 100% oxygen to the patient with minimal dilution from the entrainment of room air (Figure 2-11).

■ A nonrebreather mask is the delivery device of choice when high concentrations of oxygen are needed in the spontaneously breathing patient. Depending on the patient's respiratory pattern, oxygen concentrations of up to 100% can be delivered when an oxygen flow rate (typically 10-15 L/min) is used that prevents the reservoir bag from collapsing completely on inspiration.

■ Inflate the reservoir bag with oxygen *before* placing the nonrebreather mask on the patient (Figure 2-12).

■ Advantages and disadvantages of using a nonrebreather mask are shown in Table 2-4.

 When using a partial rebreather or nonrebreather mask, make sure that the bag does not collapse when the patient inhales. Should the bag collapse, increase the delivered oxygen by 2-L increments until the bag remains inflated. The reservoir bag must remain at least ⅔ full so that sufficient supplemental oxygen is available for each breath.

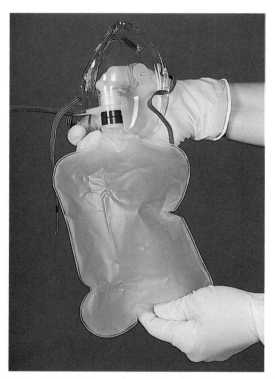

Figure 2-12 • Be sure to fill the reservoir bag of a partial rebreather or nonrebreather mask with oxygen before placing the mask on the patient. After placing the mask on the patient, adjust the flow rate so the bag does not completely deflate when the patient inhales.

TABLE 2-4	Nonrebreather Mask—Advantages and Disadvantages
Advantages	**Disadvantages**
• Delivers higher oxygen concentration than by nasal cannula, simple face mask, and partial rebreather mask • Inspired oxygen not mixed with room air	• Can only be used in a spontaneously breathing patient • Not tolerated well in severely dyspneic patients • Can be uncomfortable • Difficult to hear the patient speaking when the device is in place • Must be removed at meals • Mask must fit snugly on the patient's face to prevent room air from mixing with oxygen inhaled from the reservoir bag

VENTURI MASK

■ A Venturi mask fits over the patient's nose and mouth and contains a short corrugated hose with a jet orifice connected to oxygen supply tubing (Figure 2-13).

■ Oxygen under pressure is forced through a small jet orifice entering the mask. As the oxygen passes through the orifice, it draws room air into the mask. The resulting mixture is delivered to the patient through the face mask.

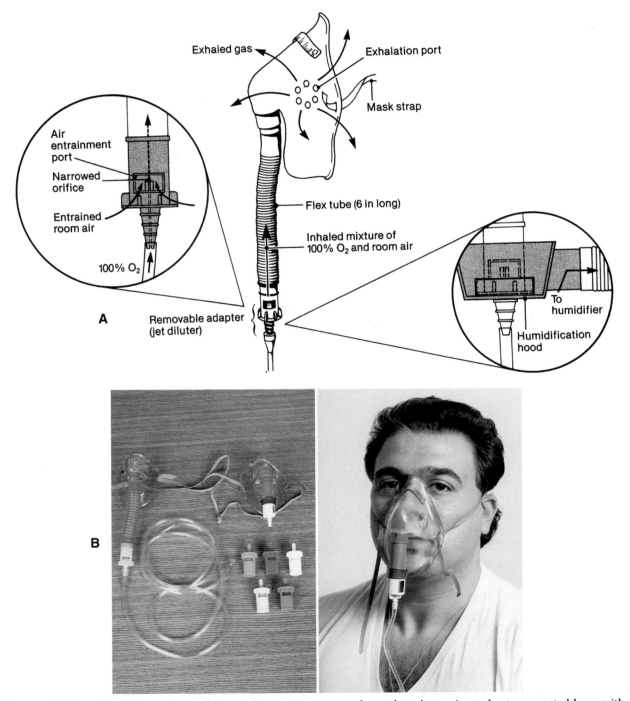

Figure 2-13 • **A,** The Venturi mask fits over the patient's nose and mouth and contains a short corrugated hose with a jet orifice that is connected to oxygen supply tubing. Oxygen under pressure is forced through a small jet orifice entering the mask. As the oxygen passes through the orifice, it draws ambient air into the mask. The resulting mixture is delivered to the patient through the face mask. **B,** The Venturi mask may be supplied with several color-coded adapters that alter the rate of oxygen flow past the air entrainment port. The mix of air and oxygen delivered to the patient is adjusted by changing either the flow of oxygen or the size of the air entrainment port.

TABLE 2-5	Venturi Mask—Advantages and Disadvantages	
Advantages		**Disadvantages**
• Provides precise inspired oxygen concentration in a selected range • Recommended for patients who rely on a hypoxic respiratory drive (such as chronic obstructive pulmonary disease)		• Can only be used in a spontaneously breathing patient • Not tolerated well in severely dyspneic patients • Can be uncomfortable • Difficult to hear the patient speaking when the device is in place • Must be removed at meals • Mask must fit snugly on the patient's face

TABLE 2-6	Oxygen Percentage Delivery by Device	
Device	**Approximate Inspired Oxygen Concentration**	**Liter Flow (L/Min)**
Nasal cannula	25%-45%	1-6
Simple face mask	40%-60%	6-10 (8-10 recommended)
Partial rebreather mask	35%-60%	6-10
Nonrebreather mask	60%-100%	10-15
Venturi mask	24%-50%	4-8

- A Venturi mask typically delivers oxygen concentrations of 24%, 28%, 35%, 40%, or 50% oxygen. The mask is usually supplied with several color-coded adapters that change the rate of oxygen flow past the air entrainment port. The mix of air and oxygen delivered to the patient is adjusted by changing the adapter attached to the base of the mask or by having an adjustable, rotating opening that changes the amount of air mixing with oxygen.
- Advantages and disadvantages of using a Venturi mask are shown in Table 2-5. A summary of oxygen percentages by oxygen delivery device is shown in Table 2-6.

OPENING THE AIRWAY—MANUAL AIRWAY MANEUVERS

- The tongue is the most common cause of airway obstruction in an unresponsive patient (Figure 2-14).
- If the patient is breathing, snoring respirations are a sign of airway obstruction due to displacement of the tongue. If the patient is not breathing, airway obstruction due to the tongue may go undetected until ventilation is attempted. Ventilating an apneic patient with an airway obstruction is difficult. If the airway obstruction is due to the tongue, repositioning of the patient's head and jaw may be all that is needed to open the airway.
- Manual airway maneuvers are summarized in Table 2-7.

The head-tilt/chin-lift and jaw thrust without head tilt maneuvers *do* cause movement of the cervical spine. Lay rescuers are now taught to open the airway using a head-tilt/chin-lift maneuver for both injured and noninjured victims. The jaw thrust is no longer recommended for lay rescuers.[1]

Healthcare professionals should open the airway with the head-tilt/chin-lift if no trauma is suspected. Use a jaw thrust without head tilt if you suspect possible trauma. However, "Because maintaining a patent airway and providing adequate ventilation is a priority in CPR, use a head-tilt/chin-lift maneuver if the jaw thrust does not open the airway."[2]

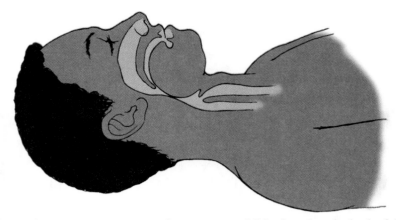

Figure 2-14 • In the unresponsive patient, the tongue may fall back against the back of the throat due to a loss of muscle control, causing an airway obstruction.

TABLE 2-7	Manual Airway Maneuvers	
	Head-Tilt/Chin-Lift	**Jaw Thrust without Head Tilt**
Indications	Unresponsive patient • No mechanism for cervical spine injury • Unable to protect own airway	Unresponsive patient • Possible cervical spine injury • Unable to protect own airway
Contraindications	• Awake patient • Possible cervical spine injury	• Awake patient
Advantages	• Simple to perform • No equipment required • Noninvasive	• No equipment required • Noninvasive
Disadvantages	• Does not protect lower airway from aspiration • May cause spinal movement	• Difficult to maintain • Second rescuer needed for BVM ventilation • Does not protect lower airway from aspiration • May cause spinal movement

HEAD-TILT/CHIN-LIFT

To perform a head-tilt/chin-lift:
■ Place the patient in a supine position.
■ Place one hand on the patient's forehead and apply firm pressure with your palm to tilt the patient's head back (Figure 2-15).
■ Place the tips of the fingers of your other hand under the bony part of the patient's chin and gently lift up and pull the jaw forward. Positioning your fingers under the bony part of the patient's chin is important because compression of the soft tissue under the patient's chin can obstruct the airway.
■ Open the patient's mouth by pulling down on the patient's lower lip using the thumb of the same hand used to lift the chin (Figure 2-16).

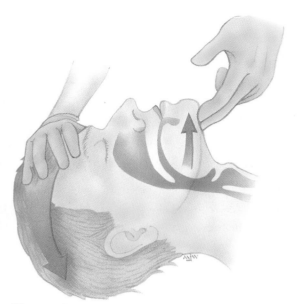

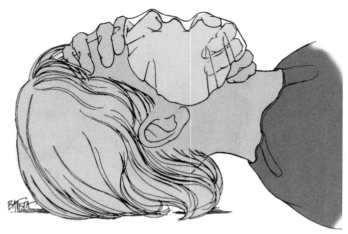

Figure 2-16 • Using the thumb of the same hand used to lift the chin, open the patient's mouth by pulling down on the patient's lower lip.

Figure 2-15 • Head-tilt/chin-lift maneuver. Place one of your hands on the patient's forehead and apply firm downward pressure with your palm to tilt the patient's head back. Place the tips of the fingers of your other hand under the bony part of the patient's chin and gently lift the jaw forward.

 The head-tilt/chin-lift and jaw thrust without head-tilt maneuvers *do* cause movement of the cervical spine.

Lay rescuers are now taught to open the airway using a head-tilt/chin-lift maneuver for both injured and noninjured victims. The jaw thrust is no longer recommended for lay rescuers.

Healthcare professionals should open the airway with the head-tilt/chin-lift if no head, neck, or spinal trauma is suspected. Use the jaw thrust without head tilt if there is the possibility of trauma. However, "because maintaining a patent airway and providing adequate ventilation is a priority in CPR, use a head-tilt/chin-lift maneuver if the jaw thrust does not open the airway."[2]

JAW THRUST WITHOUT HEAD-TILT MANEUVER

To perform a jaw thrust without head-tilt maneuver:
- Place the patient in a supine position (log-roll).
- Rest your elbows on the surface on which the patient is lying.
- While stabilizing the patient's head in a neutral position, grasp the angles of the patient's lower jaw with your fingertips.
- Displace the lower jaw forward (Figure 2-17).

 The jaw thrust without head-tilt maneuver is a difficult technique for one person to manage. In most cases, one rescuer is needed to displace the patient's lower jaw forward. A second rescuer is usually needed to ventilate the patient.

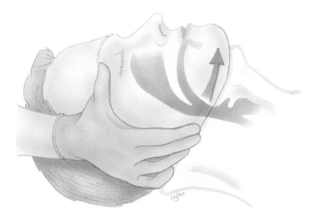

Figure 2-17 • Jaw thrust without head-tilt maneuver. While stabilizing the patient's head in a neutral position, grasp the angles of the patient's lower jaw with both hands, one on each side, and displace the mandible forward.

SUCTIONING

PURPOSE OF SUCTIONING

■ Remove vomitus, saliva, blood, and other material from the patient's airway.
■ Improve gas exchange.
■ Prevent atelectasis.
■ Obtain secretions for diagnosis.

SUCTION DEVICES

■ Fixed (stationary, installed) suction devices
  ▶ Mounted in hospitals, in extended care facilities, and in many emergency vehicles.
  ▶ Electrically operated by vacuum pumps or by the vacuum produced by a vehicle engine manifold (Figure 2-18).
  ▶ Should be capable of generating a vacuum of >300 mm Hg when the distal end of the tube is clamped and provide an airflow of >40 L/min when the tube is open.
  ▶ Amount of suction should be adjustable for use in children and intubated patients.
■ Portable suction units
  ▶ May be hand, foot, or oxygen powered; electrically powered; or battery powered.
  ▶ Hand-operated suction devices are popular because they are lightweight, compact, reliable, and inexpensive (Figure 2-19).
  ▶ Should provide a vacuum and airflow adequate for pharyngeal suction.

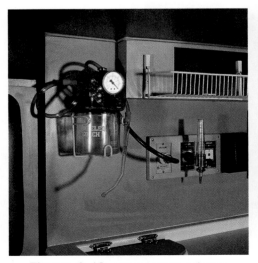

Figure 2-18 • Fixed suction device.

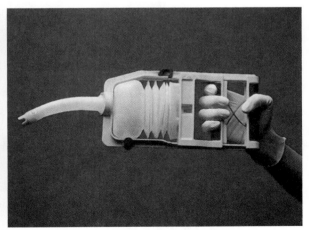

Figure 2-19 • A hand-operated portable suction device.

SUCTION CATHETERS

- Rigid catheters
  - ▶ Also called "hard," "tonsil tip," or "Yankauer" catheters.
  - ▶ Made of hard plastic and are angled to aid removal of secretions from the mouth and throat. Because of their size, rigid suction catheters are not used to suction the nares, except externally.
  - ▶ Typically, they have one large and several small holes at the distal end through which particles may be suctioned.
- Soft catheters
  - ▶ Also called "whistle-tip," "flexible," or "French" catheters.
  - ▶ Long, narrow, flexible pieces of plastic primarily used to clear blood or mucus from a tracheal tube or the nasopharynx (Figure 2-20).
  - ▶ A side opening is present at the proximal end of most catheters that is covered with the thumb to produce suction. (In some cases, suctioning is initiated when a button is pushed on the suction device.)
  - ▶ Can be inserted into the nares, oropharynx, or nasopharynx, through an oral or nasal airway, or through an ET tube or tracheostomy tube.

SUCTIONING TECHNIQUE

Suctioning the Upper Airway

- Assemble necessary equipment.
- Using personal protective equipment (PPE), preoxygenate the patient before suctioning if possible.
- Turn on the power to the suction unit.
- To determine the appropriate depth for catheter insertion, measure the catheter from the patient's earlobe to the corner of the mouth.
- Insert the catheter into the patient's mouth to the proper depth *without* applying suction (Figure 2-21).
- Withdraw the catheter while applying suction. Suction should not be applied for more than 10 to 15 seconds (adults).
- Ventilate the patient with 100% oxygen for about 30 seconds and flush the suction catheter and tubing with saline before repeating the procedure.

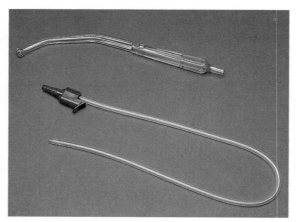

Figure 2-20 • Suction catheters. Rigid suction catheter (top) and soft suction catheter (bottom).

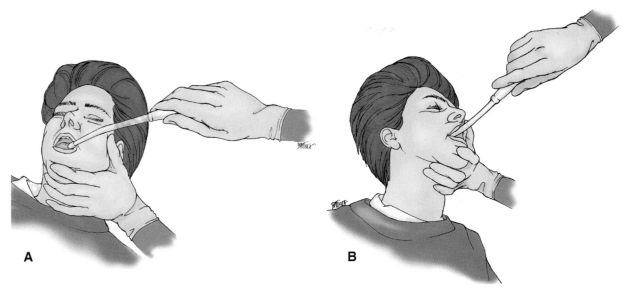

Figure 2-21 • Suctioning the upper airway. **A,** Insert the catheter into the mouth to the proper depth without applying suction. **B,** Withdraw the catheter while applying suction.

Suctioning the Lower Airway

- ■ Assemble necessary equipment.
- ■ Using PPE, preoxygenate the patient before suctioning.
- ■ Turn on the power to the suction unit.
- ■ To determine the appropriate depth for catheter insertion, measure the distance from the nose to the ear and the nose to the sternal notch.
- ■ Insert the catheter into the ET (or tracheostomy) tube WITHOUT applying suction (Figure 2-22).

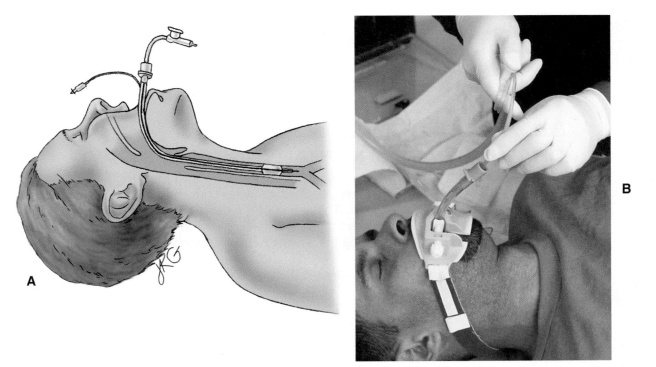

Figure 2-22 • Suctioning the lower airway. **A,** Insert the suction catheter to the proper depth. **B,** Withdraw the catheter while applying intermittent suction.

- Withdraw the catheter while applying suction. Suction should not be applied for more than 10 to 15 seconds (adults).
- Ventilate the patient with 100% oxygen for about 30 seconds and flush the suction catheter and tubing with saline before repeating the procedure.
- Possible complications of suctioning are shown in Box 2-1.

 When possible, perform tracheal suction before suctioning the throat. The mouth and throat contain more bacteria than the trachea. Suctioning the trachea first will lead to less potential for bacterial contamination of the lungs.

BOX 2-1

Suctioning—Possible Complications

- Hypoxia
- Dysrhythmias
- Increased intracranial pressure
- Local swelling
- Hemorrhage
- Tracheal ulceration
- Tracheal infection
- Bronchospasm
- Bradycardia and hypotension due to vagal stimulation

QUICK REVIEW 2-2

1. A 23-year-old man was involved in a motor vehicle crash. He is unresponsive. How should you open this patient's airway?

2. What type of suction catheter is used to clear secretions from a tracheal tube?

3. When suctioning, apply intermittent suction while _____ the catheter.

AIRWAY ADJUNCTS

ORAL AIRWAY (OROPHARYNGEAL AIRWAY)

- An oral airway is a J-shaped plastic device that, when correctly positioned, extends from the patient's lips to the pharynx. The flange of the device rests on the patient's lips or teeth. The distal tip lies between the base of the tongue and the back of the throat, preventing the tongue from blocking the airway. Air passes around and through the device (Figure 2-23).
- There are two main types of oral airways (Figure 2-24):
  - ▶ Guedel—tubular design
  - ▶ Berman—airway channels along each side of the device
- Oral airways are available in a variety of sizes (infant, child, adult). The size of the airway is based on the distance, in millimeters, from the flange to the distal tip. Proper airway size is determined by holding the device against the side of the patient's face and selecting an airway that extends from the corner of the mouth to the tip of the earlobe or the angle of the jaw.

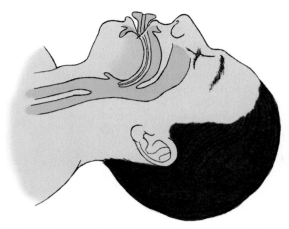

Figure 2-23 • An oral airway in proper position.

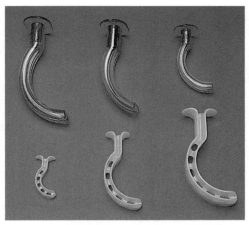

Figure 2-24 • Types of oral airways.

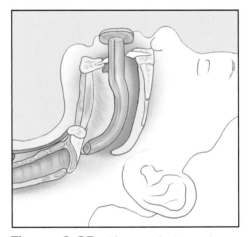

Figure 2-25 • If an oral airway is too long, it may press the epiglottis against the entrance of the larynx, resulting in a complete airway obstruction.

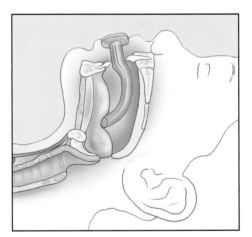

Figure 2-26 • If an oral airway is too short, the tongue may be pushed back into the throat, resulting in an airway obstruction, or the airway may advance out of the mouth.

■ Proper size is important. If the airway is too long, it may press the epiglottis against the entrance of the larynx, resulting in a complete airway obstruction (Figure 2-25). If the airway is too short, it will not displace the tongue and may advance out of the mouth (Figure 2-26).

■ Indications, contraindications, advantages, and disadvantages of oral and nasal airways are shown in Table 2-8.

TABLE 2-8	Oral and Nasal Airways	
	Oral Airway	**Nasal Airway**
Indications	• Helps maintain an open airway in an unresponsive patient who is not intubated • Helps maintain an open airway in an unresponsive patient with no gag reflex who is being ventilated with a BVM or other positive-pressure device • May be used as a bite block after insertion of an ET tube or orogastric tube	• To aid in maintaining an airway when use of an oral airway is contraindicated or impossible • Trismus (spasm of the muscles used to grind, crush, and chew food) • Biting • Clenched jaws or teeth
Contraindications	• Responsive patient	• Severe craniofacial trauma • Patient intolerance
Sizing	• Corner of mouth to tip of earlobe or angle of jaw	• Tip of nose to angle of the jaw or the tip of the ear
Advantages	• Positions the tongue forward and away from the back of the throat • Easily placed	• Provides a patent airway • Tolerated by responsive patients • Does not require mouth to be open
Disadvantages	• Does not protect the lower airway from aspiration • May produce vomiting if used in a responsive or semiresponsive patient with a gag reflex	• Does not protect the lower airway from aspiration • Improper technique may result in severe bleeding • Resulting epistaxis may be difficult to control • Suctioning through the device is difficult • Although tolerated by most responsive and semiresponsive patients, can stimulate the gag reflex in sensitive patients, precipitating laryngospasm and vomiting
Precautions	• Use of the device does not eliminate the need for maintaining proper head position	• Use of the device does not eliminate the need for maintaining proper head position

Inserting an Oral Airway

- Before inserting an oral airway:
  - Use PPE.
  - Open the patient's airway.
  - Make sure the mouth and throat are clear of secretions, blood, and vomitus.
- After selecting an oropharyngeal airway (OPA) of proper size, hold the device at its flange end and insert it into the patient's mouth with the tip pointing toward the roof of the patient's mouth (Figure 2-27). Slide the airway along the roof of the mouth. When the distal end nears the back of the throat, rotate the airway 180 degrees so that it is positioned over the tongue.
- Another method of OPA insertion requires the use of a tongue blade to depress the tongue. If this method is used, the OPA is inserted with the tip of the OPA facing the floor of the patient's mouth (curved side down). Using the tongue blade to depress the tongue, the OPA is gently advanced into place over the tongue (Figure 2-28).
- Regardless of the insertion method used, when the OPA is properly inserted, the flange of the device should rest comfortably on the patient's lips or teeth. Proper placement of the device is confirmed by ventilating the patient. If the OPA is correctly placed, chest rise should be visible and breath sounds should be present on auscultation of the lungs during ventilation.

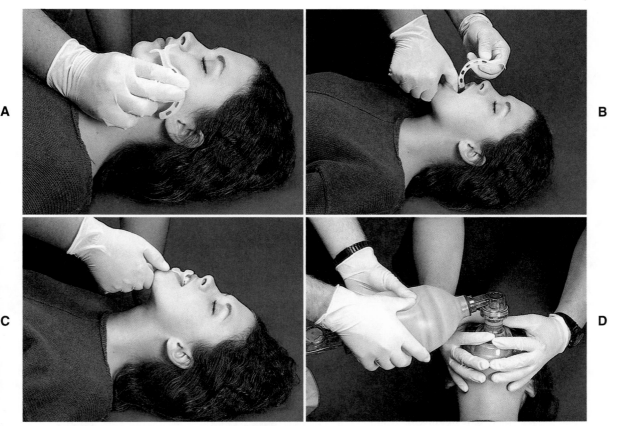

Figure 2-27 • Inserting an oral airway. **A,** Select an airway of appropriate size. **B,** Open the patient's mouth and insert the airway with the tip pointing toward the roof of the patient's mouth. When the tip of the airway nears the back of the throat, rotate the airway 180 degrees so that it is positioned over the tongue. **C,** When the airway is in proper position, the flange should rest on the patient's lips or teeth. **D,** Ventilate the patient with 100% oxygen.

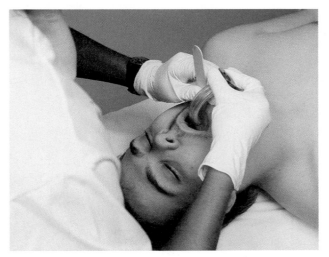

Figure 2-28 • If a tongue blade is used, the OPA is inserted with the tip pointing toward the floor of the patient's mouth and advanced until the tip is positioned at the base of the tongue.

NASAL AIRWAY (NASOPHARYNGEAL AIRWAY)

■ A nasal airway is a soft, uncuffed rubber or plastic tube designed to keep the tongue away from the back of the throat. It is placed in one nostril and advanced until the distal tip lies in the back of the throat just below the base of the tongue, while the proximal tip rests on the external nares.

■ Nasal airways are available in many sizes varying in length and internal diameter (ID) (Figure 2-29).

■ Proper airway size is determined by holding the device against the side of the patient's face and selecting an airway that extends from the tip of the nose to the angle of the jaw or the tip of the ear (Figure 2-30). An airway that is too long may stimulate the gag reflex. One that is too short may not be inserted far enough to keep the tongue away from the back of the throat. Figure 2-31 shows a nasal airway in proper position.

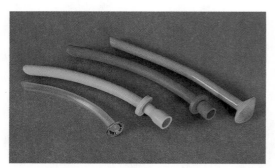

Figure 2-29 • Nasal airways are available in sizes of varying length and internal diameter.

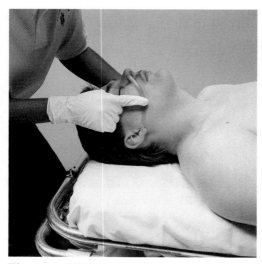

Figure 2-30 • Proper airway size is determined by holding the device against the side of the patient's face and selecting an airway that extends from the tip of the nose to the angle of the jaw or the tip of the ear.

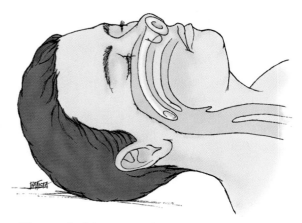

Figure 2-31 • A nasal airway in proper position.

Inserting a Nasal Airway

- Before inserting a nasopharyngeal airway (NPA), use PPE and open the airway. Lubricate the distal tip of the device liberally with a water-soluble lubricant to minimize resistance and decrease irritation to the nasal passage.

- After selecting an NPA of the proper size, hold the device at its flange end like a pencil and slowly insert it into the patient's nostril with the bevel pointing toward the nasal septum (Figure 2-32). Advance the airway along the floor of the nostril, following the natural curvature of the nasal passage, until the flange is flush with the nostril.

- The nasal cavity is very vascular. During insertion, do not force the airway because it may cut or scrape the nasal mucosa and result in significant bleeding, increasing the risk of aspiration. If resistance is encountered, a gentle back-and-forth rotation of the device between your fingers may ease insertion. If resistance continues, withdraw the NPA, reapply lubricant, and attempt insertion in the patient's other nostril.

- Proper placement of the device is confirmed by ventilating the patient. If the NPA is correctly placed, chest rise should be visible and breath sounds should be present on auscultation of the lungs during ventilation.

Some nasal airways have a slide at the flange end of the device to adjust for proper length. If present, this slide should *not* be removed. Incidents have occurred in which an NPA that was improperly sized (too small) and in which the adjustable slide had been removed was subsequently "sucked" into the patient's lower airway, necessitating removal by bronchoscopy.

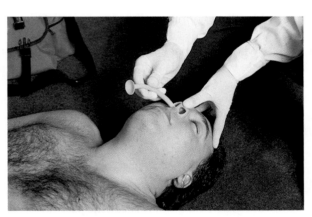
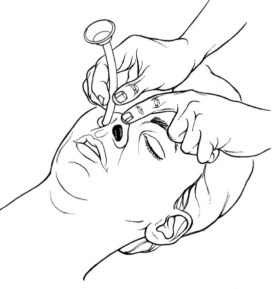

Figure 2-32 • After selecting an NPA of the proper size, hold the device at its flange end and insert it into the patient's nostril with the bevel pointing toward the nasal septum.

QUICK REVIEW 2-3

1. What is the most common cause of airway obstruction in the unresponsive patient?
2. How do you determine the proper size oral airway to use?
3. True or False. An oral airway protects the lower airway from aspiration.
4. While attempting to insert a nasal airway, you find that you are unable to advance the device. How should you proceed?
5. What is the maximum length of time for a suctioning attempt in an adult?

TECHNIQUES OF ARTIFICIAL VENTILATION

Adequate oxygenation requires an open airway *and* adequate air exchange. After the airway has been opened, determine if the patient's breathing is adequate or inadequate. If respiratory efforts are inadequate, the patient's breathing may be assisted by forcing air into the lungs (i.e., delivering positive-pressure ventilations).

Several methods may be used to deliver positive-pressure ventilation:
- Mouth-to-mask ventilation
- One-person or two-person (preferred) BVM ventilation
- ATVs
- Flow-restricted oxygen-powered ventilation devices

> ## KEEPING IT SIMPLE
>
> Regardless of the method used, effective positive-pressure ventilation requires the delivery of an adequate volume of air at an appropriate rate.

MOUTH-TO-MASK VENTILATION

- The device used for mouth-to-mask ventilation is commonly called a **pocket mask** or pocket face mask (Table 2-9). A pocket mask is a clear semirigid mask that is sealed around the mouth and nose of an adult, child, or infant.
- A pocket mask should be:
  - Made of transparent material to allow assessment of the patient's lip color and detection of vomitus, secretions, or other substances.
  - Capable of a tight seal on the face, covering the mouth and nose.
  - Equipped with a standard 15-/22-mm fitting that permits connection to a BVM (or other ventilation) device.
  - Available in one average size for adults, with additional sizes for infants and children.
  - Equipped with a one-way valve that diverts the patient's exhaled gas, reducing the risk of infection.
  - Fitted with an oxygen inlet to allow the delivery of increased oxygen concentrations to the patient. Some mouth-to-mask devices have an oxygen inlet on the mask, allowing delivery of supplemental oxygen; others do not.

> ## KEEPING IT SIMPLE
>
> Selection of a mask of proper size is necessary to ensure a good seal between the patient's face and the mask. A mask of correct size should extend from the bridge of the nose to the groove between the lower lip and chin. If the mask is not properly positioned and a tight seal maintained, air will leak from between the mask and the patient's face, resulting in less tidal volume delivery to the patient. Less tidal volume → less lung inflation → less oxygenation. If you do not have a mask of the proper size available, use a larger mask and turn it upside down. Remember: adequate ventilation is present if you ventilate with just enough volume to see gentle chest rise.

Gastric distention is a complication of positive-pressure ventilation that can lead to vomiting and subsequent aspiration. Gastric distention also restricts movement of the diaphragm, impeding ventilation.

TABLE 2-9	Mouth-to-Mask Ventilation
Inspired oxygen concentration	• Without supplemental oxygen equals about 16%-17% (exhaled air). • Mouth-to-mask breathing combined with supplemental oxygen at a minimum flow rate of 10 L/min equals about 50%.
Advantages	• Aesthetically more acceptable than mouth-to-mouth ventilation. • Easy to teach and learn. • Physical barrier between the rescuer and the patient's nose, mouth, and secretions. • Reduces (but does not prevent) the risk of exposure to infectious disease. • Use of a one-way valve at the ventilation port decreases exposure to patient's exhaled air. • If the patient resumes spontaneous breathing, the mask can be used as a simple face mask to deliver 40%-60% oxygen by giving supplemental oxygen through the oxygen inlet on the mask (if so equipped). • Can deliver a greater tidal volume with mouth-to-mask ventilation than with a BVM device. • Rescuer can feel the compliance of the patient's lungs. (Compliance refers to the resistance of the patient's lung tissue to ventilation.)
Disadvantages	• Rescuer fatigue. • Gastric distention.

Using a Pocket Mask

▦ To use a pocket mask, begin by putting on PPE.

▦ If not already attached, connect a one-way valve to the ventilation port on the mask, and connect oxygen tubing to the oxygen inlet on the mask (Figure 2-33). Set the oxygen flow rate at 10 to 12 L/min.

▦ Position yourself at the patient's head or side.

  ▶ Positioning yourself directly above the patient's head allows you to watch the patient's chest while delivering ventilations. This position is used if the patient is in respiratory arrest (but not cardiac arrest) or when two-rescuer CPR is being performed.

  ▶ If you are by yourself, positioning yourself at the patient's side allows you to maintain the same position for both rescue breathing and chest compressions.

▦ Open the patient's airway with a head-tilt/chin-lift; or, if trauma is suspected, perform the jaw thrust without head tilt maneuver. If needed, clear the patient's airway of secretions or vomitus. If the patient is unresponsive, insert an oral airway.

▦ Select a mask of appropriate size and place it on the patient's face.

  ▶ Apply the narrow portion (apex) of the mask over the bridge of the patient's nose and stabilize it in place with your thumbs.

  ▶ Lower the mask over the patient's face and mouth.

  ▶ Use the remaining fingers of both hands to stabilize the wide end (base) of the mask over the groove between the lower lip and chin and maintain proper head position.

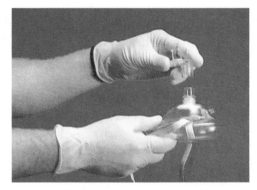

Figure 2-33 • Mouth-to-mask ventilation. If not already attached, connect a one-way valve to the ventilation port on the mask and connect oxygen tubing to the oxygen inlet on the mask.

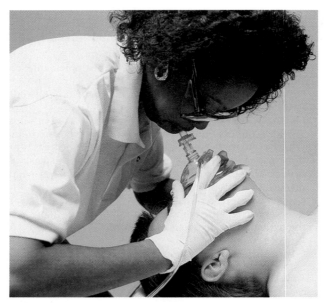

Figure 2-34 • Apply the mask to the patient's face and stabilize it in place. Ventilate the patient through the one-way valve on the top of the mask, delivering each breath over 1 second. Watch for gentle chest rise.

■ Ventilate the patient through the one-way valve on the top of the mask. If the patient is an adult, give breaths at a rate of 10 to 12 breaths per minute (1 breath every 5 to 6 seconds). Ventilate an infant or child at a rate of 12 to 20 bpm (1 breath every 3 to 5 seconds). Give each breath over 1 second, watching for gentle chest rise (Figure 2-34). Stop ventilation when adequate chest rise is observed. Allow the patient to exhale between breaths.

■ Adequate ventilation is being provided if you see the chest rise and fall gently with each breath and you hear and feel air escape during exhalation.

 You can deliver a greater tidal volume to the patient with mouth-to-mask ventilation than with a bag-mask device because both of your hands can be used to secure the mask in place while simultaneously maintaining proper head position. Your **vital capacity** can also compensate for leaks between the mask and the patient's face, resulting in greater lung ventilation.

BAG-MASK VENTILATION

■ A bag-mask device consists of a self-inflating bag; a nonrebreathing valve with an adapter that can be attached to a mask, tracheal tube, or other invasive airway device; and an oxygen inlet valve (Figure 2-35).

▶ A bag-mask device may also be referred to as a bag-mask device or bag-mask resuscitator (when the mask is used), or a bag-mask device (when the mask is not used; i.e., when ventilating a patient with an ET tube or tracheostomy tube in place).

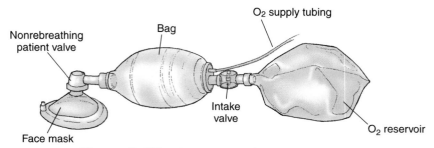

Figure 2-35 • Components of a bag-mask device.

- The bag-mask device should:
  - ▶ Consist of a self-refilling bag that is disposable (or easily cleaned and sterilized), and easy to grip and compress.
  - ▶ Have a clear mask to allow evaluation of the patient's lip color and detection of vomitus, secretions, or other substances.
  - ▶ Be capable of a tight seal on the face, covering the mouth and nose.
  - ▶ Include a nonjam valve system that can accommodate a maximum oxygen inlet flow of 30 L/min.
  - ▶ Have either no pop-off valve (pressure-release valve) or a pop-off valve that can be disabled during resuscitation.
  - ▶ Have standard 15-/22-mm fittings to allow for attachment of the device to a standard mask, tracheal tube, or other ventilation device.
  - ▶ Include a system for delivering high concentrations of oxygen with an oxygen reservoir and supplemental oxygen source.
  - ▶ Have a nonrebreathing valve that does not permit the patient's exhaled gases to escape into the bag.
  - ▶ Perform satisfactorily under all common environmental conditions and temperature extremes.
  - ▶ Be available in adult, child, and infant sizes. Most adult devices are capable of storing about 1600 mL of air.

A good tempo to remember for bag-mask ventilation is "squeeze-release-release." This provides appropriate inhalation and exhalation times.

Ventilation of patients in cardiac arrest often requires higher than usual airway pressures. Higher than usual ventilation pressures may also be needed in situations involving near-drowning, pulmonary edema, and asthma. To effectively ventilate a patient in these situations, the pressures needed for ventilation may exceed the limits of the pop-off valve. Thus, a pop-off valve may prevent generation of sufficient tidal volume to overcome the increase in airway resistance. Disabling the pop-off valve, or using a bag-mask device with no pop-off valve, helps ensure delivery of adequate tidal volumes to the patient during resuscitation. To disable a pop-off valve, depress the valve with a finger during ventilation or twist the pop-off valve into the closed position.

Oxygen Delivery

- A bag-mask device used without supplemental oxygen will deliver 21% oxygen (room air) to the patient (Figure 2-36).
- The bag-mask device should be connected to an oxygen source. To do this, attach one end of a piece of oxygen connecting tubing to the oxygen inlet on the bag-mask device and the other end to an oxygen regulator. A bag-mask device used with supplemental oxygen set at a flow rate of 15 L/min will deliver about 40% to 60% oxygen to the patient (Figure 2-37).

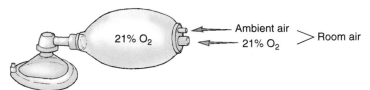
21% O_2 Ambient air
21% O_2 ⟩ Room air

Figure 2-36 • A bag-mask used without supplemental oxygen will deliver 21% oxygen (room air).

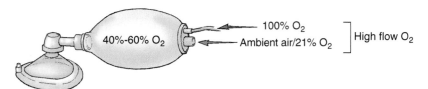

Figure 2-37 • A bag-mask device used with supplemental oxygen set at a flow rate of 15 L/min will deliver approximately 40% to 60% oxygen to the patient.

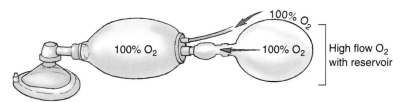

Figure 2-38 • A bag-mask device used with supplemental oxygen set at a flow rate of 15 L/min and a reservoir will deliver approximately 90% to 100% oxygen to the patient.

■ An oxygen-collecting device (reservoir) should be attached to the bag-mask device to deliver high-concentration oxygen. The reservoir collects a volume of 100% oxygen equal to the capacity of the bag. After squeezing the bag, the bag re-expands, drawing in 100% oxygen from the reservoir into the bag. A bag-mask device used with supplemental oxygen (set at a flow rate of 15 L/min) and an attached reservoir will deliver about 90% to 100% oxygen to the patient (Figure 2-38).

■ Advantages and disadvantages of bag-mask ventilation are shown in Table 2-10.

TABLE 2-10	Bag-Mask Ventilation	
Advantages	• Provides a means for delivery of an oxygen-enriched mixture to the patient • Conveys a sense of compliance of patient's lungs to the bag-mask operator • Provides a means for immediate ventilatory support • Can be used with the spontaneously breathing patient as well as the nonbreathing patient	
Disadvantages	• Requires practice to use effectively • Delivery of inadequate tidal volume • Rescuer fatigue • Gastric distention	

KEEPING IT SIMPLE

Bag-mask ventilation should be a two- or three-rescuer operation. If two rescuers are present, one should hold the mask to the patient's face (making sure there is a good mask to face seal) and maintain an open airway. The other rescuer is committed to compressing the bag. If a third rescuer is present and the patient is unresponsive, he or she should apply cricoid pressure during positive-pressure ventilation.

Ventilating with a Bag-Mask Device

■ Using PPE, position yourself at the top of the supine patient's head. Open the patient's airway using a head-tilt/chin-lift; or if trauma is suspected, perform the jaw thrust without head tilt maneuver. If needed, clear the patient's airway of secretions or vomitus. If the patient is unresponsive, insert an oral airway.

■ Select a mask of appropriate size and place it on the patient's face.

  ▶ Apply the narrow portion (apex) of the mask over the bridge of the patient's nose and the wide end (base) of the mask over the groove between the lower lip and chin. If the mask has a large, round cuff surrounding a ventilation port, center the port over the mouth.

  ▶ Stabilize the mask in place with your thumb and forefinger, creating a "C." Use the remaining fingers of the same hand to maintain proper head position by lifting the jaw along the bony portion of the mandible. The remaining fingers create an "E."

  ▶ Connect the bag to the mask, if not already done. Connect the bag to oxygen at 15 L/min and attach a reservoir.

  ▶ If you are alone, squeeze the bag with one hand, or with one hand and your arm or chest (Figure 2-39). If an assistant is available, ask the assistant to squeeze the bag until the patient's chest rises while you press the mask firmly against the patient's face with both hands and simultaneously maintain proper head position (Figure 2-40).

■ Observe the rise and fall of the patient's chest with each ventilation. Stop ventilation when you see gentle chest rise. Allow for adequate exhalation after each ventilation.

■ Ventilate the adult patient once every 5 to 6 seconds (10 to 12 ventilations per minute). Give each ventilation over 1 second.

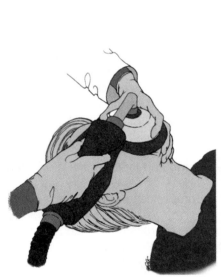

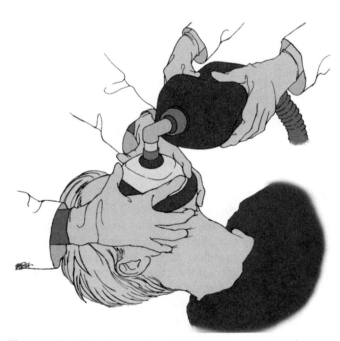

Figure 2-39 • Bag-mask ventilation—one-person technique.

Figure 2-40 • Bag-mask ventilation—two-person technique.

Troubleshooting Bag-Mask Ventilation

◼ The most frequent problem with the bag-mask is the inability to deliver adequate ventilatory volumes. This is due to the use of poor technique and/or difficulty in providing a leakproof seal to the face while maintaining an open airway at the same time.

◼ If the chest does not rise and fall with bag-mask ventilation, reassess.
- ▶ Reassess head position; reposition the airway, and try again to ventilate.
- ▶ Inadequate tidal volume delivery may be the result of an improper mask seal or incomplete bag compression.
  - • If air is escaping from under the mask, reposition your fingers and the mask.
  - • Reevaluate the effectiveness of bag compression.
- ▶ Check for an airway obstruction.
  - • Lift the jaw.
  - • Suction the airway as needed.
- ▶ If the chest still does not rise, select an alternative method of positive-pressure ventilation (such as a pocket mask or an automatic transport ventilator [ATV]).

QUICK REVIEW 2-4

1. Why is an oral airway not used in responsive or semiresponsive patients?

2. What is the purpose of suctioning?

3. How do you determine the correct size nasal airway?

Cricoid Pressure

◼ When providing positive-pressure ventilation to an unresponsive patient, apply cricoid pressure (Sellick maneuver) if an assistant is available. This technique takes advantage of the rigid cartilaginous rings of the trachea to occlude the esophagus. By pressing down on the cricoid cartilage, the esophagus is compressed between the cricoid cartilage and the fifth and sixth cervical vertebrae. This helps reduce inflation of the stomach during positive-pressure ventilation, reducing the likelihood of vomiting and aspiration.

◼ Technique
- ▶ Locate the cricoid cartilage (Figure 2-41).
- ▶ Apply firm pressure on the cricoid cartilage with the thumb and index or middle finger, just lateral to the midline (Figure 2-42).
- ▶ If active vomiting occurs while performed the procedure, release cricoid pressure to avoid rupture of the stomach or esophagus.

◼ If cricoid pressure is performed during ET intubation, cricoid pressure should be maintained until the ET tube cuff is inflated and proper tube position is verified.

◼ Complications
- ▶ Laryngeal trauma with excessive force.
- ▶ Esophageal rupture from unrelieved high gastric pressures.
- ▶ Excessive pressure may obstruct the trachea in small children.

Cricoid pressure is not intended to aid visualization of the vocal cords during intubation.

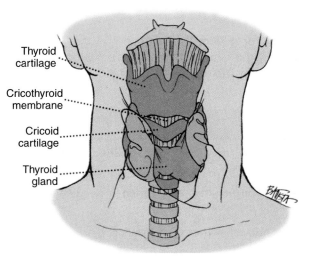

Thyroid cartilage

Cricothyroid membrane

Cricoid cartilage

Thyroid gland

Figure 2-41 • Landmarks of the cricoid cartilage.

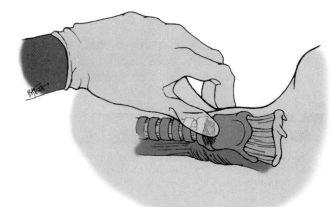

Figure 2-42 • Applying cricoid pressure.

Quick Review 2-5

1. Why is application of cricoid pressure beneficial during positive-pressure ventilation?

2. What is the most common problem with use of the bag-mask device?

3. True or False. A greater tidal volume can be delivered with mouth-to-mask ventilation than with a bag-mask device.

4. A bag-mask used with supplemental oxygen set at a flow rate of 15 L/min but no reservoir will deliver approximately __% oxygen to the patient.

AUTOMATIC TRANSPORT VENTILATOR

An ATV is a volume-cycled/rate-controlled ventilator (Figure 2-43). ATVs are used in the in-hospital and prehospital setting when transporting patients who require ventilatory support. Advantages and disadvantages of ATVs are shown in Table 2-11.

TABLE 2-11	Automatic Transport Ventilator	
Indications	• Patients requiring ventilatory assistance due to a decreased level of responsiveness or apnea • Patients requiring extended ventilation	
Contraindications	• Airway obstruction • Increased airway resistance (asthma, suspected pneumothorax, or tension pneumothorax) • Poor lung compliance (emphysema, significant pulmonary edema)	
Advantages	• Lightweight, portable, and durable • Provides a means for delivery of an oxygen-enriched mixture to the patient • Can be used for breathing and nonbreathing patients, intubated and nonintubated patients • Frees the rescuer for other tasks when used in intubated patients • In patients who are not intubated, the rescuer has both hands free to apply the mask and maintain the airway • Adjustable settings; once set, provides a specific tidal volume, respiratory rate, and minute ventilation	
Disadvantages	• Need for an oxygen source (or sometimes electric power) • Unable to detect increasing airway resistance • Hard to secure • Reliance on oxygen tank pressure • Some ATVs should not be used in children younger than 5 years of age	

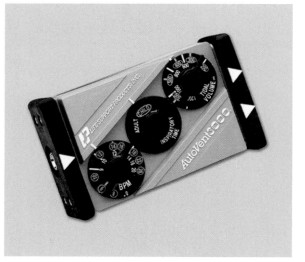
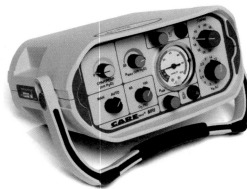

Figure 2-43 • Examples of ATVs.

Using an Automatic Transport Ventilator

ATVs should only be used by persons properly trained in the use of the device. To use an ATV:

- ▇ Test the ATV to make sure it is working properly before using it on a patient.
- ▇ If not already set, set the tidal volume and ventilation rate. Adjust the tidal volume to about 6 to 7 mL/kg (500-600 mL) to make the chest rise with breaths delivered over 1 second. If an advanced airway is not in place, set the ventilation rate at 10 to 12 per minute. If the patient is unresponsive, cricoid pressure should be applied by an assistant to reduce the risk of gastric inflation until an advanced airway is in place. Once an advanced airway is in place during CPR, adjust the ventilation rate to 8 to 10 per minute.
- ▇ Occlude the outlet adapter. An audible pressure limit alarm should sound with the next cycle (breath) to ensure that the pressure limit is intact and the lungs will not be overinflated.
- ▇ Assess lung compliance and chest rise with a bag-valve device.
- ▇ Attach the patient valve assembly to the airway device (tracheal tube, mask, or airway adjunct).
- ▇ Assess ventilations, listen for bilateral lung sounds, and look for adequate chest rise.
- ▇ Count the number of ventilator cycles for 1 minute to ensure proper correlation with the bpm setting on the ATV.
- ▇ Monitor the device to ensure delivery of adequate tidal volume and ventilation rate.

FLOW-RESTRICTED OXYGEN-POWERED VENTILATION DEVICES

- ▇ A flow-restricted oxygen-powered ventilation device (FROPVD) allows positive-pressure ventilation with 100% oxygen (Figure 2-44). It consists of high-pressure tubing connecting the oxygen supply and a valve that is activated by a lever or push button. When the valve is open, oxygen flows into the patient.
- ▇ The device can be attached to a face mask, tracheal tube, or tracheostomy tube. Indications, contraindications, advantages, and disadvantages of FROPVDs are shown in Table 2-12.

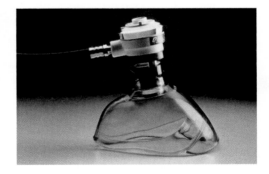

Figure 2-44 • Flow-restricted oxygen-powered ventilation device.

TABLE 2-12	Flow-Restricted Oxygen-Powered Ventilation Devices
Indications	• Patients requiring ventilatory assistance due to decreased ventilation or apnea
Contraindications	• Not for use in pediatric patients
Advantages	• Easy to use
	• Provides high oxygen concentrations and good volume delivery
	• Provides a means for delivery of an oxygen-enriched mixture to the patient
	• Can be used for breathing and nonbreathing patients
Disadvantages	• Need for an oxygen source
	• Requires high oxygen flow rate, which quickly depletes portable oxygen cylinders
	• Gastric distention in patients who are not intubated
	• Inability to monitor lung compliance
	• Barotrauma to the lungs (such as a pneumothorax)

Using a Flow-Restricted Oxygen-Powered Ventilation Device

- ■ Using PPE, attach an adult mask and obtain a mask seal.
- ■ Open the airway.
- ■ Connect the device to the mask, if not already done.
- ■ Trigger the device until the patient's chest rises. Allow the patient to exhale passively. Repeat once every 5 to 6 seconds. During CPR, avoid placing the device in automatic mode because it applies continuous positive end-expiratory pressure (PEEP) that can hinder cardiac output during chest compressions.
- ■ Observe for gastric distention. If seen, reposition the head and ensure an open airway.

QUICK REVIEW 2-6

1. You are ventilating a nonbreathing patient using the mouth-to-mask technique. The mask is connected to supplemental oxygen at 10 L/min. The inspired oxygen concentration delivered to this patient is about __%.
2. True or False. A BVM device can be used for a spontaneously breathing patient as well as a nonbreathing patient.
3. Can you name three advantages of using an automatic transport ventilator?
   1.
   2.
   3.
4. Can you name two possible complications of cricoid pressure?
   1.
   2.

KEEPING IT SIMPLE

Advanced Airways—Examples
- Combitube
- Laryngeal mask airway
- Endotracheal tube

ADVANCED AIRWAYS

Advanced airways include the esophageal-tracheal Combitube (ETC), the LMA, and the ET tube. The Combitube and LMA may be used in areas where tracheal intubation is not permitted, or in communities in which healthcare providers have little opportunity to obtain experience with the technique of tracheal intubation because of few patients.

THE ESOPHAGEAL-TRACHEAL COMBITUBE

- ■ The esophageal-tracheal Combitube (commonly called the Combitube), allows ventilation of the lungs and reduces the risk of aspiration of gastric contents. It does not require visualization of the vocal cords (blind insertion) to ventilate the trachea. Healthcare professionals who have been trained to use a Combitube can use it as an acceptable alternative to an ET tube for airway management in cardiac arrest.

■ The Combitube is a dual-lumen tube with two balloon cuffs. The proximal (pharyngeal) balloon is located near the halfway point of the tube and is considerably larger than the distal cuff. When inflated, the balloon fills the space between the base of the tongue and the soft palate, anchoring the Combitube in position. The trachea is isolated from the esophagus when the pharyngeal and esophageal balloons are inflated (Figure 2-45).

■ When the Combitube is in place, a BVM device (or other ventilation device) is then used to blow air into the tube, with the outlet between the two balloons.

■ The Combitube is available in 41 and 37 Fr sizes. The 37 Fr size is used for patients between 4 and 5 feet tall. The 41 Fr size is used for patients more than 5 feet tall.

■ Failure to confirm proper placement of a Combitube can be fatal. Esophageal trauma, including lacerations, bruising, and subcutaneous emphysema, are possible complications associated with the use of a Combitube. Indications, contraindications, advantages, and disadvantages of Combitubes are shown in Table 2-13.

TABLE 2-13	Combitube
Indications	• Difficult face mask fit (beards, absence of teeth) • Patient in whom intubation has been unsuccessful and ventilation is difficult • Patient in whom airway management is necessary but the healthcare provider is untrained in the technique of visualized orotracheal intubation
Contraindications	• Patient with an intact gag reflex • Patient with known or suspected esophageal disease • Patient known to have ingested a caustic substance • Suspected upper airway obstruction due to laryngeal foreign body or pathology • Patient less than 4 feet tall
Advantages	• Minimal training and retraining required • Visualization of the upper airway or use of special equipment not required for insertion • Reasonable technique for use in suspected neck injury because the head does not need to be hyperextended • Because of the oropharyngeal balloon, the need for a face mask is eliminated • Can provide an open airway with either esophageal or tracheal placement • If placed in the esophagus, allows suctioning of gastric contents without interruption of ventilation • Reduces risk of aspiration of gastric contents
Disadvantages	• Proximal port may be occluded with secretions • Proper identification of tube location may be difficult, leading to ventilation through the wrong lumen • Soft tissue trauma due to rigidity of tube • Impossible to suction the trachea when the tube is in the esophagus • Esophageal or tracheal trauma due to poor insertion technique or use of wrong size device • Damage to the cuffs by the patient's teeth during insertion • Inability to insert due to limited mouth opening

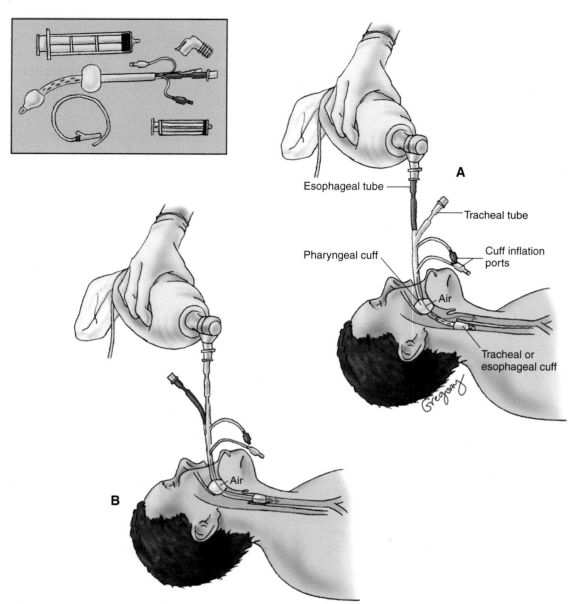

Figure 2-45 • **A,** The Combitube inserted into the esophagus. **B,** The Combitube inserted into the trachea.

Using a Combitube

- Using PPE, open the patient's mouth and clear the airway of any dentures, foreign objects, or debris. If an oral airway was inserted, remove it.
- Auscultate bilateral breath sounds to establish a baseline. Instruct an assistant to preoxygenate the patient with 100% oxygen. Assemble the proper equipment and check the cuffs for leaks.
- Insert the Combitube in the same direction as the natural curvature of the pharynx. Insert the tip into the mouth in the midline and advance it gently along the base of the tongue and into the airway until the black rings (heavy black lines) on the tube are positioned at the level of the patient's teeth (or gums, if the patient lacks teeth) (Figure 2-46A). If the tube does not insert easily, do not use force—withdraw and retry.
- Inflate the proximal (pharyngeal) cuff with 100 mL of air through the blue pilot tube marked #1 (Figure 2-46B). Once inflated, the pharyngeal balloon holds the device in place and helps prevent the escape of air through the nose or mouth.
- Inflate the distal (esophageal) cuff with 15 mL of air through the white pilot tube marked #2 (Figure 2-46C). Once inflated, the esophageal balloon seals the esophagus so that air does not enter the stomach, reducing the risk of aspiration of gastric contents.

■ Attach a bag-valve device to the longer (blue) connecting tube marked #1 (the esophageal tube) and begin ventilation (Figure 2-46D). Ventilation with the Combitube begins with the esophageal tube because of the high probability of esophageal placement after blind insertion. Confirm placement and ventilation by observing chest rise and auscultating over the epigastrium and bilaterally over each lung (Figure 2-46E). If the chest rises, breath sounds are present bilaterally, and epigastric sounds are absent, the Combitube is in the esophagus. Continue to ventilate through long (blue) tube. When esophageal tube placement has been verified, the short (clear) tube (marked #2) can be used for gastric suction with the suction catheter provided in the airway kit.

■ If the chest does not rise or sounds are only heard over the epigastrium, attach the bag-valve device to the second (ET) tube and begin ventilation to determine if the Combitube has entered the trachea. If the device is in the trachea, the chest should rise when ventilating through the second (shorter, clear) tube (see Figure 2-46). (The Combitube functions

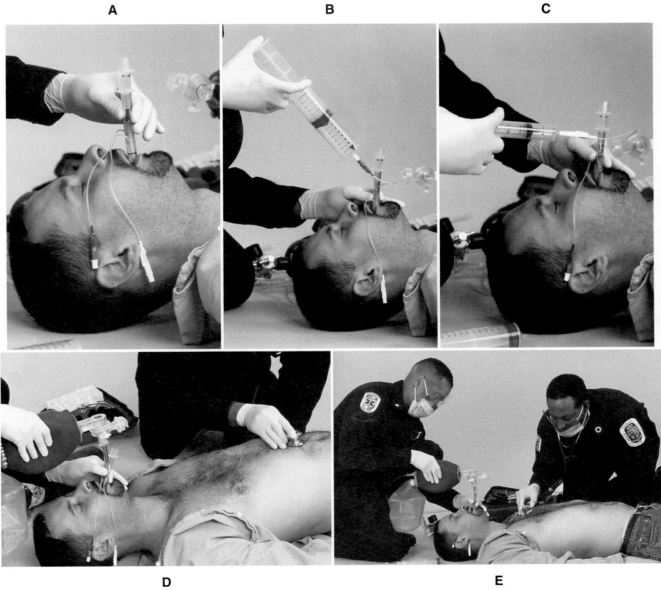

A   **B**   **C**

D   **E**

Figure 2-46 • **A,** Insert the Combitube until the black rings on the tube are positioned at the level of the patient's teeth. **B,** Inflate the pharyngeal cuff through the blue pilot tube marked #1. **C,** Inflate the esophageal cuff through the white pilot balloon. **D,** Attach a bag-valve device to the blue tube and begin ventilation. **E,** Confirm placement and ventilation by watching for chest rise and auscultating over the epigastrium and bilaterally over each lung.

as a standard ET tube when the device is placed in the trachea.) Confirm placement and ventilation by observing chest rise, auscultation over epigastrium, and bilaterally over each lung. If the Combitube is in the trachea and placement has been confirmed, continue ventilation through the second tube.

■ If breath sounds *and* epigastric sounds are absent, immediately deflate the cuffs (blue first). Slightly withdraw the tube and then reinflate the cuffs (blue first). Ventilate and reassess placement. If breath sounds and epigastric sounds are still absent, immediately deflate the cuffs and remove the tube. Suction as necessary, insert an oral or nasal airway, ventilate the patient with a BVM device, and reassess.

THE LARYNGEAL MASK AIRWAY

■ The LMA may be used as an alternative to either an ET tube or face mask with either spontaneous or positive-pressure ventilation.[3] Healthcare professionals who have been trained to use an LMA can use it as an acceptable alternative to an ET tube for airway management in cardiac arrest.

■ Because of the relative ease of learning how to use the device, healthcare workers in an emergency setting who are not trained in ET intubation can be taught to use the LMA. The LMA may be used as the primary airway, as a channel for an ET tube, or as an option in the management of a difficult airway where intubation is unsuccessful.

■ An LMA consists of a tube that is fused to an elliptical, spoon-shaped mask at a 30-degree angle. When inserted, the tube protrudes from the patient's mouth and is connected to a ventilation device via a standard 15-mm inside diameter connector. The mask resembles a miniature face mask and has an inflatable rim that is filled with air from a syringe using a pilot valve-balloon system. The tube opens into the middle of the mask by means of three vertical slits that prevent the tip of the epiglottis from falling back and blocking the lumen of the tube.

■ The LMA is inserted through the mouth and into the pharynx. The device is advanced until resistance is felt. The mask is then inflated, providing a low-pressure seal around the laryngeal inlet. The posterior aspect of the tube is marked with a longitudinal black line. When the LMA is correctly placed, the black line on the tube should rest in the midline against the patient's upper lip.

■ Indications, contraindications, advantages, and disadvantages of LMAs are shown in Table 2-14. LMA size recommendations based on weight are shown in Table 2-15.

The inflatable LMA cuff *does not* ensure an airtight seal to protect the airway from aspiration.

TABLE 2-14	Laryngeal Mask Airway
Indications	• Difficult face mask fit (beards, absence of teeth) • Patient in whom intubation has been unsuccessful and ventilation is difficult • Patient in whom airway management is necessary but the healthcare provider is untrained in the technique of visualized orotracheal intubation • Many elective surgical procedures (i.e., minimal soft tissue trauma with less patient discomfort and relatively short periods of anesthesia)
Contraindications	• Healthcare provider untrained in use of LMA • Contraindicated if a risk of aspiration exists (i.e., patients with full stomachs)
Advantages	• Can be quickly inserted to provide ventilation when BVM ventilation is not sufficient and ET intubation cannot be readily accomplished • Tidal volume delivered may be greater when using the LMA than with face mask ventilation • Less gastric insufflation than with BVM ventilation • Provides ventilation equivalent to the tracheal tube • Training simpler than with tracheal intubation • Unaffected by anatomic factors (e.g., beard, absence of teeth) • No risk of esophageal or bronchial intubation • When compared to tracheal intubation, less potential for trauma from direct laryngoscopy and tracheal intubation • Less coughing, laryngeal spasm, sore throat, and voice changes than with tracheal intubation
Disadvantages	• Does not provide protection against aspiration • Cannot be used if the mouth cannot be opened more than 0.6 in (1.5 cm) • May not be effective when respiratory anatomy is abnormal (i.e., abnormal oropharyngeal anatomy or the presence of pathology is likely to result in a poor mask fit) • May be difficult to provide adequate ventilation if high airway pressures are required

TABLE 2-15	Laryngeal Mask Airway, Disposable LMA (LMA Unique), and Intubating LMA Size Recommendation Based on Weight		
Weight	LMA	Disposable LMA	Intubating LMA
<5 kg	1.0	1.0	—
5-10 kg	1.5	1.5	—
10-20 kg	2.0	2.0	—
20-30 kg	2.5	2.5	—
30-50 kg	3.0	3.0	3.0
50-70 kg	4.0	4.0	4.0
70-100 kg	5.0	5.0	5.0
>100 kg	6.0	—	—

Modified from: Vrocher D, Hopson LR: Basic Airway Management and Decision-Making. In Roberts JR, Hedges JR (Eds): *Clinical Procedures in Emergency Medicine* (4th ed). Philadelphia: Saunders, 2004. p. 63.

Using the Laryngeal Mask Airway

■ Using PPE, open the patient's mouth and clear the airway of any foreign objects or debris. If an oral airway was inserted, remove it.

■ Auscultate bilateral breath sounds to establish a baseline and instruct an assistant to pre-oxygenate the patient with 100% oxygen.

■ Assemble the proper equipment and check the cuff and valve for leaks. Deflate the cuff and apply water-soluble lubricant. (Avoid lubricating the anterior surface of the mask, because the lubricant may be aspirated.) Position the rim of the mask so that it is facing away from the mask opening. There should be no folds near the tip.

■ Place the patient in the "sniffing" position (neck flexed and head extended). During the insertion procedure, maintain this position with your nondominant hand.

■ With the distal opening of the LMA facing anteriorly, insert the tip of the LMA into the patient's mouth (Figure 2-47). Press the tip of the mask upward against the hard palate to flatten it out. Using your index or third finger, in one smooth movement advance the mask

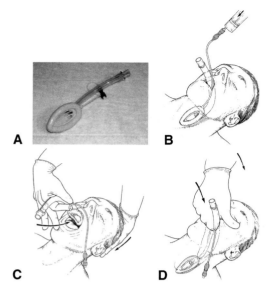

Figure 2-47 • The LMA. **A,** An LMA with the cuff inflated. **B,** LMA in place with cuff overlying larynx. **C,** LMA placement into the pharynx. **D,** LMA placement using the index finger as a guide.

over the hard palate, the soft palate, and as far as possible into the laryngopharynx until resistance is felt. When the LMA has been properly positioned, the cuff tip lies at the base of the laryngopharynx, the sides in the pyriform fossae, and the upper border of the mask at the base of the tongue, pushing it forward.

■ Make sure that the black line on the LMA is in the midline against the patient's upper lip. Failure to make sure that the black line on the LMA is correctly positioned may result in misplacement of the cuff and a partial airway obstruction. Without holding the tube, inflate the cuff with a volume of air appropriate for the mask size selected. As the cuff is inflated, there will be a slight outward movement of the tube as the cuff centers itself around the laryngeal inlet. This results in slight movement of the thyroid and cricoid cartilages.

■ Confirm placement of the LMA with auscultation, observation of chest rise, and use of an exhaled CO_2 detector. Secure the LMA and a bite-block in place.

 In the "sniffing" position, the neck is flexed at the fifth and sixth cervical vertebrae, and the head is extended at the first and second cervical vertebrae. This position aligns the axes of the mouth, pharynx, and trachea. The sniffing position is not used in cases of suspected trauma.

QUICK REVIEW 2-7

1. True or False. The laryngeal mask airway is available in only one size.
2. Can you list two indications for use of the Combitube?
   1.
   2.
3. List four contraindications to use of the Combitube.
   1.
   2.
   3.
   4.

ENDOTRACHEAL INTUBATION

■ **Endotracheal intubation** is an advanced airway procedure in which a tube is placed directly into the trachea. It may be performed for a variety of reasons including the delivery of anesthesia, assisting a patient's breathing with positive-pressure ventilation, and protection of the patient's airway from aspiration. Intubation requires special equipment and supplies (Box 2-2)

■ A laryngoscope is an instrument that consists of a handle and blade used for examining the interior of the larynx. It is used to visualize the glottic opening (the space between the vocal cords). A standard laryngoscope is made of plastic or stainless steel.

■ The laryngoscope handle contains the batteries for the light source. It attaches to a plastic or stainless steel blade that has a bulb located in the blade's distal tip. The point where the handle and the blade attach to make electrical contact is called the fitting. The bulb on the laryngoscope blade lights when the blade is attached to the laryngoscope handle and elevated to a right angle (Figure 2-48).

BOX 2-2

Endotracheal Intubation—Equipment and Supplies

- Laryngoscope handle
- Laryngoscope blades
- Extra batteries
- Endotracheal tubes of various sizes
- 10-mL syringe for inflation of the ET tube cuff (if present)
- Stylet
- BVM device with supplemental oxygen and reservoir
- Suction equipment
- Commercial tube-holder or tape
- Water-soluble lubricant
- Bite-block or oral airway
- Exhaled CO_2 detector and/or esophageal detector device

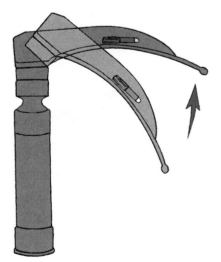

Figure 2-48 • The bulb on the laryngoscope blade lights when the blade is attached to the laryngoscope handle and elevated to a right angle.

■ Laryngoscope blades are available in a variety of sizes ranging from 0 to 4. Size #0 is used for infants; size #4 blade is used for large adults. Select the appropriate blade size with the laryngoscope blade held next to the patient's face. A blade of proper size should reach between the patient's lips and larynx. If you are unsure of the correct size, it is usually best to select a blade that is too long, rather than too short.

▶ There are two types of laryngoscope blades—straight and curved.
  • The straight blade is also referred to as the Miller, Wisconsin, or Flagg blade (Figure 2-49). During ET intubation, the tip of the straight blade is positioned under the epiglottis. When the laryngoscope handle is lifted anteriorly, the blade directly lifts the epiglottis out of the way to expose the glottic opening (Figure 2-50).
  • The curved blade is also called the Macintosh blade (Figure 2-51). The tip of the curved blade is inserted into the vallecula. When the laryngoscope handle is lifted anteriorly, the blade elevates the tongue and indirectly lifts the epiglottis, allowing visualization of the glottic opening (Figure 2-52).

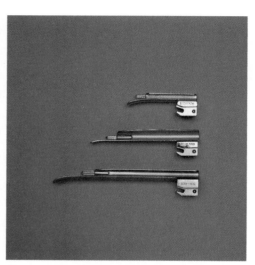

Figure 2-49 • Straight laryngoscope blades.

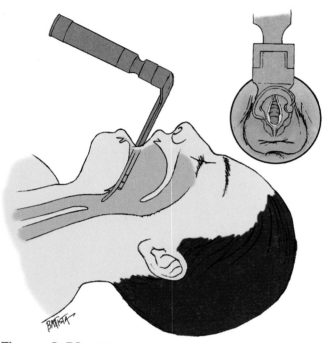

Figure 2-50 • The tip of the straight blade is positioned under the epiglottis to expose the glottic opening.

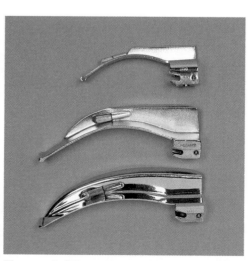

Figure 2-51 • Curved laryngoscope blades.

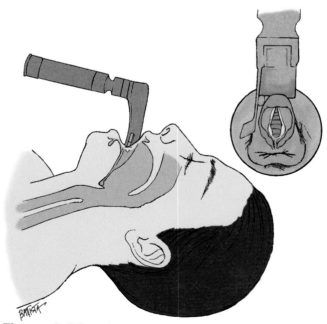

Figure 2-52 • The curved blade is inserted into the vallecula, the space or "pocket" between the base of the tongue and the epiglottis.

■ An ET tube is a curved tube that is open at both ends. A standard 15-mm connector is located at the proximal end for attachment of various devices for delivery of positive-pressure ventilation. The distal end of the tube is beveled to facilitate placement between the vocal cords.

■ Some ET tubes have an inflatable balloon cuff that surrounds the distal tip of the tube. When the distal cuff is inflated, it contacts the wall of the trachea as it expands, sealing off the trachea from the remainder of the pharynx and reducing the risk of aspiration. The cuff is attached to a one-way valve through a side tube with a pilot balloon that is used to indicate if the cuff is inflated (Figure 2-53).

■ ET tubes are measured in millimeters (mm) by their internal diameter (ID) and external diameter (OD). Centimeter markings on the tube indicate the distance from the tip.

  ▶ ET tubes are available in lengths ranging from 12 cm to 32 cm. Internal tube diameters range from 2.5 mm to 4.5 mm (uncuffed) and 5.0 mm to 10.0 mm (uncuffed).

  ▶ Selection of an ET tube of the correct size is important. An ET tube that is too small may provide too little airflow and may lead to the delivery of inadequate tidal volumes. A tube that is too large may cause tracheal edema and/or vocal cord damage. Select the largest tube size appropriate for the patient, because larger tubes facilitate suctioning of secretions and decrease the work of breathing.

  ▶ Common internal diameters of ET tubes for adults are typically from 7.0 to 8.5 mm. Most common sizes used for adults:
    • Adult female: 7.0 to 8.0 mm ID
    • Adult male: 8.0 to 8.5 mm ID

  ▶ Because of the size variation in adults, it is important to have several sizes of tubes on hand. At a minimum, have the size tube most commonly used (see above), plus a tube ½ size smaller and another ½ size larger. When immediate ET tube placement is necessary, most adults can accept an ET tube with an internal diameter of at least 7.5 mm.

  ▶ When the ET tube has been properly placed, the centimeter markings on the side of the tube should be observed and recorded. This value is typically between the 19- and 23-cm mark at the front teeth.

KEEPING IT SIMPLE

- Average ET tube depth in men = 23 cm at the lips, 22 cm at the teeth
- Average ET tube depth in women = 22 cm at the lips, 21 cm at the teeth

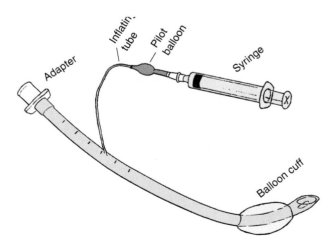

Figure 2-53 • Components of the ET tube.

■ A **stylet** is a flexible, plastic-coated wire inserted into an ET tube used for molding and maintaining the shape of the tube (Figure 2-54). When a stylet is used, the tip of the stylet must be recessed about ½ inch from the end of the ET tube to avoid trauma to the airway structures.

■ Indications, contraindications, advantages, and disadvantages of ET intubation are shown in Table 2-16.

TABLE 2-16	Endotracheal Intubation	
Indications	• Inability of the patient to protect his or her own airway due to the absence of protective reflexes (e.g., coma, respiratory and/or cardiac arrest) • Inability of the rescuer to ventilate the unresponsive patient with less invasive methods • Present or impending airway obstruction/respiratory failure (e.g., inhalation injury, severe asthma, exacerbation of chronic obstructive pulmonary disease, severe pulmonary edema, severe flail chest, or pulmonary contusion) • When prolonged ventilatory support is required	
Contraindications	• Healthcare provider untrained in ET intubation	
Advantages	• Isolates the airway • Keeps the airway open • Reduces the risk of aspiration • Ensures delivery of a high concentration of oxygen • Permits suctioning of the trachea • Provides a route for administration of some medications (see Chapter 5) • Ensures delivery of a selected tidal volume to maintain lung inflation	
Disadvantages	• Considerable training and experience required • Special equipment needed • Bypasses physiologic function of upper airway (e.g., warming, filtering, humidifying of inhaled air) • Requires direct visualization of vocal cords	

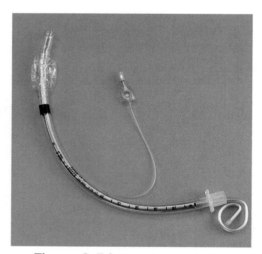

Figure 2-54 • ET tube with stylet.

■ Technique:
- ❱ Using PPE (at a minimum, use gloves, protective eyewear, and a mask), open the patient's airway. Ask an assistant to preoxygenate the patient while you auscultate bilateral lung sounds to establish a baseline.
- ❱ While your assistant continues to preoxygenate the patient, assemble and prepare the equipment needed for intubation, including suction equipment.
- ❱ Select the proper size blade and then assemble the laryngoscope. Attach the blade to the handle and check the blade for a "white, bright light." After verifying that the light is in working order, move the blade to its unlocked position to conserve battery life until the light is needed.
- ❱ Select the proper size ET tube and test it for leaks. If there are no leaks, completely deflate the cuff. Leave the syringe filled with air attached to the inflation valve. If a stylet will be used, insert it into the ET tube, making sure that the end of the stylet is recessed at least ½ inch from the tip of the ET tube. Bend the proximal end of the stylet over the ET tube to prevent it from sliding down into the tube. Lubricate the distal end of the ET tube with water-soluble lubricant.

A petroleum-based lubricant should never be used to lubricate airway devices because it may damage the airway device and cause tissue inflammation.

- ❱ Place the patient's head in the "sniffing" position to align the axes of the mouth, pharynx, and trachea (Figure 2-55). Open the patient's mouth and inspect the oral cavity. Remove dentures and/or debris, if present. Do *not* place the patient's head in this position if trauma is suspected. If trauma is suspected, an assistant should manually stabilize the cervical spine in a neutral position.
- ❱ Stop ventilations and remove the ventilation face mask and oral airway (if present). Do not exceed 30 seconds from ventilation to ventilation for each intubation attempt.
- ❱ Direct an assistant to apply cricoid pressure and maintain pressure until the airway is secured. If the patient begins to actively vomit, discontinue cricoid pressure until the vomiting stops and the airway has been cleared.
- ❱ Holding the laryngoscope in the left hand and with the tip of the blade pointing away from you, insert the blade into the right side of the patient's mouth between the teeth, sweeping the tongue to the left (Figure 2-56). Advance the laryngoscope blade until the distal end reaches the base of the tongue (Figure 2-57).

The laryngoscope is held in the left hand because most laryngoscopes are designed for right-handed individuals. This allows the dominant (right) hand to be used for handling the ET tube.

Figure 2-55 • Head positioning for tracheal intubation. **A,** Neutral position. **B,** Head elevated. **C,** "Sniffing" position. The sniffing position aligns the axes of the mouth, pharynx, and trachea, creating the shortest distance and straightest line between the teeth and vocal cords.

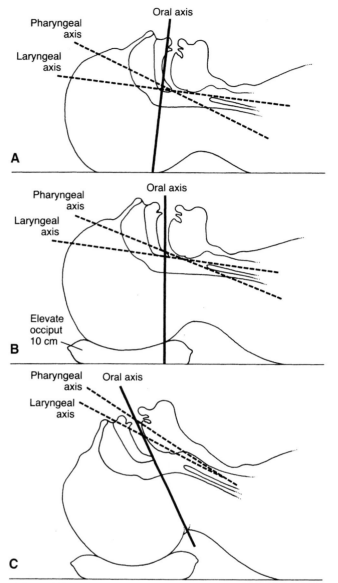

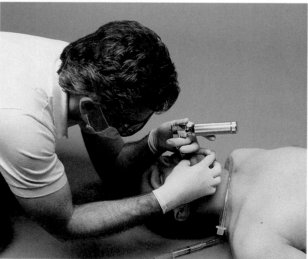

Figure 2-56 • Holding the laryngoscope in the left hand and with the tip of the blade pointing away from you, insert the blade into the right side of the patient's mouth between the teeth, sweeping the tongue to the left.

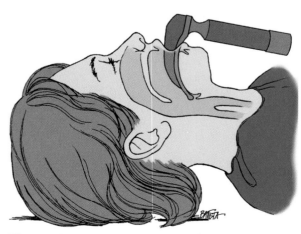

Figure 2-57 • Advance the laryngoscope blade until the distal end reaches the base of the tongue.

▶ Lift the laryngoscope to elevate the mandible without putting pressure on the front teeth (Figure 2-58) and visualize the epiglottis (Figure 2-59). Do *not* use the patient's teeth or gums as a fulcrum. Do not allow the blade to touch the patient's teeth. Suction the airway if needed.

▶ After visualizing the epiglottis, identify the vocal cords, and place the blade in the proper position. If using a curved blade, advance the tip of the blade into the vallecula. If using a straight blade, advance the tip under the epiglottis.

BURP Technique

Viewing the vocal cords may be aided with the use of the BURP (*b*ackward, *u*pward, *r*ightward *p*ressure) technique. With this maneuver, the larynx is displaced in the three specific directions (1) posteriorly against the cervical vertebrae, (2) superiorly as possible, and (3) slightly laterally to the right. This maneuver improves visualization of the larynx more easily than simple backpressure on the larynx (cricoid pressure) because the BURP technique moves the larynx back to the position from which it was displaced by a right-handed (held in operator's left hand) laryngoscope.[4]

In a Canadian study, researchers attempted to determine if the application of a BURP maneuver to the cricoid cartilage would combine the benefits of both the BURP and the Sellick maneuvers, resulting in an improved glottic view and offering the potential of protection against passive gastric regurgitation. Interestingly, their results showed that the combination of the BURP maneuver and cricoid pressure *worsened* the view obtained at laryngoscopy in 30% of cases. Cricoid pressure alone worsened the view in 12.5% of cases. No difference was seen in 65% of cases. They concluded that there was no benefit to routinely applying a modified BURP maneuver to the cricoid cartilage during rapid sequence induction of anesthesia.[5]

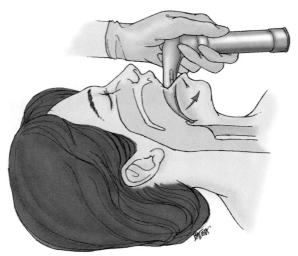

Figure 2-58 • Lift the laryngoscope to elevate the mandible without putting pressure on the front teeth.

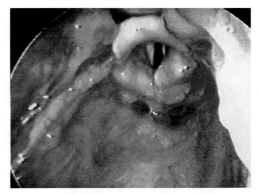

Figure 2-59 • View of the epiglottis and vocal cords.

▶ Grasp the ET tube with your right hand and introduce it into the right corner of the patient's mouth (Figure 2-60). Advance the tube through the glottic opening until the distal cuff disappears past the vocal cords (Figure 2-61). The black marker on the ET tube should be at the level of the vocal cords. Advance the ET tube until the proximal end of the cuff lies ½ to 1 inch beyond the cords.

▶ While firmly holding the ET tube, remove the stylet (if used), and inflate the distal cuff with approximately 6 to 10 mL of air (volume varies depending on cuff size). Disconnect the syringe from the inflation valve.

▶ Attach a ventilation device to the ET tube and ventilate the patient. Confirm proper placement of the tube by first auscultating over the epigastrium (should be silent) and then in the midaxillary and anterior chest line on the right and left sides of the patient's chest (Figure 2-62). Observe the patient's chest for full movement with ventilation.

▶ Use an exhaled CO_2 detector and/or esophageal detector device to verify placement (Figure 2-63). Once placement is confirmed, note and record the depth (cm marking) of the tube at the patient's teeth.

An advanced airway that is misplaced or becomes dislodged can be fatal. Make it a habit to recheck placement of an advanced airway immediately after insertion, after securing the tube, during transport, and whenever the patient is moved. Capnography (discussed later in this chapter) can be used to immediately alert you to a misplaced or dislodged tube.

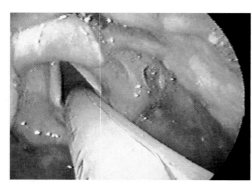

Figure 2-61 • An ET tube passing through the glottic opening.

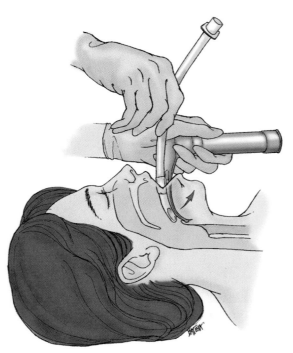

Figure 2-60 • Advance the ET tube into the larynx and then through the glottic opening.

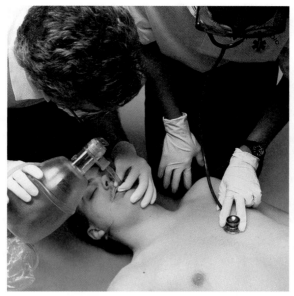

Figure 2-62 • Confirm proper placement of the tube by first auscultating over the epigastrium and then in the lateral aspects of the patient's chest at the right and left midaxillary lines.

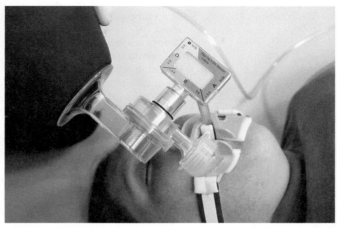

Figure 2-63 • Confirming proper endotracheal tube placement using an exhaled CO_2 detector.

❱ If breath sounds are absent bilaterally after intubation and gurgling is heard over the epigastrium, assume esophageal intubation. Deflate the ET cuff, remove the tube, and preoxygenate before reattempting intubation.

❱ If breath sounds are diminished on the left after intubation but present on the right, assume right mainstem bronchus intubation. Deflate the ET cuff, pull back the ET tube slightly, reinflate the cuff, and reevaluate breath sounds.

❱ Secure the ET tube with a commercial tube holder or tape and provide ventilatory support with supplemental oxygen. After securing the tube, recheck (and record) the tube depth at the patient's teeth.

❱ Possible complications of ET intubation are listed in Box 2-3. A summary of advanced airways is shown in Table 2-17.

BOX 2-3

Endotracheal Intubation—Possible Complications

- Bleeding
- Laryngospasm
- Vocal cord damage
- Mucosal necrosis
- Barotrauma
- Aspiration
- Cuff leak
- Esophageal intubation
- Right mainstem intubation

- Occlusion caused by patient biting the tube or secretions
- Laryngeal or tracheal edema
- Tube occlusion
- Inability to talk
- Hypoxia due to prolonged or unsuccessful intubation
- Dysrhythmias
- Trauma to the lips, teeth, tongue, or soft tissues of the oropharynx
- Increased intracranial pressure

TABLE 2-17	Advanced Airways	
Device	Indications	Sizing
Esophageal-tracheal Combitube	• Difficult face mask fit (beards, absence of teeth) • Deep unresponsiveness, cardiac, and/or respiratory arrest • Patient in whom intubation has been unsuccessful and ventilation is difficult • Patient in whom airway management is necessary but healthcare provider is untrained in the technique of visualized orotracheal intubation • When BVM ventilation is inadequate or causing excessive gastric distention	• 37 Fr size is used for patients between 4 and 5 feet tall. • 41 Fr size is used for patients over 5 feet tall.
LMA	• Difficult face mask fit (beards, absence of teeth) • Patient in whom intubation has been unsuccessful and ventilation is difficult • Patient in whom airway management is necessary but healthcare provider is untrained in the technique of visualized orotracheal intubation • Many elective surgical procedures	Because masks are available in several sizes, the LMA can be used in patients of all ages, from neonates to adults.
Endotracheal intubation	• Inability of the patient to protect his or her own airway due to the absence of protective reflexes (e.g., coma, respiratory and/or cardiac arrest) • Inability of the rescuer to ventilate the unresponsive patient with less invasive methods • Present or impending airway obstruction/respiratory failure (e.g., inhalation injury, severe asthma, exacerbation of chronic obstructive pulmonary disease, severe pulmonary edema, severe flail chest, or pulmonary contusion) • When prolonged ventilatory support is required	• Adult female: 7-8 mm ID. • Adult male: 8-8.5 mm ID.

Confirming Endotracheal Tube Placement

Methods used to verify proper placement of an ET tube include the following:
- Visualizing the passage of the ET tube between the vocal cords
- Auscultating the presence of bilateral breath sounds
- Confirming the absence of sounds over the epigastrium during ventilation
- Observing adequate chest rise with each ventilation
- Observing absence of vocal sounds after placement of the ET tube
- Monitoring for changes in the color (colorimetric device) or number (digital device) on an exhaled CO_2 detector
- Verifying tube placement by an esophageal detector device

It is important to note that auscultation for breath sounds over the lungs and abdomen and observing chest rise are not always indicative of correct ET tube placement. After visualizing the ET tube passing through the vocal cords and confirming placement of the tube by auscultation, be sure to verify tube placement using an exhaled CO_2 detector and/or an esophageal detector device.

Exhaled CO_2 monitoring has been suggested as the "sixth vital sign" that should be monitored in patients in addition to heart rate, blood pressure, respiratory rate, body temperature, and blood oxygen saturation.[6]

Exhaled Carbon Dioxide Detection

■ **Capnography:** Continuous analysis and recording of CO_2 concentrations in respiratory gases

■ **Capnograph:** A device that provides a numerical reading of exhaled CO_2 concentrations and a waveform (tracing)

■ **Capnometer:** A device used to measure the concentration of CO_2 at the end of exhalation

■ **Capnometry:** A numerical reading of exhaled CO_2 concentrations without a continuous written record or waveform

■ **Exhaled CO_2 detector** (also called an end-tidal CO_2 detector): A capnometer that provides a noninvasive estimate of alveolar ventilation, the concentration of exhaled CO_2 from the lungs, and arterial CO_2 content

■ Exhaled CO_2 monitoring is commonly used in the following situations:
  ▶ Assessment of conscious sedation safety
  ▶ Evaluation of mechanical ventilation and resuscitation efforts
  ▶ Verification of ET tube placement
  ▶ Continuous monitoring of ET tube position
  ▶ Monitoring of exhaled CO_2 levels in patients with suspected increased intracranial pressure

■ Because the air in the esophagus normally has very low levels of CO_2, capnometry is considered a rapid method of preventing unrecognized esophageal intubation.

■ Exhaled CO_2 detectors are available as disposable colorimetric devices (Figure 2-64) or electronic monitors (Figure 2-65).

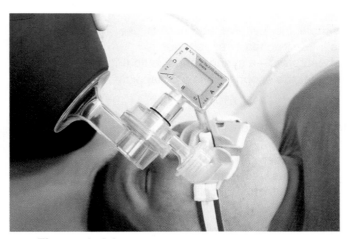

Figure 2-64 • Colorimetric exhaled CO_2 detector.

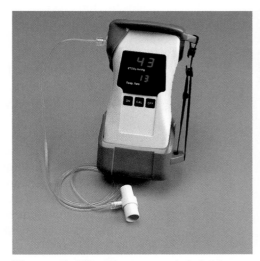

Figure 2-65 • Electronic exhaled CO_2 detector.

▶ Disposable colorimetric devices provide CO_2 readings by chemical reaction on pH-sensitive litmus paper housed in the detector. The device is placed between an ET tube or Combitube and a ventilation device. The presence of CO_2 (evidenced by a color change on the colorimetric device or number/light on the electronic monitor) suggests tracheal tube placement. A lack of CO_2 (no color change on colorimetric detector or indicator on the electronic monitor) suggests tube placement in the esophagus, particularly in patients with spontaneous circulation.

▶ Because CO_2 may inadvertently enter the stomach, ventilate the patient at least six times before evaluating ET tube placement using an exhaled CO_2 detector to quickly wash out any retained CO_2.

▶ In animals, false-positive results (CO_2 is detected despite tube placement in the esophagus) have been reported when large amounts of carbonated beverages were ingested before a cardiac arrest.

▶ False-negative results (lack of CO_2 detection despite tube placement in the trachea) may occur in cardiac arrest or in a patient who has a significant pulmonary embolus because of reduced delivery of CO_2 to the lungs.

KEEPING IT SIMPLE

Pulse oximetry provides important information about oxygenation. Capnography provides information about the effectiveness of ventilation.

Colorimetric capnography is susceptible to inaccurate results due to the age of the paper, exposure of the paper to the environment, patient secretions (e.g., vomitus), or acidic drugs, such as endotracheally administered epinephrine.

Esophageal Detector Devices

■ Esophageal detector devices are simple, inexpensive, and easy to use. They are used as an aid to determine if an ET tube is in the trachea or esophagus.

■ There are two types of esophageal detectors—a syringe and a bulb (Figure 2-66). These devices operate under the principle that the esophagus is a collapsible tube and the trachea a rigid one.

■ Syringe device
▶ The syringe device is connected to an ET tube with the plunger fully inserted into the barrel of the syringe.
▶ If the ET tube is in the trachea, the plunger can be easily withdrawn from the syringe barrel. If the ET tube is in the esophagus, resistance will be felt when the plunger is withdrawn because the walls of the esophagus will collapse when negative pressure is applied to the syringe.

■ Bulb device
▶ The bulb device is compressed before it is connected to an ET tube. A vacuum is created as the pressure on the bulb is released.
▶ If the ET tube is in the trachea, the bulb will refill easily when pressure is released, indicating proper tube placement. If the ET tube is in the esophagus, the bulb will remain collapsed, indicating improper tube placement.

■ Conditions in which the trachea tends to collapse can result in misleading findings. Examples of these conditions include morbid obesity, late pregnancy, status asthmaticus, and the presence of profuse tracheal secretions.

When using an esophageal detector device to confirm placement of the ET tube, do *not* inflate the ET tube cuff before using the esophageal detector. Inflating the cuff moves the distal end of the ET tube away from the walls of the esophagus. If the tube was inadvertently inserted into the esophagus, this movement will cause the detector bulb to reexpand, falsely suggesting that the tube was in the trachea.

QUICK REVIEW 2-8

1. What is the average ET tube size for an adult male? An adult female?

2. An advantage of ventilation with a bag-valve device is that a sense of compliance of the lungs is conveyed to the operator. What is meant by the term "compliance"?

3. A nasal cannula with a liter flow of 4 L/min will deliver what percentage of oxygen?

4. Name the three axes of the upper airway that must be aligned during orotracheal intubation.

5. Endotracheal intubation should be accomplished within _____.

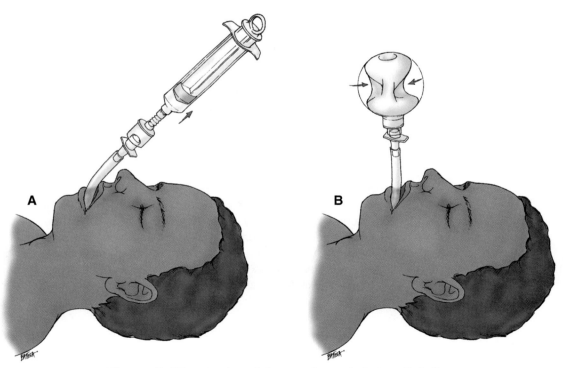

Figure 2-66 • Esophageal detector device. **A,** Syringe. **B,** Bulb.

QUICK REVIEW ANSWERS

Quick Review Number	Answers
2-1	1. False. The cricoid cartilage is the narrowest diameter of the airway in infants and children younger than 10 years of age. The glottic opening is the narrowest portion of an adult's airway. 2. Epiglottis 3. Vallecula 4. Hard palate 5. Glottis 6. The point where the trachea bifurcates into the right and left mainstem bronchi 7. The right mainstem bronchus is shorter, wider, and straighter than the left.
2-2	1. Jaw thrust without head tilt maneuver 2. Soft (whistle-tip, flexible, French) 3. Withdrawing
2-3	1. The tongue 2. Hold the device against the side of the patient's face and select an airway that extends from the corner of the mouth to the tip of the earlobe or the angle of the jaw. 3. False 4. If resistance is encountered, a gentle back-and-forth rotation of the device between your fingers may ease insertion. If resistance continues, withdraw the NPA, reapply lubricant, and attempt insertion in the patient's other nostril. 5. 10 to 15 seconds
2-4	1. Use in responsive or semiresponsive patients may stimulate the gag reflex when the back of the tongue or posterior pharynx is touched, resulting in retching, vomiting, and/or laryngospasm. 2. To remove vomitus, saliva, blood, and other material from the patient's airway 3. Align the nasal airway on the side of the patient's face. Proper size is determined by selecting a device that extends from the tip of the nose to the angle of the jaw or the tip of the ear.
2-5	1. Application of cricoid pressure helps minimize inflation of the stomach during ventilation, reducing the likelihood of vomiting and aspiration. 2. The most common problem with using the bag-mask device is the inability to provide adequate ventilatory volumes due to an inadequate face-to-mask seal. 3. True. A greater tidal volume can be delivered with mouth-to-mask ventilation than with a bag-mask device. 4. A bag-mask device used with supplemental oxygen set at a flow rate of 15 L/min but no reservoir will deliver approximately 40% to 60% oxygen to the patient.
2-6	1. 50% 2. True. A bag-mask device can be used for a spontaneously breathing patient as well as a nonbreathing patient. 3. Advantages of using an ATV include the following: lightweight, portable, and durable; provides a means for delivery of an oxygen-enriched mixture to the patient; can be used for breathing and nonbreathing patients, intubated and nonintubated patients; frees the rescuer for other tasks when used in intubated patients; in patients who are not intubated, the rescuer has both hands free to apply the mask and maintain the airway; adjustable settings; once set, provides a specific tidal volume, respiratory rate, and minute ventilation. 4. Possible complications of cricoid pressure include laryngeal trauma with excessive force, esophageal rupture from unrelieved high gas-

tric pressures, and excessive pressure may obstruct the trachea in small children.

2-7   1. False. Because masks are available in several sizes, the LMA can be used in patients of all ages, from neonates to adults. 2. Indications for use of a Combitube include the following: difficult face mask fit (beards, absence of teeth), patient in whom intubation has been unsuccessful and ventilation is difficult, patient in whom airway management is necessary but healthcare provider is untrained in technique of visualized orotracheal intubation. 3. Contraindications to the use of a Combitube include the following: patient with an intact gag reflex, patient with known or suspected esophageal disease, patient known to have ingested a caustic substance, suspected upper airway obstruction due to laryngeal foreign body or pathology, and a patient less than 4 feet tall.

2-8   1. The average ET tube size for an adult male is 8 to 8.5 ID and 7 to 8 for an adult female. 2. Compliance refers to the resistance of the patient's lung tissue to ventilation. 3. A nasal cannula at an oxygen flow rate of 4 L/min can deliver an oxygen concentration of about 37%. 4. Mouth, pharynx, and trachea 5. 30 seconds

STOP & REVIEW

Questions 1–26. Match each answer below (a through z) with its corresponding description.

a) Lower
b) Spontaneously
c) Tidal
d) Laryngeal
e) Nasal cannula
f) Epiglottis
g) Carina
h) Nonrebreather
i) Ventilation
j) Two
k) Upper
l) Vallecula
m) Soft palate

n) Simple face mask
o) Sellick
p) One
q) Uvula
r) Compliance
s) Pharynx
t) Capnometer
u) Hard palate
v) Combitube
w) Pulse
x) Glottic
y) Venturi
z) Cricoid

_____ 1. A dual-lumen airway

_____ 2. When giving rescue breaths, each breath should be delivered over __ second(s)

_____ 3. The back part of the roof of the mouth that is composed of mucous membrane, muscular fibers, and mucous glands

_____ 4. Exhaled CO_2 detectors provide information about the effectiveness of _____

_____ 5. Fleshy tissue resembling a grape that hangs down from the soft palate

_____ 6. _____ oximetry is a noninvasive method of measuring the percentage of oxygen saturated in the blood

_____ 7. The _____ cartilage is the only completely cartilaginous ring in the larynx

_____ 8. The _____ airway includes the nose and nasal cavities, pharynx, and larynx

_____ 9. Bony portion of the roof of the mouth that forms the floor of the nasal cavity

_____ 10. A small leaf-shaped cartilage located at the top of the larynx that prevents food from entering the respiratory tract during swallowing

_____ 11. Oxygen delivery devices such as a nasal cannula are used for _____ breathing patients

_____ 12. The _____ opening is the narrowest part of the adult larynx

_____ 13. The "L" in LMA

_____ 14. A _____ mask is recommended for patients who rely on a hypoxic respiratory drive, such as those who have chronic obstructive pulmonary disease

_____ 15. The _____ maneuver is another name for cricoid pressure

____16. _____ volume is the volume of air moved into or out of the lungs during a normal breath

____17. The recommended oxygen flow rate with this device is 8 to 10 L/min

____18. The space/pocket between the base of the tongue and the epiglottis

____19. The point where the trachea divides into the right and left mainstem bronchi

____20. Lung _____ refers to the resistance of the patient's lung tissue to ventilation

____21. A passageway common to both the respiratory and digestive systems

____22. A device that measures the concentration of carbon dioxide at the end of exhalation

____23. The _____ airway includes the trachea, bronchi, bronchioles, alveoli, and lungs

____24. Should a partial rebreather or nonrebreather bag collapse when the patient inhales, increase the delivered oxygen by ____-liter increments until the bag remains inflated

____25. A _____ mask is the delivery device of choice when high concentrations of oxygen are needed in the spontaneously breathing patient

____26. Delivers an oxygen concentration of 25% to 45% at a flow rate of 1 to 6 L/min

27. A 65-year-old woman is complaining of shortness of breath. You have applied a pulse oximeter and cardiac monitor. Which of the following SpO_2 readings suggests mild hypoxia?
   a. An SpO_2 reading between 98% and 100%
   b. An SpO_2 reading between 94% and 98%
   c. An SpO_2 reading between 91% and 95%
   d. An SpO_2 reading between 88% and 91%

28. Which of the following statements is correct regarding the use of a Combitube?
   a. Direct visualization of the airway is required for insertion of the device
   b. Because it is available in several sizes, the Combitube can be used in patients of all ages, from neonates to adults
   c. Once the Combitube is positioned, ventilation should begin through the tracheal tube
   d. Esophageal trauma is a possible complication of Combitube use

29. An oral airway:
   a. May result in an airway obstruction if improperly inserted
   b. Should be lubricated with a petroleum-based lubricant before insertion
   c. Is usually well tolerated in the responsive or semiresponsive patient
   d. Is considered the optimal method of managing the airway during cardiac arrest

30. With an oxygen flow rate of 1 to 6 L/minute, a nasal cannula can deliver an estimated oxygen concentration of:
    a. 17% to 21%
    b. 25% to 45%
    c. 40% to 60%
    d. 60% to 100%

The wife of a 72-year-old man reports that her husband "just stopped breathing" moments ago. As you approach the patient, you see that he is supine in bed and note that his eyes are closed. He is unaware of your approach. You do not see any chest movement. His skin looks pale.

31. From the information provided, complete the following about your first impression of this patient.
    a. Appearance:
    b. Breathing:
    c. Circulation:

32. Based on the information provided, is this patient "sick" or "not sick?" How should you proceed?

33. You have arrived at the patient's side. The patient does not respond to your voice or to application of a painful stimulus. After determining that the patient is unresponsive, what is your next course of action?
    a. Open the patient's airway using a head-tilt/chin-lift maneuver
    b. Apply a pulse oximeter and cardiac monitor
    c. Begin chest compressions
    d. Obtain a detailed medical history from the patient's wife

34. Assessment reveals gurgling respirations at a rate of 4/min. What should be done next?
    a. An airway obstruction is present. Begin chest compressions.
    b. Check the patient's oxygen saturation with a pulse oximeter.
    c. Suction the patient's upper airway.
    d. Apply the AED pads to the patient's bare chest.

35. The patient's respirations continue at a rate of 4/min. Chest movement is barely visible with each breath. Which of the following oxygen delivery devices would be most appropriate to use in this situation?
    a. A nonrebreather mask at 15 L/min
    b. A nasal cannula at 4 L/min
    c. A simple face mask at 4 L/min
    d. A bag-mask device with supplemental oxygen at 15 L/min and a reservoir

36. Complete the following table.

Device	Approximate Inspired Oxygen Concentration	Liter Flow (L/min)
Nasal cannula		
Simple face mask		6 to 10 (8 to 10 recommended)
Partial rebreather mask	35% to 60%	6 to 10
Nonrebreather mask		
Venturi mask		4 to 8

You and a coworker arrive to find a 78-year-old woman unresponsive in bed.

37. After opening the patient's airway, you should check for breathing for
    a. 2 to 3 seconds
    b. Up to 5 seconds
    c. Up to 10 seconds
    d. 30 seconds

38. The patient is not breathing. You have a pocket mask on hand that is equipped with an oxygen inlet. After quickly connecting oxygen tubing to the inlet on the mask, you should set the oxygen flow rate at:
    a. 1 to 2 L/min
    b. 4 to 6 L/min
    c. 8 to 10 L/min
    d. 10 to 12 L/min

39. Which of the following statements is correct regarding ventilating this patient with a pocket mask?
    a. Take a deep breath before each ventilation, and then ventilate at a rate of 15 to 20 breaths per minute
    b. Take a normal breath before each ventilation, and then ventilate at a rate of 10 to 12 breaths per minute
    c. Take a normal breath before each ventilation, and then ventilate at a rate of 12 to 20 breaths per minute
    d. Take a deep breath before each ventilation, and then ventilate at a rate of 12 to 15 breaths per minute

40. The patient has no pulse. Chest compressions are being performed by a coworker while you continue positive-pressure ventilation with the pocket mask. Which of the following statements is correct?
    a. The recommended compression to ventilation ratio in this situation is 30 to 2
    b. The recommended compression to ventilation ratio in this situation is 15 to 2
    c. During two-rescuer adult CPR, the rate of ventilations should be slowed to a rate of 6 to 8/min
    d. The rate of chest compressions should be at least 120 to 150/min

41. The AED indicates "no shock advised." A coworker has intubated the patient. Proper placement of the ET tube has been confirmed, the tube has been secured in place, and the tube marking at the patient's teeth recorded. Which of the following statements is correct regarding ventilation of this patient?
    a. It is important that the rescuer performing chest compressions pause periodically to permit adequate ventilation of the patient with a bag-valve device
    b. Chest compressions should be given without interruption and the rate of ventilations altered to 8 to 10 bpm
    c. Chest compressions should be interrupted about every 30 seconds to deliver ventilations through the ET tube with the bag-valve device
    d. Chest compressions should be given without interruption and the rate of ventilations changed to 20 to 24 bpm

42. True or False. Intubation of the left mainstem bronchus is more common than intubation of the right mainstem bronchus

43. Which of the following statements is *incorrect* regarding the nasal airway?
    a. The nasal airway is the airway adjunct of choice in patients who have severe craniofacial trauma
    b. The nasal airway may cause a nosebleed if forcefully inserted
    c. Most responsive and semiresponsive patients can tolerate a nasal airway
    d. A nasal airway should be lubricated with a water-soluble lubricant before insertion

44. Endotracheal intubation:
    a. Is contraindicated in unresponsive patients
    b. Eliminates the risk of aspiration of gastric contents
    c. Should be preceded by efforts to ventilate by another method
    d. When attempted, should be performed in less than 60 seconds

45. Which of the following is *not* a desirable feature of a bag-valve device used during cardiac arrest?
    a. Nonrebreathing valve
    b. Compressible, self-refilling bag
    c. Clear mask in adult and pediatric sizes
    d. Functional pop-off (pressure release) valve

STOP & REVIEW ANSWERS

1. v	14. y
2. p	15. o
3. m	16. c
4. i	17. n
5. q	18. l
6. w	19. g
7. z	20. r
8. k	21. s
9. u	22. t
10. f	23. a
11. b	24. j
12. x	25. h
13. d	26. e

27. c. An SpO_2 reading between 96% and 100% generally indicates adequate oxygenation. A reading between 91% and 95% suggests mild hypoxia. An SpO_2 reading less than 91% generally represents severe hypoxia.

28. d. Esophageal traumas, including lacerations, bruising, and subcutaneous emphysema, are possible complications of Combitube use. A Combitube is inserted blindly (does not require visualization of the vocal cords). Ventilation begins with the esophageal tube because of the high probability of esophageal placement after blind insertion. Combitubes are available in two sizes. The 37 Fr size is used for patients between 4 and 5 feet tall. The 41 Fr size is used for patients more than 5 feet tall.

29. a. An oral airway should only be used in unresponsive patients who have no cough or gag reflex, because it may stimulate vomiting or laryngospasm in responsive or semi-responsive patients. If the airway is too long, it may press the epiglottis against the entrance of the larynx, resulting in a complete airway obstruction. If the airway is too short, it will not displace the tongue and may advance out of the mouth. A petroleum-based lubricant should never be used because it may damage the airway device and cause tissue inflammation. Although an oral airway may aid in the delivery of adequate ventilation with a bag-mask device, it is not considered the optimal method of managing the airway during cardiac arrest.

30. b. At an oxygen flow rate of 1 to 6 L/min, a nasal cannula can deliver about 25% to 45% oxygen.

31. Based on the information provided, your first impression of this patient revealed the following information:
Appearance: unaware of your approach
Breathing: no obvious signs of breathing
Circulation: pale skin color

32. This patient appears "sick." Proceed immediately with a rapid assessment of his level of responsiveness, airway, breathing, and circulation. Ask your coworker to get the AED. If you identify a problem during the primary survey, perform necessary emergency care ("treat as you find").

33. a. After finding that the patient is unresponsive, open his airway. Because trauma is not suspected in this situation, open the patient's airway with a head-tilt/chin-lift. Assess for sounds of airway compromise (such as gurgling). Look in the mouth for blood, broken teeth, loose dentures, gastric contents, and foreign objects. Clear the airway and insert an oral airway if needed to maintain an open airway.

34. c. A patient who has gurgling respirations needs *immediate* suctioning. Suction the patient's airway using a rigid (Yankauer) suction catheter.

35. d. Remember that an open airway does not ensure adequate ventilation. This patient's breathing is inadequate as evidenced by his rate and depth of respirations. The patient with inadequate breathing requires positive-pressure ventilation with 100% oxygen. Of the choices listed, the only device that can provide positive-pressure ventilation is the bag-mask. If readily available, an oral airway should be inserted before beginning bag-mask ventilation (if the patient does not have a gag or cough reflex).

36.

Device	Approximate Inspired Oxygen Concentration	Liter Flow (L/min)
Nasal cannula	25% to 45%	1 to 6
Simple face mask	40% to 60%	6 to 10 (8 to 10 recommended)
Partial rebreather mask	35% to 60%	6 to 10
Nonrebreather mask	60% to 100%	10 to 15
Venturi mask	24% to 50%	4 to 8

37. c. Look, listen, and feel for breathing for up to 10 seconds.

38. d. If not already attached, connect a one-way valve to the ventilation port on the pocket mask and connect oxygen tubing to the oxygen inlet on the mask. Set the oxygen flow rate at 10 to 12 L/min.

39. b. When giving rescue breaths, you are more likely to get dizzy or lightheaded if you take deep breaths before each delivering each rescue breath. Take a normal breath before each ventilation and ventilate at a rate of 10 to 12 bpm (1 breath every 5 to 6 seconds).

40. a. The recommended compression to ventilation ratio in adult one and two rescuer CPR is 30 to 2. The recommended rate of chest compressions for adults, infants, and children is about 100/min.

41. b. Once an advanced airway is in place, chest compressions should be given without interruption and the rate of ventilations altered to 8 to 10 bpm.

42. False. ET tubes that are advanced too far tend to enter the right mainstem bronchus because it is shorter, wider, and straighter than the left.

43. a. Because of the possibility of intracranial placement in patients who have a basilar skull fracture, nasal airways should be avoided in patients with severe craniofacial trauma.

44. c. ET intubation should be preceded by attempts to ventilate by another method. ET intubation is indicated in situations where the patient is unable to protect his or her own airway. ET intubation reduces (but does not eliminate) the risk of aspiration of gastric contents and, when attempted, should be performed in less than 30 seconds.

45. d. Pop-off valves are not recommended during resuscitation attempts since higher than usual airway pressures are often needed to ventilate patients in cardiac arrest. Pop-off valves may prevent the creation of airway pressures sufficient to overcome the increase in airway resistance.

REFERENCES

1. 2005 American Heart Association guidelines for cardiopulmonary resuscitation and emergency cardiovascular care, part 4: Adult basic life support. *Circulation* 2005;112(suppl IV):IV-20.
2. ACLS 2005 American Heart Association guidelines for cardiopulmonary resuscitation and emergency cardiovascular care, part 4: Adult basic life support. *Circulation* 2005;112(suppl IV):IV-22.
3. Brain AI:T AI:T he laryngeal mask—A new concept in airway management. *Br J Anaesth* 1983;55(8):801-805.
4. Takahata O, Kubota M, Mamiya K, et al: the efficacy of the "BURP" maneuver during a difficult laryngoscopy. *Anesth Analg* 1997;84(2):419-421.
5. Snider DD, Clarke D, Finucane BT: The "BURP" maneuver worsens the glottic view when applied in combination with cricoid pressure. *Can J Anaesth* 2005;52(1):100-104.
6. Vardi A, Levin I, Paret G, Barzilay Z: The sixth vital sign: end-tidal CO_2 in pediatric trauma patients during transport. *Harefuah* 2000;139(3-4):85-87, 168.

Rhythm Recognition

CHAPTER 3

OBJECTIVES

Upon completion of this chapter, you will be able to:

1. Name the primary branches of the right and left coronary arteries.
2. Describe the two types of myocardial cells and the function of each.
3. Describe the significance of each waveform in the cardiac cycle.
4. Describe the normal duration of the PR interval and QRS complex.
5. Describe at least two methods of determining heart rate.
6. Name the primary and escape pacemakers of the heart and the normal rates of each.
7. Define the absolute and relative refractory periods and their location in the cardiac cycle.
8. Describe the electrocardiogram (ECG) characteristics of narrow-QRS tachycardias.
9. Describe the ECG characteristics of wide-QRS tachycardias.
10. Describe differentiation of right and left bundle branch block (BBB) using lead V_1 or modified chest lead (MCL_1).
11. Describe the ECG characteristics of irregular tachycardias.
12. Describe the ECG characteristics of sinus bradycardia, junctional escape rhythm, and ventricular escape rhythm.
13. Describe the ECG characteristics of first-, second-, and third-degree atrioventricular (AV) blocks.
14. Name and describe four dysrhythmias that may be observed during cardiac arrest.
15. Describe the appearance of the waveform on the ECG produced as a result of atrial pacing and ventricular pacing.

INTRODUCTION

A prerequisite to participation in most advanced cardiac life support (ACLS) courses is completion of a basic ECG recognition course. This requirement exists because there simply isn't time in an ACLS course to cover information about rhythm recognition in detail. A basic ECG course teaches you how to identify cardiac rhythms. An ACLS course quickly reviews cardiac rhythms, but it focuses on teaching how to recognize serious signs and symptoms related to those rhythms and how to treat them.

Cardiac rhythms can be classified into four main groups: normal, absent/pulseless (cardiac arrest rhythms), slower than normal for age (bradycardia), or faster than normal for age (tachycardia). Disturbances in cardiac rhythm (dysrhythmias) are common. Some dysrhythmias do not cause serious signs and symptoms, while others can be life-threatening.

To help you understand and recognize cardiac dysrhythmias, this chapter reviews the heart's blood supply, conduction pathways, lead systems, and methods used to measure heart rate and rhythm. Cardiac dysrhythmias and their identifying features are also discussed.

QUICK REVIEW 3-1

1. Can you name the four main groups of cardiac rhythms?
   1.
   2.
   3.
   4.

Answers can be found at the end of this chapter.

ANATOMY REVIEW

CORONARY ARTERIES

Right Coronary Artery

■ The right coronary artery (RCA) originates from the right side of the aorta. It travels along the groove between the right atrium and right ventricle (Figure 3-1).
  ◗ Blockage of the RCA can result in inferior wall myocardial infarction (MI) and/or disturbances in AV nodal conduction.

Left Coronary Artery

■ The left coronary artery (LCA) originates from the left side of the aorta.
■ The first part of the LCA is called the left main coronary artery. It is about the width of a soda straw and less than an inch long. The left main coronary artery supplies oxygen-rich blood to its two primary branches: the left anterior descending (LAD) (also called the anterior interventricular) artery and the left circumflex (LCx) artery. These vessels are slightly smaller than the left main coronary artery.
■ The major branches of the LAD are the septal and diagonal arteries.
  ◗ Blockage of the septal branch of the LAD can result in a septal MI.
  ◗ Blockage of the diagonal branch of the LAD can result in an anterior wall MI.
  ◗ Blockage of the LAD can result in pump failure and/or intraventricular conduction delays.

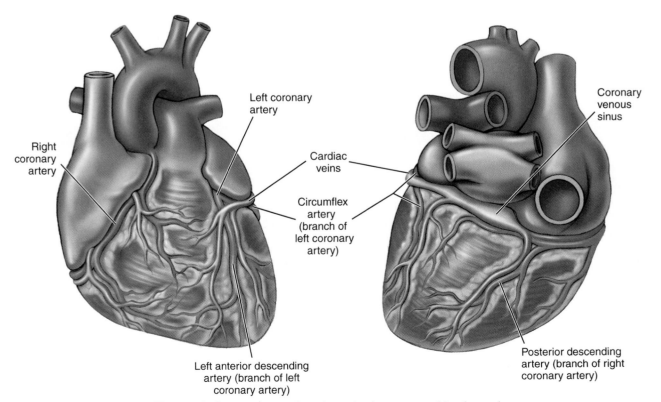

Figure 3-1 • The heart's blood supply: the coronary blood vessels.

■ The LCx coronary artery circles around the left side of the heart. It is embedded in the epicardium on the back of the heart.

▶ Blockage of the LCx artery can result in a lateral wall MI.

▶ In some patients, the circumflex artery may also supply the inferior portion of the left ventricle. A posterior wall MI may occur because of blockage of the RCA or the LCx artery (Table 3-1).

 Blockage of the left main coronary artery has been referred to as the "widow maker" because of its association with sudden death.

A common cause of MI is a blocked coronary artery. When viewing the patient's 12-lead ECG, an understanding of the coronary artery anatomy makes it possible to predict which coronary artery is blocked.

TABLE 3-1	Coronary Arteries	
Coronary Artery and Its Branches	**Portion of Myocardium Supplied**	**Portion of Conduction System Supplied**
Right Posterior descending Right marginal	• Right atrium • Right ventricle • Inferior surface of left ventricle (about 85%)* • Posterior surface of left ventricle (about 85%)*	• Sinoatrial node (about 60%)* • AV node (85%-90%)* • Proximal portion of bundle of His • Part of posterior-inferior fascicle of left bundle branch
Left Anterior descending	• Anterior surface of left ventricle • Part of lateral surface of left ventricle • Most of the interventricular septum	• Most of right bundle branch • Anterior-superior fascicle of left bundle branch • Part of posterior-inferior fascicle of left bundle branch
Circumflex	• Left atrium • Part of lateral surface of left ventricle • Inferior surface of left ventricle (about 15%)* • Posterior surface of left ventricle (15%)*	• SA node (about 40%)* • AV node (10%-15%)*

*Of population.

QUICK REVIEW 3-2

1. An inferior wall MI is usually the result of blockage of the _____ coronary artery.
2. An anterior wall MI is usually the result of blockage of the _____ _____ _____ coronary artery.
3. Blockage of the LCx coronary artery usually results in a(n) _____ wall MI.
4. True or false. A septal MI is usually the result of blockage of the RCA.

BASIC ELECTROPHYSIOLOGY

MYOCARDIAL CELL TYPES

The heart has two main types of cells—myocardial cells and pacemaker cells (Table 3-2).

■ Myocardial cells
- ▶ Also called working or mechanical cells
- ▶ Contain contractile filaments
- ▶ When electrically stimulated, these filaments slide together and the myocardial cell contracts
- ▶ Do not normally spontaneously generate electrical impulses, depending on pacemaker cells for this function

■ Pacemaker cells
- ▶ Specialized cells of the electrical conduction system
- ▶ Responsible for the spontaneous generation and conduction of electrical impulses

TABLE 3-2	Myocardial Cell Types		
Kinds of Cardiac Cells	**Where Found**	**Primary Function**	**Primary Property**
Myocardial cells	Myocardium	Contraction and relaxation	Contractility
Pacemaker cells	Electrical conduction system	Generation and conduction of electrical impulses	Automaticity Conductivity

Modified from Huszar RJ: *Basic Dysrhythmias: Interpretation and Management,* 2nd ed. St. Louis: 1994, Mosby-Year Book.

PROPERTIES OF CARDIAC CELLS

■ **Automaticity**
- ▶ Ability of pacemaker cells to spontaneously initiate an electrical impulse without being stimulated from another source (such as a nerve).
- ▶ Sinoatrial (SA) node, AV junction, and Purkinje fibers normally possess this characteristic.

■ **Excitability** (or **irritability**)
- ▶ Ability of cardiac muscle cells to respond to an external stimulus, such as that from a chemical, mechanical, or electrical source.
- ▶ All cardiac cells possess this characteristic.

■ **Conductivity**
- ▶ Ability of a cardiac cell to receive an electrical stimulus and conduct that impulse to the next cardiac cell.
- ▶ All cardiac cells possess this characteristic.

■ **Contractility**
- ▶ Ability of cardiac cells to shorten, causing cardiac muscle contraction in response to an electrical stimulus.
- ▶ Contractility can be enhanced with certain medications, such as digitalis, dopamine, and epinephrine.

CARDIAC ACTION POTENTIAL

■ Cell membranes contain membrane channels. These channels are pores through which specific ions or other small, water-soluble molecules can cross the cell membrane from outside to inside (Figure 3-2).

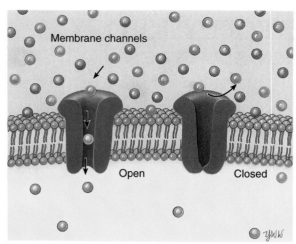

Figure 3-2 • Cell membranes contain membrane channels. These channels are pores through which specific ions or other small, water-soluble molecules can cross the cell membrane from outside to inside.

■ Electrical impulses are the result of the rapid flow of charged ions back and forth across the cell membrane. The cardiac action potential is an illustration of these events in a single cardiac cell during polarization, depolarization, and repolarization (Figure 3-3). The stimulus that changes the gradient across the cell membrane may be electrical, mechanical, or chemical.

Polarization

■ **Polarization** is the resting state during which no electrical activity occurs in the heart. It is also called the resting membrane potential or "ready state" because the cells are waiting to respond to a stimulus.
■ When a cardiac muscle cell is polarized, the inside of the cell is more negative than the outside (Figure 3-4).

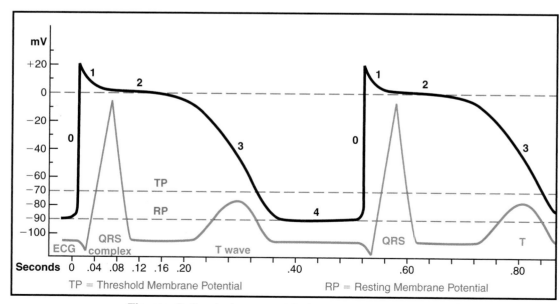

Figure 3-3 • Action potential of a ventricular muscle cell.

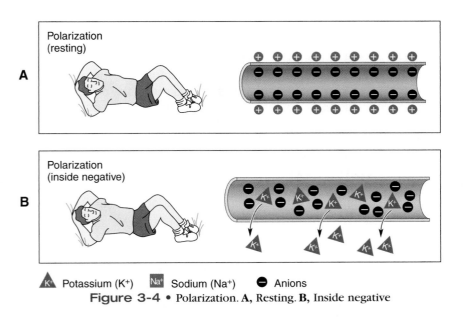

Potassium (K+)   Sodium (Na+)   ● Anions

Figure 3-4 • Polarization. **A,** Resting. **B,** Inside negative

Depolarization

▪ Before the heart's working cells can contract and pump blood, they must first be electrically stimulated. When a cardiac muscle cell is stimulated, the cell is said to **depolarize.** During depolarization, changes in the cell membrane allow sodium (Na^+) ions to rush into the cell through fast Na^+ membrane channels (Figure 3-5). Calcium (Ca^{2+}) moves slowly into the cell through Ca^{2+} channels. Movement of these charged particles causes the inside of the cell to become more positive.

▪ When the cell depolarizes, cardiac contraction begins. Depolarization proceeds from the innermost layer of the heart (**endocardium**) to the outermost layer (**epicardium**).

Depolarization is *not* the same as contraction. Depolarization is an electrical event *expected* to result in contraction (a mechanical event). It is possible to view organized electrical activity on the cardiac monitor, yet assessment of the patient reveals no palpable pulse. This clinical situation is termed **pulseless electrical activity (PEA).**

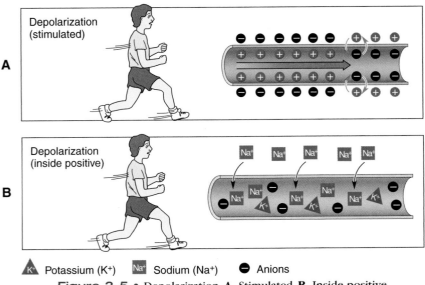

Potassium (K+)   Sodium (Na+)   ● Anions

Figure 3-5 • Depolarization. **A,** Stimulated. **B,** Inside positive.

Repolarization

■ After the cell depolarizes, changes occur again in the cell membrane. Changes in the cell membrane cause the fast Na^+ channels to close. This stops the rapid flow of Na^+ into the cell. Ca^{2+} channels close and potassium rapidly flows out of the cell.

■ Active transport via the sodium-potassium pump begins restoring potassium to the inside of the cell and sodium to the outside of the cell. The cell returns to its negative state due to the outflow of potassium (Figure 3-6). This recovery stage is called **repolarization.** The cell gradually becomes more sensitive to external stimuli until its original sensitivity has been restored. The cell can then be stimulated again if another electrical impulse arrives at the cell membrane.

■ Repolarization proceeds from the epicardium to the endocardium.

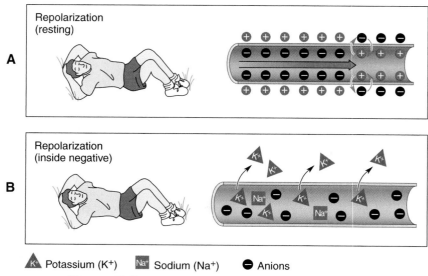

Figure 3-6 • Repolarization. **A,** Resting. **B,** Inside negative.

KEEPING IT SIMPLE

Polarization = ready state
Depolarization = stimulation
Repolarization = recovery

THE CONDUCTION SYSTEM

- Primary pacemaker
  - ▶ Normally, the pacemaker cells with the fastest rate control the heart at any given time. Because it fires more quickly than other pacemaker sites in the heart, the **sinoatrial node** (SA node or "sinus") is normally the heart's primary pacemaker (Figure 3-7).
  - ▶ Built-in firing rate = 60 to 100 bpm.
- Escape (back up) pacemakers
  - ▶ AV junction
    - • The **AV junction** is the AV node and the nonbranching portion of the bundle of His (Figure 3-8). The pacemaker cells in the AV junction are located near the non-branching portion of the bundle of His.

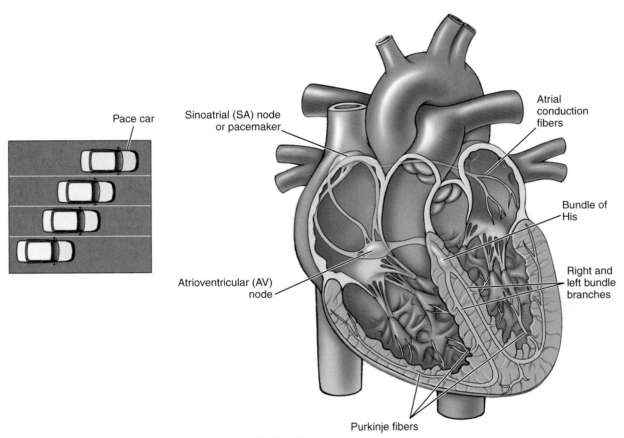

Figure 3-7 • The conduction system.

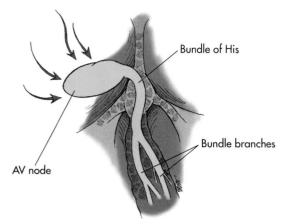

Figure 3-8 • The AV junction consists of the AV node and the nonbranching portion of the bundle of His.

- If the SA node fails to produce an impulse at its normal rate, or stops functioning entirely, pacemaker cells in the AV junction will usually assume the role of the heart's pacemaker (but at a slower rate).
- Built-in firing rate = 40 to 60 bpm.
  ▶ Ventricles
- If the SA node and AV junction fail, an escape pacemaker below it (the bundle branches and the Purkinje fibers) may take over at an even slower rate.
- Built-in firing rate = 20 to 40 bpm.
■ Normal pathway followed by a cardiac impulse
  ▶ SA node → right and left atria → AV node → bundle of His → right and left bundle branches → Purkinje fibers → ventricular myocardium.
  ▶ A summary of the conduction system is shown in Table 3-3.

TABLE 3-3	Summary of the Conduction System	
Structure	**Location**	**Function**
SA node	Right atrial wall just below opening of superior vena cava	Primary pacemaker; initiates impulse that is normally conducted throughout the left and right atria. Built-in rate 60–100 bpm.
AV node	Posterior septal wall of the right atrium immediately behind the tricuspid valve and near the opening of the coronary sinus	Receives impulse from SA node and delays relay of the impulse to the bundle of His, allowing time for the atria to empty their contents into the ventricles before the onset of ventricular contraction.
Bundle of His	Upper portion of interventricular septum	Receives impulse from AV node and relays it to right and left bundle branches. Built in pacemaker ability of 40–60 bpm.
Right and left bundle branches	Interventricular septum	Receives impulse from bundle of His and relays it to Purkinje fibers in ventricular myocardium.
Purkinje fibers	Ventricular myocardium	Receives impulse from bundle branches and relays it to ventricular myocardium. Built in pacemaker ability of 20–40 bpm.

THE ELECTROCARDIOGRAM

■ A cardiac monitor can be thought of as a sophisticated voltmeter. By using electrodes and cables, a cardiac monitor records the electrical voltages (potentials) generated by depolarization of a large mass of atrial and ventricular cells. An **electrocardiogram (ECG)** is a recording of this electrical activity, which appears on ECG paper as specific waveforms and complexes.

■ ECG monitoring may be used to monitor a patient's heart rate, assess the effects of disease or injury on heart function, assess pacemaker function, assess the response to medications (such as antiarrhythmics), and/or get a baseline recording before, during, and after a medical procedure.

■ An ECG can provide information about the following:
  ▶ The orientation of the heart in the chest
  ▶ Conduction disturbances
  ▶ Electrical effects of medications and electrolytes
  ▶ The mass of cardiac muscle
  ▶ The presence of ischemic damage

An ECG records the *electrical* activity of a large mass of atrial and ventricular cells as waveforms and complexes. The ECG does *not* provide information about the mechanical (contractile) condition of the myocardium. To assess the effectiveness of the heart's mechanical activity, assess the patient's pulse and blood pressure.

ELECTRODES

■ An **electrode** is a paper, plastic, or metal device that contains conductive gel and is applied to the patient's skin. An ECG cable is a wire that attaches to the electrode and conducts current back to the cardiac monitor.

■ Electrodes are applied at specific places on the patient's chest and limbs in combinations of two, three, four, or five to view the heart's electrical activity from different angles and planes (Figure 3-9).

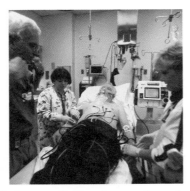

Figure 3-9 • Electrodes are applied at specific locations on the patient's chest wall and limbs to view the heart's electrical activity from different angles and planes.

LEADS

■ The word "lead" is used in two ways: (1) the position of the positive electrode on the patient's body and (2) the actual ECG record (tracing) obtained. For example, V_1 position represents the proper location of the positive electrode on the patient's chest. "Lead V_1" refers to the tracing obtained from that position.[1]

■ Each lead records the average current flow at a specific time in a part of the heart.

■ Leads II and modified chest lead (MCL_1) are commonly used for continuous ECG monitoring.

■ Moving the lead selector on the ECG machine allows us to make any of the electrodes positive or negative. The position of the positive electrode on the body determines the portion of the heart "seen" by each lead (Figure 3-10).

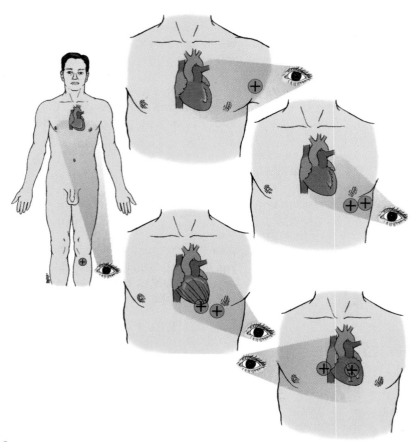

Figure 3-10 • The position of the positive electrode on the body determines the portion of the heart "seen" by each lead.

There are three types of leads—standard limb leads, augmented leads, and precordial (chest) leads. Leads allow viewing of the heart's electrical activity in two different planes: frontal or horizontal (transverse).

■ Frontal plane leads view the heart from the front of the body.

■ Horizontal plane leads view the heart as if the body were sliced in half.

■ A 12-lead ECG provides views of the heart in both the frontal and horizontal planes and views the surfaces of the left ventricle from 12 different angles.

> ❯ Six leads view the heart in the frontal plane as if the body were flat: three bipolar leads and three unipolar leads. Leads I, II, III, aVL, and aVF are obtained from electrodes placed on the patient's arms and legs. The "a" in aVR, aVL, and aVF refers to augmented. The "V" refers to voltage. The "R" refers to right arm, the "L" to left arm, and the "F" to left foot (leg). The position of the positive electrode corresponds to the last letter of each of these leads.[1]

> ❯ As their names suggest, the six chest leads, V_1 to V_6, are obtained from electrodes placed on the patient's chest. The chest leads view the heart in the horizontal plane, allowing a view of the front and left side of the heart.

Standard Limb Leads

■ Leads I, II, and III are called "standard limb leads" or "bipolar" leads (Table 3-4). A **bipolar lead** consists of a positive and negative electrode. Each lead records the difference in electrical potential between two selected electrodes.

TABLE 3-4	Summary of Standard Limb Leads		
Lead	**Positive Electrode**	**Negative Electrode**	**Heart Surface Viewed**
Lead I	Left arm	Right arm	Lateral
Lead II	Left leg	Right arm	Inferior
Lead III	Left leg	Left arm	Inferior

Augmented Limb Leads

■ An augmented limb lead consists of a single positive electrode and a reference point. The reference point for these leads lies in the center of the heart's electrical field (left of the interventricular septum and below the AV junction).

■ The electrical potential produced by the augmented leads is normally relatively small. The ECG machine augments (magnifies) the amplitude of the electrical potentials detected at each extremity by about 50% over those recorded at the bipolar leads.

■ Leads aVR, aVL, and aVF are augmented limb leads (Table 3-5, Figure 3-11). The position of the positive electrode corresponds to the last letter in each of these leads.

  ▶ The positive electrode in lead aVR is located on the right arm.
  ▶ aVL has a positive electrode at the left arm.
  ▶ aVF has a positive electrode positioned on the left leg.

TABLE 3-5	Summary of Augmented Leads	
Lead	**Positive Electrode**	**Heart Surface Viewed**
Lead aVR	Right arm	None
Lead aVL	Left arm	Lateral
Lead aVF	Left leg	Inferior

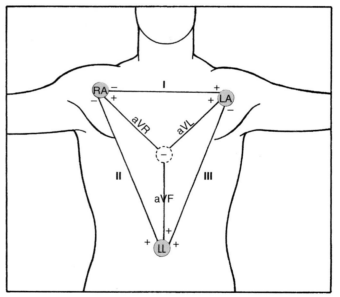

Figure 3-11 • View of the standard limb leads and augmented leads.

Chest Leads

■ The six chest leads (also known as precordial or "V" leads) are identified as V_1, V_2, V_3, V_4, V_5, and V_6 (Table 3-6, Figure 3-12).

■ Because the chest leads are unipolar, the positive electrode for each lead is placed at a specific location on the chest; the heart is the theoretical negative electrode.

Right-Sided and Posterior Leads

■ Other chest leads that are not part of a standard 12-lead ECG may be used to view specific surfaces of the heart.

■ Use right chest leads when a right ventricular MI is suspected.

  ▶ Placement of right chest leads is identical to placement of the standard chest leads except it is done on the right side of the chest (Figure 3-13).

TABLE 3-6	Summary of Chest Leads	
Lead	**Positive Electrode Position**	**Heart Surface Viewed**
Lead V_1	Right side of sternum, 4th intercostal space	Septum
Lead V_2	Left side of sternum, 4th intercostal space	Septum
Lead V_3	Midway between V_2 and V_4	Anterior
Lead V_4	Left midclavicular line, 5th intercostal space	Anterior
Lead V_5	Left anterior axillary line at same level as V_4	Lateral
Lead V_6	Left midaxillary line at same level as V_4	Lateral

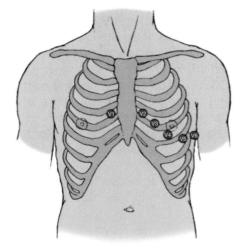

Figure 3-12 • The position of the six chest leads.

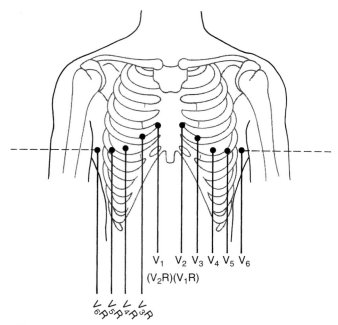

Figure 3-13 • Placement of the left and right chest leads.

▶ Obtain a standard 12-lead first. The cables for the standard chest leads are then moved to the electrodes for the additional leads.
▶ If time does not permit obtaining all of the right chest leads, the lead of choice is V_4R.
▶ The right chest leads and their placement are as follows:
  • Lead V_1R = Lead V_2
  • Lead V_2R = Lead V_1
  • Lead V_3R = Midway between V_2R and V_4R
  • Lead V_4R = Right midclavicular line, fifth intercostal space
  • Lead V_5R = Right anterior axillary line at same level as V_4R
  • Lead V_6R = Right midaxillary line at same level as V_4R
▧ On a standard 12-lead ECG, no leads directly face the posterior surface of the heart.
  ▶ The leads corresponding to the posterior wall of the left ventricle are V_7, V_8, and V_9. These three leads are positioned horizontally level with V_4. Lead V_7 is placed at the posterior axillary line. Lead V_8 is placed at the angle of the scapula (posterior scapular line), and lead V_9 is placed over the left border of the spine. The position for these leads is shown in Figure 3-14.
▧ Any chest lead cable can be moved to obtain the right and/or posterior leads. However, once these leads are printed, the correct lead must be handwritten onto the ECG to indicate the origin of the tracing.[1]

Modified Chest Leads

▧ Modified chest leads are bipolar chest leads that are variations of the unipolar chest leads.
  ▶ Each modified chest lead consists of a positive and negative electrode applied to a specific location on the chest. Accurate placement of the positive electrode is important.
  ▶ Modified chest leads are useful in detecting bundle branch blocks (BBBs), differentiating right and left premature beats, and differentiating supraventricular tachycardia (SVT) from ventricular tachycardia (VT).
▧ Lead MCL_1 is a variation of the chest lead V_1. MCL stands for modified chest lead.
  ▶ Views the ventricular septum.
  ▶ The negative electrode is placed below the left clavicle toward the left shoulder.
  ▶ The positive electrode is placed to the right of the sternum in the fourth intercostal space (Figure 3-15A).

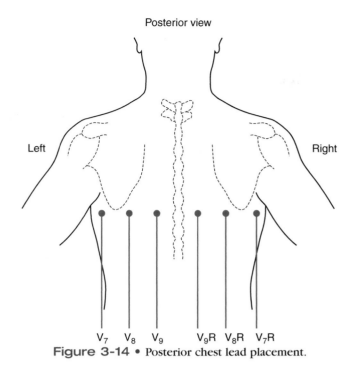

Posterior view

Left

Right

V_7 V_8 V_9 V_9R V_8R V_7R

Figure 3-14 • Posterior chest lead placement.

QUICK REVIEW 3-4

1. Complete the following table.

Lead	Heart Surface Viewed	Lead	Heart Surface Viewed
Lead I		V_1	
Lead II		V_2	
Lead III		V_3	
aVR		V_4	
aVL		V_5	
aVF		V_6	

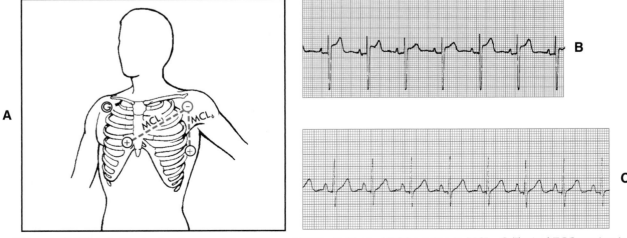

Figure 3-15 • **A,** Electrode placement for MCL_1 and MCL_6. **B,** Typical ECG tracing in MCL_1. **C,** Typical ECG tracing in MCL_6.

▶ In this lead, the positive electrode is in a position to the right of the left ventricle. Because the primary wave of depolarization is directed toward the left ventricle, the QRS complex recorded in this lead will normally appear negative (Figure 3-15B).

■ Lead MCL_6 is a variation of the chest lead V_6.
  ▶ Lead MCL_6 views the low lateral wall of the left ventricle.
  ▶ The negative electrode is placed below the left clavicle toward the left shoulder.
  ▶ The positive electrode is placed at the fifth intercostal space, left midaxillary line. An example of a typical ECG tracing recorded in this lead is shown in Figure 3-15C.

Leads MCL_1 and V_1 are similar but not identical. In V_1, the negative electrode is calculated by the ECG machine at the center of the heart. In MCL_1, the negative electrode is located just below the left clavicle.[1]

QUICK REVIEW 3-5

1. The position of the _____ electrode on the body determines the portion of the heart "seen" by each lead.
2. Name three leads that look at the inferior wall of the left ventricle.
   1.
   2.
   3.
3. Name two leads that look at the anterior wall of the left ventricle.
   1.
   2.
4. Name four leads that look at the lateral wall of the left ventricle.
   1.
   2.
   3.
   4.
5. _____ plane leads view the heart as if the body were sliced in half.

ELECTROCARDIOGRAM PAPER

■ ECG paper is graph paper made up of small and large boxes.
■ Smallest boxes are 1 mm wide and 1 mm high.
■ The horizontal axis of the paper corresponds with *time* (Figure 3-16). Time is stated in seconds.
■ ECG paper normally records at a constant speed of 25 mm/sec. Each horizontal unit (1-mm box) represents 0.04 second (25 mm/sec (0.04 sec = 1 mm).
  ▶ The rate at which the paper goes through the printer is adjustable. Standard paper speed is 25 mm/sec.

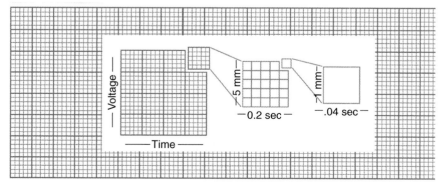

Figure 3-16 • The horizontal axis represents time. The vertical axis represents amplitude or voltage.

- ▶ A faster paper speed makes the rhythm appear slower and the QRS wider. In patients who have a fast heart rate, a faster paper speed makes it easier to see the waveforms and analyze the tachycardia. A slower paper speed makes the rhythm appear faster and the QRS narrower.[1]
- ▪ There are five small boxes in each large box on the paper.
  - ▶ A large box represents 0.20 second.
  - ▶ Five large boxes, each consisting of five small boxes, represent 1 second.
  - ▶ Fifteen large boxes equal an interval of 3 seconds; 30 large boxes represent 6 seconds.
- ▪ The vertical axis of the paper represents **voltage** or **amplitude** of the ECG waveforms or deflections.
  - ▶ Voltage may appear as a positive or negative value.
  - ▶ Size or amplitude of a waveform is measured in millivolts or millimeters.

QUICK REVIEW 3-6

1. In lead II, where is the positive electrode located?
2. On the horizontal axis, each small square on ECG graph paper represents _____.
3. There are _____ small boxes in each large box on ECG graph paper.
4. Each small square on ECG paper is _____ mm in height and width.

WAVEFORMS AND COMPLEXES

An ECG waveform is movement away from the baseline in either a positive (upward) or negative (downward) direction (Table 3-7). Waveforms are named alphabetically, beginning with P, QRS, T, and U. A waveform that is partly positive and partly negative is **biphasic.**

TABLE 3-7	Terminology
Waveform	Movement away from the baseline in either a positive or negative direction
Segment	A line between waveforms; named by the waveform that precedes or follows it
Interval	A waveform and a segment
Complex	Several waveforms

P Wave

- First wave in the cardiac cycle (Figure 3-17).
- Represents atrial depolarization and the spread of the electrical impulse throughout the right and left atria.
- Normally smooth, rounded, and no more than 0.11 second in duration (width).
- Positive (upright) in leads I, II, aVF, and V_2 through V_6.

QRS Complex

- The QRS complex consists of the Q wave, R wave, and S wave.
- Q wave is the first deflection of the QRS complex—*always* negative (below the baseline).
  - With the exception of leads III and aVR, a normal Q wave in the limb leads is less than 0.04 second (one small box) in duration and less than one third the height of the R wave in that lead.
  - An abnormal (pathologic) Q wave is more than 0.04 second (one small box) in duration or more than one third the height of the following R wave in that lead.
- R wave is the first positive deflection (above the baseline) in the QRS complex.
- S wave is a negative deflection following the R wave.
- It represents the spread of the electrical impulse through the ventricles (ventricular depolarization).
- In adults, it normally measures between 0.06 and 0.10 second.
  - If the impulse originates in a bundle branch, the duration of the QRS may be only slightly greater than 0.10 second. For example, a QRS measuring 0.10 to 0.12 second is called an *incomplete* BBB. A QRS measuring more than 0.12 second is called a *complete* BBB.
- One or even two of the three waveforms that make up the QRS complex may not always be present.

If an electrical impulse does not follow the normal ventricular conduction pathway, it will take longer to depolarize the myocardium. This delay in conduction through the ventricle produces a wider QRS complex than normal.

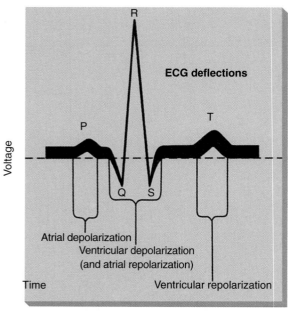

Figure 3-17 • ECG waveforms—P, QRS, and T.

T Wave

■ The T wave represents ventricular repolarization.

■ Normally slightly asymmetrical.

■ Not normally more than 5 mm in height in any limb leads or 10 mm in any chest lead.

■ Generally upright in all leads except lead aVR; may be positive or negative in leads III and V_1.

■ Negative (inverted) T waves suggest myocardial ischemia.

■ Tall, pointed (peaked) T waves are commonly seen in hyperkalemia.

■ Low amplitude T waves may be seen in hypokalemia.

QUICK REVIEW 3-7

1. What does the T wave represent?
2. What is the normal duration of the QRS complex in adults?
3. In a patient complaining of chest discomfort, what would the presence of a negative (inverted) T wave suggest?
4. True or False. P waves are normally upright in lead II.
5. True or False. The R wave is the first negative deflection in the QRS complex.

SEGMENTS AND INTERVALS

PR-Segment

■ Horizontal line between the end of the P wave and the beginning of the QRS complex.

■ Part of the PR interval.

■ Normally isoelectric (flat).

■ His-Purkinje system is activated during the PR-segment.

PR Interval

■ P wave plus the PR-segment equals the PR interval (PRI) (Figure 3-18).

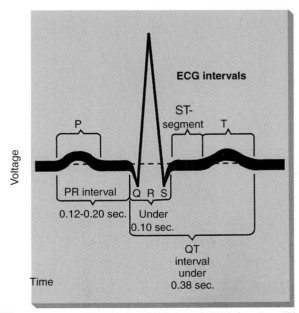

Figure 3-18 • ECG-segments and intervals—PR interval, QRS duration, ST-segment, QT interval.

- PR interval reflects depolarization of the right and left atria (the P wave) and the spread of the impulse through the AV node, bundle of His, right and left bundle branches, and the Purkinje fibers (the PR-segment).
- Measured from the point where the P wave leaves the baseline to the beginning of the QRS complex.
- Normally measures 0.12 to 0.20 second in adults.

QUICK REVIEW 3-8

1. A _____ is a line between waveforms.
2. The ____ _____ reflects atrial depolarization.
3. A waveform and a segment is called a(n) _____.
4. What is the normal duration of the PR interval?
5. How is a PR interval measured?

ST-Segment

- The ST-segment is a portion of the ECG tracing between the QRS complex and the T wave.
- It represents the early part of repolarization of the right and left ventricles.
- The ST-segment begins with the end of the QRS complex (S wave) and ends with the onset of the T wave.
  - In the limb leads, the normal ST-segment is isoelectric (flat) but may normally be slightly elevated or depressed (usually by less than 1 mm).
  - In the chest leads, ST-segment deviation may vary from −0.5 to +2 mm.
- The point where the QRS complex and the ST-segment meet is called the junction or J-point (Figure 3-19).
- Various conditions may cause displacement of the ST-segment from the isoelectric line in either a positive or negative direction.
  - Myocardial ischemia, injury, and infarction are among the causes of ST-segment displacement. The ST-segment is considered elevated if the segment is deviated above the baseline. It is considered depressed if the segment is deviated below it.
    - ST-segment elevation in the shape of a "smiley" face (upward concavity) is usually benign, particularly when it occurs in an otherwise healthy, asymptomatic patient (Figure 3-20).

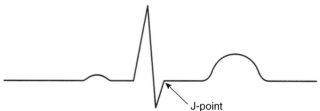

Figure 3-19 • The point where the QRS complex and the ST-segment meet is called the "junction" or "J" point.

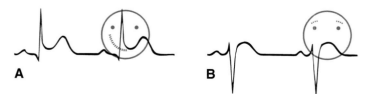

Figure 3-20 • **A,** ST-segment elevation in the shape of a "smiley" face (upward concavity) is usually benign, particularly when it occurs in an otherwise healthy, asymptomatic patient. **B,** ST-segment elevation in the shape of a "frowny" face (downward concavity) is more often associated with an acute injury pattern.

- The appearance of coved ("frowny face") ST-segment elevation is called an *acute injury pattern.*

▶ Other possible shapes of ST-segment elevation seen with acute MI are shown in Figure 3-21.

▶ A horizontal ST-segment (forming a sharp angle with the T wave) is suggestive of ischemia.

▶ Digitalis causes a depression (scoop) of the ST-segment sometimes referred to as a "dig dip."

In a patient experiencing an acute coronary syndrome, myocardial injury refers to myocardial tissue that has been cut off from or experienced a severe reduction in its blood and oxygen supply. The tissue is not yet dead and may be salvageable if the blocked vessel can be quickly opened, restoring blood flow and oxygen to the injured area. ST-segment elevation provides the strongest ECG evidence for the early recognition of MI.[1]

Although some deviation of the ST-segment from the isoelectric line can be a normal finding, the following ECG findings are considered significant if they are seen in two or more leads facing the same anatomic area of the heart (also known as contiguous leads):

- ST-segment depression of more than .5 mm (suggests myocardial ischemia)
- ST-segment elevation of more than 1 mm (suggests myocardial injury)

QT Interval

■ Represents total ventricular activity—the time from ventricular depolarization (stimulation) to repolarization (recovery).

■ Normally measures 0.36 to 0.44 second but varies with the patient's age, gender, and heart rate (as heart rate increases, QT interval decreases; as heart rate decreases, QT interval increases).

■ A prolonged QT interval indicates a lengthened relative refractory period (vulnerable period)—which puts the ventricles at risk for life-threatening dysrhythmias if a premature impulse occurs during this period.

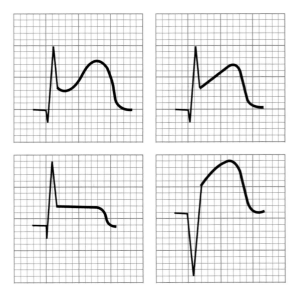

Figure 3-21 • Variable shapes of ST-segment elevation seen with acute MI.

TP-Segment

- The TP-segment is the portion of the ECG tracing between the end of the T wave and the beginning of the following P wave (Figure 3-22).
- When the heart rate is within normal limits, the TP-segment is usually isoelectric. With rapid heart rates, the TP-segment is often unrecognizable because the P wave encroaches on the preceding T wave.

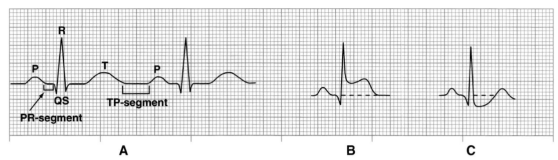

Figure 3-22 • **A,** The PR- and TP-segments are used as the baseline from which to determine the presence of ST-segment elevation or depression. **B,** ST-segment elevation. **C,** ST-segment depression.

QUICK REVIEW 3-9

1. What does the QRS complex represent?
2. What is the name of the portion of an ECG tracing between the end of the QRS complex and the beginning of the T wave?
3. What portion of an ECG tracing is used as the baseline from which to evaluate the degree of displacement of the ST-segment from the isoelectric line?
4. What does the QT interval represent?

5. A 68-year-old man is complaining of chest pain. ST-segment elevation of 4 mm is present in leads II, III, and aVF. The ST-segment elevation observed on the ECG suggests the presence of _____ _____.

REFRACTORY PERIODS

- **Refractoriness** is the extent to which a cell is able to respond to a stimulus.
- *Absolute* **refractory period** (also known as the effective refractory period)
  - The absolute refractory period corresponds with the onset of the QRS complex to the peak of the T wave.
  - During this period, the myocardial cell will not respond to further stimulation, no matter how strong the stimulus.
- *Relative* **refractory period** (also known as the vulnerable period)
  - The relative refractory period corresponds with the downslope of the T wave.
  - During this period, some cardiac cells have repolarized to their threshold potential and can be stimulated to respond (depolarize) if subjected to a stronger than normal stimulus.
- Supernormal period
  - After the relative refractory period is a **supernormal period** during which a weaker than normal stimulus can cause depolarization of cardiac cells.
  - Corresponds with the end of the T wave. It is possible for cardiac dysrhythmias to develop during this period (Figure 3-23).

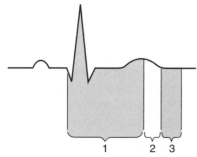

Figure 3-23 • Refractory periods. **1,** The absolute refractory period; **2,** relative refractory period; and **3,** the supernormal period.

ANALYZING A RHYTHM STRIP

■ Assess the rate. A tachycardia exists if the rate is more than 100 bpm. A bradycardia exists if the rate is less than 60 bpm.
  ▶ Six-second method
    • Most ECG paper is printed with 1-second or 3-second markers on the top or bottom of the paper.
    • To determine the ventricular rate, count the number of R-R intervals within a period of 6 seconds and multiply that number by 10 to find the number of complexes in 1 minute (Figure 3-24). To determine the atrial rate, count the number of P-P intervals in 6 seconds and multiple by 10.
  ▶ Large boxes
    • To determine the ventricular rate, count the number of large boxes between two R-R intervals and divide into 300.
    • To determine the atrial rate, count the number of large boxes between two consecutive P waves (P-P interval) and divide into 300.
  ▶ Small boxes
    • Each 1-mm box on the graph paper represents 0.04 second. There are 1500 boxes in one minute. 60 seconds/minute divided by 0.04 seconds/box = 1500 boxes/minute.
    • To calculate the ventricular rate, count the number of small boxes between two consecutive R waves and divide into 1500.
    • To determine the atrial rate, count the number of small boxes between two consecutive P waves and divide into 1500.

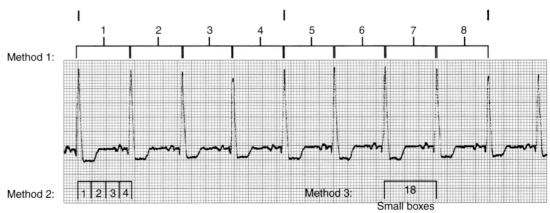

Figure 3-24 • Calculating heart rate. **Method 1,** Number of R-R intervals in 6 sec × 10 (e.g., 8 × 10 = 80/min). **Method 2,** Number of large boxes between QRS complexes divided into 300 (e.g., 300 ÷ by 4 = 75/min). **Method 3,** Number of small boxes between QRS complexes divided into 1500 (e.g., 1500 ÷ 18 = 84/min).

> ▶ Sequence method
>   • To determine ventricular rate, select an R wave that falls on a dark vertical line. Number the next six consecutive dark vertical lines as follows: 300, 150, 100, 75, 60, and 50.
>   • Note where the next R wave falls in relation to the six dark vertical lines already marked. This is the heart rate (Figure 3-25).

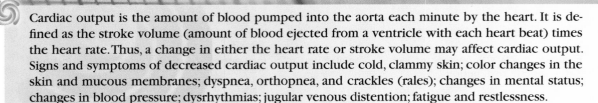

Cardiac output is the amount of blood pumped into the aorta each minute by the heart. It is defined as the stroke volume (amount of blood ejected from a ventricle with each heart beat) times the heart rate. Thus, a change in either the heart rate or stroke volume may affect cardiac output. Signs and symptoms of decreased cardiac output include cold, clammy skin; color changes in the skin and mucous membranes; dyspnea, orthopnea, and crackles (rales); changes in mental status; changes in blood pressure; dysrhythmias; jugular venous distention; fatigue and restlessness.

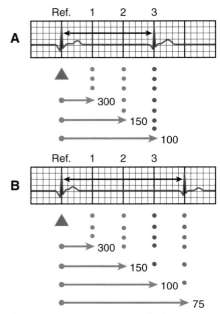

Figure 3-25 • Determining heart rate—sequence method. To measure the ventricular rate, find a QRS complex that falls on a heavy dark line. Count 300, 150, 100, 75, 60, and 50 until a second QRS complex occurs. This will be the heart rate. **A,** Heart rate = 100. **B,** Heart rate = 75.

QUICK REVIEW 3-10

1. You are viewing a rhythm strip and note that an R wave falls on a dark vertical line. The next R wave falls on a dark vertical line three boxes to the right of the first. What is the ventricular rate?
2. What is the ventricular rate if there are 12 QRS complexes in a 6-second strip?

▪ Assess rhythm/regularity.
  ▶ To determine if the ventricular rhythm is regular or irregular, measure the distance between two consecutive R-R intervals and compare that distance with the other R-R intervals.
  ▶ To determine if the atrial rhythm is regular or irregular, measure the distance between two consecutive P-P intervals and compare that distance with the other P-P intervals.
▪ Identify and examine P waves.
  ▶ To locate P waves, look to the left of each QRS complex.

- Normally, one P wave precedes each QRS complex; they occur regularly; and they appear similar in size, shape, and position.
- If no P wave is present, the rhythm originated in the AV junction or the ventricles.
- Assess intervals (evaluate conduction).
  - PR interval.
    - Measure the PR interval from the point where the P wave leaves the baseline to the beginning of the QRS complex. Normal is 0.12 to 0.20 second.
    - If the PR intervals are the same, they are said to be constant.
    - If the PR intervals are different, is there a pattern?
  - Identify the QRS complexes and measure their duration.
    - A QRS is narrow (normal) if it measures 0.10 second or less and is considered wide if it measures more than 0.10 second.
  - Measure the QT interval in the leads that show the largest amplitude T waves.
    - If the measured QT interval is less than half the R-R interval, it is probably normal. This method of QT interval measurement works well as a general guideline until the ventricular rate exceeds 100 bpm.
- Evaluate the overall appearance of the rhythm.
  - Is the ST segment elevated or depressed?
  - Are the T waves upright and of normal height? The T wave following an abnormal QRS complex is usually opposite in direction from the QRS.
- Interpret the rhythm and evaluate its clinical significance.
  - Interpret the rhythm specifying the site of the origin (pacemaker site) of the rhythm (sinus), the mechanism (bradycardia), and the ventricular rate (i.e., "sinus bradycardia at 38/min").
  - Evaluate the patient's clinical presentation to determine how he or she is tolerating the rate and rhythm.

QUICK REVIEW 3-11

1. List the six steps in analyzing a rhythm strip.
   1.
   2.
   3.
   4.
   5.
   6.

DYSRHYTHMIA RECOGNITION

SINUS RHYTHM

Sinus rhythm is the name given to a normal heart rhythm. Sinus rhythm reflects normal electrical activity—that is, the rhythm starts in the SA node and then heads down the normal conduction pathway through the atria, AV junction, bundle branches, and ventricles. This results in depolarization of the atria and ventricles. The SA node normally produces electrical impulses faster than any other part of the heart's conduction system. As a result, the SA node is normally the heart's primary pacemaker. A person's heart rate varies with age. In adults and adolescents, the SA node normally fires at a regular rate of 60 to 100 bpm (Table 3-8, Figure 3-26).

TABLE 3-8	Characteristics of Sinus Rhythm	
Rate	Within normal limits for age; in adults, 60-100 bpm	
Rhythm	Regular	
P waves	Uniform in appearance, positive (upright) in lead II, one precedes each QRS complex	
PR interval	Within normal limits for age and constant from beat to beat; in adults, 0.12-0.20 sec	
QRS duration	0.10 sec or less unless an intraventricular conduction delay exists	

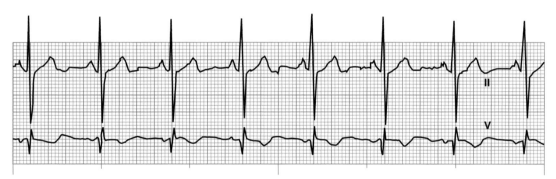

Figure 3-26 • Sinus rhythm.

SINUS ARRHYTHMIA

The SA node fires quite regularly most of the time. When it fires irregularly, the resulting rhythm is called a sinus arrhythmia. Sinus arrhythmia begins in the SA node and follows the normal pathway of conduction through the atria, AV junction, bundle branches, and ventricles, resulting in atrial and ventricular depolarization. Sinus arrhythmia that is associated with the phases of respiration and changes in intrathoracic pressure is called *respiratory sinus arrhythmia.* Sinus arrhythmia that is not related to the respiratory cycle is called *nonrespiratory sinus arrhythmia.*

A sinus arrhythmia usually occurs at a rate of 60 to 100 bpm. If sinus arrhythmia is associated with a slower than normal rate, it is called *sinus bradyarrhythmia.* If the rhythm is associated with a faster than normal rate, it is known as *sinus tachyarrhythmia.*

What Causes It?

Respiratory sinus arrhythmia is a normal phenomenon that occurs with changes in intrathoracic pressure. The heart rate increases with inspiration (R-R intervals shorten) and decreases with expiration (R-R intervals lengthen). Sinus arrhythmia is most commonly observed in children and adults younger than 30 years of age.

In respiratory sinus arrhythmia, the changes in rhythm disappear when the patient holds his or her breath.

Nonrespiratory sinus arrhythmia can be seen in people with normal hearts but is more likely in older individuals and in those with heart disease. It is common after acute inferior wall MI and may be seen with increased intracranial pressure. Nonrespiratory sinus arrhythmia may be the result of effects of medications (such as digitalis and morphine) or carotid sinus pressure.

What Do I Do About It?

Sinus arrhythmia does not usually require treatment unless it is accompanied by a slow heart rate that causes hemodynamic compromise. If hemodynamic compromise is present, intravenous (IV) atropine may be indicated (Table 3-9, Figure 3-27).

TABLE 3-9	Characteristics of Sinus Arrhythmia
Rate	Usually 60-100 bpm but may be slower or faster
Rhythm	Irregular, phasic with respiration; heart rate increases gradually during inspiration (R-R intervals shorten) and decreases with expiration (R-R intervals lengthen)
P waves	Uniform in appearance, positive (upright) in lead II, one precedes each QRS complex
PR interval	0.12-0.20 sec and constant from beat to beat
QRS duration	0.10 sec or less unless an intraventricular conduction delay exists

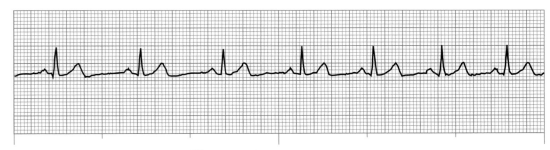

Figure 3-27 • Sinus arrhythmia.

QUICK REVIEW 3-12

1. True or False. Depolarization is the movement of ions across a cell membrane causing the inside of the cell to become more positive.
2. What is the built-in (intrinsic) rate of the SA node?
3. _____ is measured on the vertical axis of ECG paper.
4. What is a common dysrhythmia associated with changes in respiratory rate?

5. If the SA node fails to generate an impulse, what is the next (escape) pacemaker that should generate an impulse?
6. Describe the appearance of a normal P wave that originates from the SA node.

SECTION 2
Tachydysrhythmias: Too Fast Rhythms

NARROW-QRS TACHYCARDIAS

Supraventricular arrhythmias (SVA) begin above the bifurcation of the bundle of His. This means that SVA include rhythms that begin in the SA node, the atrial tissue, or the AV junction.

SINUS TACHYCARDIA

Normal heart rates vary with age. In adults, the rate associated with sinus tachycardia is usually between 101 and 180 bpm (Table 3-10, Figure 3-28). Because an infant or child's heart rate can transiently increase during episodes of crying or pain, or in the presence of a fever, the term tachycardia is used to describe a significant and persistent increase in heart rate. In infants, a tachycardia is a heart rate of more than 200 bpm. In a child older than 5 years of age, a tachycardia is a heart rate of more than 160 bpm.

What Causes It?

Sinus tachycardia is a normal response to the body's demand for increased oxygen because of many conditions (Box 3-1). The patient is often aware of an increase in heart rate. Some patients complain of palpitations, a racing heart, or "pounding" in their chest. Sinus tachycardia is seen in some patients with acute MI, especially those with an anterior infarction.

TABLE 3-10	Characteristics of Sinus Tachycardia
Rate	101-180 bpm
Rhythm	Regular
P waves	Uniform in appearance, positive (upright) in lead II, one precedes each QRS complex; at very fast rates it may be difficult to distinguish a P wave from a T wave
PR interval	0.12-0.20 sec and constant from beat to beat
QRS duration	0.10 sec or less unless an intraventricular conduction delay exists

BOX 3-1
Causes of Sinus Tachycardia

- Exercise
- Fever
- Pain
- Fear and anxiety
- Hypoxia
- Congestive heart failure
- Acute MI
- Infection
- Sympathetic stimulation
- Shock
- Dehydration, hypovolemia
- Pulmonary embolism
- Hyperthyroidism
- Medications such as epinephrine, atropine, dopamine, and dobutamine
- Caffeine-containing beverages
- Nicotine
- Drugs such as cocaine, amphetamines, "ecstasy," and cannabis

What Do I Do About It?

In a patient with coronary artery disease, sinus tachycardia can cause problems. The heart's demand for oxygen increases as the heart rate increases. As the heart rate increases, there is less time for the ventricles to fill and less blood for the ventricles to pump out with each contraction. This can lead to decreased cardiac output. Because the coronary arteries fill when the ventricles are at rest, rapid heart rates decrease the time for coronary artery filling. This decreases the heart's blood supply. Chest discomfort can result if the supply of blood and oxygen to the heart is inadequate. Sinus tachycardia in a patient who is having an acute MI may be an early warning signal for heart failure, cardiogenic shock, and more serious dysrhythmias.

Treatment for sinus tachycardia is directed at correcting the underlying cause (i.e., fluid replacement, relief of pain, removal of offending medications or substances, and reducing fever and/or anxiety). Sinus tachycardia in a patient experiencing an acute MI may be treated with beta-blockers. Beta-blockers such as atenolol (Tenormin) or metoprolol (Lopressor) are given to slow the heart rate and decrease myocardial oxygen demand, provided there are no signs of heart failure or other contraindications to beta-blocker therapy.

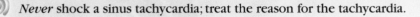

Never shock a sinus tachycardia; treat the reason for the tachycardia.

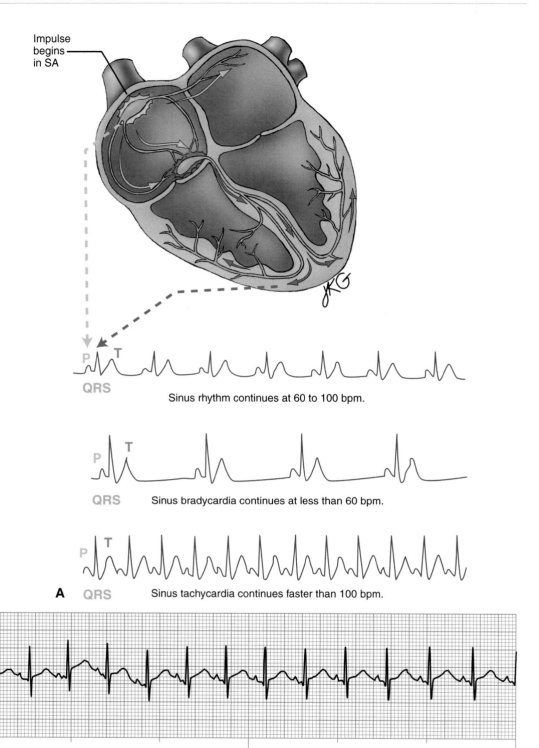

Impulse begins in SA

P T
QRS
Sinus rhythm continues at 60 to 100 bpm.

P T
QRS Sinus bradycardia continues at less than 60 bpm.

P T
A QRS Sinus tachycardia continues faster than 100 bpm.

B

Figure 3-28 • **A,** Sinus rhythm, sinus bradycardia, and sinus tachycardia. **B,** Sinus tachycardia.

The term SVT includes three main types of fast rhythms, which are shown in Figure 3-29.

■ **Atrial tachycardia (AT).** In AT, an irritable site in the atria fires automatically at a rapid rate.

■ **Atrioventricular nodal reentrant tachycardia (AVNRT).** In AVNRT, fast and slow pathways in the AV node form an electrical circuit or loop. The impulse spins around the AV nodal (junctional) area.

■ **Atrioventricular reentrant tachycardia (AVRT).** In AVRT, the impulse begins above the ventricles but travels via a pathway other than the AV node and bundle of His.

A *nonsustained* rhythm lasts from three beats up to 30 seconds. A *sustained* rhythm lasts more than 30 seconds.

Keeping It Simple

Some SVTs need the AV node to sustain the rhythm and some don't. For example, AVNRT and AVRT require the AV node as part of the reentry circuit to continue the tachycardia. Other SVTs use the AV node only to conduct the rhythm to the ventricles. For example, atrial tachycardia, atrial flutter, and atrial fibrillation arise from a site (or sites) within the atria. They do not need the AV node to sustain the rhythm.

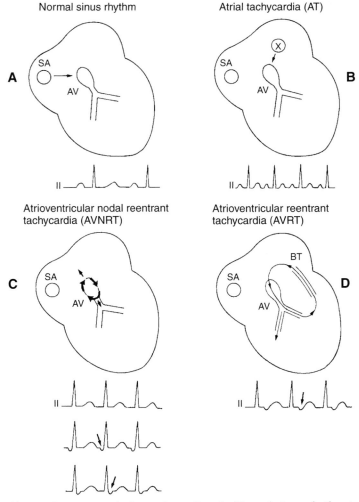

Figure 3-29 • Types of supraventricular tachycardias. **A,** Normal sinus rhythm is presented here as a reference. **B,** Atrial tachycardia. **C,** AV nodal reentrant tachycardia. **D,** AV reentrant tachycardia.

ATRIAL TACHYCARDIA

AT is usually the result of altered automaticity or triggered activity. It consists of a series of rapid beats from an irritable site in the atria. This rapid atrial rate overrides the SA node and becomes the pacemaker. Conduction of the atrial impulse to the ventricles is often 1:1. This means that every atrial impulse is conducted to the ventricles (Figure 3-30).

There is more than one type of AT. Multifocal AT is discussed later in this chapter with irregular tachycardias.

KEEPING IT SIMPLE

AT is often confused with sinus tachycardia. Although atrial looks similar to sinus tachycardia, atrial P waves differ in shape from sinus P waves.

- AT that begins in a small area (focus) within the heart is called focal atrial tachycardia. There are several types of focal atrial tachycardia. Focal AT may be due to an automatic, triggered, or reentrant mechanism. A patient with focal AT often presents with paroxysmal AT. The atrial rate is usually between 100 and 250 bpm and rarely 300 bpm.
- Automatic AT (also called ectopic AT) is another type of AT in which a small cluster of cells with altered automaticity fire. The impulse is spread from the cluster of cells to the surrounding atrium and then to the ventricles via the AV node. This type of AT often has a "warm up" period. This means there is a progressive shortening of the P-P interval for the first few beats of the arrhythmia. Automatic AT gradually slows down as it ends. This has been called a "cool down" period. The atrial rate is usually between 100 and 250 bpm (Table 3-11). P waves look different from sinus P waves but are still related to the QRS complex. Vagal maneuvers do not usually stop the tachycardia, but they may slow the ventricular rate.

What Causes It?

AT can occur in persons with normal hearts or in patients with organic heart disease. Atrial tachycardia associated with automaticity or triggered activity is often related to an acute event including:

- Stimulant use (such as caffeine, albuterol, theophylline, cocaine)
- Infection
- Electrolyte imbalance
- Acute illness with excessive catecholamine release
- MI

TABLE 3-11	Characteristics of Atrial Tachycardia
Rate	150-250 bpm
Rhythm	Regular
P waves	One positive P wave precedes each QRS complex in lead II but the P waves differ in shape from sinus P waves. With rapid rates, it is difficult to distinguish P waves from T waves.
PR interval	May be shorter or longer than normal and may be difficult to measure because P waves may be hidden in T waves
QRS duration	0.10 sec or less unless an intraventricular conduction delay exists

What Do I Do About It?

If episodes of AT are short, the patient may be asymptomatic. If AT is sustained and the patient is symptomatic because of the rapid rate, treatment usually includes oxygen, IV access, and vagal maneuvers. Although AT will rarely stop with vagal maneuvers, they are used to try to stop the rhythm or slow conduction through the AV node. If this fails, antiarrhythmic medications should be tried. Adenosine is the drug of choice, except for patients with severe asthma. A significant percentage of ATs will terminate with administration of adenosine.[2] If needed, Ca^{2+} channel blockers or beta-blockers may be used to slow the ventricular rate (if no contraindications exist). Synchronized cardioversion seldom stops automatic ATs but may be successful for ATs due to reentry or triggered automaticity. Synchronized cardioversion should be considered for patients with drug-resistant arrhythmia.[2] Synchronized cardioversion is discussed in Chapter 4.

The signs and symptoms experienced by a patient with a tachycardia depend on the following:
- Ventricular rate
- How long the tachycardia lasts
- General health, presence of underlying heart disease

The faster the heart rate, the more likely the patient is to have signs and symptoms due to the rapid rate.

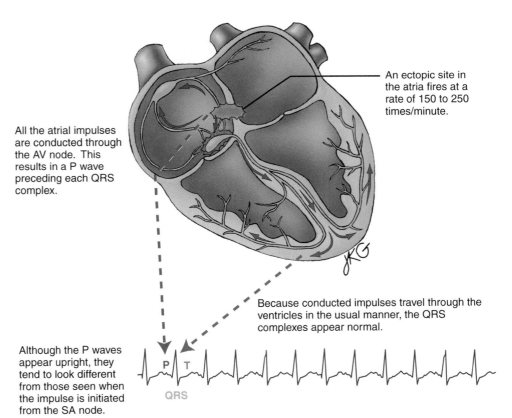

An ectopic site in the atria fires at a rate of 150 to 250 times/minute.

All the atrial impulses are conducted through the AV node. This results in a P wave preceding each QRS complex.

Because conducted impulses travel through the ventricles in the usual manner, the QRS complexes appear normal.

Although the P waves appear upright, they tend to look different from those seen when the impulse is initiated from the SA node.

Figure 3-30 • Atrial tachycardia.

ATRIOVENTRICULAR NODAL REENTRANT TACHYCARDIA

AVNRT is the most common type of SVT. It is caused by reentry in the area of the AV node. In the normal AV node, there is only one pathway through which an electrical impulse is conducted from the SA node to the ventricles. Patients with AVNRT have two conduction pathways within the AV node that conduct impulses at different speeds and recover at different rates. The fast pathway conducts impulses rapidly but has a long refractory period (slow recovery time). The slow pathway conducts impulses slowly but has a short refractory period (fast recovery time) (Figure 3-31). Under the right conditions, the fast and slow pathways can form an electrical circuit or loop. As one side of the loop is recovering, the other is firing.

AVNRT is usually caused by a premature atrial complex (PAC) that is spread by the electrical circuit. This allows the impulse to spin around in a circle indefinitely, reentering the normal electrical pathway with each pass around the circuit. The result is a very rapid and regular rhythm that ranges from 150 to 250 bpm (Table 3-12, Figure 3-32).

What Causes It?

AVNRT can occur at any age. Whether a person is born with a tendency to have AVNRT or whether it develops later in life for an unknown reason has not been clearly determined. AVNRT is common in young, healthy persons with no structural heart disease. It occurs more often in women than in men. AVNRT also occurs in persons with chronic obstructive pulmonary disease (COPD), coronary artery disease, valvular heart disease, heart failure, and digitalis toxicity. AVNRT can cause angina or MI in patients with coronary artery disease. Possible triggers of AVNRT include the following:

- Hypoxia
- Stress
- Overexertion
- Anxiety
- Caffeine
- Smoking
- Sleep deprivation
- Medications

TABLE 3-12	Characteristics of AVNRT	
Rate	150-250 bpm; typically 170-250 bpm.	
Rhythm	Ventricular rhythm is usually very regular.	
P waves	P waves are often hidden in the QRS complex. If the ventricles are stimulated first and then the atria, a negative (inverted) P wave will appear after the QRS in leads II, III, and aVF. When the atria are depolarized after the ventricles, the P wave typically distorts the end of the QRS complex.	
PR interval	P waves are not seen before the QRS complex, therefore the PR interval is not measurable.	
QRS duration	0.10 sec or less unless an intraventricular conduction delay exists	

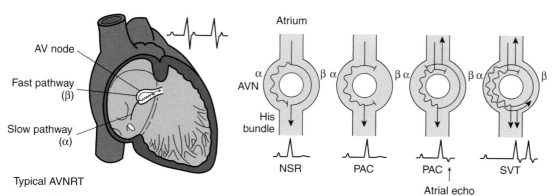

Figure 3-31 • Schematic for SVT due to AV nodal reentry. *NSR,* Normal sinus rhythm.

What Do I Do About It?

Treatment depends on the severity of the patient's signs and symptoms. Signs and symptoms that may be associated with rapid ventricular rates include:

- Palpitations (common)
- Lightheadedness
- Neck vein pulsations
- Syncope or near-syncope
- Dyspnea
- Weakness
- Nausea
- Nervousness, anxiety
- Chest pain or pressure
- Signs of shock
- Congestive heart failure

If the patient is stable but symptomatic (and symptoms are due to the rapid heart rate), treatment usually includes oxygen, IV access, and vagal maneuvers. If vagal maneuvers do not slow the rate or cause conversion of the tachycardia to a sinus rhythm, the first drug given is usually adenosine. If the patient is unstable, treatment usually includes oxygen, IV access, and sedation (if the patient is awake and time permits), followed by synchronized cardioversion.

A regular, narrow-QRS tachycardia that starts or ends suddenly is called **paroxysmal supraventricular tachycardia (PSVT)** (Figure 3-33). (PSVT is discussed here because most SVTs are due to AVNRT.) P waves are seldom seen because they are hidden in T waves of preceding beats. The QRS is narrow unless there is a problem with conduction of the impulse through the ventricles, as in a BBB.

ST-segment changes (usually depression) are common in patients with SVTs. In most patients, these ST-segment changes are thought to be the result of repolarization changes. However, in elderly patients and those with a high likelihood of ischemic heart disease, ST-segment changes may represent ECG changes consistent with an acute coronary syndrome. The patient should be watched closely. Appropriate laboratory tests and a 12-lead ECG should be obtained to rule out infarction as needed.

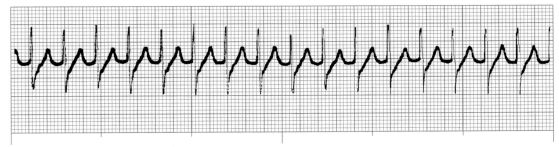

Figure 3-32 • AVNRT.

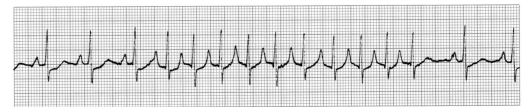

Figure 3-33 • PSVT.

ATRIOVENTRICULAR REENTRANT TACHYCARDIA

AVRT is the second most common type of SVT. Remember that the AV node is normally the only electrical connection between the atria and ventricles. **Preexcitation** is a term used to describe rhythms that originate from above the ventricles but in which the impulse travels via a pathway other than the AV node and bundle of His. Thus, the supraventricular impulse excites the ventricles earlier than would be expected if the impulse traveled by way of the normal conduction system. Patients with preexcitation syndromes are prone to AVRT.

What Causes It?

During fetal development, strands of myocardial tissue form connections between the atria and ventricles, outside the normal conduction system. These strands normally become nonfunctional shortly after birth; however, in patients with preexcitation syndrome, these connections persist as congenital malformations of working myocardial tissue. Because these connections bypass part or all of the normal conduction system, they are called **accessory pathways.** The term **bypass tract** is used when one end of an accessory pathway is attached to normal conductive tissue. This pathway may connect the right atrial and ventricular walls, the left atrial and ventricular walls, or the atrial and ventricular septa on either the right or the left side.

There are three major forms of preexcitation syndrome, each differentiated by their accessory pathways or bypass tracts[3] (Figure 3-34).

■ In **Wolff-Parkinson-White (WPW) syndrome,** the accessory pathway is called the Kent bundle. This bundle connects the atria directly to the ventricles, completely bypassing the normal conduction system. WPW is the most common preexcitation syndrome. It is more common in men than women. Between 60% and 70% of people with WPW have no associated heart disease. WPW is one of the most common causes of tachydysrhythmias in infants and children. Although the accessory pathway in WPW is believed to be congenital in origin, symptoms associated with preexcitation often do not appear until young adulthood (Table 3-13).

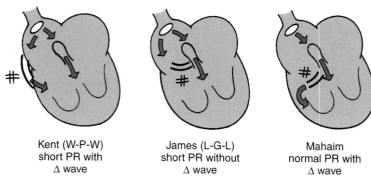

| Kent (W-P-W) short PR with Δ wave | James (L-G-L) short PR without Δ wave | Mahaim normal PR with Δ wave |

Figure 3-34 • The three major forms of preexcitation. Location of the accessory pathways and corresponding ECG characteristics.

TABLE 3-13	Characteristics of Wolff-Parkinson-White Syndrome
Rate	Usually 60-100 bpm, if the underlying rhythm is sinus in origin
Rhythm	Regular, unless associated with atrial fibrillation
P waves	Upright in lead II unless WPW is associated with atrial fibrillation
PR interval	If P waves are observed, <0.12 sec because the impulse travels very quickly across the accessory pathway, bypassing the normal delay in the AV node
QRS duration	Usually >0.12 sec. Slurred upstroke of the QRS complex (delta wave) may be seen in one or more leads.

■ In **Lown-Ganong-Levine (LGL) syndrome,** the accessory pathway is called the James bundle. This bundle connects the atria directly to the lower portion of the AV node, thus partially bypassing the AV node. In LGL syndrome, one end of the James bundle is attached to normal conductive tissue. This congenital pathway may be called a bypass tract.

■ Another unnamed preexcitation syndrome involves the Mahaim fibers. These fibers do not bypass the AV node but originate below the AV node and insert into the ventricular wall, bypassing part or all of the ventricular conduction system.

Delta waves are produced with accessory pathways that insert directly into ventricular muscle. A **delta wave** is the initial slurred deflection at the beginning of the QRS complex. It results from initial activation of the QRS by conduction over the accessory pathway (Figures 3-35, 3-36).

KEEPING IT SIMPLE

Recognizing WPW
- Short PR interval
- Delta wave
- Widening of the QRS

V₃

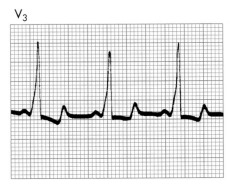

Figure 3-35 • Lead V₃. Typical WPW pattern showing the short PR interval, delta wave, wide QRS complex, and secondary ST and T-wave changes.

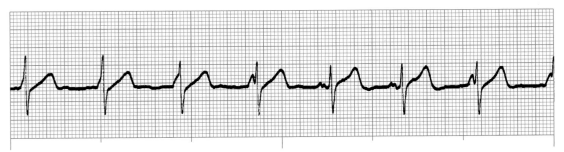

Figure 3-36 • Sinus rhythm with a ventricular rate of about 70 bpm. Patient with known WPW; note delta waves. WPW confirmed by 12-lead ECG.

What Do I Do About It?

Persons with WPW are predisposed to tachydysrhythmia (most commonly atrial fibrillation, atrial flutter, or PSVT). This is because the accessory pathway bypasses the protective blocking mechanism provided by the AV node and provides a mechanism for reentry. Some people with WPW never have symptoms. Common signs and symptoms associated with WPW and a rapid ventricular rate include palpitations, lightheadedness, shortness of breath, anxiety, weakness, dizziness, chest discomfort, and signs of shock.

If the patient is symptomatic because of the rapid ventricular rate, treatment will depend on how unstable the patient is, the width of the QRS complex (wide or narrow), and the regularity of the ventricular rhythm. Consultation with a cardiologist is recommended. A stable but symptomatic patient with narrow QRS AVRT is usually treated with O₂, an IV, and attempts to slow or convert the rhythm with vagal maneuvers. If vagal maneuvers fail, IV medications such as amiodarone may be used. Don't give drugs that slow or block conduction through the AV node, such as adenosine, digoxin, diltiazem, or verapamil. They may speed up conduction through the accessory pathway.

Junctional Tachycardia

Junctional tachycardia is an ectopic rhythm that begins in the pacemaker cells found in the bundle of His. When three or more sequential premature junctional complexes (PJCs) occur at a rate of more than 100 bpm, a junctional tachycardia exists. Nonparoxysmal (gradual onset) junctional tachycardia usually starts as an accelerated junctional rhythm, but the heart rate gradually increases to more than 100 bpm. The usual ventricular rate for nonparoxysmal junctional tachycardia is 101 to 140 bpm (Table 3-14). Paroxysmal junctional tachycardia starts and ends suddenly and is often precipitated by a PJC. The ventricular rate for paroxysmal junctional tachycardia is generally faster, 140 bpm or more.

If the AV junction paces the heart, the electrical impulse must travel in a backward (retrograde) direction to activate the atria. If a P wave is seen, it will be upside down in leads II, III, and aVF because the impulse is traveling away from the positive electrode (Figure 3-37).

TABLE 3-14	Characteristics of Junctional Tachycardia
Rate	101-180 bpm.
Rhythm	Very regular.
P waves	May occur before, during, or after the QRS. If visible, the P wave is inverted in leads II, III, and aVF.
PR interval	If a P wave occurs before the QRS, the PR interval will usually be ≤0.12 sec. If no P wave occurs before the QRS, there will be no PR interval.
QRS duration	Usually 0.10 sec or less unless an intraventricular conduction delay exists.

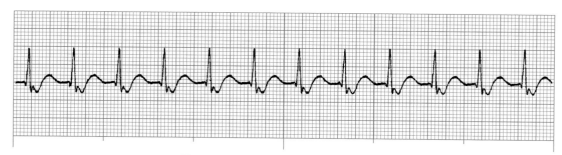

Figure 3-37 • Junctional tachycardia.

What Causes It?

Junctional tachycardia may occur because of an acute coronary syndrome, heart failure, theophylline administration, or digitalis toxicity (common cause).

What Do I Do About It?

With sustained ventricular rates of 150 bpm or more, the patient may complain of a "racing heart" and severe anxiety. Because of the fast ventricular rate, the ventricles may be unable to fill completely, resulting in decreased cardiac output. Junctional tachycardia associated with an acute coronary syndrome may

- Increase myocardial ischemia
- Increase the frequency and severity of chest pain
- Extend the size of an MI
- Cause heart failure, hypotension, or cardiogenic shock
- Predispose the patient to ventricular dysrhythmias

Treatment depends on the severity of the patient's signs and symptoms. If the patient tolerates the rhythm, observation is often all that is needed. If the patient is symptomatic as a result of the rapid rate, initial treatment should include oxygen and IV access. Because it is often difficult to distinguish junctional tachycardia from other narrow-QRS tachycardias, vagal maneuvers and, if necessary, IV adenosine may be used to help determine the origin of the rhythm (Table 3-15). A beta-blocker or Ca^{2+} channel blocker may be ordered (if no contraindications exist). If the rhythm is the result of digitalis toxicity, the drug should be withheld. If the rhythm is the result of theophylline administration, the infusion should be slowed or stopped.

Vagal Maneuvers

Vagal maneuvers are methods used to stimulate baroreceptors located in the internal carotid arteries and the aortic arch. Stimulation of these receptors results in reflex stimulation of the vagus nerve and release of acetylcholine. Acetylcholine slows conduction through the AV node, resulting in slowing of the heart rate. Although there is some overlap of the right and left vagus nerves, it is thought that the right vagus nerve has more fibers to the SA node and atrial muscle and the left vagus more fibers to the AV node and some ventricular muscle.

Examples of vagal maneuvers include the following:

- Coughing.
- Squatting.
- Breath-holding.
- Carotid sinus pressure. This procedure is performed with the patient's neck extended. Firm pressure is applied just underneath the angle of the jaw for up to 5 seconds. Carotid pressure should be avoided in older patients and in patients with carotid artery bruits. Simultaneous, bilateral carotid pressure should *never* be performed.
- Application of a cold stimulus to the face (such as a washcloth soaked in iced water, cold pack, or crushed ice mixed with water in a plastic bag or glove) for up to 10 seconds. This technique is often effective in infants and young children. When using this method, do not obstruct the patient's mouth or nose or apply pressure to the eyes.
- Valsalva's maneuver. Ask the patient to blow through an occluded straw or take a deep breath and bear down as if having a bowel movement for up to 10 seconds. This strains the abdominal muscles and increases intrathoracic pressure.
- Gagging. Use a tongue depressor or culturette swab to briefly touch the back of the throat.

When using vagal maneuvers, keep the following points in mind:

- Make sure oxygen, suction, a defibrillator, and emergency medications are available before attempting the procedure.
- A 12-lead ECG recording is desirable when a vagal maneuver is performed.
- Continuous monitoring of the patient's ECG is *essential*. Note the onset and end of the vagal maneuver on the ECG rhythm strip.
- In general, a vagal maneuver should not be continued for more than 10 seconds.
- Application of external ocular pressure may be dangerous and should not be used because of the risk of retinal detachment.
- Carotid massage is less effective in children than in adults and is not recommended.

TABLE 3-15	Effects of Vagal Maneuvers in Different Types of Tachycardias
Dysrhythmia	**Effects of Vagal Maneuvers**
Sinus tachycardia	Gradual slowing and return to previous rate upon cessation of maneuver
AVNRT	Abrupt cessation of the tachycardia or no effect
AVRT	Abrupt cessation of the tachycardia or no effect
Atrial flutter	Ventricular rate unchanged or temporarily slowed; flutter waves may be revealed during maneuver
Atrial fibrillation	Ventricular rate unchanged or temporarily slowed
Ventricular tachycardia	No effect

WIDE-QRS TACHYCARDIAS

 The width of a QRS complex is most accurately determined when it is viewed and measured in more than one lead. The measurement should be taken from the QRS complex with the longest duration and clearest onset and end.

INTRAVENTRICULAR CONDUCTION DEFECTS

A delay or block can occur in any part of the intraventricular conduction system. If a delay or block occurs in one of the bundle branches, the ventricles will not depolarize at the same time. The impulse travels first down the unblocked branch and stimulates that ventricle. Because of the block, the impulse must then travel from cell to cell through the myocardium (rather than through the normal conduction pathway) to stimulate the other ventricle. This means of conduction is slower than normal, and the QRS complex appears widened on the ECG. The ventricle with the blocked bundle branch is the last to be depolarized.

A QRS measuring 0.10 to 0.12 second is called an *incomplete* right or left BBB. A QRS measuring more than 0.12 second is called a *complete* right or left BBB. If the QRS is wide but there is no BBB pattern, the term "wide QRS" or "intraventricular conduction delay" is used to describe the QRS.

ECG criteria for identification of a right or left BBB are

■ A QRS duration of more than 0.12 second (if a complete BBB).
■ QRS complexes produced by supraventricular activity (i.e., the QRS complex is not a paced beat nor did it originate in the ventricles).

To determine right versus left BBB

■ Look at lead V_1 or MCL_1.
■ Move from the J-point back into the QRS complex and determine if the terminal portion (last 0.04 second) of the QRS complex is a positive (upright) or negative (downward) deflection (Figures 3-38, 3-39).
■ If the two criteria for BBB are met and the terminal portion of the QRS is positive, a right BBB is most likely present. If the terminal portion of the QRS is negative, a left BBB is most likely present.

 In left bundle branch block (LBBB), activation of the septum is altered and the right ventricle depolarizes before the left. Thus, abnormal Q waves originating from the left ventricle may be obscured. Further, ST-segment and T-wave changes are often present with LBBB, making the diagnosis of acute MI even more difficult.[1]

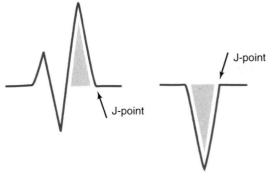

Figure 3-38 • Move from the J-point back into the QRS complex and determine if the terminal portion (last 0.04 second) of the QRS complex is a positive (upright) or negative (downward) deflection. If the two criteria for BBB are met and the terminal portion of the QRS is positive, a right BBB is most likely present. If the terminal portion of the QRS is negative, a left BBB is most likely present.

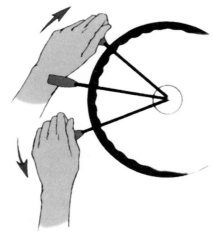

Figure 3-39 • Differentiating right versus left BBB. The "turn signal theory"—right is up, left is down.

ACCELERATED IDIOVENTRICULAR RHYTHM

An **accelerated idioventricular rhythm (AIVR)** exists when three or more ventricular escape beats occur in a row at a rate of 41 to 100 bpm (Figure 3-40, Table 3-16). Although this heart rate is not considered a tachycardia, AIVR is discussed here because some cardiologists consider the upper end of the rate range to be about 120 bpm.

AIVR is usually considered a benign escape rhythm that appears when the sinus rate slows and disappears when the sinus rate speeds up. Episodes of AIVR usually last a few seconds to a minute. Because AIVR usually begins and ends gradually, it is also called **nonparoxysmal VT.**

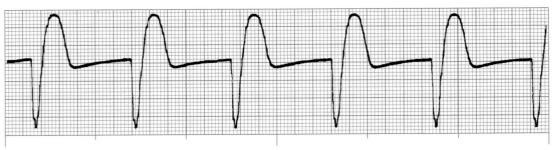

Figure 3-40 • AIVR.

TABLE 3-16	Characteristics of Accelerated Idioventricular Rhythm	
Rate	41-100 bpm (41-120 bpm per some cardiologists)	
Rhythm	Essentially regular	
P waves	Usually absent or, with retrograde conduction to the atria, may appear after the QRS (usually upright in the ST-segment or T wave)	
PR interval	None	
QRS duration	>0.12 sec, T wave usually in opposite direction of the QRS complex	

What Causes It?

AIVR occurs most often in the setting of acute MI, most often during the first 12 hours. It is particularly common after successful reperfusion therapy. AIVR has been observed in patients with the following:

- Digitalis toxicity
- Cocaine toxicity
- Subarachnoid hemorrhage
- Acute myocarditis
- Hypertensive heart disease
- Dilated cardiomyopathy

What Do I Do About It?

AIVR generally requires no treatment because the rhythm is protective and often transient, spontaneously resolving on its own. However, possible dizziness, lightheadedness, or other signs of hemodynamic compromise may occur because of the loss of atrial kick.

VENTRICULAR TACHYCARDIA

VT exists when three or more PVCs occur in immediate succession at a rate greater than 100 bpm. VT may occur as a short run lasting less than 30 seconds (nonsustained) (Figure 3-41), but it more commonly persists for more than 30 seconds (sustained). VT may occur with or without pulses, and the patient may be stable or unstable with this rhythm.

VT, like PVCs, may originate from an ectopic focus in either ventricle. When the QRS complexes of VT are of the same shape and amplitude, the rhythm is called **monomorphic VT** (Figure 3-42, Table 3-17). When the QRS complexes of VT vary in shape and amplitude from beat to beat, the rhythm is called polymorphic VT. In polymorphic VT, the QRS complexes appear to twist from upright to negative or negative to upright and back. Polymorphic VT is discussed later in this chapter, with irregular tachycardias.

 Monomorphic VT with a ventricular rate greater than 200 bpm is called ventricular flutter by some cardiologists.

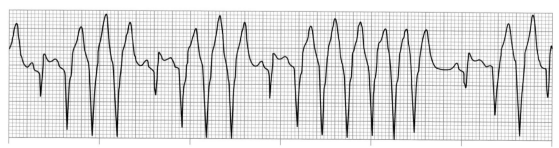

Figure 3-41 • Nonsustained VT.

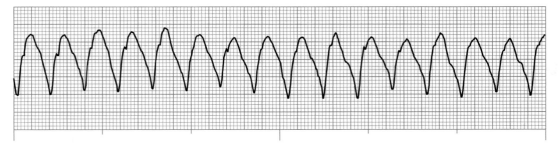

Figure 3-42 • Sustained VT. When the QRS complexes of VT are of the same shape and amplitude, the rhythm is called monomorphic VT.

TABLE 3-17	Characteristics of Monomorphic Ventricular Tachycardia
Rate	101-250 bpm
Rhythm	Essentially regular
P waves	Usually not seen; if present, they have no set relationship to the QRS complexes, appearing between them at a rate different from that of the VT
PR interval	None
QRS duration	>0.12 sec; often difficult to differentiate between the QRS and T wave

What Causes It?

Sustained monomorphic VT is often associated with underlying heart disease, particularly myocardial ischemia. It rarely occurs in patients without underlying heart disease. Common causes of VT include the following:

- Acute coronary syndromes
- Cardiomyopathy
- Tricyclic antidepressant overdose
- Digitalis toxicity
- Valvular heart disease
- Cocaine abuse
- Mitral valve prolapse
- Acid-base imbalance
- Trauma (such as myocardial contusion, invasive cardiac procedures)
- Electrolyte imbalance (such as hypokalemia, hyperkalemia, hypomagnesemia)

What Do I Do About It?

Signs and symptoms associated with VT vary. VT may occur with or without pulses. The patient who has sustained monomorphic VT may be stable for long periods of time. However, when the ventricular rate is very fast, or when myocardial ischemia is present, monomorphic VT can degenerate to polymorphic VT or ventricular fibrillation (VF). Syncope or near-syncope may occur because of an abrupt onset of VT. The patient's only warning symptom may be a brief period of lightheadedness.

Treatment is based on the patient's signs and symptoms and the type of VT. If the rhythm is monomorphic VT (and the patient's symptoms are due to the tachycardia):

- CPR and defibrillation are used to treat the pulseless patient in VT.
- Stable but symptomatic patients are treated with oxygen, IV access, and ventricular anti-arrhythmics (such as amiodarone) to suppress the rhythm.
- Unstable patients (usually a sustained heart rate of 150 bpm or more) are treated with oxygen, IV access, and sedation (if awake and time permits) followed by synchronized cardioversion.
- In all cases, an aggressive search must be made for the cause of the VT.

Sustained VT does not always produce signs of hemodynamic instability.

SVT with an intraventricular conduction delay may be difficult to distinguish from VT. Keep in mind that VT is considered a potentially life-threatening dysrhythmia. If you are unsure whether a regular, wide-QRS tachycardia is VT or SVT with an intraventricular conduction delay, treat the rhythm as VT until proven otherwise. Obtaining a 12-lead ECG may help differentiate VT from SVT, but do not delay treatment if the patient is symptomatic.

IRREGULAR TACHYCARDIAS
MULTIFOCAL ATRIAL TACHYCARDIA

Wandering atrial pacemaker is rhythm in which the size, shape, and direction of the P waves vary, sometimes from beat to beat. The difference in the look of the P waves is a result of the gradual shifting of the dominant pacemaker between the SA node, the atria, and/or the AV junction (Figure 3-43). When a wandering atrial pacemaker is associated with a ventricular rate greater than 100 bpm, the rhythm is called multifocal atrial tachycardia (MAT) (Figure 3-44, Table 3-18). MAT is also called **chaotic atrial tachycardia.**

Lead II (continuous)

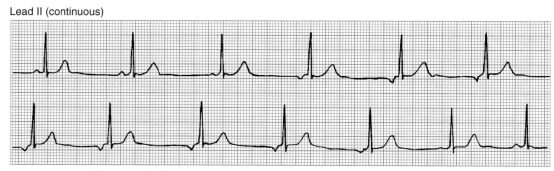

Figure 3-43 • Wandering atrial pacemaker. Continuous strip (lead II).

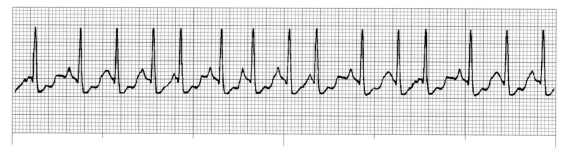

Figure 3-44 • MAT.

TABLE 3-18	Characteristics of Multifocal Atrial Tachycardia
Rate	Ventricular rate is >100 bpm.
Rhythm	May be irregular as the pacemaker site shifts from the SA node to ectopic atrial locations and the AV junction.
P waves	Size, shape, and direction may change from beat to beat; at least three different P-wave configurations (seen in the same lead) are required for a diagnosis of wandering atrial pacemaker or multifocal atrial tachycardia.
PR interval	Variable.
QRS duration	Usually 0.10 sec or less unless an intraventricular conduction delay exists.

What Causes It?

In MAT, multiple ectopic sites stimulate the atria. MAT is most often seen in
- Severe COPD
- Hypoxia
- Acute coronary syndromes
- Digoxin toxicity
- Rheumatic heart disease
- Theophylline toxicity
- Electrolyte imbalances

What Do I Do About It?

Treatment of MAT is directed at the underlying cause. If the patient is stable and symptomatic but you are uncertain if the rhythm is MAT, you can try a vagal maneuver. If vagal maneuvers are ineffective, you can try adenosine IV. Remember that MAT is the result of random and chaotic firing of multiple sites in the atria. MAT does not involve reentry through the AV node. Therefore, it is unlikely that vagal maneuvers or giving adenosine will terminate the rhythm. However, they may momentarily slow the rate enough so that you can look at the P waves and determine the specific type of tachycardia. By determining the type of tachycardia, treatment specific to that rhythm can be given.

If you know the rhythm is MAT and the patient is symptomatic, treatment may include medications such as Ca^{2+} channel blockers. Beta-blockers are usually contraindicated because of the presence of severe underlying pulmonary disease.

ATRIAL FLUTTER

Atrial flutter is an ectopic atrial rhythm in which an irritable site fires regularly at a very rapid rate. Because of this extremely rapid stimulation, waveforms are produced that resemble the teeth of a saw, or a picket fence, called "flutter" waves (Figure 3-45). Flutter waves are best observed in leads II, III, aVF, and V_1. If each impulse were sent to the ventricles, the ventricular rate would equal 300 bpm. The healthy AV node protects the ventricles from these extremely fast atrial rates.

Atrial flutter with an atrial rate of 300 bpm and a ventricular rate of 150 bpm = 2:1 conduction; 100 bpm = 3:1 conduction; 75 bpm = 4:1 conduction; 50 bpm = 6:1 conduction, and so on. Although conduction ratios in atrial flutter are often even (2:1, 4:1, 6:1), variable conduction can also occur, producing an irregular ventricular rhythm (Table 3-19).

TABLE 3-19	Characteristics of Atrial Flutter
Rate	In type I atrial flutter (also called typical rapid atrial flutter), the atrial rate ranges from 250-350 bpm. In type II atrial flutter (also called atypical or very rapid atrial flutter), the atrial rate ranges from 350-450 bpm.
Rhythm	Atrial regular, ventricular regular or irregular depending on AV conduction/blockade.
P waves	No identifiable P waves; saw-toothed "flutter" waves are present.
PR interval	Not measurable.
QRS duration	Usually 0.10 sec or less but may be widened if flutter waves are buried in the QRS complex or if an intraventricular conduction delay exists.

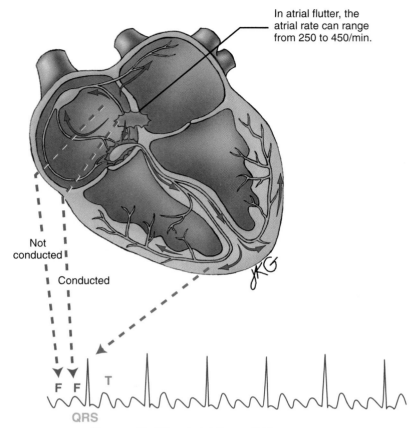

In atrial flutter, the atrial rate can range from 250 to 450/min.

Not conducted

Conducted

F F T

QRS

Figure 3-45 • Atrial flutter. *F,* Flutter wave.

What Causes It?

Atrial flutter is usually caused by a reentry circuit in which an impulse circles around a large area of tissue, such as the entire right atrium. It is usually a paroxysmal rhythm that is precipitated by a premature atrial complex. It may last for seconds to hours and occasionally 24 hours or more. Chronic atrial flutter is unusual. This is because the rhythm usually converts to sinus rhythm or atrial fibrillation, either on its own or with treatment. Conditions associated with atrial flutter are shown in Box 3-2.

What Do I Do About It?

Treatment decisions are based on the ventricular rate, the duration of the rhythm, the patient's general health, and how he or she is tolerating the rhythm. When atrial flutter is present with 2:1 conduction, it may be difficult to tell the difference between atrial flutter and sinus tachy-

---

BOX 3-2

Conditions Associated with Atrial Flutter

- Hypoxia
- Pulmonary embolism
- Chronic lung disease
- Mitral or tricuspid valve stenosis or regurgitation
- Pneumonia
- Ischemic heart disease
- Complication of MI
- Cardiomyopathy
- Hyperthyroidism
- Digitalis or quinidine toxicity
- Cardiac surgery
- Pericarditis/myocarditis

cardia, atrial tachycardia, AVNRT, AVRT, or PSVT. Vagal maneuvers may help identify the rhythm by temporarily slowing AV conduction and revealing the underlying flutter waves (Figure 3-46). If atrial flutter is associated with a rapid ventricular rate and the patient is stable but symptomatic, treatment may be directed toward controlling the ventricular rate or converting the rhythm to a sinus rhythm. In the prehospital and emergency department setting, treatment is usually aimed at controlling the ventricular rate. Consider synchronized cardioversion if a patient is in atrial flutter with a rapid ventricular rate and has serious signs and symptoms (such as low blood pressure, signs of shock, or heart failure).

Atrial flutter or atrial fibrillation that has a ventricular rate of more than 100 bpm is described as "uncontrolled." The ventricular rate is considered "rapid" when it is 150 bpm or more. New-onset atrial flutter or atrial fibrillation (AFib) is often associated with a rapid ventricular rate. Atrial flutter or AFib with a rapid ventricular response is commonly called "aflutter with RVR" or "AFib with RVR."

Atrial flutter or AFib that has a ventricular rate of less than 100 bpm, is described as "controlled." A controlled ventricular rate may be the result of a healthy AV node protecting the ventricles from very fast atrial impulses or drugs used to control (block) conduction through the AV node, decreasing the number of impulses reaching the ventricles.

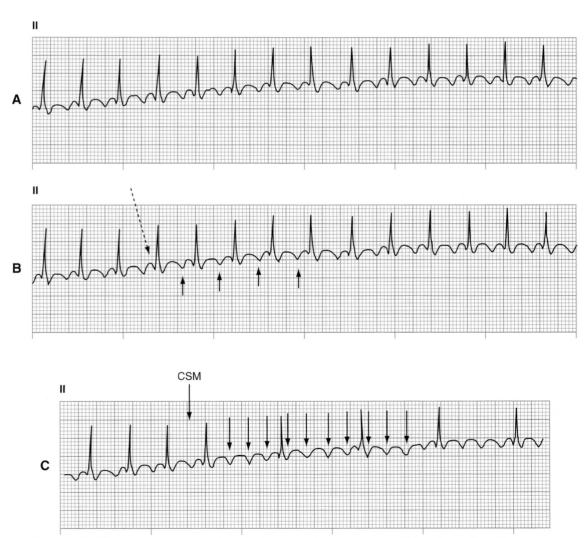

Figure 3-46 • Atrial flutter. **A,** This rhythm strip shows a narrow-QRS tachycardia with a ventricular rate just under 150 bpm. **B,** The same rhythm shown in A with arrows added indicating possible atrial activity. **C,** When carotid sinus massage is performed, the rate of conduction through the AV node slows, revealing atrial flutter. *CSM,* Carotid sinus massage.

ATRIAL FIBRILLATION

AFib occurs because of altered automaticity in one or several rapidly firing sites in the atria or reentry involving one or more circuits in the atria (Figure 3-47). These rapid impulses cause the muscles of the atria to quiver (fibrillate). This results in ineffectual atrial contraction, decreased stroke volume, a subsequent decrease in cardiac output, and loss of atrial kick (Table 3-20).

What Causes It?

Atrial fibrillation can occur in patients with or without detectable heart disease or related symptoms. Conditions associated with AFib are shown in Box 3-3.

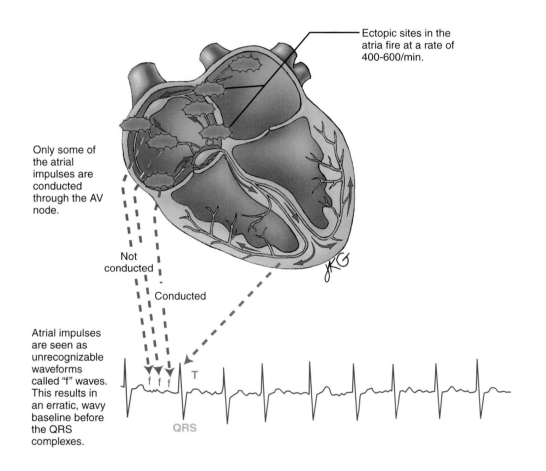

Ectopic sites in the atria fire at a rate of 400-600/min.

Only some of the atrial impulses are conducted through the AV node.

Not conducted

Conducted

Atrial impulses are seen as unrecognizable waveforms called "f" waves. This results in an erratic, wavy baseline before the QRS complexes.

Figure 3-47 • Atrial fibrillation. *f,* Fibrillatory wave.

TABLE 3-20	Characteristics of Atrial Fibrillation
Rate	Atrial rate usually 400-600 bpm; ventricular rate variable
Rhythm	Ventricular rhythm usually irregularly irregular
P waves	No identifiable P waves; fibrillatory waves present; erratic, wavy baseline
PR interval	Not measurable
QRS duration	Usually 0.10 sec or less but may be widened if an intraventricular conduction delay exists

BOX 3-3

Conditions Associated with Atrial Fibrillation

- Idiopathic (no clear cause)
- Hypertension
- Ischemic heart disease
- Advanced age
- Rheumatic heart disease (especially mitral valve disease)
- Cardiomyopathy
- Congestive heart failure
- Congenital heart disease
- Sick sinus syndrome/degenerative conduction system disease
- WPW syndrome
- Pericarditis
- Pulmonary embolism
- Chronic lung disease
- After surgery
- Diabetes
- Stress
- Sympathomimetics
- Excessive caffeine
- Hypoxia
- Hypokalemia
- Hypoglycemia
- Systemic infection
- Hyperthyroidism
- Electrocution

What Do I Do About It?

Treatment decisions are based on the ventricular rate, the duration of the rhythm, the patient's general health, and how he or she is tolerating the rhythm. If AFib is associated with a rapid ventricular rate and the patient is stable but symptomatic, treatment may be directed toward controlling the ventricular rate or converting the rhythm to a sinus rhythm (Figure 3-48). In the prehospital and emergency department settings, treatment is usually aimed at controlling the ventricular rate. Consider synchronized cardioversion if a patient is in AFib with a rapid ventricular rate and has serious signs and symptoms (such as low blood pressure, signs of shock, or heart failure).

Patients who experience AFib are at increased risk of having a stroke. Because the atria do not contract effectively and expel all of the blood within them, blood may pool within them and form clots. A stroke can result if a clot moves from the atria and lodges in an artery in the brain.

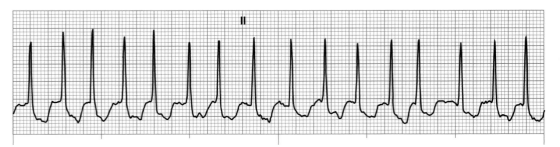

Figure 3-48 • Atrial fibrillation with a rapid ventricular response.

POLYMORPHIC VENTRICULAR TACHYCARDIA

In polymorphic VT, the QRS complexes appear to twist from upright to negative or negative to upright and back (Figure 3-49). Polymorphic VT that occurs in the presence of a long QT interval is called *torsades de pointes.* Polymorphic VT that occurs in the presence of a normal QT interval is simply referred to as *polymorphic VT* or *polymorphic VT resembling torsades de pointes* (Table 3-21).

What Causes It?

Polymorphic VT may be precipitated by slow heart rates or associated with medications or electrolyte disturbances that prolong the QT interval. A prolonged QT interval may be congenital or acquired.

What Do I Do About It?

Symptoms are usually related to the decreased cardiac output that occurs because of the fast ventricular rate. Signs of shock are often present. The patient may experience a syncopal episode or seizures. The rhythm may occasionally terminate spontaneously and recur after several seconds or minutes, or it may deteriorate to VF.

If the rhythm is polymorphic VT, it is important to determine if the patient's QT interval just before the tachycardia is normal or prolonged. If the QT interval is normal and the patient is symptomatic due to the tachycardia, treat ischemia if present, correct electrolyte abnormalities, and proceed with electrical therapy or antiarrhythmic medications if necessary. If the QT interval is prolonged and the patient is symptomatic due to the tachycardia, discontinue any medications the patient may be taking that prolong the QT interval, correct electrolyte abnormalities, and proceed with electrical therapy or antiarrhythmic medications if necessary. If the rhythm is sustained polymorphic VT and the patient is unstable or has no pulse, defibrillate.

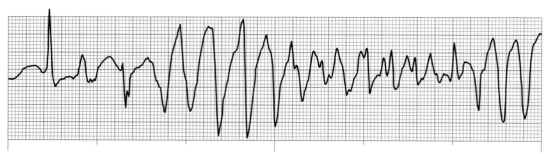

Figure 3-49 • When the QRS complexes of VT vary in shape and amplitude, the rhythm is termed polymorphic VT.

TABLE 3-21	Characteristics of Polymorphic Ventricular Tachycardia	
Rate	150-300 bpm, typically 200-250 bpm	
Rhythm	May be regular or irregular	
P waves	None	
PR interval	None	
QRS duration	>0.12 sec; gradual alteration in amplitude and direction of the QRS complexes; a typical cycle consists of 5-20 QRS complexes	

QUICK REVIEW 3-13

1. What dysrhythmia is characterized by waveforms resembling teeth of a saw or picket fence before each QRS?

2. What is the significance of the relative refractory period?

3. How do you determine if the ventricular rhythm on a rhythm strip is regular or irregular?

4. Describe the appearance of atrial activity in atrial fibrillation on the ECG.

5. Name a consequence of decreased ventricular filling time.

6. What is the most common preexcitation syndrome?

SECTION 3

Bradydysrhythmias: Too Slow Rhythms

SINUS BRADYCARDIA

If the SA node fires at a rate slower than normal for the patient's age, the rhythm is called sinus bradycardia (Figure 3-50). The rhythm starts in the SA node and then heads down the normal pathway of conduction through the atria, AV junction, bundle branches, and ventricles. This results in atrial and ventricular depolarization. In adults and adolescents, a sinus brady-cardia has a heart rate of less than 60 bpm (Table 3-22). The term *severe sinus bradycardia* is sometimes used to describe a sinus bradycardia with a rate of less than 40 bpm.

WHAT CAUSES IT?

Sinus bradycardia occurs in adults during sleep and in well-conditioned athletes. It is also present in up to 35% of people younger than 25 years of age while at rest. Sinus bradycardia is common in some MIs. Stimulation of the vagus nerve can also result in slowing of the heart rate. For example, coughing, vomiting, straining to have a bowel movement, or sudden expo-sure of the face to cold water can result in slowing of the heart rate. Carotid sinus pressure can also slow the heart rate. In people who have a sensitive carotid sinus, slowing of the heart rate can occur when a tight collar is worn or with the impact of the stream of water on the neck while in the shower. Other causes of sinus bradycardia are shown in Box 3-4.

WHAT DO I DO ABOUT IT?

Assess how the patient tolerates the rhythm at rest and with activity. If the patient has no symp-toms, no treatment is necessary. If the patient is symptomatic because of the slow rate, initial treatment may include O_2, starting an IV, giving IV atropine, and/or transcutaneous pacing.

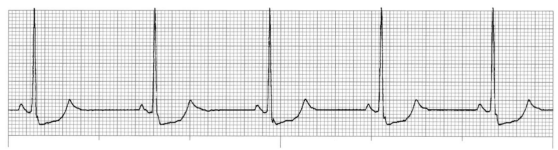

Figure 3-50 • Sinus bradycardia.

TABLE 3-22	Characteristics of Sinus Bradycardia
Rate	<60 bpm
Rhythm	Regular
P waves	Uniform in appearance, positive (upright) in lead II, one precedes each QRS complex
PR interval	0.12-0.20 sec and constant from beat to beat
QRS duration	0.10 sec or less unless an intraventricular conduction delay exists

BOX 3-4

Causes of Sinus Bradycardia

- Inferior MI
- Posterior MI
- Disease of the SA node
- Vagal stimulation
- Hypoxia
- Hypothermia
- Increased intracranial pressure
- Hypothyroidism
- Hypokalemia
- Postheart transplant
- Hyperkalemia
- Obstructive sleep apnea
- Medications such as Ca^{2+} channel blockers, digitalis, beta-blockers, amiodarone, and sotalol

In the setting of an MI, sinus bradycardia is often temporary. A slow heart rate can be beneficial in the patient who has had an MI (and has no symptoms due to the slow rate). This is because the heart's demand for oxygen is less when the heart rate is slow.

JUNCTIONAL ESCAPE RHYTHM

Remember that the SA node is normally the heart's pacemaker. The AV junction may assume responsibility for pacing the heart if
- The SA node fails to discharge (such as sinus arrest).
- An impulse from the SA node is generated but blocked as it exits the SA node (such as SA block).
- The rate of discharge of the SA node is slower than that of the AV junction (such as a sinus bradycardia or the slower phase of a sinus arrhythmia).
- An impulse from the SA node is generated and is conducted through the atria but is not conducted to the ventricles (such as an AV block).

The built-in rate of the AV junction is 40 to 60 bpm. Because a junctional rhythm starts from above the ventricles, the QRS complex is usually narrow and its rhythm is very regular (Figures 3-51, 3-52). If the AV junction paces the heart at a rate slower than 40 bpm, the resulting rhythm is called a *junctional bradycardia.* This may seem confusing because the AV junction's normal pacing rate (40 to 60 bpm [Table 3-23]) *is* bradycardic. However, the term junctional bradycardia refers to a rate slower than normal for the AV junction.

TABLE 3-23	Characteristics of Junctional Escape Rhythm
Rate	40-60 bpm.
Rhythm	Very regular.
P waves	May occur before, during, or after the QRS. If visible, the P wave is inverted in leads II, III, and aVF.
PR interval	If a P wave occurs before the QRS, the PR interval will usually be ≤0.12 sec. If no P wave occurs before the QRS, there will be no PR interval.
QRS duration	Usually 0.10 sec or less unless an intraventricular conduction delay exists.

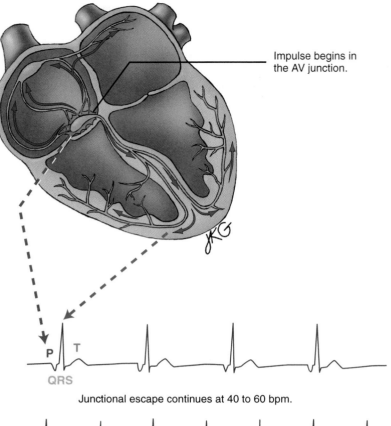

Impulse begins in the AV junction.

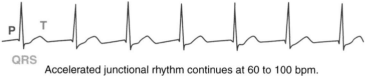

Junctional escape continues at 40 to 60 bpm.

Accelerated junctional rhythm continues at 60 to 100 bpm.

Junctional tachycardia continues at 100 to 180 bpm.

Figure 3-51 • Junctional rhythms.

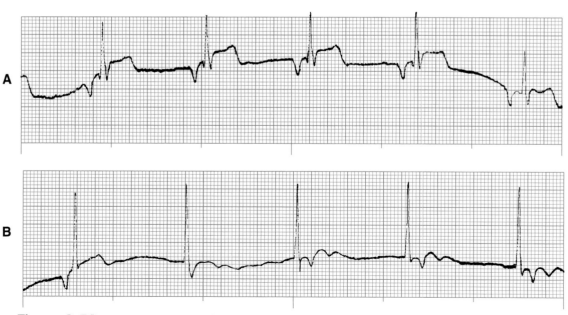

A

B

Figure 3-52 • Junctional escape rhythm. Lead II—continuous strips. **A,** Note the retrograde P waves before the QRS complexes. **B,** Note the change in the location of the P waves. In the first beat, the retrograde P wave is observed before the QRS. In the second beat, no P wave is observed. In the remaining beats, the P wave is observed after the QRS complexes.

WHAT CAUSES IT?

Causes of a junctional rhythm include the following:

- Acute coronary syndromes (particularly inferior wall MI)
- Hypoxia
- Rheumatic heart disease
- Valvular disease
- SA node disease
- Increased parasympathetic tone
- Immediately after cardiac surgery
- Effects of medications including digitalis, quinidine, beta-blockers, and Ca^{2+} channel blockers

WHAT DO I DO ABOUT IT?

The patient may be asymptomatic with a junctional escape rhythm or may experience signs and symptoms that may be associated with the slow heart rate and decreased cardiac output. Treatment depends on the cause of the dysrhythmia and the patient's presenting signs and symptoms. If the dysrhythmia is caused by digitalis toxicity, this medication should be withheld. If the patient's signs and symptoms are related to the slow heart rate, atropine and/or transcutaneous pacing should be considered. Other medications that may be used in the treatment of symptomatic bradycardia include dopamine and epinephrine IV infusions.

VENTRICULAR ESCAPE RHYTHM

A ventricular escape or idioventricular rhythm (IVR) exists when three or more ventricular beats occur in a row at a rate of 20 to 40 bpm (Figure 3-53, Table 3-24).

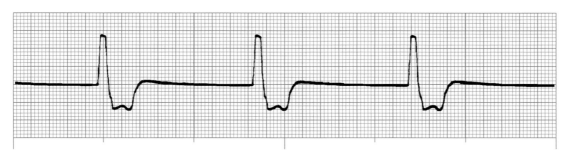

Figure 3-53 • IVR.

TABLE 3-24	Characteristics of Ventricular Escape (Idioventricular) Rhythm
Rate	20-40 bpm
Rhythm	Essentially regular
P waves	Usually absent or, with retrograde conduction to the atria, may appear after the QRS (usually upright in the ST-segment or T wave)
PR interval	None
QRS duration	>0.12 sec, T wave frequently in opposite direction of the QRS complex

WHAT CAUSES IT?

A ventricular escape rhythm may occur in the following situations:

- The SA node and the AV junction fail to initiate an electrical impulse.
- The rate of discharge of the SA node or AV junction becomes less than the intrinsic rate of the ventricles.
- Impulses generated by a supraventricular pacemaker site are blocked.

A ventricular escape rhythm may also occur because of MI, digitalis toxicity, or metabolic imbalances.

WHAT DO I DO ABOUT IT?

Because the ventricular rate associated with a ventricular escape rhythm is very slow (20 to 40 bpm), the patient may experience serious signs and symptoms because of decreased cardiac output. If the patient has a pulse and is symptomatic because of the slow rate, transcutaneous pacing should be attempted right away. If the patient is not breathing and has no pulse despite the appearance of organized electrical activity on the cardiac monitor, PEA exists. Management of PEA includes CPR, giving oxygen, possible placement of an advanced airway, starting an IV, giving epinephrine (and atropine if the rate is slow), and an aggressive search for the underlying cause of the arrest.

QUICK REVIEW 3-14

1. _____ toxicity/excess is a common cause of junctional dysrhythmias.
2. In a junctional rhythm, where is the location of the P wave on the ECG if atrial depolarization precedes ventricular depolarization?

ATRIOVENTRICULAR BLOCKS

AV blocks are divided into three main types: first-, second-, and third-degree AV block (Figure 3-54).

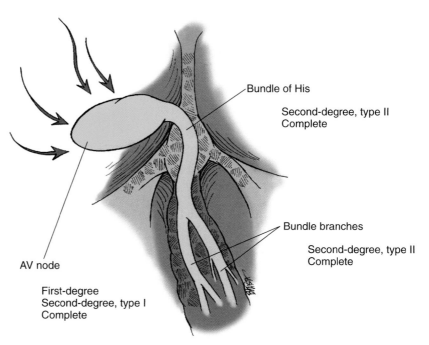

Figure 3-54 • Locations of AV block.

FIRST-DEGREE ATRIOVENTRICULAR BLOCK

First-degree AV block is not a dysrhythmia itself. It is a condition describing the consistent prolonged PR interval viewed on the ECG rhythm strip. In first-degree AV block, impulses from the SA node to the ventricles are *delayed* (not blocked). First-degree AV block usually occurs at the AV node (Figure 3-55).

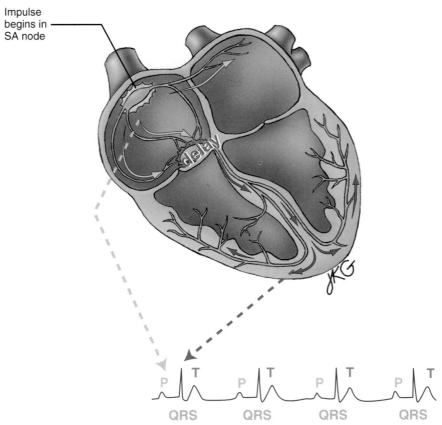

Figure 3-55 • First-degree AV block.

What Causes It?

First-degree AV block may be a normal finding in individuals with no history of cardiac disease, especially in athletes. In some people, mild prolongation of the PR interval may be a normal variant, especially with sinus bradycardia during rest or sleep. First-degree AV block may also occur because of the following:

- Ischemia or injury to the AV node or junction
- Medications
- Rheumatic heart disease
- Hyperkalemia
- Acute MI (often inferior wall MI)
- Increased vagal tone

What Do I Do About It?

The patient with a first-degree AV block is often asymptomatic; however, marked first-degree AV block can lead to symptoms even in the absence of higher degrees of AV block.[4] First-degree AV block that occurs with acute MI should be monitored closely. If first-degree AV block accompanies a symptomatic bradycardia, treat the bradycardia (Figure 3-56, Table 3-25).

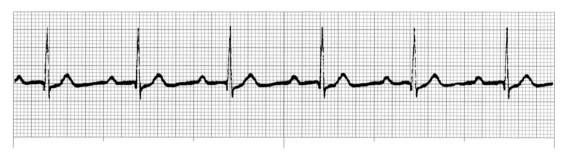

Figure 3-56 • Sinus rhythm at 60 bpm with a first-degree AV block.

TABLE 3-25	Characteristics of First-Degree AV Block
Rate	Usually within normal range, but depends on underlying rhythm
Rhythm	Regular
P waves	Normal in size and shape, one positive (upright) P wave before each QRS in leads II, III, and aVF
PR interval	Prolonged (>0.20 sec) but constant
QRS duration	Usually 0.10 sec or less unless an intraventricular conduction delay exists

KEEPING IT SIMPLE

A Quick Look at P Waves and AV Blocks

AV Block	P-Wave Conduction
First Degree	All P waves conducted but delayed
Second Degree	Some P waves conducted, others blocked
Third Degree	No P waves conducted

SECOND-DEGREE ATRIOVENTRICULAR BLOCK

Second-Degree AV Block, Type I (Wenckebach, Mobitz Type I)

Second-degree AV block type I is also known as Mobitz type I and Wenckebach. The Wenckebach pattern is the progressive lengthening of the PR interval followed by a P wave with no QRS complex (Table 3-26). The conduction delay in second-degree AV block type I usually occurs at the level of the AV node (Figure 3-57).

What Causes It?

Second-degree AV block type I is usually caused by a conduction delay within the AV node. Remember that the RCA supplies the AV node in 90% of the population. Thus, RCA occlusions are associated with AV block occurring in the AV node. If the RCA is blocked, ischemia may develop in the AV node. As a result of this ischemia, there can be a disturbance in the balance between the parasympathetic and sympathetic divisions of the autonomic nervous system, resulting in an increase in parasympathetic tone. Once parasympathetic tone increases, conduction through the AV node is slowed. This slowing may manifest itself as a prolonged PR interval or as dropped beats (Figure 3-58).

What Do I Do About It?

The patient with this type of AV block is usually asymptomatic because the ventricular rate often remains nearly normal, and cardiac output is not significantly affected. If the patient is symptomatic and the rhythm is a result of medications, these substances should be withheld. If the heart rate is slow and serious signs and symptoms occur because of the slow rate, consider atropine and/or temporary pacing. When associated with an acute inferior wall MI, this dysrhythmia is usually transient. It usually resolves within 48 to 72 hours as the effects of parasympathetic stimulation disappear. When this rhythm occurs in conjunction with acute MI, the patient should be observed for increasing AV block.

TABLE 3-26	Characteristics of Second-Degree AV Block Type I
Rate	Atrial rate is greater than the ventricular rate.
Rhythm	Atrial regular (Ps plot through on time), ventricular irregular.
P waves	Normal in size and shape. Some P waves are not followed by a QRS complex (more Ps than QRSs).
PR interval	**Lengthens with each cycle** (although lengthening may be very slight), until a P wave appears without a QRS complex. The PRI *after* the nonconducted beat is shorter than the interval preceding the nonconducted beat.
QRS duration	Usually 0.10 sec or less but is periodically dropped.

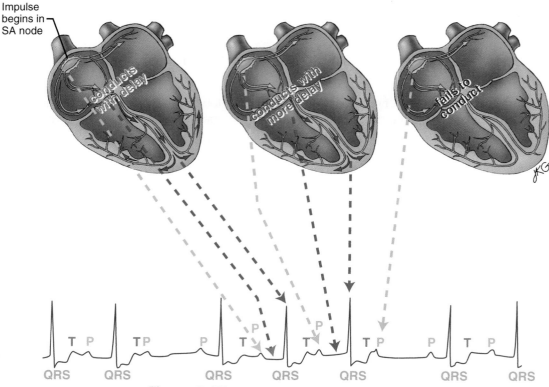

Impulse begins in SA node

Figure 3-57 • Second-degree AV block, type I.

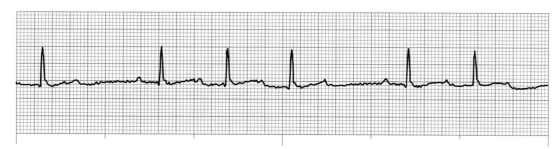

Figure 3-58 • Second-degree AV block, type I.

KEEPING IT SIMPLE

AV blocks that occur in the AV node usually produce a narrow QRS complex (just as a junctional rhythm does) and an AV block in the bundle branches usually produces a wide QRS complex (just as a ventricular rhythm does). Although there are exceptions to this rule, it is a useful hint when determining the site of an AV block.[1]

Second-Degree AV Block, Type II (Mobitz Type II)

Second-degree AV block type II is also called Mobitz Type II AV block. The conduction delay in second-degree AV block type II occurs below the AV node, either at the bundle of His or, more commonly, at the level of the bundle branches (Figure 3-59). This type of block is more serious than second-degree AV block type I and often progresses to third-degree AV block (Table 3-27).

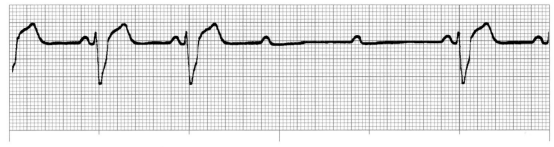

Figure 3-59 • Second-degree AV block, type II.

TABLE 3-27	Characteristics of Second-Degree AV Block, Type II
Rate	Atrial rate is greater than the ventricular rate. Ventricular rate is often slow.
Rhythm	Atrial regular (Ps plot through on time), ventricular irregular.
P waves	Normal in size and shape. Some P waves are not followed by a QRS complex (more Ps than QRSs).
PR interval	Within normal limits or slightly prolonged but *constant* for the conducted beats. There may be some shortening of the PR interval that follows a nonconducted P wave.
QRS duration	Usually 0.10 sec or greater, periodically absent after P waves.

What Causes It?

The bundle branches receive their primary blood supply from the LCA. Thus, disease of the LCA or an anterior MI is usually associated with blocks that occur within the bundle branches. Second-degree AV block type II may also occur because of acute myocarditis or other types of organic heart disease.

What Do I Do About It?

Preparations should be made for pacing when this rhythm is recognized. The use of atropine should be avoided. In this situation, atropine will usually not improve the block but will increase the rate of discharge of the SA node. This may trigger a situation in which even fewer impulses are conducted through to the ventricles and the ventricular rate is further slowed.

Second-Degree AV Block, 2:1 Conduction (2:1 AV Block)

In 2:1 AV block, two P waves occur for every one QRS complex (2:1 conduction). Because there are no two-PQRST cycles in a row from which to compare PR intervals, the decision as to what to term the rhythm is based on the width of the QRS complex. A 2:1 AV block associated with a narrow QRS complex (0.10 sec or less) usually represents a form of second-degree AV block, type I (Figure 3-60, Table 3-28). A 2:1 AV block associated with wide QRS complexes (greater than 0.10 sec) is usually associated with a delay in conduction below the bundle of His; thus, it is usually a type II block (Figure 3-61). The causes are those of type I or type II block previously described. A comparison of the types of second-degree AV blocks is shown in Figure 3-62.

TABLE 3-28	Characteristics of Second-Degree AV Block 2:1 Conduction (2:1 AV Block)
Rate	Atrial rate is twice the ventricular rate.
Rhythm	Atrial regular (Ps plot through). Ventricular regular.
P waves	Normal in size and shape; every other P wave is followed by a QRS complex (more Ps than QRSs).
PR interval	Constant.
QRS duration	Within normal limits, if the block occurs above the bundle of His (probably type I); wide if the block occurs below the bundle of His (probably type II); absent after every other P wave.

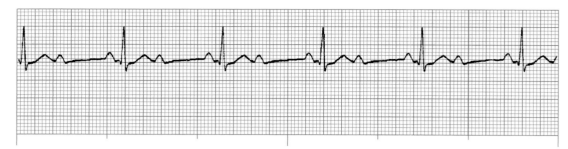

Figure 3-60 • Second-degree AV block, 2:1 conduction, probably type I.

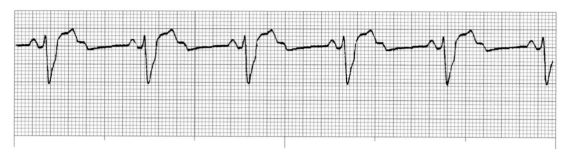

Figure 3-61 • Second-degree AV block, 2:1 conduction, probably type II.

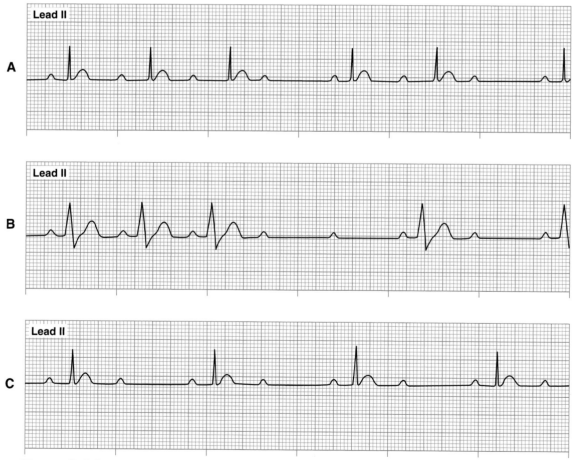

Figure 3-62 • Types of second-degree AV block. **A,** Second-degree AV block type I. **B,** Second-degree AV block type II. **C,** 2:1 AV block.

THIRD-DEGREE ATRIOVENTRICULAR BLOCK

In third-degree AV block, impulses generated by the SA node are blocked before reaching the ventricles so no P waves are conducted (Table 3-29). The atria and ventricles beat independently of each other. Thus, third-degree AV block is also called *complete AV block.* The block may occur at the AV node, bundle of His, or bundle branches (Figure 3-63). A secondary pacemaker (either junctional or ventricular) stimulates the ventricles; therefore, the QRS may be narrow or wide, depending on the location of the escape pacemaker and the condition of the intraventricular conduction system.

What Causes It?

Third-degree AV block associated with an inferior MI is thought to be the result of a block above the bundle of His. It often occurs after progression from first-degree AV block or second-degree AV block type I. The resulting rhythm is usually stable because the escape pacemaker is usually junctional (narrow QRS complexes) with a ventricular rate of more than 40 bpm (Figure 3-64).

TABLE 3-29	Characteristics of Third-Degree AV Block
Rate	Atrial rate is greater than the ventricular rate. The ventricular rate is determined by the origin of the escape rhythm.
Rhythm	Atrial regular (Ps plot through). Ventricular regular. There is no relationship between the atrial and ventricular rhythms.
P waves	Normal in size and shape.
PR interval	*None*—the atria and ventricles beat independently of each other, thus there is no true PR interval.
QRS duration	Narrow or wide depending on the location of the escape pacemaker and the condition of the intraventricular conduction system. Narrow = junctional pacemaker, wide = ventricular pacemaker.

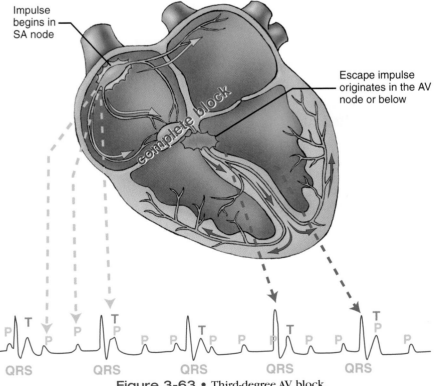

Figure 3-63 • Third-degree AV block.

Third-degree AV block associated with an anterior MI is usually preceded by second-degree AV block type II or an intraventricular conduction delay (right or left BBB). The resulting rhythm is usually unstable because the escape pacemaker is usually ventricular (wide QRS complexes) with a ventricular rate of less than 40 bpm (Figure 3-65).

What Do I Do About It?

The patient's signs and symptoms will depend on the origin of the escape pacemaker (junctional versus ventricular) and the patient's response to a slower ventricular rate. If the QRS is narrow and the patient is symptomatic due to the slow rate, initial management consists of atropine and/or transcutaneous pacing. If the QRS is wide and the patient is symptomatic due to the slow rate, transcutaneous pacing should be instituted while preparations are made for insertion of a transvenous pacemaker.

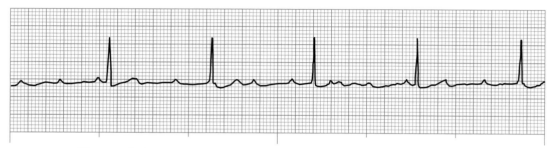

Figure 3-64 • Third-degree AV block with a junctional escape pacemaker.

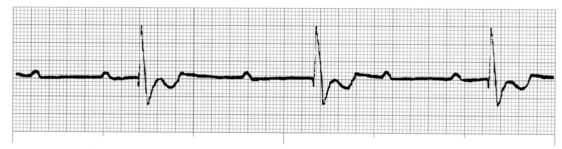

Figure 3-65 • Third-degree AV block with a ventricular escape pacemaker.

QUICK REVIEW 3-15

1. Describe the most significant ECG characteristics of second-degree AV block type I.

2. True or False. In a third-degree AV block, the QRS may be wide or narrow depending on the location of the escape pacemaker and the condition of the intraventricular conduction system.

3. Second-degree AV block type I is most commonly associated with a(n) _____ MI.

4. Which AV block is characterized by a PR interval greater than 0.20 second and one P wave for each QRS complex?

5. Which AV block may progress to a third-degree AV block without warning?

SECTION 4

Cardiac Arrest: Absent/Pulseless Rhythms

KEEPING IT SIMPLE

Cardiac Arrest Rhythms
- VF
- (Pulseless) ventricular tachycardia
- Asystole
- PEA

VENTRICULAR FIBRILLATION

VF is a chaotic rhythm that begins in the ventricles. In VF, there is no organized depolarization of the ventricles (Figures 3-66, 3-67). The ventricular muscle quivers. As a result, there is no effective myocardial contraction and no pulse (Table 3-30).

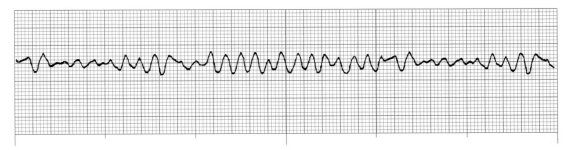

Figure 3-66 • VF with waves that are 3 mm high or more is called "coarse" VF.

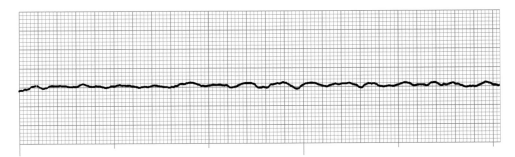

Figure 3-67 • VF with low-amplitude waves (<3 mm) is called "fine" VF.

TABLE 3-30	Characteristics of Ventricular Fibrillation
Rate	Cannot be determined because there are no discernible waves or complexes to measure
Rhythm	Rapid and chaotic with no pattern or regularity
P waves	Not discernible
PR interval	Not discernible
QRS duration	Not discernible

WHAT CAUSES IT?

Factors that increase the susceptibility of the myocardium to fibrillate include the following:
- Increased sympathetic nervous system activity
- Vagal stimulation
- Electrolyte imbalance
- Antiarrhythmics and other medications
- Environmental factors (e.g., electrocution)
- Hypertrophy
- Acute coronary syndromes
- Heart failure
- Dysrhythmias

WHAT DO I DO ABOUT IT?

Because no drugs used in cardiac arrest have been shown to improve survival to hospital discharge, the priorities of care in cardiac arrest due to pulseless VT or VF are CPR and defibrillation (see Chapters 4 and 8).

VENTRICULAR TACHYCARDIA

Monomorphic VT and polymorphic VT have already been discussed. If either of these rhythms presents without a pulse, the rhythm is treated as VF.

ASYSTOLE (CARDIAC STANDSTILL)

Asystole is a total absence of ventricular electrical activity (Figure 3-68). There is no ventricular rate or rhythm, no pulse, and no cardiac output. Some atrial electrical activity may be evident. If atrial electrical activity is present, the rhythm is called "P-wave" asystole or ventricular standstill (Figure 3-69, Table 3-31).

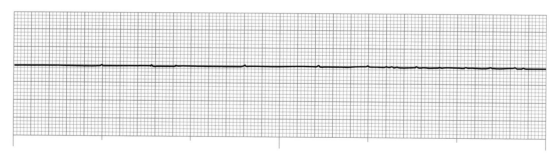

Figure 3-68 • Asystole.

TABLE 3-31	Characteristics of Asystole	
Rate	Ventricular usually not discernible but atrial activity may be observed ("P-wave" asystole)	
Rhythm	Ventricular not discernible, atrial may be discernible	
P waves	Usually not discernible	
PR interval	Not measurable	
QRS duration	Absent	

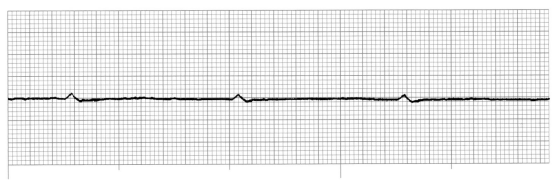

Figure 3-69 • "P-wave" asystole.

WHAT CAUSES IT?

Use the memory aids "PATCH-4-MD" and "The 5 H's and 5 T's" to recall possible treatable causes of cardiac arrest. In addition, ventricular asystole may occur temporarily following termination of a tachycardia with medications, defibrillation, or synchronized cardioversion (Figure 3-70).

WHAT DO I DO ABOUT IT?

Confirm there is no pulse, begin immediate CPR, and confirm the rhythm in two leads. If the rhythm is confirmed as asystole, additional care includes starting an IV, considering the possible causes of the arrest, possible insertion of an advanced airway, epinephrine, and atropine.

PULSELESS ELECTRICAL ACTIVITY

Pulseless electrical activity (PEA) is a clinical situation, not a specific dysrhythmia. PEA exists when organized electrical activity (other than VT) is observed on the cardiac monitor, but the patient is unresponsive, not breathing, and a pulse cannot be felt (Figure 3-71). PEA was formerly called EMD (electromechanical dissociation). The term was changed from EMD to PEA because research using ultrasonography and indwelling pressure catheters revealed that the electrical activity seen in some of these situations *is* associated with mechanical contractions—the contractions are simply too weak to produce a palpable pulse or measurable blood pressure.

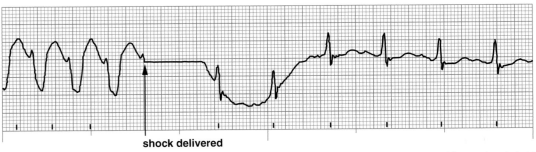

shock delivered

Figure 3-70 • This rhythm strip is from a 62-year-old man complaining of palpitations. The patient's initial rhythm was monomorphic VT. A synchronized shock was delivered, resulting in a sinus rhythm with a prolonged PR interval.

KEEPING IT SIMPLE

PATCH-4-MD

Pulmonary embolism
Acidosis
Tension pneumothorax
Cardiac tamponade
Hypovolemia
Hypoxia
Heat/cold (hypo-/hyperthermia)
Hypo-/hyperkalemia (and other electrolytes)
Myocardial infarction
Drug overdose / accidents

Five H's and Five T's

Hypovolemia	Tamponade, cardiac
Hypoxia	Tension pneumothorax
Hypothermia	Thrombosis: lungs (massive pulmonary embolism)
Hypo-/hyperkalemia	Thrombosis: heart (acute coronary syndromes)
Hydrogen ion (acidosis)	Tablets/toxins: drug overdose

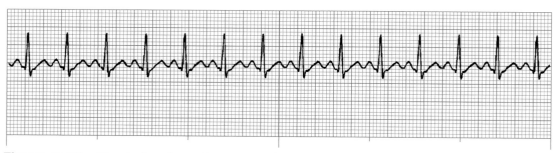

Figure 3-71 • The rhythm shown is a sinus tachycardia; however, if no pulse is associated with the rhythm, the clinical situation is termed *PEA*.

WHAT CAUSES IT?

Use the memory aids "PATCH-4-MD" and "The 5 H's and 5 T's" to recall possible treatable causes of cardiac arrest.

WHAT DO I DO ABOUT IT?

PEA has a poor prognosis unless the underlying cause can be rapidly identified and appropriately managed. Treatment includes CPR, O₂, IV access, possible insertion of an advanced airway, giving epinephrine (and atropine if the rate is slow), and an aggressive search for possible causes of the situation.

QUICK REVIEW 3-16

1. What is the name given to the clinical situation in which organized electrical activity (other than VT) is observed on the cardiac monitor, but the patient has no pulse?

2. True or False. VT is an essentially regular ventricular rhythm with a ventricular rate of more than 100 bpm.

3. _____ _____ _____ is a type of polymorphic VT associated with a prolonged QT interval.

SECTION 5
Premature Beats and Pacemaker Rhythms

PREMATURE BEATS
PREMATURE ATRIAL COMPLEXES

What Causes It?

Common causes of PACs include emotional stress, heart failure, myocardial ischemia or injury, mental and physical fatigue, atrial enlargement, digitalis toxicity, hypokalemia, hypomagnesemia, hyperthyroidism, and excessive intake of caffeine or tobacco (Figure 3-72, Table 3-32).

What Do I Do About It?

PACs usually do not require treatment if they are infrequent. In susceptible individuals, frequent PACs may set off episodes of atrial fibrillation, atrial flutter, or PSVT. Frequent PACs are treated by correcting the underlying cause.

The term *complex* is used instead of *contraction* to correctly identify an early beat because the ECG depicts electrical activity, not mechanical function of the heart. Some prefer the term *conduction* instead of complex.

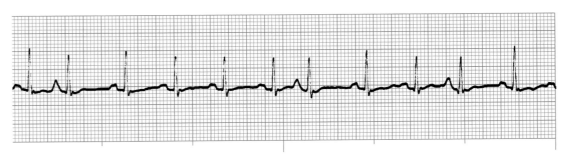

Figure 3-72 • Sinus tachycardia with three PACs. From the left, beats 2, 7, and 10 are PACs.

TABLE 3-32	Characteristics of Premature Atrial Complexes
Rate	Usually within normal range, but depends on underlying rhythm.
Rhythm	Regular with premature beats.
P waves	Premature (occurring earlier than the next expected sinus P wave), positive (upright) in lead II, one before each QRS complex, often differ in shape from sinus P waves—may be flattened, notched, pointed, biphasic, or lost in the preceding T wave.
PR interval	May be normal or prolonged depending on the prematurity of the beat.
QRS duration	Usually 0.10 sec or less but may be wide (aberrant) or absent, depending on the prematurity of the beat. The QRS of the PAC is similar in shape to those of the underlying rhythm unless the PAC is abnormally conducted.

PREMATURE JUNCTIONAL COMPLEXES

What Causes It?

There are many causes of PJCs, including excessive caffeine, tobacco, or alcohol intake; valvular disease, ischemia, heart failure, digitalis toxicity, increased vagal tone, acute MI, hypoxia, electrolyte imbalance (particularly magnesium and potassium), exercise, and rheumatic heart disease (Figure 3-73, Table 3-33).

What Do I Do About It?

Most people with PJCs do not have symptoms. However, PJCs may lead to symptoms of palpitations or the feeling of skipped beats. Lightheadedness, dizziness, and other signs of decreased cardiac output can occur if PJCs are frequent.

PJCs do not normally require treatment. If PJCs occur because of ingestion of stimulants or digitalis toxicity, these substances should be withheld.

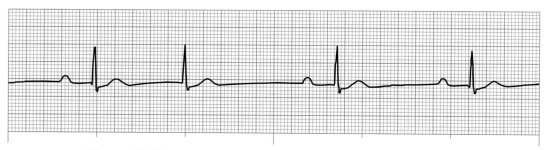

Figure 3-73 • Sinus bradycardia with first-degree AV block and a PJC.

TABLE 3-33	Characteristics of Premature Junctional Complexes
Rate	Usually within normal range, but depends on underlying rhythm.
Rhythm	Regular with premature beats.
P waves	May occur before, during, or after the QRS. If visible, the P wave is inverted in leads II, III, and aVF.
PR interval	If a P wave occurs before the QRS, the PR interval will usually be ≤0.12 sec. If no P wave occurs before the QRS, there will be no PR interval.
QRS duration	Usually 0.10 sec or less unless an intraventricular conduction delay exists.

PREMATURE VENTRICULAR COMPLEXES

What Causes It?

PVCs may be a normal variant or due to hypoxia, stress, anxiety, exercise. digitalis toxicity, acid-base imbalance, myocardial ischemia, electrolyte imbalance, heart failure, increased sympathetic tone, acute coronary syndromes, stimulants (caffeine, tobacco), or medications (sympathomimetics, cyclic antidepressants, phenothiazines) (Table 3-34).

TABLE 3-34	Characteristics of Premature Ventricular Complexes
Rate	Usually within normal range, but depends on underlying rhythm
Rhythm	Essentially regular with premature beats
P waves	Usually absent or, with retrograde conduction to the atria, may appear after the QRS (usually upright in the ST-segment or T wave)
PR interval	None with the PVC because the ectopic originates in the ventricles
QRS duration	>0.12 sec, wide, and bizarre, T wave frequently in opposite direction of the QRS complex

What Do I Do About It?

Patients experiencing PVCs may be asymptomatic or complain of palpitations, a "racing heart," skipped beats, or chest or neck discomfort. Treatment of PVCs focuses on treatment of the underlying cause. In the setting of an acute coronary syndrome, treatment is directed at ensuring adequate oxygenation, relieving pain, and rapidly identifying and correcting hypoxia, heart failure, and electrolyte or acid-base abnormalities. Examples of PVCs are shown in Figures 3-74 through 3-77.

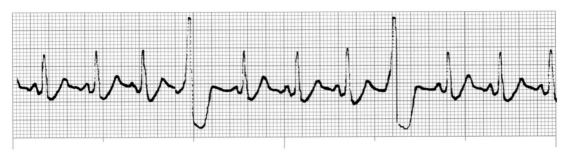

Figure 3-74 • Premature ventricular beats that look alike in the same lead and begin from the same anatomic site (focus) are called uniform PVCs. This rhythm strip shows a sinus tachycardia with frequent uniform PVCs.

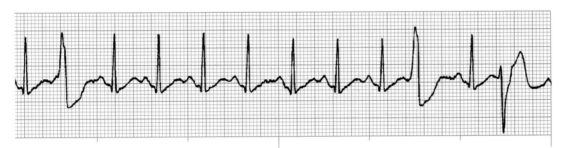

Figure 3-75 • PVCs that look different from one another in the same lead are called multiform PVCs. This rhythm strip shows a sinus tachycardia with multiform PVCs.

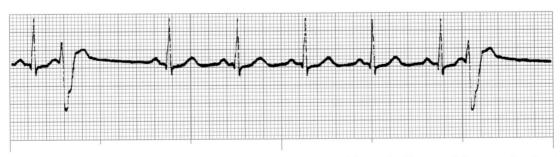

Figure 3-76 • R-on-T PVCs occur when the R wave of a PVC falls on the T wave of the preceding beat. This rhythm strip shows a sinus rhythm with two R-on-T PVCs.

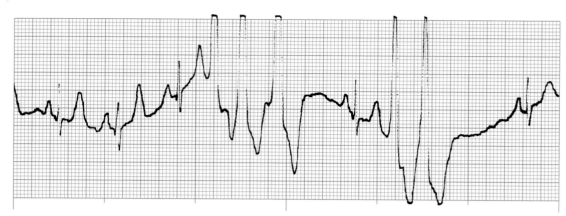

Figure 3-77 • Two PVCs in a row are called a couplet or paired PVCs. The appearance of couplets indicates that the ventricular ectopic site is very irritable. Three or more PVCs in a row at a rate of more than 100 bpm are considered a "salvo," "run," or "burst" of VT. This rhythm shows a sinus rhythm with a run of VT and one episode of couplets.

 PVCs may occur in patterns:
- Pairs (couplets): two PVCs in a row.
- "Runs" or "bursts": three or more PVCs in a row.
- Bigeminal PVCs (ventricular bigeminy): every other beat is a PVC.
- Trigeminal PVCs (ventricular trigeminy): every third beat is a PVC.
- Quadrigeminal PVCs (ventricular quadrigeminy): every fourth beat is a PVC.

PREMATURE BEATS—COMPARISON

A comparison of premature beats is shown in Fig. 3-78.

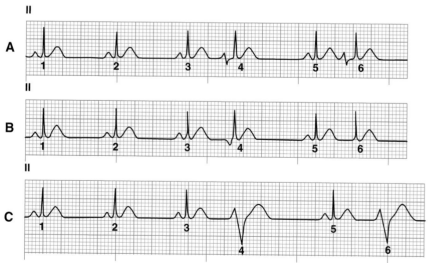

Figure 3-78 • Premature beats. **A,** Sinus rhythm with PACs. The fourth and sixth beats are preceded by premature P waves that look different from the normally conducted sinus beats. Note that the QRS complex that follows each of these PACs is narrow and identical in appearance to that of the sinus-conducted beats. **B,** Sinus rhythm with PJCs. The fourth and sixth beats are PJCs. Beat 4 is preceded by an inverted P wave with a short PR interval. There is no identifiable atrial activity associated with beat 6. **C,** Sinus rhythm with PVCs. The fourth and sixth beats do not have P waves and look very different from the sinus beats. Beats 4 and 6 are PVCs.

PACEMAKER RHYTHMS

ATRIAL PACING

■ A pacing electrode is placed in the right atrium.
■ Produces a pacemaker spike followed by a P wave (Figure 3-79).
■ May be used when the SA node is diseased or damaged but conduction through the AV junction and ventricles is normal.
■ Ineffective if an AV block develops because it cannot pace the ventricles.

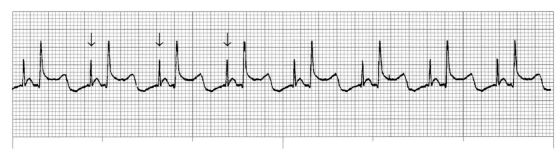

Figure 3-79 • Atrial pacing. *Arrows* indicate pacer spikes.

VENTRICULAR PACING

■ Accomplished by placing a pacing electrode in the right ventricle.
■ Stimulation of the ventricles produces a pacemaker spike on the ECG followed by a wide QRS, resembling a ventricular ectopic beat (Figure 3-80).
■ QRS complex is wide because a paced impulse does not follow the normal conduction pathway in the heart.

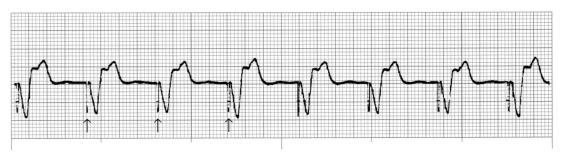

Figure 3-80 • Ventricular pacing. *Arrows* indicate pacer spikes.

DUAL-CHAMBER PACING

- A dual-chamber pacemaker paces both the atrium and the ventricle.
- Two-lead system placed in the heart
  - One lead is placed in the right atrium.
  - A second lead is placed in the right ventricle.
- AV sequential pacemaker is an example of a dual-chamber pacemaker.
  - This stimulates the right atrium and right ventricle sequentially (stimulating first the atrium, then the ventricle) (Figure 3-81).
  - This mimics normal cardiac physiology and preserves the atrial contribution to ventricular filling (atrial kick).

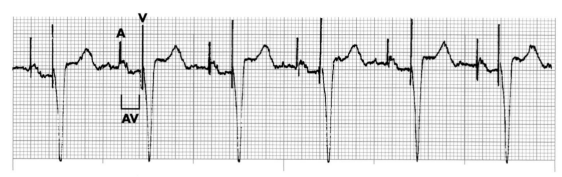

Figure 3-81 • AV sequential pacing. *A,* Atrial pacing; *V,* ventricular pacing; *AV,* AV interval.

QUICK REVIEW ANSWERS

Quick Review Number	Answers
3-1	Cardiac rhythms can be classified into four main groups: normal, absent (cardiac arrest rhythms), slower than normal for age (bradycardia), or faster than normal for age (tachycardia).
3-2	1. Right 2. Left anterior descending 3. Lateral 4. False. Blockage of the septal branch of the left anterior descending can result in a septal MI.
3-3	1. Myocardial (working) cells (also known as mechanical cells) are found in the myocardium. These cells contain contractile filaments that contract when the cells are electrically stimulated. Electrical (pacemaker) cells are found in the electrical conduction system. Their primary function is generation and conduction of electrical impulses. 2. Automaticity is the ability of pacemaker cells to spontaneously initiate an electrical impulse without being stimulated from another source (such as a nerve). 3. No. Depolarization is an electrical event. Contraction is a mechanical event.

3-4

Lead	Heart Surface Viewed	Lead	Heart Surface Viewed
Lead I	Lateral	V_1	Septum
Lead II	Inferior	V_2	Septum
Lead III	Inferior	V_3	Anterior
aVR	None	V_4	Anterior
aVL	Lateral	V_5	Lateral
aVF	Inferior	V_6	Lateral

3-5	1. Positive 2. Leads II, III, and aVF 3. V_3 and V_4 4. Lead I, aVL, V_5, V_6 5. Horizontal/transverse
3-6	1. Left leg 2. 0.04 second 3. Five 4. One millimeter
3-7	1. Ventricular repolarization 2. 0.06 to 0.10 second 3. Myocardial ischemia 4. True 5. False. The R wave is always a positive waveform.
3-8	1. Segment 2. P wave 3. Interval 4. 0.12 to 0.20 second 5. The PR interval is measured from the beginning of the P wave to the beginning of the QRS complex.
3-9	1. Ventricular depolarization 2. ST-segment 3. TP or PR-segment 4. Total ventricular activity—the time from ventricular depolarization (stimulation) to repolarization (recovery) 5. Myocardial injury
3-10	1. 100 2. 120

3-11

1. Assess the rate 2. Assess rhythm/regularity 3. Identify and examine P waves 4. Assess intervals (evaluate conduction— PR interval, QRS duration, QT interval) 5. Evaluate overall appearance of the rhythm (ST-segment elevation/depression, T-wave inversion) 6. Interpret rhythm and evaluate clinical significance

3-12

1. True 2. 60 to 100 bpm 3. Amplitude/voltage 4. Sinus arrhythmia 5. AV junction 6. Positive (upright) in lead II, one precedes each QRS

3-13

1. Atrial flutter 2. During this period, most (but not all) cardiac cells have repolarized and can be stimulated to depolarize if a stimulus is strong enough. Should a stimulus precipitate depolarization during this period, chaos may result. 3. Measure the distance between two consecutive R-R intervals and compare that distance with another R-R interval. If the ventricular rhythm is regular, the R-R intervals will measure the same. 4. In atrial fibrillation, the atria are not contracting, they are quivering. This produces an erratic, wavy baseline (fibrillatory waves) on the ECG. P waves are not visible. 5. Decreased stroke volume, decreased cardiac output 6. WPW syndrome

3-14

1. Digitalis 2. Inverted P wave precedes the QRS complex in leads II, III, and aVF

3-15

1. Irregular ventricular rhythm, more P waves than QRSs, P waves occur on time, progressive lengthening of the PR interval until a P wave appears without a QRS after it. Cycle repeats. 2. True 3. Inferior wall 4. First degree 5. Second-degree AV block type II

3-16

1. PEA 2. True 3. Torsades de pointes

STOP & REVIEW

1. Which of the following are the main branches of the LCA?
   a. Circumflex and marginal arteries
   b. Anterior descending and oblique arteries
   c. Circumflex and anterior descending arteries
   d. Marginal and oblique arteries

2. The most common type of paroxysmal SVA is
   a. AV reentrant tachycardia
   b. AV nodal reentrant tachycardia
   c. Atrial tachycardia
   d. Ventricular escape rhythm

3. Complete the following table:

	Sinus Bradycardia	Junctional Rhythm	Ventricular Escape Rhythm
Rate			
Rhythm			
P Waves (lead II)			
PR Interval			
QRS			

4. The R wave
   a. Is the first negative deflection after the P wave
   b. Is the second negative deflection after the P wave
   c. May be a positive or negative waveform that follows the P wave
   d. Is the first positive deflection after the P wave

5. Three or more PVCs occurring in a row at a rate of more than 100/min is called:
   a. Ventricular bigeminy
   b. A run of VT
   c. Accelerated idioventricular rhythm
   d. A run of ventricular trigeminy

6. Select the *incorrect* statement regarding vagal maneuvers.
   a. Simultaneous bilateral carotid pressure is applied to make sure the heart rate slows
   b. Carotid sinus pressure should be avoided in older patients
   c. Carotid sinus pressure should be avoided if carotid bruits are present
   d. An ECG monitor should be used when carotid sinus pressure is performed

7. Which of the following dysrhythmias has the greatest potential for sudden, third-degree AV block?
   a. Junctional rhythm
   b. Second-degree AV block, type II
   c. First-degree AV block
   d. Sinus bradycardia

8. On the ECG, the P wave represents _____ depolarization and the QRS complex represents _____ depolarization

9. Complete the following table about types of cardiac cells

Kinds of Cardiac Cells	Where Found	Primary Function	Primary Property
Myocardial Cells			
Pacemaker Cells			

10. Match the following parts of the cardiac cycle with its description.

Component of the Cardiac Cycle

___ R wave
___ PR-segment

___ PR interval

___ QT interval

___ P wave

___ TP-segment
___ S wave

___ QRS complex

___ ST-segment

Description

a) This is *always* negative (below the baseline)
b) Portion of the ECG tracing between the end of the T wave and the beginning of the following P wave
c) Horizontal line between the end of the P wave and the beginning of the QRS complex
d) Portion of the ECG tracing between the QRS complex and the T wave
e) First positive deflection (above the baseline) in the QRS complex
f) Normally measures 0.12 to 0.20 second in adults
g) Represents the spread of an electrical impulse through the ventricles (ventricular depolarization)
h) Represents total ventricular activity—the time from ventricular depolarization (stimulation) to repolarization (recovery)
i) Represents atrial depolarization and the spread of an electrical impulse throughout the right and left atria

11. ST-segment elevation of more than ___ mm in the limb leads or more than ____ mm in the chest leads suggests myocardial injury

12. A delta wave is frequently seen with
   a. Atrial tachycardia
   b. Atrial fibrillation
   c. WPW syndrome
   d. Sinus tachycardia

13. In most adults, the normal QRS complex measures no more than ___ in duration.
   a. 0.04 second
   b. 0.06 second
   c. 0.10 second
   d. 0.14 second

Identify each of the following rhythm strips. All rhythms recorded in lead II unless otherwise noted.

14.

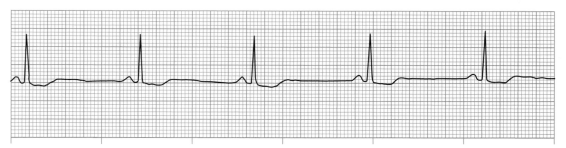

Figure 3-82

Identification _____

15. This rhythm strip is from an 80-year-old woman with chest pain. Her blood pressure is 140/78. She states she had a new pacemaker "installed" 13 days ago.

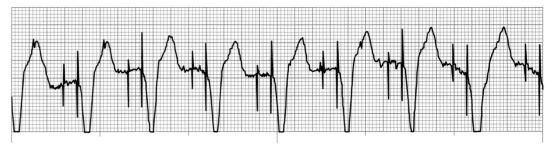

Figure 3-83

Identification _____

16.

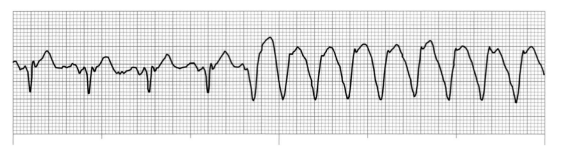

Figure 3-84

Identification _____

17.

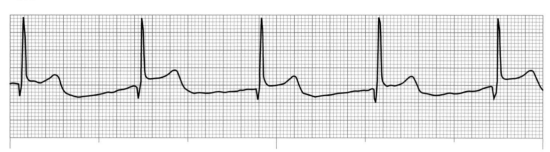

Figure 3-85

18.

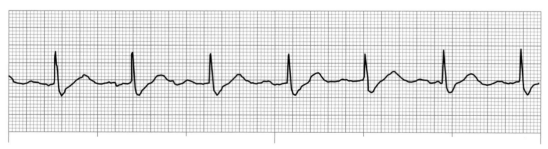

Figure 3-86

Identification _____

19.

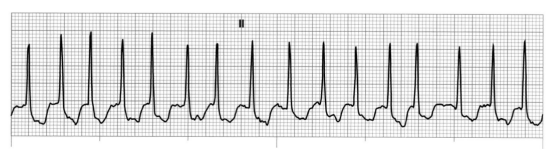

Figure 3-87

Identification _____

20.

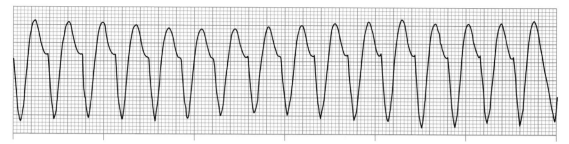

Figure 3-88

Identification _____

21. This rhythm strip is from a 29-year-old woman with a kidney stone.

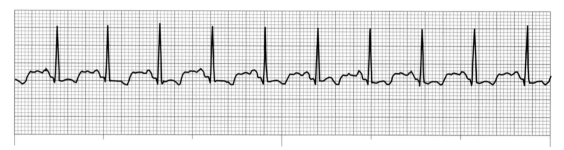

Figure 3-89

Identification _____

22. This rhythm strip is from a 90-year-old unresponsive woman. She has a history of heart failure. Her medications include furosemide and albuterol.

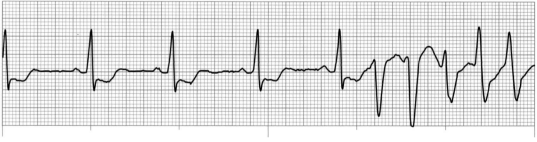

Figure 3-90

Identification _____

23.

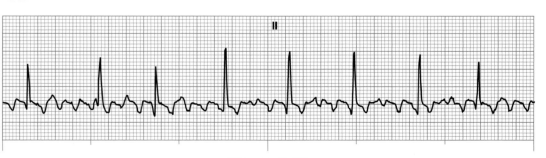

Figure 3-91

Identification _____

24. Complete the following table. Next to each of the numbered leads, indicate the part of the left ventricle that each lead "sees."

I	aVR None	V$_1$	V$_4$
II	aVL	V$_2$	V$_5$
III	aVF	V$_3$	V$_6$

25. Match the following dysrhythmias with their respective ECG characteristics.

Rhythm	ECG Characteristics
___ Third-degree AV block	a) Ventricular rhythm may be regular or irregular, waveforms resembling teeth of a saw or picket fence before QRS
___ Polymorphic VT	b) Regular ventricular rate between 150 and 250 bpm; narrow QRS
___ VF	c) More P waves than QRSs, P waves occur regularly, irregular ventricular rhythm, lengthening PR intervals, QRS usually narrow
___ Idioventricular (ventricular escape) rhythm	d) Early complex characterized by no P wave or an inverted P wave before or after the QRS; QRS usually narrow
___ PAC	e) Rapid rhythm in which the QRS complex is wide and usually regular; QRS complexes are of same shape and amplitude
___ Atrial fibrillation	f) Early complex characterized by no P wave before the QRS; QRS usually wide
___ AVNRT	g) More P waves than QRSs, P waves occur regularly, regular ventricular rhythm, no pattern to PR intervals, QRS narrow or wide
___ Second-degree AV block type I	h) Irregularly irregular rhythm with no normal-looking waveforms; chaotic deflections vary in shape and amplitude
___ PVC	i) One upright P wave before each QRS, ventricular rate 101-180 bpm
___ PJC	j) More P waves than QRSs, P waves occur regularly, irregular ventricular rhythm, constant PR intervals, QRS usually wide
___ Atrial flutter	k) Early complex characterized by an upright P wave before the QRS; QRS usually narrow
___ Monomorphic VT	l) Irregularly irregular ventricular rhythm, no identifiable P waves
___ Second-degree AV block type II	m) Rapid rhythm in which the QRS complexes are wide and appear to twist from upright to negative or negative to upright and back
___ Sinus tachycardia	n) Absent P waves, wide QRS, ventricular rate 40 bpm or less

STOP & REVIEW ANSWERS

1. c. The circumflex and anterior descending are the main branches of the left coronary artery.

2. b. Atrial tachycardia, AVNRT, and AVRT are types of SVT. The most common type of paroxysmal SVT is AVNRT. The next most common is AVRT. A ventricular escape rhythm is a bradycardia (20-40 bpm), not a tachycardia and it is a ventricular (not a supraventricular) rhythm.

3.

	Sinus Bradycardia	Junctional Rhythm	Ventricular Escape Rhythm
Rate	<60 bpm	40-60 bpm	20-40 bpm
Rhythm	Regular.	Regular.	Essentially regular.
P Waves (lead II)	Upright.	May occur before, during, or after the QRS. If visible, the P wave is inverted in leads II, III, and aVF.	Usually absent or, with retrograde conduction to the atria, may appear after the QRS (usually upright in the ST-segment or T wave).
PR Interval	0.12-0.20 sec.	If a P wave is present before the QRS, usually less than or equal to 0.12 sec. If no P wave occurs before the QRS, there will be no PR interval.	None.
QRS	≤0.10 sec unless an intraventricular conduction delay exists.	0.10 sec or less unless an intraventricular conduction delay exists.	>0.12 sec.

4. d. The QRS complex consists of the Q wave, R wave, and S wave and represents the spread of the electrical impulse through the ventricles (ventricular depolarization). The QRS complex begins as a downward deflection, the Q wave. A Q wave is *always* a negative waveform. The QRS complex continues as a large, upright, triangular waveform called the R wave. The S wave is the negative waveform following the R wave. An R wave is *always* positive and an S wave is *always* negative. Thus, the R wave is the first positive deflection after the P wave on the ECG.

5. b. Three or more PVCs occurring in a row at a rate of more than 100/minute is called a salvo, burst, or run of VT.

6. a. When using vagal maneuvers, make sure oxygen, suction, a defibrillator, and emergency medications are available before attempting the procedure. Continuous monitoring of the patient's ECG is essential, and a 12-lead ECG recording is desirable. Carotid sinus pressure should be avoided in older patients and in patients with carotid artery bruits. Simultaneous, bilateral carotid pressure should *never* be performed.

7. b. Second-degree AV block type II is often associated with anteroseptal MI and may progress rapidly to a third-degree AV block.

8. On the ECG, the P wave represents **atrial** depolarization and the QRS complex represents **ventricular** depolarization.

9.

Kinds of Cardiac Cells	Where Found	Primary Function	Primary Property
Myocardial cells	Myocardium	Contraction and relaxation	Contractility
Pacemaker cells	Electrical conduction system	Generation and conduction of electrical impulses	Automaticity Conductivity

10.

Component of the Cardiac Cycle

e   R wave

c   PR-segment

f   PR interval

h   QT interval

i   P wave

b   TP-segment

a   S wave

g   QRS complex

d   ST-segment

11. ST-segment elevation of more than <u>1 mm</u> in the limb leads or more than <u>2 mm</u> in the chest leads suggests myocardial injury.

12. c. A delta wave is often seen with WPW syndrome.

13. c. The normal duration of the QRS complex in an adult varies between 0.06 and 0.10 sec. About half of adults have a QRS duration of 0.08 second. A 0.11-second duration may sometimes be observed in healthy individuals.

14. Sinus bradycardia

15. 100% paced rhythm—AV sequential pacemaker

16. Sinus rhythm to monomorphic VT

17. Junctional rhythm with ST-segment elevation

18. Sinus rhythm with first-degree AV block, ST-segment depression

19. Atrial fibrillation with a rapid ventricular response, ST-segment depression

20. Monomorphic VT

21. Sinus tachycardia with inverted T waves

22. Sinus rhythm with ST-segment depression → polymorphic VT

23. Atrial flutter (controlled ventricular response)

24.

I	Lateral	aVR	------------	V1	Septum	V4	Anterior
II	Inferior	aVL	Lateral	V2	Septum	V5	Lateral
III	Inferior	aVF	Inferior	V3	Anterior	V6	Lateral

25.

Rhythm

g   Third-degree AV block

m   Polymorphic VT

h   VF

n   Idioventricular (ventricular escape) rhythm

k   PAC

l   Atrial fibrillation

b   AVNRT

c   Second-degree AV block type I

f   PVC

d   PJC

a   Atrial flutter

e   Monomorphic VT

j   Second-degree AV block type II

i   Sinus tachycardia

REFERENCES

1. Phalen T, Aehlert B: *The 12-lead ECG in Acute Coronary Syndromes.* St. Louis: 2006, Mosby.
2. Blomström-Lundqvist C, Scheinman MM, Aliot EM, et al: ACC/AHA/ESC guidelines for the management of patients with supraventricular arrhythmias—executive summary: A report of the American College of Cardiology/American Heart Association Task Force on Practice Guidelines, and the European Society of Cardiology Committee for Practice Guidelines (Writing Committee to Develop Guidelines for the Management of Patients with Supraventricular Arrhythmias). *J Am Coll Cardiol* 2003;42:1493-1531.
3. Crawford MV, Spence MI: *Common Sense Approach to Coronary Care,* 6th ed. St. Louis: 1995, Mosby-Year Book.
4. Barold SS: Indications for permanent cardiac pacing in first-degree AV block: Class I, II, or III? *Pacing Clin Electrophysiol* 1996;19:747-751.

Electrical Therapy

OBJECTIVES

Upon completion of this chapter, you will be able to:

1. Explain defibrillation and name three indications for this procedure.
2. Describe four factors affecting transthoracic resistance.
3. Describe proper placement of hand-held defibrillator paddles or self-adhesive monitoring/defibrillation pads.
4. Discuss monophasic and biphasic defibrillation.
5. Describe the procedure for defibrillation.
6. Explain synchronized cardioversion and name three indications for this procedure.
7. Describe the differences in the delivery of energy relative to the cardiac cycle with synchronized cardioversion and defibrillation.
8. Describe the procedure for synchronized cardioversion.
9. For each of the following rhythms, identify the energy levels currently recommended and indicate if the shock delivered should be a synchronized or unsynchronized countershock:
   - Pulseless ventricular tachycardia (VT)/ventricular fibrillation (VF)
   - Monomorphic VT
   - Polymorphic VT
   - Narrow-QRS tachycardia
   - Atrial fibrillation with a rapid ventricular response
   - Atrial flutter with a rapid ventricular response
10. Differentiate between a fully automated external defibrillator (AED) and a semiautomated external defibrillator.
11. List the steps in the operation of an automated external defibrillator.
12. Explain the precautions that should be taken when defibrillating a patient with a permanent pacemaker or an implantable cardioverter-defibrillator.
13. Discuss indications for transcutaneous pacing.
14. List possible complications of transcutaneous pacing.

INTRODUCTION

Electrical therapies used in the management of a cardiac emergency may include defibrillation, synchronized cardioversion, and transcutaneous pacing. Defibrillation may be performed using an automated external defibrillator (AED) or a manual defibrillator. Using an AED is an important part of basic life support that may be performed by laypersons and healthcare professionals. Using a manual defibrillator and performing synchronized cardioversion or transcutaneous pacing are advanced life support skills.

In this chapter, we discuss types of electrical therapies, when electrical therapy is indicated, and the steps needed to safely perform each procedure.

INTERVENTIONS BEFORE DEFIBRILLATION
PRECORDIAL THUMP

A **precordial thump** (also called "thump version") is a forceful blow delivered to the lower half of an adult's sternum (but above the xiphoid process) to terminate ventricular tachycardia (VT) or ventricular fibrillation (VF). Use of this technique is controversial. There is some evidence that VT has been converted to a sinus rhythm with this technique.[1,2] However, there are also reports that the rate of VT accelerated,[3] VT converted to asystole or pulseless electrical activity (PEA),[2] or the precordial thump had no effect.[4]

Precordial Thump—Possible Complications
- Rate acceleration of VT
- Conversion of VT into VF
- Complete AV block
- Asystole

The 2005 American Heart Association guidelines make no recommendation for or against the use of the precordial thump by ACLS providers.[5] However, the 2005 International Liaison Committee on Resuscitation (ILCOR) guidelines indicate that one precordial thump may be considered after a monitored cardiac arrest if a defibrillator is not immediately available.[6] (A monitored cardiac arrest means that the patient is on a cardiac monitor.)

When performed, a single precordial thump is delivered to the lower half of the sternum (but above the xiphoid process) of an adult. A clenched fist delivers the thump from a height of about 8 inches (Figure 4-1). After delivery of a precordial thump, recheck the patient's pulse and rhythm.

KEEPING IT SIMPLE

A precordial thump
- Should *never* delay defibrillation.
- May be considered in a monitored cardiac arrest if a defibrillator is not immediately available.
- Should only be performed by healthcare professionals trained in the technique.
- Should not be performed in infants and children.
- Should not be taught to lay rescuers.

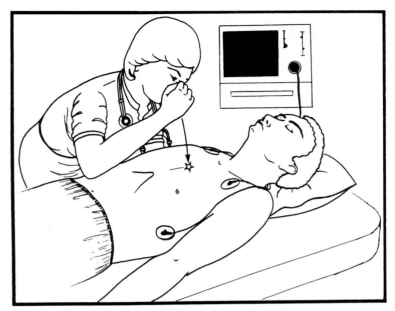

Figure 4-1 • Precordial thump.

COUGH VERSION

Cough version (also called "cough CPR") is forceful and repetitive coughing. A small number of case reports have shown that repeated coughing every 1 to 3 seconds during episodes of sustained torsades de pointes, VT, VF, and asystole can maintain a mean arterial pressure of more than 100 mm Hg and maintain consciousness for up to 90 seconds.[7,8] At the onset of the abnormal rhythm (and before consciousness is lost), the patient is instructed to cough hard and keep coughing.

At this time, no data support the usefulness of cough CPR in any setting other than the cardiac catheterization laboratory, and there is no specific evidence for or against use of cough CPR by laypersons in unsupervised settings.[9]

DEFIBRILLATION

KEEPING IT SIMPLE

Defibrillation—Indications
- Pulseless VT
- VF
- Sustained polymorphic VT

DEFINITION AND PURPOSE

Defibrillation is delivery of an electrical current across the heart muscle over a very brief period to terminate an abnormal heart rhythm. Defibrillation is also called unsynchronized countershock or asynchronous countershock because the delivery of current has no relationship to the cardiac cycle. Indications for defibrillation include sustained polymorphic VT, pulseless VT, and VF.

Manual defibrillation refers to the placement of paddles or pads on a patient's chest, interpretation of the patient's cardiac rhythm by a trained healthcare professional, and the healthcare professional's decision to deliver a shock (if indicated). **Automated external defibrillation** refers to the placement of paddles or pads on a patient's chest and interpretation of the patient's cardiac rhythm by the defibrillator's computerized analysis system. Depending on the type of AED used, the machine will deliver a shock (if a shockable rhythm is detected) or instruct the operator to deliver a shock. AEDs are discussed in more detail later in this chapter.

Defibrillation does not "jump start" the heart. The shock attempts to deliver a uniform electrical current of sufficient intensity to depolarize ventricular cells (including fibrillating cells) at the same time, causing momentary asystole. This provides an opportunity for the heart's natural pacemakers to resume normal activity. When the cells repolarize, the pacemaker with the highest degree of automaticity should assume responsibility for pacing the heart. Although the goal of defibrillation is to restore spontaneous circulation, the shock delivered is considered successful if there is an absence of VF/VT for at least 5 seconds after shock delivery.[10,11]

KEEPING IT SIMPLE

Defibrillation and CPR are the most important treatments for the patient in cardiac arrest due to pulseless VT or VF.

ENERGY, VOLTAGE, AND CURRENT

A **defibrillator** is a device used to deliver a shock to eliminate an abnormal heart rhythm (Figure 4-2). It consists of the following:

- A capacitor that stores energy (electrons) at a particular voltage. Think of voltage as the electrical pressure that drives a flow of electrons (current) through a defibrillator circuit (such as the chest).
- An energy select button or dial. The shocks used for defibrillation and cardioversion are expressed in **joules (J)** of energy.
- A charge switch/button that allows the capacitor to charge.
- Discharge buttons that allow the capacitor to discharge.
- Hand-held paddles or combination pads through which current is delivered from the defibrillator to the patient (Figure 4-3). Combination pads consist of a flexible metal "paddle," a layer of conductive gel, and an adhesive ring that holds them in place on the patient's chest.
  - ▶ If available, use combination pads instead of hand-held paddles for electrical therapy. Combination pads are disposable and have multiple functions. They are applied to a patient's bare chest for electrocardiogram (ECG) monitoring and then used for defibrillation and synchronized cardioversion (and in some cases, pacing) if necessary.
  - ▶ Not all combination pads are alike. Some pads can be used for defibrillation, synchronized cardioversion, ECG monitoring, and pacing. Others can be used for defibrillation, synchronized cardioversion, and ECG monitoring but not for pacing. Be sure you are familiar with the capabilities of the pads you are using.

◗ Combination pads enhance operator safety by physically separating the operator from the patient. Instead of leaning over the patient with hand-held paddles, the operator delivers a shock to the patient by means of discharge buttons (one for each pad) located on a remote cable, an adapter, or the defibrillator itself.

KEEPING IT SIMPLE

Energy (joules) = Current (amperes) × Voltage (volts) × Time (seconds)

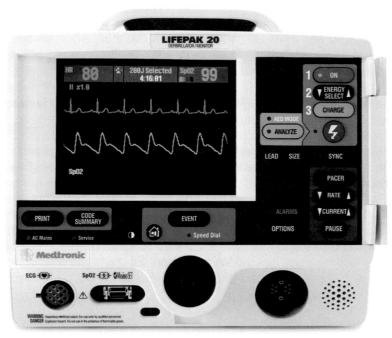

Figure 4-2 • A defibrillator is used to deliver an electrical shock to terminate an abnormal heart rhythm.

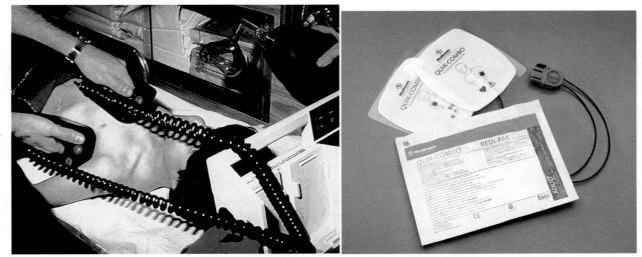

Figure 4-3 • **A,** Hand-held paddles. **B,** Combination pads have multiple functions. They are applied to a patient's bare chest for ECG monitoring and then used to deliver pacing, defibrillation, and synchronized cardioversion if necessary.

When the charge button on the defibrillator is pushed, the capacitor charges. Once the capacitor is charged and the shock control is pressed, voltage pushes a flow of electrons (current) to the patient by means of hand-held paddles or combination pads. Current passes through the heart in "waveforms" that travel from one paddle/pad, through the chest, and back to the other paddle/pad over a brief period.

Combination pads have multiple names including "combo pads," "multi-purpose pads," "combination electrodes," "therapy electrodes," and "self-adhesive monitoring/defibrillation pads."

TRANSTHORACIC RESISTANCE (IMPEDANCE)

Factors Known To Affect Transthoracic Resistance
- Paddle/electrode size
- Paddle/electrode position
- Use of conductive material (when using hand-held paddles)
- Phase of patient's respiration
- Paddle pressure (when using hand-held paddles)
- Selected energy

Although the energy selected for defibrillation or cardioversion is expressed in joules, it is *current* that delivers energy to the patient and depolarizes the myocardium. **Impedance** refers to the resistance to the flow of current. **Transthoracic impedance** (resistance) refers to the natural resistance of the chest wall to the flow of current. Impedance is measured in **ohms**. Transthoracic resistance varies greatly among individuals. Factors that affect transthoracic resistance are discussed next.

Body Tissue and Hair

The skin surface, fat, bone, and hair can cause significant increases in resistance. It may be difficult to ensure good electrode-to-skin contact on a patient who has a hairy chest. However, if good contact is not ensured, transthoracic resistance will be high and the effectiveness of defibrillation reduced.[12] There will also be an increased risk of burns and a risk of arcing (sparks) from electrode to skin and electrode to electrode.

If excessive chest hair is present, use a razor to quickly remove hair in the areas of intended electrode placement. If this is not feasible (or if a razor is unavailable), check to see if an extra set of electrodes is available. If so, apply one set to the patient's chest and then quickly remove them. This should remove some hair and improve electrode-to-skin contact when you apply a second set of pads. *Do not delay defibrillation.*

Paddle/Pad Size

To a point, transthoracic resistance decreases with increased paddle size. For adults, the optimal paddle/electrode size ranges from 8 to 12 cm in diameter. Adult paddles/pads should be used for patients more than 10 kg (older than 1 year of age). Use 4.5 cm diameter (pediatric) paddles/pads for infants and children weighing less than 10 kg. As a general rule, use the largest pads that will fit the patient's chest without overlapping. Avoid using pediatric electrodes for adult defibrillation because myocardial injury can occur.[13]

When applying defibrillation paddles or pads, remove clothing and expose the patient's chest. Be sure to look for transdermal patches or disks, which may be used to deliver nitroglycerin, nicotine, analgesics, hormones, or antihypertensives. Do not apply paddles or pads directly over the medication patch or disk because the patch may prevent good electrode contact, hindering the delivery of energy from the defibrillation electrode to the heart. A lack of good contact can cause arcing and may cause skin burns.[14] If a medication patch, disk, or ointment is located at or near the site of paddle/pad placement, remove it and wipe the area clean (do not use alcohol or alcohol-based cleansers) before applying defibrillation paddles or pads.[15]

Paddle/Pad Position

Hand-held paddles or combination pads should be placed on the patient's bare chest according to the manufacturer's instructions. Paddles or pads may be labeled according to their position on the chest (sternum/apex, front/back) or according to their polarity (positive, negative).

The typical paddle/pad position used during resuscitation is the sternum-apex position (also called the anterolateral or apex-anterior position). This position is often used because the anterior chest is usually easy to get to and placement of the paddles/pads in this position approximates ECG electrode positioning in lead II. Place the right (sternum) paddle/pad to the right of the sternum, just below the clavicle. Place the center of the left (apex) paddle/pad in the midaxillary line, about level with the V_6 ECG electrode position (about the fifth intercostal space) (Figure 4-4).

Proper paddle/pad position is important. If the paddles/pads are placed too close together on the anterior surface of the chest, a substantial amount of current shunts between them and an insufficient amount reaches the left ventricle (Figure 4-5). Placement of the paddles/pads farther apart allows a sufficient amount of current to reach the left ventricle (Figure 4-6).

Electrical Therapy in Women

Elevate the left breast and place the apex paddle or pad lateral to or underneath the breast. Placing defibrillation paddles or pads directly on breast tissue results in higher transthoracic resistance, reducing current flow.[16]

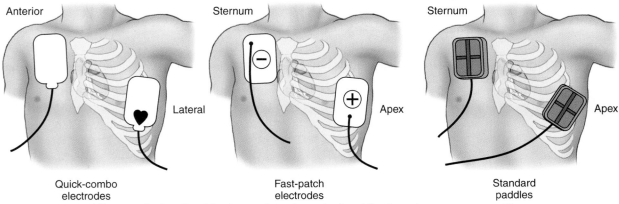

Quick-combo electrodes　　Fast-patch electrodes　　Standard paddles

Figure 4-4 • Combination pads and standard paddles in a sternum-apex position.

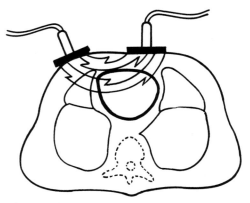 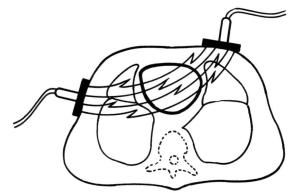

Figure 4-5 • If the paddles/pads are placed too close together on the anterior surface of the chest, a substantial amount of current shunts between them and an insufficient amount reaches the left ventricle.

Figure 4-6 • Placement of the paddles/pads farther apart allows a sufficient amount of current to reach the left ventricle.

Other acceptable positions may include the following:

- Anterior-posterior (paddles and pads). In this position, one paddle/pad is placed over the heart on the left chest. The other is placed on the back, just below the right or left scapula (Figure 4-7). Some defibrillators are equipped with a special posterior paddle attachment.
- Apex-posterior (pads). In this position, one pad is placed over the heart on the left chest. The other pad is placed behind the heart, just below the left scapula (Figure 4-8).
- Biaxillary (paddles and pads). In this position, one paddle/pad is placed on the right lateral chest wall and the other paddle/pad is placed on the left lateral chest wall (Figure 4-9).

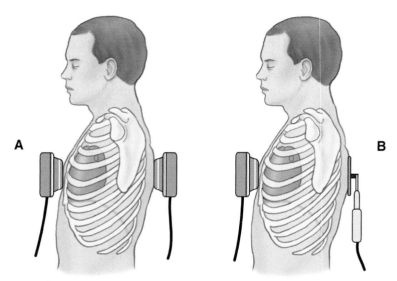

Figure 4-7 • Anterior-posterior paddle positioning. **A,** Standard paddles. **B,** Standard anterior paddle and special posterior paddle.

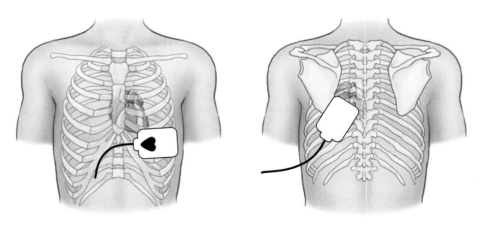

Anterior   Posterior

Figure 4-8 • Combination pads in an apex-posterior position.

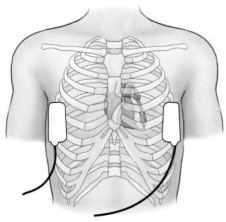

Figure 4-9 • Combination pads in a biaxillary position.

When preparing the skin for paddle or pad placement, do not use alcohol, tincture of benzoin, or antiperspirant. When positioning paddles or pads, be sure that they do not overlap bone (such as the sternum, spine, or scapulae) because bone is not a good conductor of current.

Some manual defibrillators should not be placed in AED mode when the paddles/pads are placed in other than a sternum-apex position. Because the ECG signal obtained through paddles/pad in positions other than a sternum-apex position do not approximate a standard ECG lead, a shock or no shock decision may be inappropriately advised by the AED.

KEEPING IT SIMPLE

In resuscitation situations, precious seconds can be lost when rescuers try to make sure that the "sternum" pad is placed on the sternum and the "apex" pad is placed over the apex of the heart. Delays sometimes occur when rescuers realize that paddles or pads have been placed in reversed positions and then attempt to reposition them to their "proper" location. Reversal of the position of the electrodes is not important during defibrillation, provided the heart is located between them.[17]

Use of Conductive Material

When using hand-held paddles, the use of gels, pastes, or pregelled defibrillation pads aids the passage of current at the interface between the defibrillator paddles/electrodes and the body surface. Failure to use conductive material results in increased transthoracic resistance, a lack of penetration of current, and burns to the skin surface. Combination pads are pregelled and do not require the application of additional gel to the patient's chest.

When using pregelled pads with hand-held paddles, make sure the pads cover the entire paddle surface to avoid arcing current and potential burns. When hand-held paddles are used with pregelled pads, the electrolyte gel becomes polarized and a poor conductor after defibrillation. After the delivery of a shock, ECG monitoring through gel pads may result in the display of false asystole that may continue for 3 to 4 minutes.[18,19] When paddles and gel pads are used and asystole is observed after delivering a shock, confirm that asystole is present by using ECG electrodes rather than the paddles.

Do not use saline-soaked gauze or alcohol-soaked pads for defibrillation. Excess saline on the chest may cause arcing and burns. Alcohol-soaked pads may ignite. Do not use gels or pastes that are not specifically made for defibrillation (such as ultrasound gel). Use of improper pastes, creams, gels, or pads can cause burns or sparks and pose a risk of fire in an oxygen-enriched environment.[20] If too much gel is used, the material may spread across the chest wall during resuscitation. This can lead to arcing of the current from one paddle to another and away from the heart. This can also produce a potentially dangerous spark or burns.

Phase of Respiration

The phase of the patient's respiration is another determinant of transthoracic resistance.[21] Inspiration increases transthoracic resistance, and resistance is lowered during exhalation. Because air is a poor conductor of electricity, the greater the volume of air in the lungs when a shock is delivered, the greater the resistance to the flow of current.[22] Resistance may be lowest when a shock is delivered during the expiratory phase of respiration because the distance between the paddles and the heart is decreased.

Paddle Pressure

When using hand-held paddles for adult defibrillation, apply firm pressure (about 25 pounds) to each paddle. This lowers transthoracic resistance by improving contact between the skin surface and the paddles and decreasing the amount of air in the lungs. When using hand-held paddles for pediatric defibrillation:[23,24]

- Apply firm pressure of about 7 pounds (3 kg) for children weighing less than 10 kg.
- Apply firm pressure of about 11 pounds (5 kg) for larger children when using adult paddles.

No pressure is applied when using combination pads. Despite the absence of pressure, the pads appear to be as effective as hand-held paddles.[25]

Selected Energy

When electrical therapy is used to treat an abnormal heart rhythm, it is important to select the appropriate energy level (joules). If the energy level selected and current delivered are too low, the shock will not eliminate the abnormal rhythm. If excessive energy and current are used, myocardial injury may result.

KEEPING IT SIMPLE

The amount of current delivered to a patient is determined by the energy level you select and the patient's transthoracic resistance. Increased resistance = decreased current delivery.

MONOPHASIC VERSUS BIPHASIC DEFIBRILLATION

There are three general types or classes of defibrillation waveforms: monophasic, biphasic, and triphasic.[26] Waveforms are classified by whether the current flow delivered is in one direction, two directions, or multiple directions.

When a monophasic waveform is used, current passes through the heart in one (mono) direction (Figure 4-10). Although few monophasic waveform defibrillators are manufactured today, many are in use. When using a monophasic waveform defibrillator to treat pulseless VT/VF, use 360 J for all shocks.[27]

Before the 2005 resuscitation guidelines, the initial shocks delivered for pulseless VT/VF were delivered in a series of three shocks (assuming the rhythm didn't change). This was referred to as the delivery of "stacked" or "serial" shocks. This technique is no longer recommended. In the 2005 guidelines, the recommended treatment is to give *one* shock and then immediately resume CPR, starting with chest compressions. The reason for this change is that lengthy interruptions in chest compressions (such as that to perform three shocks) are associated with a decreased probability of conversion of VF to another rhythm. Furthermore, if one shock fails to stop pulseless VT or VF, the likelihood of a second or third "stacked" shock being beneficial is low. Resuming CPR immediately after a shock is more likely to be beneficial than another shock.[28]

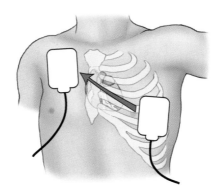

Figure 4-10 • When a monophasic waveform is used, current passes through the heart in one direction.

With biphasic waveforms, energy is delivered in two (bi) phases. The current moves in one direction for a specified period, stops, and then passes through the heart a second time in the opposite direction in a very short period (milliseconds) (Figure 4-11). Biphasic waveforms include biphasic truncated exponential, rectilinear, and pulsed biphasic versions. At this time, there is no certain evidence of clinical superiority of one waveform over another in terms of either efficacy or myocardial injury.[29] Most AEDs and manual defibrillators sold today use biphasic waveform technology. Manufacturers of biphasic defibrillators recommend slightly different energy levels specific for their device. Both escalating (increasing energy levels) and nonescalating (no increase in energy level) biphasic waveform defibrillators are available; however, there are insufficient data to recommend one type of device over another.

When using a biphasic waveform defibrillator to treat pulseless VT/VF, use the energy levels recommended by the manufacturer for the initial and subsequent shocks. If you do not know what the recommended energy levels are, the 2005 resuscitation guidelines state that it is reasonable to use 200 J for the first shock. Use either an equal or higher dose for the second or subsequent shocks, depending on the capabilities of the device.[27]

Triphasic and quadriphasic waveforms deliver multidirectional shocks. Future generations of defibrillators may implement this technology.

If a shock delivered successfully terminates pulseless VT/VF but the rhythm recurs, begin defibrillation at the last energy level used that resulted in successful defibrillation.

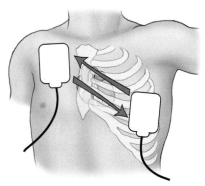

Figure 4-11 • With biphasic waveforms, energy is delivered in two phases. The current moves in one direction for a specified period, stops, and then passes through the heart a second time in the opposite direction.

QUICK REVIEW 4-1

1. What is the purpose of defibrillation?

2. List four factors that affect transthoracic resistance.
   1.
   2.
   3.
   4.
3. List three indications for defibrillation.
   1.
   2.
   3.

Answers can be found at the end of this chapter.

DEFIBRILLATION PROCEDURE

The procedure described below assumes that the patient is an adult and confirmed to be unresponsive, not breathing, and pulseless. It also assumes that the patient's cardiac rhythm is pulseless VT or VF and that a four-person team is available to assist with procedures during the resuscitation effort.

KEEPING IT SIMPLE

Critical Resuscitation Tasks
- Airway management
- Chest compressions
- Monitoring and defibrillation
- Vascular access and medication administration

■ Be sure that the CPR team member continues chest compressions as the defibrillator is readied for use. The airway management team member should insert an oral airway, assemble a bag-valve-mask device with supplemental oxygen, and then coordinate rescue breaths with the CPR team member until an advanced airway is placed and its position confirmed.

■ Instruct the defibrillation team member to expose the patient's chest and remove any transdermal patches or ointment from the patient's chest, if present. Be sure that CPR is continued until the defibrillator is ready.
  ▶ If hand-held paddles are used, apply conductive material to the defibrillator paddles (gel) or apply disposable pregelled defibrillator pads to the patient's bare chest.
  ▶ If combination pads are used, remove the pads from their sealed package. Check the pads for the presence of adequate gel. Attach the pads to the hands-free defibrillation cable. Attach the combination pads to the patient's chest in the position recommended by the manufacturer. When applying the adhesive pads, press from one edge of the pad across the entire surface to remove all air and avoid the development of air pockets (Figure 4-12). Attach the hands-free defibrillation cable to the monitor/defibrillator.

■ Turn the power on to the monitor/defibrillator and verify the presence of a shockable rhythm on the monitor. Select an appropriate energy level.
  ▶ Use 360 J for all shocks if a monophasic defibrillator is used.
  ▶ Use the energy levels recommended by the manufacturer for the initial and subsequent shocks if a biphasic defibrillator is used. If you do not know what the recommended energy levels are, it is reasonable to use 200 J for the first shock.

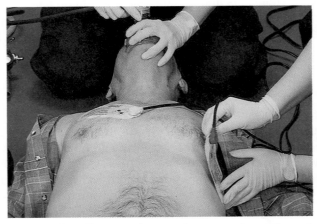

Figure 4-12 • When applying the adhesive pads, press from one edge of the pad across the entire surface to remove all air and avoid the development of air pockets.

- ▶ While the defibrillator is readied, instruct the intravenous (IV)/medication team member to prepare the initial drugs that will be used and start an IV after the first shock is delivered.
- ▦ If hand-held paddles are used, instruct the defibrillation team member to place the paddles in their proper positions on the patient's chest. Be sure that firm downward pressure (about 25 pounds) is applied to each paddle. Do not lean on the paddles—they may slip!
- ▦ Charge the defibrillator. If hand-held paddles are used, press the CHARGE button on the machine or the button located on the apex paddle. If combination pads are used, press the CHARGE button on the machine.
  - ▶ All team members with the exception of the chest compressor should *immediately* clear the patient as the machine charges. As the airway team member clears the patient, he or she should be reminded to turn off the oxygen flow.
  - ▶ Listen as the machine charges. The sound usually changes when it reaches its full charge. The chest compressor should continue CPR while the machine is charging. Once the defibrillator is charged, the chest compressor should *immediately* clear the patient.
- ▦ Recheck the ECG rhythm. If the rhythm is unchanged call, "Clear!" Look (360 degrees) to be sure that everyone (including you) is clear of the patient, the bed, and any equipment connected to the patient and that the oxygen flow is off.
- ▦ Press the SHOCK buttons to discharge energy to the patient. After the shock has been delivered, release the buttons.
- ▦ Instruct the team to immediately resume CPR, beginning with chest compressions. Instruct the airway team member to turn on the oxygen. Instruct the IV/medications team member to start an IV and give a vasopressor. Remember: CPR should not be interrupted to start an IV, to give medications, or to check a rhythm immediately after defibrillation.
- ▦ After five cycles of CPR (about 2 minutes), recheck the rhythm.
  - ▶ If a shockable rhythm is present, charge the defibrillator and then call, "Clear!" Check to be certain that everyone is clear and the oxygen flow is off. Deliver a second shock and then immediately resume CPR. Instruct the airway team member to turn on the oxygen.
    - • Use 360 J for the second and subsequent shocks if a monophasic defibrillator is used.
    - • Use the energy levels recommended by the manufacturer if a biphasic defibrillator is used. If you do not know what the recommended energy levels are, use 200 J or a higher dose for the second or subsequent shocks, depending on the capabilities of the defibrillator.
    - • Instruct the IV/medications team member to give an antiarrhythmic IV. Consider placement of an advanced airway and possible causes of the arrest.
  - ▶ If a shockable rhythm is not present:
    - • Check a pulse if an organized rhythm is present on the monitor. If there is an organized rhythm on the monitor and a pulse *is* present, check the patient's blood pressure and other vital signs and begin postresuscitation care.
    - • If there is an organized rhythm on the monitor but there is no pulse (PEA) or if the rhythm is asystole, resume CPR, consider possible causes of the arrest, and give medications and other emergency care as indicated.

What If . . . ?

- ▦ What if you charge the defibrillator and the patient spontaneously converts to a rhythm that is not shockable or an organized rhythm before the shock is delivered?
  - ▶ Check the operating instructions that accompany the defibrillator you are using for a definitive answer. In most cases, the machine will disarm (internally remove the stored energy) if the discharge buttons are not pressed within 60 seconds. The machine will also disarm if you change the selected energy or press the energy selector to remove the charge.

■ What energy should be used if you deliver a shock that eliminates pulseless VT/VF and then the rhythm recurs?

  ❱ If defibrillation eliminates pulseless VT/VF and then recurs, defibrillate at the last successful energy setting.

■ What if the rhythm on the monitor looks like a "flat line"?

  ❱ If the rhythm appears to be asystole, confirm the rhythm in the second lead. This is done because it is possible (although rare) that VF may be present in some leads (called "occult VF").[30]

  ❱ A 1988 study noted that a flat line produced by technical errors such as no power, leads unconnected, gain set too low, or incorrect lead selection ("false asystole") was far more frequent than occult VF.[31]

  ❱ If the rhythm appears to be asystole and hand-held paddles are used, confirm the rhythm in another lead by rotating the paddles 90 degrees from their original position and then reassess the rhythm.

  ❱ If the rhythm appears to be asystole and combination pads have been applied to the chest, it is unnecessary to remove the pads and reposition them to confirm the rhythm. Treat the rhythm as asystole.

  ❱ If electrodes and lead wires are already connected to the patient, confirming the rhythm in another lead simply requires changing the lead selector switch on the monitor to view at least one other lead.

■ What if the patient has a permanent pacemaker or implantable cardioverter-defibrillator (ICD)?

  ❱ An ICD is typically placed subcutaneously in the left upper quadrant of the patient's abdomen or the left pectoral area. It can deliver a range of therapies (also called "tiered-therapy") including defibrillation, antitachycardia ("overdrive") pacing, synchronized cardioversion, and bradycardia pacing, depending on the dysrhythmia detected and how the device is programmed. A physician determines the appropriate therapies for each patient.

  ❱ Depending on the manufacturer, the ICD may deliver a maximum of six shocks for VF. About 2 J are delivered at the body surface when the ICD discharges internally. Rescuers in contact with the patient may feel a tingling sensation when the ICD delivers a shock. Although the energy is enough to be felt by the rescuer, it is not enough to cause physiologic harm.

  ❱ When defibrillating (or cardioverting) a patient with a permanent (implanted) pacemaker or ICD, be careful not to place the defibrillator paddles or combination pads directly over the device.

  ❱ Place defibrillator paddles or combination pads at least 1 inch (2.5 cm) from the pulse generator (bulge under the patient's skin). If the device is located in the patient's left pectoral area, standard sternum-apex paddle/pad placement for defibrillation is acceptable. If the device is located in the right pectoral area, anterior-posterior paddle/pad placement can be used.

  ❱ Because some of the defibrillation current flows down the pacemaker leads, a patient who has a permanent pacemaker or ICD should have the device checked to ensure proper function after defibrillation.

KEEPING IT SIMPLE

When a "flat line" is observed on a cardiac monitor
- Make sure power to the monitor is on.
- Check the lead/cable connections.
- Make sure the correct lead is selected.
- Turn up the gain (ECG size) on the monitor.

AUTOMATED EXTERNAL DEFIBRILLATORS

AUTOMATED EXTERNAL DEFIBRILLATOR FEATURES

- An AED is an external defibrillator that has a computerized cardiac rhythm analysis system. AEDs are easy to use. Voice prompts and visual indicators guide the user through a series of steps that may include defibrillation.
- When the adhesive electrodes are attached to the patient's chest, the AED examines the patient's cardiac rhythm and analyzes it. Some AEDs require the operator to press an "analyze" control to initiate rhythm analysis, whereas others automatically begin analyzing the patient's cardiac rhythm when the electrode pads are attached to the patient's chest.
  - Safety filters check for false signals (e.g., radio transmissions, poor electrode contact, 60-cycle interference, and loose electrodes).
- When the AED analyzes the patient's cardiac rhythm, it "looks" at multiple features of the rhythm, including the QRS width, rate, and amplitude. If the AED detects a shockable rhythm, it then charges its capacitors. In addition to VF, AEDs will recommend a shock for monomorphic VT and polymorphic VT. The preset rate for "shockable" VT varies depending on the AED. For instance, some manufacturers set the shockable VT rate (for adults) at greater than 150 bpm. Others set the rate at greater than 120 bpm.
  - If the machine is a fully automated AED and a shockable rhythm is detected, it will signal everyone to stand clear of the patient and then deliver a shock by means of the adhesive pads that were applied to the patient's chest.
  - If the machine is a semiautomated AED and a shockable rhythm is detected, it will instruct the AED operator (by means of voice prompts and visual signals) to press the shock control to deliver a shock.
- Some AEDs:
  - Can be configured to allow advanced life support personnel to switch to a manual mode, allowing more decision-making control.
  - Have CPR pads available that are equipped with a sensor. The sensor detects the depth of chest compressions. If the depth of chest compressions is inadequate, the machine provides voice prompts to the rescuer.
  - Provide voice instructions in adult and infant/child CPR at the user's option. A metronome function encourages rescuers to perform chest compressions at the recommended rate of 100 compressions per minute.
  - Are programmed to detect spontaneous movement by the patient or others.
  - Have adapters available for many popular manual defibrillators, enabling the AED pads to remain on the patient when patient care is transferred.
  - Can detect the patient's transthoracic resistance through the adhesive pads applied to the patient's chest. The AED automatically adjusts the voltage and length of the shock, thus customizing how the energy is delivered to that patient.
  - Are equipped with a pediatric pad-cable system or key. When the pediatric cable system is attached to the AED, the machine recognizes the pediatric cable connection and automatically adjusts its defibrillation energy to pediatric levels (Figure 4-13).

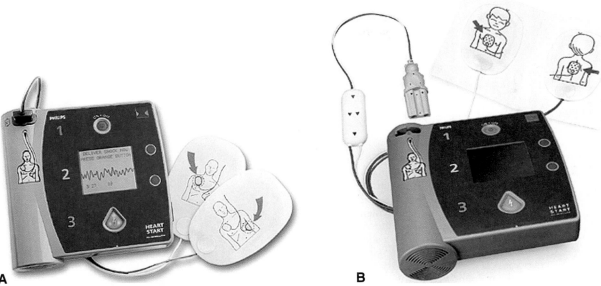

A   **B**

Figure 4-13 • **A,** AED. **B,** This defibrillation pad and cable system reduces the energy delivered by a standard AED to that appropriate for a child.

■ Use a standard AED for a patient who is unresponsive, not breathing, pulseless, and 8 years of age or older (about 55 pounds or >25 kg). If the patient is between 1 and 8 years of age and a pediatric pad-cable system is unavailable for the AED, use a standard AED. Although AEDs exist for use in infants, resuscitation guidelines currently make no recommendation for or against AED use in infants.

AUTOMATED EXTERNAL DEFIBRILLATOR OPERATION

KEEPING IT SIMPLE

AED Operation
- Turn on the power
- Attach the device
- Analyze the rhythm
- Deliver a shock if indicated and safe

■ Assess responsiveness. Open the airway and check for breathing. If the patient is not breathing, deliver two breaths. Assess for the presence of a pulse. If the patient is pulseless, begin chest compressions until the AED is ready.

■ Turn the power on to the AED (Figure 4-14). Depending on the brand of AED, this is achieved by either pressing the "on" button or lifting up the monitor screen or lid.

■ Open the package containing the adhesive pads. If the gel in the pads is dried out, use a new set of pads. Connect the pads to the AED cables (if not preconnected), and then apply the pads to the patient's chest in the locations specified by the AED manufacturer. Most models require connection of the AED cable to the AED before use.

■ Analyze the ECG rhythm. If several "looks" confirm the presence of a shockable rhythm, the AED will signal that a shock is indicated. Listen for the voice prompts.

  ▶ Artifact due to motion or 60-cycle interference may simulate VF and interfere with accurate rhythm analysis.

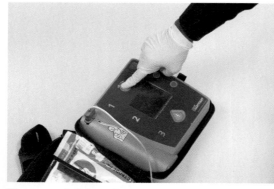
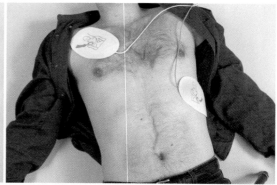
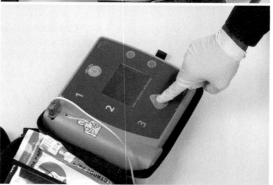

Figure 4-14 • AED operation. **A,** Turn the power on to the AED. **B,** Attach the AED pads to the patient's bare chest as directed on the pads. Allow the AED to analyze the patient's rhythm. Do not touch the patient while the rhythm is being analyzed. **C,** If the AED detects a shockable rhythm, clear the area surrounding the patient. Make sure everyone is clear of the patient, bed, and any equipment connected to the patient. If oxygen is in use, make sure it is turned off when defibrillating. Press the SHOCK button when prompted to do so by the AED.

> ◗ While the AED is analyzing the patient's cardiac rhythm, all movement (including chest compressions, artificial ventilations, and movement associated with patient transport) must stop.

- Clear the area surrounding the patient. Be sure to look around you. Ensure that everyone is clear of the patient, bed, and any equipment connected to the patient. If oxygen is in use, make sure it is turned off when defibrillating.
- If the area is clear and the AED advises a shock, press the shock control to deliver the energy to the patient. After delivering the shock, immediately resume CPR, beginning with chest compressions.
- After about 2 minutes of CPR, reanalyze the rhythm. Continue to provide care as indicated by the AED's voice and screen prompts.

 Always follow the AED manufacturer's guidelines for the application, use, and maintenance of the AED.

SPECIAL CONSIDERATIONS

- If the patient has a pacemaker or ICD, an AED may be used; but the AED pads should be placed at least 1 inch from the implanted device. If an ICD is in the process of delivering shocks to the patient, allow it about 30 to 60 seconds to complete its cycle.
- If a transdermal medication patch is present on the patient's chest, do not attempt to defibrillate through it. Remove the patch and wipe the area clean before applying the AED pads.
- If the patient's chest is dirty or wet, wipe the chest clean and dry it with a towel or cloth before applying the AED pads.
- If the patient has excessive chest hair, the AED pads may not adhere to the patient's chest resulting in a "check electrodes" message from the AED. If pressing down firmly on each AED pad does not correct the problem, quickly remove the AED pads, and apply a second set of AED pads. If the problem persists, remove the AEDs pads, quickly shave the areas of the chest where the AED pads will be placed, and then apply a new set of AED pads.

MAINTENANCE

■ Specific maintenance should be performed according to the manufacturer's recommendations.

■ Newer AEDs require minimal maintenance because they perform automated self-checks. AEDs usually self-test their internal circuitry, battery status, ECG electronics, defibrillator electronics, and microprocessor electronics.

■ The frequency with which automatic self-tests occur varies by the device. Some AEDs perform daily self-tests, whereas others occur weekly. Additional self-tests usually occur when batteries are installed and when the AED is powered on. Manual self-tests can be performed at any time.

QUICK REVIEW 4-3

1. Where is the pulse generator of an ICD typically located?

2. An 80-year-old man has experienced a cardiac arrest. The cardiac monitor displays VF. You have exposed the patient's chest and are preparing to defibrillate when you note the patient has a permanent pacemaker in place. What distance from the pacemaker generator should the defibrillator paddles/pads be placed?

3. What is an AED?

SYNCHRONIZED CARDIOVERSION

KEEPING IT SIMPLE

Synchronized Cardioversion—Indications
• Unstable supraventricular tachycardia
• Unstable atrial fibrillation with a rapid ventricular response
• Unstable atrial flutter with a rapid ventricular response
• Unstable wide-complex tachycardia
• Unstable VT with a pulse

DESCRIPTION AND PURPOSE

Synchronized cardioversion is a type of electrical therapy in which a shock is "timed" or "programmed" for delivery during the QRS complex. A synchronizing circuit in the machine searches for the highest (R-wave deflection) or deepest (QS deflection) part of the QRS complex and delivers the shock a few milliseconds after this portion of the QRS. Delivery of a shock during this portion of the cardiac cycle reduces the potential for the delivery of current during the vulnerable period of the T wave (relative refractory period).

Because the machine must be able to detect a QRS complex in order to "sync," synchronized cardioversion is used to treat rhythms that have a clearly identifiable QRS complex and a rapid ventricular rate (such as some narrow-QRS tachycardias and VT). Synchronized cardioversion is not used to treat disorganized rhythms (such as polymorphic VT) or those that do not have a clearly identifiable QRS complex (such as VF).

PROCEDURE

- If the patient is awake and time permits, give sedation.
- Turn the power on to the monitor/defibrillator.
- If combination pads are used, attach the pads to the hands-free defibrillation cable. Attach the combination pads to the patient's chest in the position recommended by the manufacturer. Attach the hands-free defibrillation cable to the monitor/defibrillator. If using hand-held paddles, apply conductive gel to the defibrillator paddles or place pregelled defibrillator pads on the patient's bare chest.
- Select a lead with an optimum QRS complex amplitude and no distortion.
- Identify the rhythm. Record an ECG strip to document the patient's rhythm.
- Press the "sync" button on the defibrillator. Look at the monitor and make sure that the machine is "marking" or "flagging" each QRS complex. If sync markers do not appear, or appear elsewhere on the ECG display, adjust the ECG size until the markers occur within the QRS complex. If adjusting the ECG size does not result in sync markers within the QRS complex, select another lead.
- Select an appropriate energy level for the rhythm. If cardioversion is needed and it is impossible to synchronize a shock (e.g., the patient's rhythm is irregular), use high-energy unsynchronized shocks.[32]
- If using hand-held paddles, place the paddles on the patient's chest and apply firm downward pressure.
- Charge the defibrillator. Recheck the ECG rhythm and check to make sure the machine is in "sync" mode.
- If the rhythm is unchanged call, "Clear!" and look (360 degrees) to be sure everyone is clear of the patient, bed, and any equipment connected to the patient, and the oxygen flow is turned off.
- Press and *hold* the discharge buttons (one for each paddle/pad) until the shock is delivered. You may notice a slight delay from the time you depress the discharge buttons and hear the machine actually discharge the energy. This occurs because the machine waits to discharge until it detects the next QRS complex. The more rapid the patient's ventricular rate, the less the delay until the machine discharges. After the shock has been delivered, release the buttons.
- Reassess the ECG rhythm. If the tachycardia persists, increase the energy level according to the appropriate algorithm. Make sure the machine is in sync mode before delivering another shock.
- If VF occurs during synchronized cardioversion, check the patient's pulse and rhythm (verify that all electrodes and cable connections are secure), turn off the sync control, and defibrillate.

 Some defibrillators revert to the defibrillation (unsynchronized) mode after the delivery of a synchronized shock. This is done to allow immediate defibrillation in case synchronized cardioversion produces VF. Other defibrillators remain in sync mode after a synchronized shock. If VF occurs during synchronized cardioversion, make sure the sync button is off before attempting to defibrillate.

DEFIBRILLATION AND CARDIOVERSION
SPECIAL CONSIDERATIONS

- Remove supplemental oxygen sources from the area of the patient's bed before defibrillation and cardioversion attempts and place them at least 3½ to 4 feet away from the patient's chest. Examples of supplemental oxygen sources include masks, nasal cannulae, resuscitation bags, and ventilator tubing. Case reports exist that describe instances of fires ignited by sparks from poorly applied defibrillator paddles/pads in the presence of an oxygen-enriched atmosphere.[33] Severe fires have resulted when ventilator tubing was disconnected from an endotracheal tube and then left next to the patient's head while defibrillation was attempted.

■ To prevent fires during defibrillation attempts:

▶ Be sure to use defibrillator paddles/pads of the appropriate size. Adult paddles/pads should be used for patients less than 10 kg. Use pediatric paddles/pads for patients less than 10 kg.

▶ Make sure there are no air pockets between the paddle/pads and the patient's skin. When applying combination pads to a patient's bare chest, press from one edge of the pad across the entire surface to remove all air.

▶ When using hand-held paddles, use appropriate conductive gel or disposable gel pads and apply firm, even pressure during defibrillation attempts.

■ Keep monitoring electrodes and wires well away from the area where defibrillator pads or combination pads will be placed. Contact may cause electrical arcing and patient skin burns during defibrillation or cardioversion.

■ Remove transdermal patches, bandages, necklaces, or other materials from the sites used for paddle placement—do not attempt to defibrillate through them. Wipe residue from a medication patch or ointment from the patient's chest. Do not use alcohol or alcohol-based cleansers.

■ If the patient is lying in water or on a wet surface, remove the patient from contact with the water and quickly dry the patient's chest before applying paddles or pads.

■ When using hand-held paddles, do not discharge the defibrillator with the paddles pressed together or into the open air. Discharging the defibrillator with the paddles together may pit or damage the surface of the paddle plates, possibly resulting in patient skin burns during defibrillation.

POSSIBLE COMPLICATIONS

■ Skin burns due to lack of conductive material, gel "bridging" (i.e., the gel forms a "bridge" on the skin)

■ Risk of fire from combination of electrical and oxygen sources

■ Myocardial damage/dysfunction

■ Embolic episodes

■ Dysrhythmias including asystole, atrioventricular (AV) block, bradycardia, or VF following cardioversion

■ Injury to the operator and/or team members if improper technique used

POSSIBLE ERRORS

■ Treating the monitor, not the patient

■ Operator unfamiliar with equipment

■ Failure to properly maintain equipment (i.e., battery maintenance, paddle cleaning)

■ Failure to remove transdermal patches, bandages, or other materials from the site used for paddle placement

■ Other procedures performed (establishing an IV, placing an advanced airway) before CPR and/or defibrillation in the patient with pulseless VT/VF

■ Prolonged or frequent interruptions of chest compressions

■ Improper paddle/electrode position (insufficient current reaches the left ventricle)

■ Excessive use of conductive gel on the patient's chest or paddles

■ Inappropriate energy level or type of shock (i.e., defibrillation versus synchronized cardioversion) selected for dysrhythmia/clinical situation

■ Failure to "clear" self and team members before delivery of each shock

■ Failure to assess for the presence of a pulse when an organized rhythm is observed on the monitor

■ Failure to assess the patient's vital signs upon return of a pulse

(See Table 4-1 for a summary of defibrillation and cardioversion.)

TABLE 4-1	Defibrillation and Cardioversion—Summary	
Type of Shock	**Rhythm**	**Recommended Energy Levels**
Defibrillation	Pulseless VT/VF Sustained polymorphic VT	Varies depending on device used • Biphasic defibrillator effective dose typically 120 J to 200 J • If effective dose range of device unknown, use 200 J for first shock, equal or higher shock dose for second and subsequent shocks • If using monophasic defibrillator, 360 J for all shocks
Synchronized cardioversion	Unstable narrow-QRS tachycardia Unstable atrial flutter Unstable atrial fibrillation Unstable wide complex tachycardia/ VT with a pulse	50 J, 100 J, 200 J, 300 J, 360 J* 50 J, 100 J, 200 J, 300 J, 360 J* 100 to 120 J, 200 J, 300 J, 360 J* 100 J, 200 J, 300 J, 360 J*

*Or equivalent biphasic energy.

QUICK REVIEW 4-4

1. What are the four main steps in the operation of an AED?
   1.
   2.
   3.
   4.
2. You just delivered a synchronized shock with 50 J to an unstable patient whose cardiac monitor shows AV nodal reentrant tachycardia. The cardiac monitor now shows VF. What course of action should you take at this time?

TRANSCUTANEOUS PACING

KEEPING IT SIMPLE

Transcutaneous Pacing—Indications
Symptomatic bradycardia
• Narrow-QRS bradycardia that does not respond to atropine
• Wide-QRS bradycardia

■ A **pacemaker** is an artificial pulse generator that delivers an electrical current to the heart to stimulate depolarization. Transcutaneous pacing (TCP) delivers pacing impulses to the heart using electrodes placed on the patient's chest. TCP is also called temporary external pacing or noninvasive pacing.

■ TCP is recommended as the initial pacing method of choice in emergency cardiac care because it is effective, quick, safe, and noninvasive.

■ TCP is indicated for significant bradycardias unresponsive to atropine therapy or when atropine is not immediately available. It may also be used as a "bridge" until transvenous pacing can be accomplished or the cause of the bradycardia is reversed (as in cases of drug overdose or hyperkalemia).

■ Although TCP is a type of electrical therapy, the current delivered is considerably less than that used for cardioversion or defibrillation. The energy levels selected for cardioversion or defibrillation are indicated in joules. The stimulating current selected for TCP is indicated in milliamperes (mA). The range of output current of a transcutaneous pacemaker varies, depending on the manufacturer. For example, the range of output current for one brand of transcutaneous pacemaker is 0 mA to 140 mA. The range for another brand is 0 mA to 200 mA.

PROCEDURE

■ Pacing may be performed in either demand or nondemand (asynchronous) mode. The demand mode is used for most patients. When the pacemaker is in demand mode, pacing is inhibited when the pacemaker "senses" the patient's own (intrinsic) beats.

▶ To detect the patient's own beats (QRS complexes), the pacemaker must be connected to ECG electrodes and an ECG cable. In addition, the QRS complexes must be of adequate size to be sensed by the pacemaker.

▶ If the gain (ECG size) on the monitor is set too low to detect the patient's beats (or if an ECG lead is off), the pacemaker will produce pacing stimuli asynchronously. In other words, the pacemaker will generate a pacing stimulus at the selected rate regardless of the patient's own rhythm.

■ Place adhesive pacing pads on the patient's bare chest according to the manufacturer's instructions (Figure 4-15). The pads should fit completely on the patient's chest with a minimum of 1 inch of space between them. The pads should not overlap the sternum, spine, or scapula. In women, make sure the anterior pacer pad is positioned *under* (not on) the left breast.

A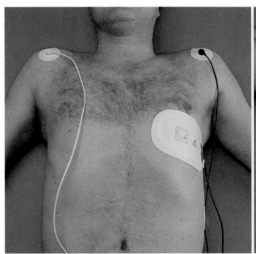

B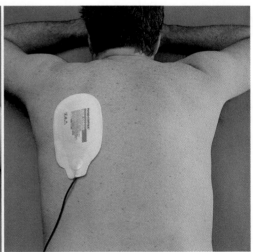

C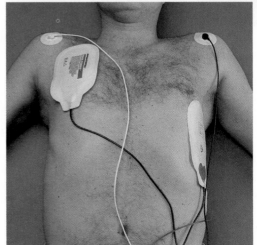

Figure 4-15 • TCP. **A** and **B,** Anterior-posterior pacing pad placement. **C,** Anterior-lateral pacing pad placement.

- Connect the patient to an ECG monitor, obtain a rhythm strip, and verify the presence of a paceable rhythm. Connect the pacing cable to the adhesive electrodes on the patient and the pulse generator.
- Turn the power on to the pacemaker and set the pacing rate (Figure 4-16). When TCP is used to treat a symptomatic bradycardia, the rate is set at a nonbradycardic rate, generally between 60 and 80 pulses per minute (ppm).
- After the rate has been regulated, set the stimulating current. This control is usually labeled CURRENT, PACER OUTPUT, and/or mA. Increase the current slowly but steadily until capture is achieved. Sedation and/or analgesia may be needed to minimize the discomfort associated with this procedure (common with currents of 50 mA or more).
- Watch the cardiac monitor closely for *electrical* capture. This is usually evidenced by a wide QRS and a T wave that appears in a direction opposite the QRS (Figure 4-17). In some patients, electrical capture is not as obvious and appears only as a change in the shape of the QRS.
- Assess *mechanical* capture by checking the patient's right upper extremity or femoral pulses. Avoid assessment of pulses in the patient's neck or on the patient's left side. This helps minimize confusion between the presence of an actual pulse and skeletal muscle contractions caused by the pacemaker.
- Once capture is achieved, continue pacing at an output level slightly higher (about 2 mA) than the threshold of initial electrical capture. For example, if capture is achieved at 90 mA, set the output level at 92 mA.
- Assess the patient's blood pressure (BP) and level of responsiveness. Monitor the patient closely and record the ECG rhythm.
- Documentation should include the date and time pacing was initiated (including baseline and pacing rhythm strips), the current required to obtain capture, the pacing rate selected, the patient's responses to electrical and mechanical capture, medications administered during the procedure, and the date and time pacing was terminated.

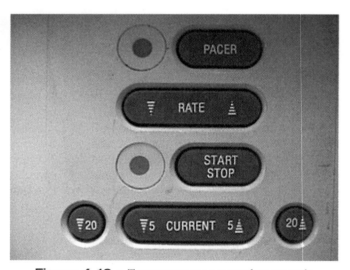

Figure 4-16 • Transcutaneous pacemaker controls.

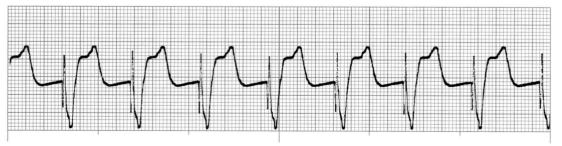

Figure 4-17 • 100% ventricular-paced rhythm.

LIMITATIONS

■ The main limitation of TCP is patient discomfort. Discomfort is proportional to the intensity of skeletal muscle contraction and the direct electrical stimulation of cutaneous nerves (Box 4-1). The degree of discomfort varies with the device used and the stimulating current required to achieve capture.

BOX 4-1		
Patient Responses to Current with Transcutaneous Pacing		
Output (mA)*	**Response**	
20	Prickly sensation on skin	
30	Slight thump on chest	
40	Definite thump on chest	
50	Coughing	
60	Diaphragm pacing and coughing	
70	Coughing and knock on chest	
80	More uncomfortable than 70 mA	
90	Strong, painful knock on chest	
100	Leaves bed because of pain	

*Responses with Zoll-NTP
From Flynn, JB: *Introduction to critical care skills.* St. Louis, 1993, Mosby-Year Book.

■ Capture may be difficult to achieve or increased stimulating current may be required in patients with increased chest wall muscle mass, chronic obstructive pulmonary disease (COPD), pleural effusions, dilated cardiomyopathy, hypoxia, or metabolic acidosis because of the extremely high current thresholds required.[34]

POSSIBLE COMPLICATIONS

■ Coughing
■ Skin burns
■ Interference with sensing due to patient agitation or muscle contractions
■ Pain from electrical stimulation of the skin and muscles
■ Failure to recognize that the pacemaker is not capturing
■ Failure to recognize the presence of underlying treatable VF
■ Tissue damage, including third-degree burns, has been reported in pediatric patients with improper or prolonged TCP[35]
■ Prolonged pacing has been associated with pacing threshold changes, leading to capture failure

PACEMAKER MALFUNCTION

Failure to Pace

■ **Failure to pace** is a pacemaker malfunction that occurs when the pacemaker fails to deliver an electrical stimulus or when it fails to deliver the correct number of electrical stimulations per minute. It is recognized on the ECG as an absence of pacemaker spikes (even though the patient's intrinsic rate is less than that of the pacemaker) and a return of the underlying rhythm for which the pacemaker was implanted.
■ Patient signs and symptoms may include syncope, chest pain, bradycardia, and hypotension.
■ Causes of failure to pace include battery failure, fracture of the pacing lead wire, displacement of the electrode tip, pulse generator failure, a broken or loose connection between

the pacing lead and the pulse generator, electromagnetic interference, and/or the sensitivity setting set too high.

- Treatment may include adjusting the sensitivity setting, replacing the pulse generator battery, replacing the pacing lead, replacing the pulse generator unit, tightening connections between the pacing lead and pulse generator, performing an electrical check, and/or removing the source of electromagnetic interference.

Failure to Capture

- **Failure to capture** is the inability of a pacemaker stimulus to depolarize the myocardium. It is recognized on the ECG by visible pacemaker spikes that are not followed by P waves (atrial pacing) or QRS complexes (ventricular pacing) (Figure 4-18).
- Patient signs and symptoms may include fatigue, bradycardia, and hypotension.
- Causes of failure to capture include battery failure, fracture of the pacing lead wire, displacement of pacing lead wire (common cause), perforation of the myocardium by a lead wire, edema or scar tissue formation at the electrode tip, output energy (mA) set too low (common cause), and/or increased stimulation threshold because of medications, electrolyte imbalance, or increased fibrin formation on the catheter tip.
- Treatment may include repositioning the patient, slowly increasing the output setting (mA) until capture occurs or the maximum setting is reached, replacing the pulse generator battery, replacing or repositioning of the pacing lead, or surgery.

(See Table 4-2 for a summary of electrical therapy.)

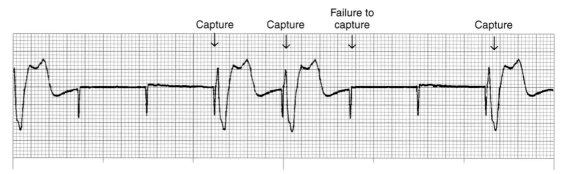

Figure 4-18 • Failure to capture.

TABLE 4-2	Electrical Therapy—Summary	
Type of Shock	**Rhythm**	**Recommended Energy Levels**
Defibrillation	Pulseless VT/VF Sustained polymorphic VT	Varies depending on device used • Biphasic defibrillator effective dose typically 120 J to 200 J • If effective dose range of device unknown, use 200 J for first shock, equal or higher shock dose for second and subsequent shocks • If using monophasic defibrillator, 360 J for all shocks
Synchronized cardioversion	Unstable narrow-QRS tachycardia	50 J, 100 J, 200 J, 300 J, 360 J*
	Unstable atrial flutter	50 J, 100 J, 200 J, 300 J, 360 J*
	Unstable atrial fibrillation	100 to 120 J, 200 J, 300 J, 360 J*
	Unstable VT with a pulse	100 J, 200 J, 300 J, 360 J*
Transcutaneous pacing	Symptomatic bradycardia	• Set initial rate at 60 to 80 pulses/min • Increase current (output/mA) until pacer spikes visible before each QRS complex; verify electrical and mechanical capture • Final mA setting should be slightly above (about 2 mA) where capture is obtained to help prevent loss of capture

* Or equivalent biphasic energy.

QUICK REVIEW ANSWERS

Quick Review Number	Answers
4-1	1. The purpose of defibrillation is to produce momentary asystole. The shock attempts to completely depolarize the myocardium at once and provide an opportunity for the natural pacemaker centers of the heart to resume normal activity. 2. Factors that affect transthoracic resistance include paddle/electrode size, paddle/electrode position, use of conductive material (when using hand-held paddles), phase of patient's respiration, paddle pressure (when using hand-held paddles), and selected energy. 3. Defibrillation is indicated for sustained polymorphic VT, pulseless VT, and VF.
4-2	Possibilities include no power, loose leads, true asystole, no connection to the patient, no connection to the defibrillator/monitor.
4-3	1. An ICD is usually located subcutaneously in the left upper quadrant of the patient's abdomen or the left pectoral region. 2. At least 1 inch from the pacemaker generator. 3. An AED is an external defibrillator with an ECG analysis system that detects and analyzes a patient's cardiac rhythm. If a shockable rhythm is detected, it delivers (if a fully automated machine) or advises the operator to deliver (if a semiautomated machine) a shock. The shock is delivered by means of two adhesive pads applied to the patient's chest.
4-4	1. The four main steps in the operation of an AED are: (1) Turn on the power, (2) Attach the device, (3) Analyze the rhythm, and (4) Deliver a shock if indicated and safe. 2. Make sure that the leads are securely in place, verify that the patient is pulseless and apneic, assure that the synchronizer switch is off, and then defibrillate immediately.

STOP & REVIEW

Questions 1-20. Match each answer below (a through t) with its corresponding description.

a) Anterior descending
b) Biphasic
c) Septum
d) Monophasic
e) Firm
f) Demand
g) Epigastrium
h) Milliamperes
i) Thump version
j) Clavicle
k) Capture
l) Mechanical
m) Epinephrine
n) Bigeminy
o) Anterolateral
p) Jaw
q) Synchronized
r) Electrical
s) Joules
t) Hyperkalemia

_____ 1. The energy selected for TCP is indicated in _____

_____ 2. Proper oral airway size is determined by measuring from the corner of the mouth to the angle of the _____

_____ 3. Another name for sternum-apex paddle/pad position

_____ 4. A common vasopressor used in cardiac arrest

_____ 5. _____ cardioversion: The timed delivery of a shock during the QRS complex

_____ 6. During pacing, assessment of _____ capture requires assessment of the patient's pulse

_____ 7. TCP is usually performed in _____ mode

_____ 8. Tall, pointed (peaked) T waves are commonly seen in this condition

_____ 9. Another name for a precordial thump

_____10. Every other beat comes from a site other than the SA node

_____11. When a _____ waveform is used for defibrillation, current passes through the heart in one direction

_____12. Leads V_1 and V_2 view this portion of the heart

_____13. During pacing, assessment of _____ capture requires observation of the cardiac monitor

_____14. The energy selected for defibrillation or cardioversion is indicated in _____

_____15. When hand-held paddles are used for defibrillation, _____ pressure must be applied to each paddle

_____16. Failure to _____ is the inability of a pacemaker stimulus to depolarize the myocardium

_____17. The sternum pad or paddle is placed just below the right _____

___18. When using _____ electrical therapy, energy is delivered in two phases

___19. One of the branches of the left coronary artery

___20. The first place to listen to confirm placement of an endotracheal tube

21. A 62-year-old man is complaining of chest pain. His level of responsiveness is rapidly decreasing. BP 50/P, P 188, R 6. The cardiac monitor reveals monomorphic VT. Your best course of action will be to:
    a. Defibrillate with 360 J
    b. Begin immediate TCP
    c. Perform synchronized cardioversion with 25 J
    d. Perform synchronized cardioversion with 100 J

22. Synchronized cardioversion:
    a. Is used only to treat rhythms with a ventricular rate of less than 60/minute
    b. Is used only for atrial dysrhythmias
    c. Delivers a shock during the QRS complex
    d. Delivers a shock between the peak and end of the T wave

23. Defibrillation is indicated in the management of:
    a. VF and asystole
    b. Pulseless VT and VF
    c. PEA and asystole
    d. Pulseless VT and PEA

24. A 62-year-old woman has experienced a cardiac arrest. You are preparing to apply combination pads to the patient's chest in the sternum-apex position. Where should the apex pad be placed?
    a. Place the center of the apex pad to the right of the sternum, just below the clavicle
    b. Place the center of the apex pad in the left midaxillary line, fifth intercostal space
    c. Place the lower edge of the apex pad to the right of the sternum, fourth intercostal space
    d. Place the upper edge of the apex pad on the patient's back, just below the left scapula

25. TCP is indicated in which of the following situations?
    a. Second-degree AV block, type II; blood pressure 64/42, altered mental status
    b. Sinus tachycardia; blood pressure 108/70, unresponsive
    c. Asystole
    d. VF

26. When performing synchronized cardioversion, you must:
    a. Depress and release one discharge button to deliver the shock
    b. Depress one or both buttons. The energy will be delivered at the appropriate time
    c. Depress and immediately release the buttons to deliver the shock
    d. Depress and *hold* both buttons depressed until the shock is delivered

27. Possible complications of TCP include:
    a. Flail chest and burns
    b. Failure to recognize that the pacemaker is not capturing
    c. Coughing and emboli
    d. Tension pneumothorax and flail chest

28. Which of the following statements is true regarding an AED?
    a. After taking multiple "looks" at the patient's rhythm, a semiautomated AED will charge its capacitors and then prompt the operator to shock the patient
    b. AEDs are programmed to recognize VF, monomorphic VT, and asystole as shockable rhythms if the rate exceeds a preset value
    c. CPR must be performed for at least 5 minutes before pressing the "analyze" control
    d. To minimize interruptions in chest compressions, CPR should be continued while the device analyzes the patient's cardiac rhythm

29. A 49-year-old man is found unresponsive, not breathing, and pulseless. The cardiac monitor reveals VT. The most important actions in the management of this patient are:
    a. CPR and defibrillation
    b. Synchronized cardioversion and resuscitation medications
    c. CPR and prompt insertion of an advanced airway
    d. Defibrillation and resuscitation medications

30. A 25-year-old man is found lying in water on the deck of a backyard pool. He is unresponsive, not breathing, and pulseless. CPR is being performed as you prepare to use an AED. Which of the following statements is correct about the use of an AED in this situation?
    a. Remove the patient from the water, wipe the chest dry, and then attach the AED pads firmly to the chest.
    b. Defibrillation cannot be performed in this situation. Continue CPR.
    c. No special precautions are necessary. Apply the AED pads to the chest and defibrillate immediately.
    d. This situation requires that both AED pads be placed directly over the sternum to minimize the risk of rescuer injury.

STOP & REVIEW ANSWERS

1. h	11. d
2. p	12. c
3. o	13. r
4. m	14. s
5. q	15. e
6. l	16. k
7. f	17. j
8. t	18. b
9. i	19. a
10. n	20. g

21. d. The patient's chest pain, decreasing level of responsiveness, and hypotension indicate that he is clearly unstable. Your best course of action is to perform synchronized cardioversion with 100 J (or an equivalent biphasic shock). TCP is not indicated. Defibrillation with an initial shock of 360 J is warranted for pulseless VT, VF, and unstable (sustained) polymorphic VT (when using a monophasic defibrillator).

22. c. Synchronized cardioversion is the timed delivery of a shock during the QRS complex. It is indicated in the management of a patient who is exhibiting serious signs and symptoms related to a tachycardia. It is used to treat rhythms that have a clearly identifiable QRS complex and a rapid ventricular rate (such as some narrow-QRS tachycardias and VT).

23. b. Defibrillation is indicated in the management of pulseless VT and VF. It is not indicated in the management of PEA. Remember: Defibrillation is performed in order to depolarize the myocardial cells at one time and provide an opportunity for one of the heart's natural pacemakers to take over. In PEA, an organized rhythm is present on the monitor. Thus, pacemaker activity is already present but there is inadequate cardiac output and no pulse. PEA is not shocked because a shock could disrupt the organized rhythm and cause chaos (VF). Defibrillation is not indicated in asystole.

24. b. Proper paddle/pad position is important. If the paddles/pads are placed too close together on the anterior surface of the chest, a substantial amount of current shunts between them and an insufficient amount reaches the left ventricle. Placement of the paddles/pads farther apart allows a sufficient amount of current to reach the left ventricle. In the sternum-apex position, the right (sternum) paddle/pad is placed to the right of the sternum, just below the clavicle. The center of the apex paddle/pad is placed in the left midaxillary line, about level with the V_6 ECG electrode position (about the fifth intercostal space).

25. a. TCP is indicated for symptomatic *bradycardias* when the patient's signs and symptoms are due to the slow heart rate. TCP is not indicated for any of the other rhythms listed.

26. d. When performing synchronized cardioversion, press and *hold* the discharge buttons (one for each paddle/pad) until the shock is delivered. It is necessary to hold the buttons in a depressed position until the machine detects the next QRS complex. Once the QRS is detected, the machine will discharge the energy. After the shock has been delivered, release the buttons.

27. b. Coughing, burns, and failure to recognize that the pacemaker is not capturing are possible complications of TCP. Once pacing has begun, it is important to reassess the patient and his or her cardiac rhythm often. Because burns are possible with prolonged pacing, check the condition of the patient's skin at the site of pacing pads at least every 30 minutes. Flail chest is a possible contraindication to TCP.

28. a. After confirming that the patient is unresponsive, not breathing, and has no pulse, CPR should be performed while the AED is being readied for use. Turn the power on to the AED, apply the pads to the patient's chest, and then analyze the patient's rhythm. All movement around the patient must stop when the AED is analyzing the patient's rhythm. For example, positive-pressure ventilation, chest compressions, and vehicle movement must temporarily stop during rhythm analysis. If movement is detected, the AED will stop analyzing the rhythm. This is a safety feature because movement can cause distortion of the patient's cardiac rhythm. Distortion can cause a nonshockable rhythm to look like a shockable rhythm, and a shockable rhythm to look like a nonshockable rhythm. A semiautomated AED prompts the operator to shock the patient. A fully automated AED charges its capacitors and delivers a shock (if a shockable rhythm is detected) without any intervention from the operator.

29. a. Defibrillation and CPR are the most important treatments for the patient in cardiac arrest due to pulseless VT or VF. Insertion of advanced airways and resuscitation medications have not been shown to increase the rate of survival to hospital discharge. Although synchronized cardioversion may be used in the treatment of an unstable patient in monomorphic VT with a pulse, it is not indicated for pulseless VT.

30. a. An AED can be used in this situation if you take safety precautions. For example, remove the patient from the water. Remove clothing from the chest and wipe the chest dry before attaching the AED pads and attempting defibrillation. Make certain that the AED pads are attached firmly to the chest with no air pockets to prevent arcing. As in other situations involving defibrillation, make sure you and other rescuers are clear of the patient before delivering a shock. Because bone is a poor conductor of electricity, paddles or pads should not be placed over the sternum, spine, or scapula.

REFERENCES

1. Caldwell G, Millar G, Quinn E, et al: Simple mechanical methods for cardioversion: Defence of the precordial thump and cough version. *Br Med J* (Clin Res Ed) Sep 7, 1985;291(6496):627-630.
2. Miller J, Tresch D, Horwitz L, et al: The precordial thump. *Ann Emerg Med* 1984;13(9, pt 2): 791-794.
3. Krijne R: Rate acceleration of ventricular tachycardia after a precordial chest thump. *Am J Cardiol* Mar 15, 1984;53(7):964-965.
4. Miller J, Addas A, Akhtar M: Electrophysiology studies: Precordial thumping patients paced into ventricular tachycardia. *J Emerg Med* 1985;3(3):175-179.
5. 2005 American Heart Association Guidelines for Cardiopulmonary Resuscitation and Emergency Cardiovascular Care, Part 7.2: Management of cardiac arrest. *Circulation* 2005;112(suppl IV):IV-64.
6. 2005 International Consensus Conference on Cardiopulmonary Resuscitation and Emergency Cardiovascular Care Science with Treatment Recommendations, January 23-30, 2005, Dallas. *Resuscitation* Dec 2005;67:203.
7. Miller B, Cohen A, Serio A, Bettock D: Hemodynamics of cough cardiopulmonary resuscitation in a patient with sustained torsades de pointes/ventricular flutter. *J Emerg Med* Sep-Oct 1994;12(5):627-632.

8. Saba SE, David SW: Sustained consciousness during ventricular fibrillation: Case report of cough cardiopulmonary resuscitation. *Cathet Cardiovasc Diagn* Jan 1996;37(1):47-48.

9. 2005 International Consensus Conference on Cardiopulmonary Resuscitation and Emergency Cardiovascular Care Science with Treatment Recommendations, January 23-30, 2005, Dallas. *Resuscitation* Dec 2005;67:192.

10. White RD: External defibrillation: The need for uniformity in analyzing and reporting results. *Ann Emerg Med* Aug 1998;32(2):234-236.

11. Gliner BE, White RD: Electrocardiographic evaluation of defibrillation shocks delivered to out-of-hospital sudden cardiac arrest patients. *Resuscitation* Jul 1999;41(2):133-144.

12. Bissing JW, Kerber RE: Effect of shaving the chest of hirsute subjects on transthoracic impedance to self-adhesive defibrillation electrode pads. *Am J Cardiol* Sep 1, 2000;86(5):587-589, A10.

13. Dahl CF, Ewy GA, Warner ED, Thomas ED: Myocardial necrosis from direct current countershock. Effect of paddle electrode size and time interval between discharges. *Circulation* Nov 1974;50(5):956-961.

14. Panacek EA, Munger MA, Rutherford WF, Gardner SF: Report of nitropatch explosions complicating defibrillation. *Am J Emerg Med* Mar 1992;10(2):128-129.

15. Wrenn K: The hazards of defibrillation through nitroglycerin patches. *Ann Emerg Med* Nov 1990;19(11):1327-1328.

16. Pagan-Carlo LA, Spencer KT, Robertson CE, et al: Transthoracic defibrillation: Importance of avoiding electrode placement directly on the female breast. *J Am Coll Cardiol* Feb 1996;27(2):449-452.

17. Olsovsky MR, Shorofsky SR, Gold MR: The effect of shock configuration and delivered energy on defibrillation impedance. *Pacing Clin Electrophysiol* Jan 1999;22(1, pt 2):165-168.

18. Bradbury N, Hyde D, Nolan J: Reliability of ECG monitoring with a gel pad/paddle combination after defibrillation. *Resuscitation* May 2000;44(3):203-206.

19. Chamberlain D: Gel pads should not be used for monitoring ECG after defibrillation. *Resuscitation* Jan 2000;43(2):159-160.

20. Hummel RS III, Ornato JP, Weinberg SM, Clarke AM: Spark-generating properties of electrode gels used during defibrillation. A potential fire hazard. *JAMA* Nov 25, 1988;260(20):3021-3024.

21. Ewy GA, Hellman DA, McClung S, Taren D: Influence of ventilation phase on transthoracic impedance and defibrillation effectiveness. *Crit Care Med* Mar 1980;8(3):164-166.

22. Sirna SJ, Ferguson DW, Charbonnier F, Kerber RE: Factors affecting transthoracic impedance during electrical cardioversion. *Am J Cardiol* Nov 15, 1988;62(16):1048-1052.

23. Bennetts SH, Deakin CD, Petley GW, Clewlow F: Is optimal paddle force applied during paediatric external defibrillation? *Resuscitation* Jan 2004;60(1):29-32.

24. Deakin CD, Bennetts SH, Petley GW, Clewlow F: What is the optimal paddle force during paediatric external defibrillation? *Resuscitation* Oct 2003;59(1):83-88.

25. Stults KR, Brown DD, Cooley F, Kerber RE: Self-adhesive monitor/defibrillation pads improve prehospital defibrillation success. *Ann Emerg Med* Aug 1987;16(8):872-877.

26. Huang J, KenKnight BH, Rollins DL, et al: Ventricular defibrillation with triphasic waveforms. *Circulation* Mar 21, 2000;101(11):1324-1328.

27. 2005 American Heart Association Guidelines for Cardiopulmonary Resuscitation and Emergency Cardiovascular Care, Part 5: Electrical Therapies: Automated External Defibrillators, Defibrillation, Cardioversion, and Pacing. *Circulation* 2005;112(suppl IV):IV-40.

28. 2005 American Heart Association Guidelines for Cardiopulmonary Resuscitation and Emergency Cardiovascular Care, Part 5: Electrical Therapies: Automated External Defibrillators, Defibrillation, Cardioversion, and Pacing. *Circulation* 2005;112(suppl IV):IV-36.

29. White RD: Waveforms for defibrillation and cardioversion: Recent experimental and clinical studies. *Curr Opin Crit Care* Jun 2004;10(3):202-207.

30. Ewy GA, Dahl CF, Zimmermann M, Otto C: Ventricular fibrillation masquerading as ventricular standstill. *Crit Care Med* 1981;9:841-844.

31. Cummins RO, Austin D Jr: The frequency of "occult" ventricular fibrillation masquerading as a flat line in prehospital cardiac arrest. *Ann Emerg Med* 1988;17:813-817.

32. 2005 American Heart Association Guidelines for Cardiopulmonary Resuscitation and Emergency Cardiovascular Care, Part 5: Electrical Therapies: Automated External Defibrillators, Defibrillation, Cardioversion, and Pacing. *Circulation* 2005;112(suppl IV):IV-41.

33. Theodorou AA, Gutierrez JA, Berg RA: Fire attributable to a defibrillation attempt in a neonate. *Pediatrics* Sep 2003;112(3, pt 1):677-679.

34. Wilson JG, Macgregor DC, Goldman BS, et al: Factors affecting patient recovery following pacemaker implantation. *Clin Prog Pacing Electrophysiology* 1984;2(6):554.

35. Beland MJ, Hesslein PS, Finlay CD, et al: Noninvasive transcutaneous cardiac pacing in children. *Pacing Clin Electrophysiol* Nov 1987;10(6):1262-1270.

Vascular Access and Medications

OBJECTIVES

Upon completion of this chapter, you will be able to:

1. Describe the indications for intravenous (IV) therapy.
2. Describe the sites of first choice for cannulation if no IV is in place at the time of cardiac arrest.
3. Describe the advantages of peripheral venipuncture over central venous access.
4. Describe the indications for central venous access.
5. List four local complications common to all IV techniques.
6. List four systemic complications common to all IV techniques.
7. Describe the use of the intraosseous (IO) and endotracheal routes as alternate routes of medication delivery in cardiac arrest.
8. Describe the location and effects of stimulation of alpha, beta, and dopaminergic receptors.
9. Define the following terms: afterload, agonist, antagonist, chronotrope, dromotrope, inotrope, parasympatholytic, preload, and sympathomimetic.
10. Identify the mechanism of action, indications, dosage, and precautions for each of the following medications:
    - Oxygen
    - Nitroglycerin
    - Morphine sulfate
    - Aspirin
    - Fibrinolytics
    - Heparin
    - Adenosine
    - Amiodarone
    - Atropine
    - Beta-blockers
    - Diltiazem
    - Epinephrine
    - Lidocaine
    - Magnesium sulfate
    - Procainamide
    - Sotalol
    - Verapamil
    - Calcium chloride
    - Dobutamine
    - Dopamine
    - Norepinephrine
    - Sodium nitroprusside
    - Vasopressin
    - Furosemide
    - Sodium bicarbonate

INTRODUCTION

Caring for a patient who is experiencing a cardiac emergency requires knowledge of vascular access and commonly used medications that affect the cardiovascular system. This chapter provides a brief overview of vascular access techniques, the autonomic nervous system (ANS), and common medications used in the care of a patient experiencing a cardiac emergency.

INTRAVENOUS THERAPY

Intravenous (IV) cannulation is the placement of a catheter into a vein to gain access to the body's venous circulation. IV access may be achieved by cannulating a peripheral or central vein.

INDICATIONS

- Maintain hydration
- Restore fluid and electrolyte balance
- Provide fluids for resuscitation
- Administration of medications, blood and blood components, and nutrient solutions
- Obtain venous blood specimens for laboratory analysis

PERIPHERAL VENOUS ACCESS

Advantages

- Effective route for medications during cardiopulmonary resuscitation (CPR).
- Does not require interruption of CPR.
- Easier to learn than central venous access.
- If an IV attempt is unsuccessful, the site is easily compressible to reduce bleeding.
- Results in fewer complications than central venous access.

Disadvantages

- In circulatory collapse, vein may be difficult to access.
- Phlebitis common with saphenous vein use.
- Should be used only for administration of isotonic solutions; hypertonic or irritating solutions may cause pain and phlebitis.
- In cardiac arrest, drugs given from a peripheral vein require 1 to 2 minutes to reach the central circulation.

Needle Size

- Gauge—outside diameter of the venipuncture device (Table 5-1).
- Provides a "rough" indication of flow rate.
- Thickness of the wall of the IV catheter varies from manufacturer to manufacturer, affecting actual flow rate.

 Fluid flow rates are proportional to the length of the catheter and its diameter. When rapid volume expansion is needed, use the shortest and smallest gauge, largest diameter catheter possible.

TABLE 5-1	Intravenous Cannula Selection	
Gauge	Use	Approximate Flow Rate (mL/min)
14 ("large-bore")	• Trauma, surgery, blood administration, administration of viscous medications • Adolescents and adults	315
16 ("large-bore")	• Trauma, surgery, blood administration, administration of viscous medications • Adolescents and adults	210
18	• Trauma, surgery, blood administration • Older children, adolescents, adults	110
20	• Suitable for most IV infusions • Older children, adolescents, adults	65
22	• Children and elderly patients	38
24	• Neonates, infants, children, and adults with fragile veins	24

Needle Types

Over-the-Needle Catheter (Figure 5-1)

■ Widely used.

■ Soft catheter commonly made of plastic or plastic-like material.

■ Rigid, plastic hub is color coded.

■ Hollow metal needle is preinserted into the catheter; the needle is used to perform the venipuncture. After venipuncture, the catheter is slid into the vein and the needle withdrawn, leaving the catheter in place through which fluid is administered.

■ Length of catheter limited by length of needle.

■ Puncture site in vein exactly size of catheter, which reduces possibility of bleeding around venipuncture site.

Hollow Needle (Figure 5-2)

■ "Butterfly" or "scalp vein" needle (also called a winged-infusion set) a common type of hollow needle—steel needle with flexible plastic wings.

■ May be easier to insert than other types of IV devices because there are no parts to manipulate.

■ Risk of infiltration higher than with other devices because steel needle tip may puncture vasculature after placement.

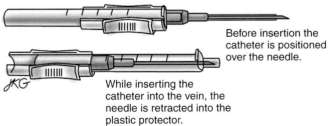

Before insertion the catheter is positioned over the needle.

While inserting the catheter into the vein, the needle is retracted into the plastic protector.

Figure 5-1 • An over-the-needle catheter.

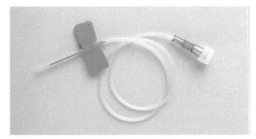

Figure 5-2 • Hollow needle—butterfly type.

Sites

Factors to consider when selecting an IV site:

- Purpose of the infusion
- Amount and type of IV fluid or medications to infuse
- Expected duration of IV therapy
- Accessibility of the vein
- Size and condition of the vein
- Patient's age, size, general condition, and preference
- Presence of disease or prior surgery, such as mastectomy
- Presence of dialysis shunt or graft
- Your experience/skill at venipuncture

External Jugular Vein

- Lies superficially along the lateral portion of the neck (Figure 5-3).
- Extends from behind the angle of the jaw and passes downward across the sternocleido-mastoid muscle and under the middle of the clavicle to join the subclavian vein.
- Considered a peripheral vein.
- Usually easy to cannulate because the vein is superficial and easy to see (Figure 5-4).
- Pressure and tension applied to the external jugular vein just above the clavicle causes the vessel to distend, making cannulation easier.
- Provides rapid access to the central circulation.
- May not be readily accessible during an arrest situation due to rescuers working to manage the airway.
- Easily dislodged and is often positional with head movement.

Upper Extremity

- Cephalic vein is located on the lateral (thumb) side and the axillary vein on the medial (little finger) side of the forearm (Figure 5-5).
  - ◗ The cephalic vein is a large vein, easy to stabilize, and easily accessible. However, wrist motion may increase patient discomfort, and irritation to the inner lining of the vessel may result from cannula movement.
- Median veins (cephalic, cubital, and basilic) lie in the antecubital fossa (Figure 5-6).
- Antecubital vein.
  - ◗ Usually easily accessible.
  - ◗ Does not interfere with ventilations and chest compressions.
  - ◗ Provides an effective route for administration of IV fluids and medications during cardiac arrest.

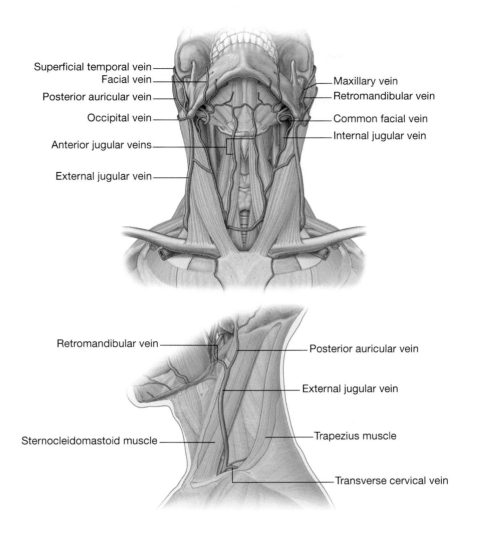

Figure 5-3 • Veins of the neck.

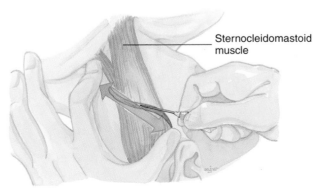

Figure 5-4 • Cannulation of the external jugular vein.

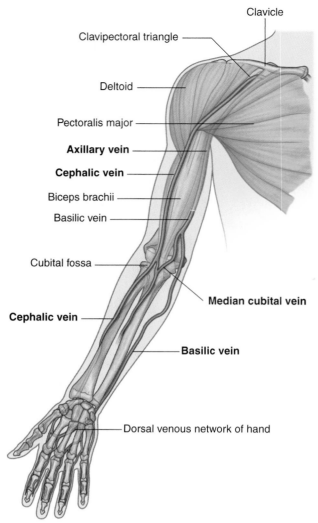

Figure 5-5 • Veins of the upper extremity.

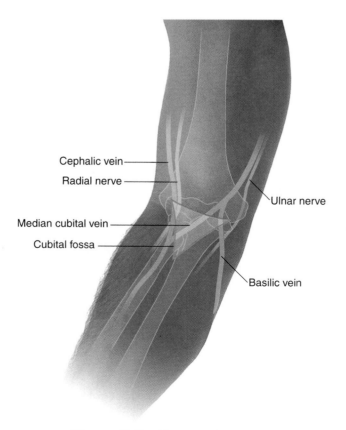

Figure 5-6 • The antecubital fossa.

During circulatory collapse or cardiac arrest, the preferred vascular access site is the largest, most accessible vein that does not require the interruption of resuscitation efforts. If no IV is in place before the arrest, establish IV access using a peripheral vein—preferably the antecubital or external jugular vein. During cardiac arrest, give IV drugs rapidly by bolus injection. Follow each drug with a 20-mL bolus of IV fluid and raise the extremity for 10 to 20 seconds to aid delivery of the drug(s) to the central circulation.

Lower Extremity

- ■ Veins of the lower extremity are not generally used during resuscitation.
    - ▶ Distance from the central circulation.
    - ▶ Cannulation of the veins of the legs, feet, and ankles may compromise lower extremity circulation and cause thrombophlebitis or embolism.
- ■ If the lower extremity must be cannulated, the long saphenous vein is the preferred site for IV therapy (Figure 5-7).

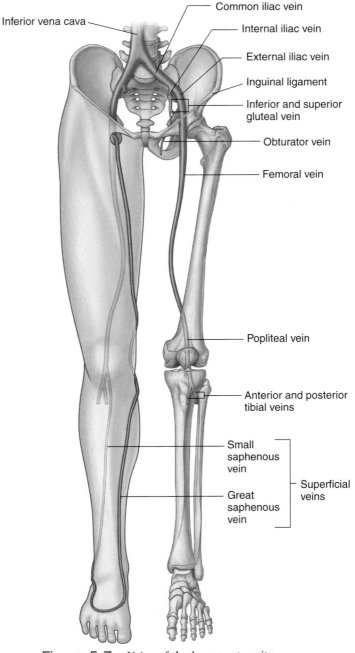

Inferior vena cava

Common iliac vein

Internal iliac vein

External iliac vein

Inguinal ligament

Inferior and superior gluteal vein

Obturator vein

Femoral vein

Popliteal vein

Anterior and posterior tibial veins

Small saphenous vein

Great saphenous vein

Superficial veins

Figure 5-7 • Veins of the lower extremity.

QUICK REVIEW 5-1

1. Can you describe the indications for IV therapy?
   1.
   2.
   3.
2. Can you describe the sites of first choice for cannulation if no IV is in place at the time of cardiac arrest?

3. Name three advantages of peripheral venipuncture over central venous access.

4. Where is the external jugular vein located?

Answers can be found at the end of this chapter.

CENTRAL VENOUS ACCESS

- To access the central circulation, a central venous catheter (also called a central line) is inserted into the vena cava from the subclavian, jugular, or femoral vein.

Indications

- Emergency access to venous circulation when peripheral sites are not readily available
- Need for long-term IV therapy
- Administration of large volume of fluid
- Administration of hypertonic solutions, caustic medications, or parenteral feeding solutions
- Placement of transvenous pacemaker electrodes
- Placement of central venous pressure or right heart catheters

Advantages

- Peak medication concentrations are higher and circulation times shorter when medications are administered via a central route compared with peripheral sites.

Disadvantages

- Special equipment (syringe, catheter, needle) required
- Excessive time (5 to 10 minutes) for placement
- High complication rate
- Skill deterioration (frequent practice required to maintain proficiency)
- Inability to initiate procedure while other patient care activities in progress

 If peripheral IV access is unsuccessful during cardiac arrest, consider an IO infusion before considering placement of a central line.

COMPLICATIONS COMMON TO ALL INTRAVENOUS TECHNIQUES

Local Complications

Local complications of IV therapy are most often seen at or near the IV insertion site and are more common than systemic complications. Some local complications can lead to more serious systemic complications. Local complications include the following:

■ Pain and irritation
■ Hematoma formation (Figure 5-8)
   ▶ Possible causes: advancing the needle completely through the vein or inadequate application of pressure to prevent leakage of blood from the vein when the catheter is removed.
   ▶ Signs and symptoms: ecchymosis over and around the insertion site, pain at the site, swelling and hardness at the insertion site, inability to flush the IV line, inability to advance the cannula all the way into the vein during insertion.
■ Infiltration and extravasation
   ▶ **Infiltration** is the intentional or unintentional process in which a substance enters or infuses into another substance or a surrounding area (Figure 5-9).
   ▶ **Extravasation** is the actual (unintentional) escape or leakage of an agent that is irritating and causes blistering (a vesicant) from a vessel into the surrounding tissue (Figure 5-10).

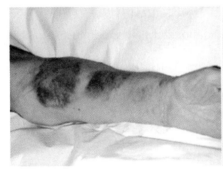

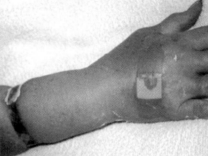

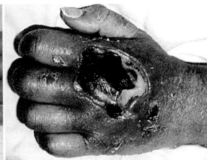

Figure 5-8 • Bruising/hematoma formation.

Figure 5-9 • Infiltration.

Figure 5-10 • Extravasation.

▶ Possible causes are shown in Box 5-1.
▶ Signs and symptoms: coolness of skin around IV site; swelling at the IV site, with or without pain; sluggish or absent flow rate; infusion continues to infuse when pressure is applied to the vein above the tip of the cannula; no backflow of blood into IV tubing when clamp fully opened and solution container lowered below IV site.

BOX 5-1

Extravasation—Possible Causes

- Venipuncture device dislodged from vein
- Puncture of distal vein wall during venipuncture
- Leakage of solution into the surrounding tissue from the cannula's insertion site
- Poorly secured IV
- Poor vein or site selection
- Irritating solution or medication that inflames the intima of the vein and causes it to weaken
- Improper cannula size
- High delivery rate or pressure of the solution or medication

---

▪ Thrombosis and thrombophlebitis (Figure 5-11)
  ▶ Possible causes: clotting at catheter tip and inflammation, injury to endothelial cells of vein wall allowing platelet aggregation and thrombus formation.
  ▶ Signs and symptoms: slowed or stopped infusion rate, aching or burning sensation at infusion site, skin warm and red around IV site, swelling of the extremity, and/or throbbing pain in the limb.
▪ Venous spasm
  ▶ Possible causes: severe irritation from irritating medications or fluids, administration of cold fluids, or blood.
  ▶ Examples: substances with a high or low pH, diazepam (Valium), phenytoin (Dilantin), and dextrose solutions with concentrations higher than 12.5%.
  ▶ Signs and symptoms: sluggish or stopped infusion rate when the clamp is completely open, severe pain from the IV site radiating up the extremity, blanching of the skin over the IV site, or redness over and around the IV site.
▪ Vessel collapse. Signs and symptoms: inability to see and/or feel a vein, loss of vessel elasticity, vessel feels flat or flaccid, or reduced or stopped infusion flow.
▪ Inadvertent arterial puncture. If administered arterially, some medications crystallize and may completely occlude the arterial blood supply distal to the point of injection, resulting in permanent interruption of the blood supply to the affected area.

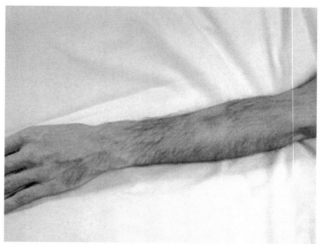

Figure 5-11 • Infusion phlebitis.

■ Cellulitis
  ▶ **Cellulitis** is a diffuse inflammation and infection of cellular and subcutaneous connective tissue that can lead to abscess formation and ulceration of deeper tissues.
  ▶ Signs and symptoms: pain, tenderness, warmth, edema, red streaking on skin (if spread to lymphatics), roughened appearance of the skin (like that of an orange peel), fever, and chills.
■ Nerve, tendon, ligament, and/or limb damage
  ▶ Possible causes: improper venipuncture technique, improper securing and stabilization of the cannula and IV line after insertion, extravasated IV solution, cellulitis.
  ▶ Signs and symptoms: tingling, numbness and loss of sensation, loss of movement, cyanosis, pallor, deformity, or paralysis.

Systemic Complications

Systemic complications of IV therapy occur within the vascular system, usually distant from the IV insertion site. Systemic complications include the following:
■ Sepsis
■ Contamination and infection
■ Hypersensitivity reactions
  ▶ Can occur as a response to the IV solution, its preservatives, or IV medications.
  ▶ Patient may have an allergy to the cannula, antiseptic preparation, or tape.
  ▶ Signs and symptoms: range from mild to severe, affect several body systems, and may develop rapidly, gradually, or be delayed hours after the allergen has been administered.
■ Speed shock
  ▶ **Speed shock** is a systemic reaction to the rapid or excessive infusion of medication or solution into the circulation.
  ▶ Signs and symptoms: flushing of head and neck, apprehension, hypertension, pounding headache, dyspnea, chest pain, chills, loss of responsiveness, and cardiac arrest.
■ Emboli (blood clot, catheter, air)
  ▶ Pulmonary embolism
    • May result from a thrombus that forms from trauma to the intima of a vein.
    • Blood flow past the thrombus can cause a portion of the clot to break off and become an embolus.
    • Signs and symptoms: dyspnea, tachypnea, dysrhythmias, hypotension, diaphoresis, anxiety, and/or a cough.
  ▶ Catheter embolism
    • May occur because of catheter shear in which a portion of the catheter is sheared off, usually because of a back-and-forth movement through the needle.
    • Signs and symptoms: sudden, severe pain at the IV site, and/or a reduced or absent blood return when checking placement of the IV catheter. If the catheter does not travel, patient may be asymptomatic. If the catheter lodges in a heart chamber or the pulmonary circulation, patient may experience hypotension, tachycardia, chest pain, cyanosis, and/or a loss of responsiveness.
  ▶ Air embolism
    • Possible causes: IV solution container empty; air enters bloodstream by means of the IV catheter tubing. It is possible for air to enter the circulation during catheter insertion or when the tubing is disconnected to replace IV solutions or IV tubing.
    • Risk of an air embolus is greatest when central venous cannulation is performed because negative pressure during cannulation may actually pull air into the vein.
    • Signs and symptoms: hypotension, extreme anxiety, lightheadedness and confusion, tachypnea, cyanosis, a weak and rapid pulse, and/or a loss of responsiveness.

ALTERNATIVE ROUTES

INTRAOSSEOUS INFUSION

When IV cannulation is unsuccessful or taking too long, an intraosseous (IO) infusion is an alternative method of gaining access to the vascular system. An **intraosseous infusion** is the process of infusing medications, fluids, and blood products into the bone marrow cavity for subsequent delivery to the venous circulation. Any medication or fluid that can be administered IV can be administered IO.

Site

Traditionally, IO infusion has been accepted as a rapid, reliable method of achieving vascular access in children under emergency conditions. Various sites have been studied to evaluate the effectiveness of IO infusion in adults including the clavicle, ilium, and tibia,[1] an area proximal to the medial malleolus,[2,3] and the manubrium (the top bone of the sternum).[4]

The sternum can be used for IO infusion in adults because it is large, thin, and flat; contains a high proportion of vascular red marrow; is easy to penetrate and less likely to be fractured; and is closer to the central circulation. Substances infused into the sternum reach the central circulation via the internal mammary and azygos venous systems within seconds. Alternate sites that may be used in adults include the tibia and humeral head.

The First Access for Shock and Trauma (F.A.S.T.) 1 device is an example of a sternal IO infusion system (Figure 5-12A). With this device, a handheld introducer is used to insert a flexible infusion tube with a stainless-steel tip to a predetermined depth in the manubrium. Fluids and medications are administered through the tube into the marrow space. Generally, vascular access can be achieved in 60 seconds with a 95% success rate using the device. It can remain in place for a maximum of 24 hours (or until conventional IV access is established). CPR can be performed while fluids are being infused.

The EZ-IO is another IO device. It consists of a small, battery-powered, IO driver (reusable) and needle set (disposable) (Figure 5-12B). For tibial insertion in adults, the EZ-IO is positioned two finger widths bellow the patella and one finger width medial (toward the inside) of the tibial tuberosity. An alternate site that may be used is the humeral head. The manufacturer, VidaCare, has extensive materials available explaining their products, supporting research, identification of anatomic landmarks, insertion technique, and related information. The EZ-IO requires no special tool for removal.

Indications

- Emergency administration of fluids and/or medications, especially in the setting of circulatory collapse where rapid vascular access is essential
- Difficult, delayed, or impossible IV access
- Burns or other injuries preventing venous access at other sites

To improve flow rates during an IO infusion, the use of a pressure bag or infusion pump may be necessary.

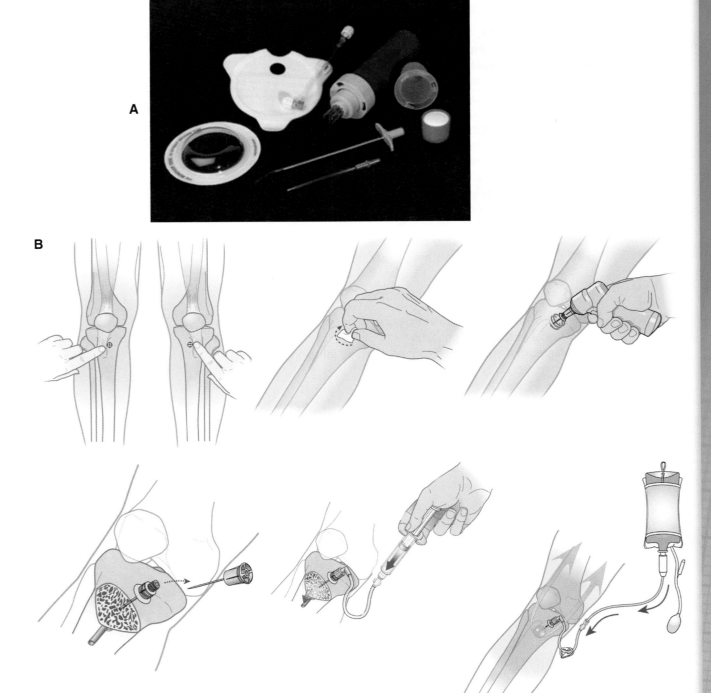

Figure 5-12 • **A,** The F.A.S.T. 1 IO infusion system. **B,** The EZ-IO device.

Precautions

Use of the F.A.S.T. 1 device is not recommended in the following situations:
- Patient is of small stature:
  - ▶ Weight less than 50 kg
  - ▶ Pathologic small size
- Chest trauma with a suspected fractured sternum
- Significant tissue damage at IO insertion site
- Severe osteoporosis or bone-softening conditions
- Previous sternotomy and/or scar

Use of the EZ-IO device is not recommended in the following situations:
- Fracture of the tibia or femur
- Previous orthopedic procedures
- Preexisting medical condition
- Infection at the insertion site
- Inability to locate landmarks
- Excessive tissue over the insertion site

Possible Complications

- Extravasation of fluids into subcutaneous tissue
- Local abscess or cellulitis
- Osteomyelitis (related to long-term IO infusion)

ENDOTRACHEAL DRUG ADMINISTRATION

■ If IV or IO access cannot be achieved to give drugs during a cardiac arrest, the endotracheal route can be used to give selected medications. The endotracheal route of drug administration is not preferred because multiple studies have shown that giving resuscitation drugs endotracheally results in lower blood concentrations than the same dose given IV.

■ An important and beneficial effect of IV epinephrine administration during cardiac arrest is its ability to increase coronary and cerebral perfusion pressures. This action is a result of epinephrine's vasoconstrictive effect due to alpha-adrenergic receptor stimulation (discussed later in this chapter).

■ Some studies suggest that endotracheal epinephrine can produce a transient *decrease* in blood pressure (BP).[5-7] This effect is presumed to be due to beta$_2$-adrenergic receptor stimulation. This can cause hypotension and lower coronary artery perfusion pressure, which may lessen the potential for a return of spontaneous circulation. In contrast, research has shown that endotracheal vasopressin produced an immediate increase in diastolic blood pressure (DBP) that lasted more than 1 hour.[8] Elevated DBP is important because it directly influences coronary perfusion pressure.

■ Previous resuscitation guidelines have recommended using a catheter to administer drugs via an endotracheal tube. Studies have shown that there are no benefits from endobronchial administration of drugs compared with administration directly into an endotracheal tube.

■ The recommended dose of some drugs that can be given via the endotracheal route is generally 2 to 2.5 times the IV dose, but the optimal endotracheal dose of most drugs is unknown. For example, some studies have shown that the endotracheal dose of epinephrine should probably be between 3 and 10 times the currently recommended IV dose.

KEEPING IT SIMPLE

Endotracheal Medications

N = Naloxone
A = Atropine
V = Vasopressin
E = Epinephrine
L = Lidocaine

A REVIEW OF THE AUTONOMIC NERVOUS SYSTEM

■ The ANS consists of sympathetic and parasympathetic divisions. The sympathetic division mobilizes the body, allowing the body to function under stress ("fight or flight" response). The parasympathetic division is responsible for the conservation and restoration of body resources ("feed and breed" or "resting and digesting" response) (Table 5-2).

TABLE 5-2	Overview of the Divisions of the Autonomic Nervous System
Sympathetic Division	**Parasympathetic Division**
"Fight or Flight" response	**"Feed and Breed" or "Resting and Digesting" response**
• Mobilizes the body	• Conservation of body resources
• Allows the body to function under stress	• Restoration of body resources

■ Nerve impulses are carried from the sensory receptors to the brain by means of the vagus and glossopharyngeal nerves (afferent pathways). The medulla of the brain serves as the integration center and interprets the sensory information received. It determines what body parameters need adjustment (if any) and transmits that information to the heart and blood vessels by means of motor nerves (efferent pathways).

■ Motor pathways of the ANS use two neurons to transmit information from the central nervous system (CNS) to various organs (effectors). The first (preganglionic) neuron conducts impulses from the CNS to the ganglion (cell body) of a second (postganglionic) neuron. The postganglionic neuron extends from the ganglion to the organ. The junction between these two neurons is called a **synapse.**

■ Sympathetic preganglionic neurons are relatively short, and the postganglionic neurons relatively long.
   ▶ One sympathetic preganglionic neuron may synapse with many postganglionic neurons in many organs. Thus, sympathetic effects are often widespread, affecting many organs.
   ▶ Parasympathetic preganglionic neurons are relatively long. The postganglionic neurons that lead to a single organ are relatively short. Thus, parasympathetic stimulation often involves a response by only one organ (Figure 5-13).

■ Preganglionic nerve fibers of both the sympathetic and parasympathetic divisions of the ANS release acetylcholine (ACh), a **neurotransmitter.**

■ Postganglionic fibers that release norepinephrine (NE) are called *adrenergic* fibers. Those that release ACh are called *cholinergic* fibers (Figure 5-14).

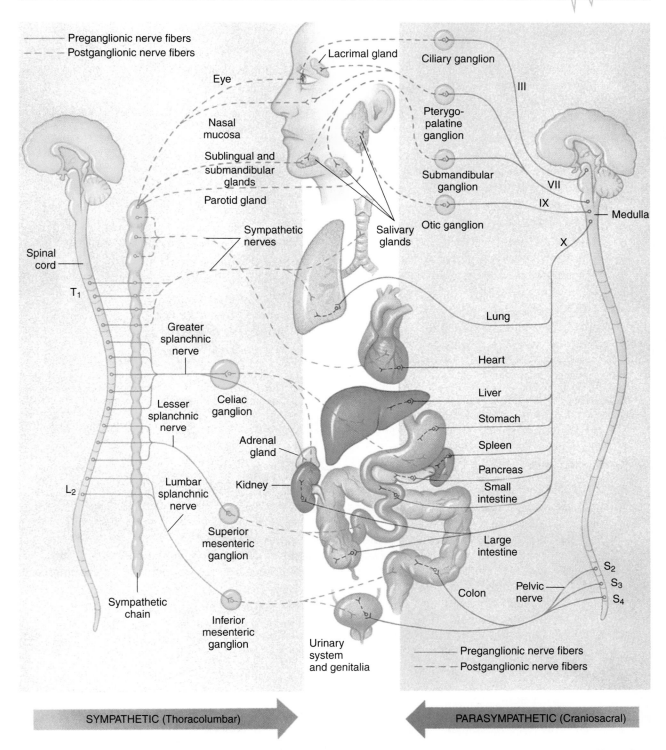

Figure 5-13 • Innervation of major target organs by the ANS. Preganglionic fibers (solid lines), postganglionic fibers (broken lines).

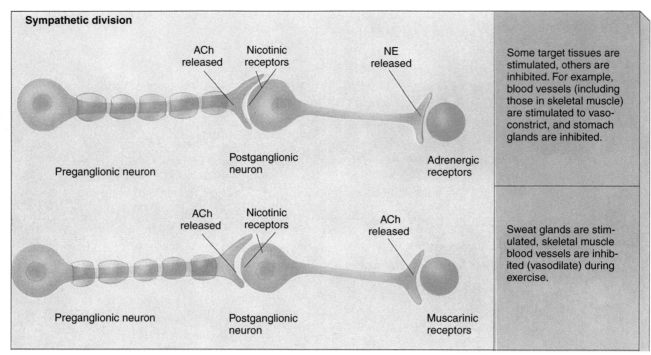

Figure 5-14 • Preganglionic fibers release ACh, which stimulates nicotinic receptors in the postganglionic neuron. Most sympathetic postganglionic fibers secrete NE, resulting in alpha- or beta-receptor stimulation. A few postganglionic fibers are cholinergic (e.g., sweat glands and some blood vessels), resulting in stimulation of muscarinic receptors.

SYMPATHETIC DIVISION

Activation of the sympathetic division of the ANS results in the following:

■ Increased heart rate, force of contraction, conduction velocity, BP, and cardiac output (Figure 5-15)
■ Dilation of smooth muscles of bronchi to improve oxygenation
■ Shunting of blood from skin and blood vessels of internal organs to skeletal muscle
■ Mobilization of stored energy to ensure an adequate supply of glucose for the brain and fatty acids for muscle activity
■ Dilation of pupils
■ Increased sweating

Sympathetic (adrenergic) receptors are located in different organs and have different physiologic actions when stimulated. There are five main types of sympathetic receptors:

1. Alpha$_1$
2. Alpha$_2$
3. Beta$_1$
4. Beta$_2$
5. Dopamine (also called dopaminergic)

■ Alpha$_1$ receptors are found in the eyes, blood vessels, bladder, and male reproductive organs. Stimulation of alpha$_1$ receptor sites results in constriction.
■ Alpha$_2$ receptor sites are found in parts of the digestive system and on presynaptic nerve terminals in the peripheral nervous system. Stimulation results in decreased secretions, peristalsis, and suppression of NE release.
■ Beta receptor sites are divided into beta$_1$ and beta$_2$. Beta$_1$ receptors are found in the heart and kidneys. Stimulation of beta$_1$ receptor sites in the heart results in increased heart rate,

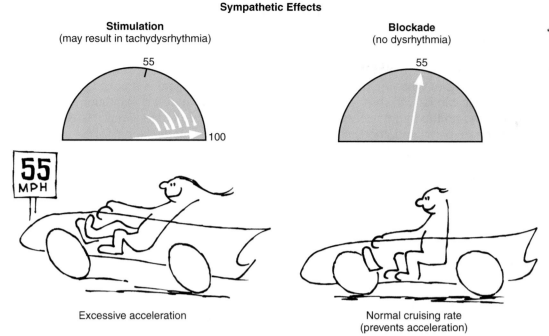

Sympathetic Effects

Stimulation
(may result in tachydysrhythmia)

Blockade
(no dysrhythmia)

Excessive acceleration

Normal cruising rate
(prevents acceleration)

Figure 5-15 • Effects of sympathetic stimulation on the heart.

contractility, and, ultimately, irritability of cardiac cells. Stimulation of beta$_1$ receptor sites in the kidneys results in the release of renin into the blood. Renin promotes the production of angiotensin, a powerful vasoconstrictor. Beta$_2$ receptor sites are found in the arterioles of the heart, lungs, and skeletal muscle. Stimulation results in dilation. Stimulation of beta$_2$ receptor sites in the smooth muscle of the bronchi results in dilation.

■ Dopamine receptors are found in the renal, mesenteric, and visceral blood vessels. Stimulation results in dilation. A summary of sympathetic receptors is shown in Table 5-3.

TABLE 5-3	Sympathetic (Adrenergic) Receptors	
Receptor Type	**Location**	**Effects of Stimulation**
Alpha$_1$	Eye	Radial muscle contraction of iris causes increased pupil size
	Arterioles of skin, viscera, mucous membranes	Constriction, ↑ peripheral vascular resistance
	Veins	Constriction
	Bladder sphincters	Constriction
	Male reproductive organs	Ejaculation
Alpha$_2$	Digestive system	Decreased secretions, peristalsis
	Presynaptic nerve terminals in peripheral nervous system	Inhibits NE release
Beta$_1$	Heart	• ↑ Heart rate • ↑ Force of contraction • ↑ Speed of conduction through AV node • ↑ Oxygen consumption
	Kidneys	Renin release
Beta$_2$	Arterioles of heart, lungs, skeletal muscle	Dilation, ↑ organ perfusion
	Bronchi	Dilation
	Uterus	Relaxation
	Liver	Glycogenolysis (breakdown of glycogen to glucose)
Dopamine	Renal, mesenteric, and visceral blood vessels	Dilation

AV, Atrioventricular.

PARASYMPATHETIC DIVISION

- Stimulation results in the release of ACh. Acetylcholine binds to parasympathetic receptors. The two main types of cholinergic receptors are nicotinic and muscarinic receptors.
- Nicotinic receptors are located in skeletal muscle. Muscarinic receptors are located in smooth muscle. When ACh binds to nicotinic receptors, there is an excitatory response. When ACh binds with muscarinic receptors, the result may be excitation or inhibition, depending on the target tissues in which the receptors are found (Figure 5-16).
- In the heart, parasympathetic (inhibitory) nerve fibers supply the sinoatrial (SA) node, atrial muscle, and the atrioventricular (AV) junction by means of the vagus nerves. The net effect of parasympathetic stimulation is slowing of the heart rate (Figure 5-17).
- Organ responses to sympathetic and parasympathetic stimulation are shown in Table 5-4. Common terms used when discussing the ANS are shown in Table 5-5. Important terms to commit to memory are listed in Table 5-6.

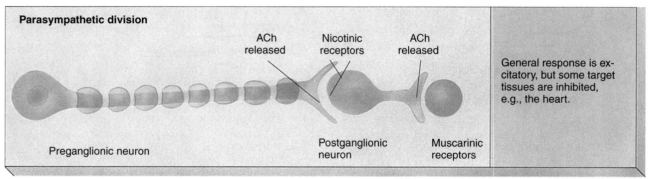

Figure 5-16 • ACh binds to muscarinic or nicotinic receptor sites. When ACh binds to nicotinic receptors, there is an excitatory response. When ACh binds with muscarinic receptors, the result may be excitation or inhibition, depending on the target tissues in which the receptors are found.

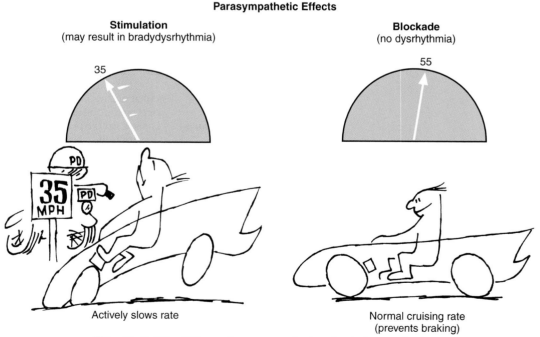

Figure 5-17 • Effects of parasympathetic stimulation on the heart.

TABLE 5-4	Organ Responses to Sympathetic and Parasympathetic Stimulation	
	Sympathetic	Parasympathetic
Eyes	Pupillary dilation	Accommodation for near vision
Saliva	↓ Secretions	↑ Secretions
Bronchial Smooth Muscle	Dilation	Constriction, ↑ secretion
Heart	↑ Rate and force of contraction (beta receptors)	↓ Rate; minimal effect on force of contraction
Liver	Glucose release (glycogenolysis) (beta receptors)	No effect
Gastrointestinal Tract	• ↓ Peristalsis (beta receptors) • Sphincter constriction (alpha receptors) • ↓ Blood flow	• ↑ Peristalsis • Sphincter relaxation • ↑ secretion
Bladder	• Relaxation (beta receptors) • Sphincter constriction (alpha receptors)	• Contraction • Relaxation
Sweat Glands	↑	No effect
Smooth Muscle of Blood Vessels		
Abdominal	Constriction (alpha receptors)	No effect
Coronary	• Constriction (alpha receptors) • Dilation (beta receptors)	Dilation
Skeletal muscle	Dilation (beta receptors)	No effect
Skin	Constriction (alpha receptors)	No effect

TABLE 5-5	Autonomic Nervous System Terminology	
	Terms That Indicate Stimulation	Terms That Indicate Inhibition
Sympathetic Division	• Sympathomimetic • Sympathetic agonist • Adrenergic • Adrenergic agonist	• Sympatholytic • Adrenergic blocker • Sympathetic blocker • Antiadrenergic • Sympathetic antagonist
Parasympathetic Division	• Parasympathomimetic • Parasympathetic agonist • Cholinergic • Cholinergic agonist	• Parasympatholytic • Cholinergic blocker • Parasympathetic blocker • Anticholinergic • Parasympathetic antagonist • Vagolytic

TABLE 5-6	Important Terms to Commit to Memory
Chronotrope	A substance that affects the heart rate • Positive chronotrope = ↑ heart rate • Negative chronotrope = ↓ heart rate
Inotrope	A substance that affects myocardial contractility • Positive inotrope = ↑ force of contraction • Negative inotrope = ↓ force of contraction
Dromotrope	A substance that affects AV conduction velocity • Positive dromotrope = ↑ AV conduction velocity • Negative dromotrope = ↓ AV conduction velocity
Preload	Pressure/volume in the left ventricle at the end of diastole
Afterload	Pressure or resistance against which the heart must pump
Agonist	A drug or substance that produces a predictable response (stimulates action)
Antagonist	An agent that exerts an action opposite to another (blocks action)

QUICK REVIEW 5-2

1. Name the primary target organs affected by stimulation of the following receptor sites: alpha$_1$, beta$_1$, and beta$_2$.

   Alpha$_1$:

   Beta$_1$:

   Beta$_2$:

2. A positive inotropic effect refers to a(n) _____ in _____ _____.

3. A negative chronotropic effect refers to a(n) _____ in _____ _____.

MEDICATIONS USED IN ACUTE CORONARY SYNDROMES

MONA is a memory aid that may be used to recall medications used in the management of acute coronary syndromes (although not in the order they are given).

M = *Morphine*
O = *Oxygen*
N = *Nitroglycerin*
A = *Aspirin*

TABLE 5-7	Oxygen
Mechanism of Action	• Increases oxygen tension • Increases hemoglobin saturation if ventilation is supported • Improves tissue oxygenation when circulation is maintained
Indications	• Cardiac or respiratory arrest • Suspected hypoxemia of any cause • Any suspected cardiopulmonary emergency, especially complaints of shortness of breath and/or suspected ischemic chest pain
Dosing	Spontaneously breathing patient: best guided by pulse oximetry,* blood gases, and patient tolerance to oxygen delivery device • Nasal cannula (1 to 6 L/min) • Simple face mask (8 to 10 L/min) • Partial rebreather mask (6 to 10 L/min) • Nonrebreather mask (10 to 15 L/min) Cardiac arrest: positive-pressure ventilation with 100% oxygen
Precautions	Toxicity possible with prolonged administration of high flow oxygen

*Note: Pulse oximetry is inaccurate in low cardiac output states or with vasoconstriction.

TABLE 5-8	Nitroglycerin	

Generic Name	nitroglycerin
Trade Names	Nitrostat, Nitro-Bid (SL forms); Tridil (IV)
Classification	Vasodilator, organic nitrate, antianginal
Mechanism of Action	• Relaxes vascular smooth muscle; including dilation of the coronary arteries (particularly in the area of plaque disruption), the peripheral arterial bed, and venous capacitance vessels • Dilation of postcapillary vessels → peripheral pooling of blood → decreases venous return to the heart → decreases preload • Arteriolar relaxation reduces systemic vascular resistance and arterial pressure (afterload)
Indications	SL tablets or spray: • Prophylaxis, treatment, and management of patients with angina pectoris • Pulmonary congestion due to LV failure IV: • Ongoing ischemic chest discomfort • Management of hypertensive emergencies, particularly if related to volume overload • Management of pulmonary congestion due to LV failure
Dosing (Adult)	SL or spray • Give a nitroglycerin tablet (or spray) every 5 minutes up to 3 doses if the patient's SBP remains >90 mm Hg or no more than 30 mm Hg below baseline and the heart rate remains between 50 and 100 bpm.* • Spray on or under the tongue for 0.5 to 1 second at 5-minute intervals. Each metered dose delivers 0.4 mg of nitroglycerin per spray. IV infusion • Initial dosage should be 5 mcg/min delivered through an infusion pump capable of exact and constant delivery of the drug. Subsequent titration must be adjusted to the clinical situation, with dose increments becoming more cautious as partial response is seen. Initial titration should be in 5 mcg/min increments, with increases every 3-5 minutes until some response is noted. If no response is seen at 20 mcg/min, increments of 10 and later 20 mcg/min can be used. Once a partial BP response is observed, the dose increase should be reduced and the interval between increments should be lengthened.† • Low doses (30 to 40 mcg/min) predominantly produce venodilation; high doses (≥150 mcg/min) provide arteriolar dilation.‡
Precautions	• Primary side effect is hypotension. Other side effects include tachycardia, bradycardia, headache, palpitations, and syncope.
Contraindications	• Viagra (or other phosphodiesterase inhibitor) use within 24 to 48 hours • Suspected inferior wall MI with possible right ventricular MI • Hypotension (SBP <90 mm Hg or <30 mm Hg below baseline) • Extreme bradycardia (<50 bpm) • Tachycardia (>100 bpm) • Increased intracranial pressure (e.g., head trauma or cerebral hemorrhage) • Uncorrected hypovolemia • Inadequate cerebral circulation • Constrictive pericarditis and pericardial tamponade
Special Considerations	• Hypotension may worsen myocardial ischemia. Hypotension usually responds to administration of IV fluids. *Establishing an IV before giving SL nitroglycerin is strongly recommended.* • When giving nitroglycerin for ischemic chest discomfort, assess the patient's pain, duration, time started, activity being performed, quality, etc. Document the patient's response to the medication. • Monitor vital signs and cardiac rhythm closely before, during, and after giving. • Significant hypotension may occur in the presence of right ventricular infarction. • Nitroglycerin tablets are light, moisture, and heat sensitive. Keep tablets in their original, brown glass bottles. Replace metal cap on bottle quickly after opening. Tablets usually lose potency within 3 to 4 months. • When giving nitroglycerin spray, do not shake the canister before use. Shaking may produce bubbles within the canister, altering delivery of the medication.
Onset of Action	SL: Typically within 1 to 3 minutes; IV: Immediate—within 1.5 minutes
Duration	SL: 10 to 30 minutes; IV: 1 to 10 minutes after IV discontinued

*2005 American Heart Association guidelines for cardiopulmonary resuscitation and emergency cardiovascular care, part 8: Stabilization of the patient with acute coronary syndromes. *Circulation* 2005;112(suppl IV):IV-91–IV-98.

†*Mosby's drug consult,* St. Louis: Mosby, 2006.

‡2005 American Heart Association guidelines for cardiopulmonary resuscitation and emergency cardiovascular care, part 7.4: Monitoring and medications. *Circulation* 2005;112(suppl IV):IV-80–IV-81.

IV, Intravenous; *BP,* blood pressure; *LV,* left ventricular; *MI,* myocardial infarction; *SBP,* systolic blood pressure; *SL,* sublingual.

TABLE 5-9	Morphine Sulfate
Generic Name	morphine sulfate
Trade Names	Duramorph, Infumorph, MS Contin, MSIR, Oramorph, Roxanol
Classification	Narcotic (opioid) analgesic (Schedule II controlled substance)
Mechanism of Action	The principal actions of a therapeutic dosage of morphine are analgesia, sedation, and alterations of mood. Opioids of this class do not usually eliminate pain, but they do reduce the perception of pain by the CNS. • Reduces pain of ischemia • Reduces anxiety • Increases venous capacitance (venous pooling) and decreases venous return (preload; sometimes called "chemical phlebotomy") • Decreases systemic vascular resistance (afterload) • Decreases myocardial oxygen demand (Pain $\uparrow$ sympathetic response $\rightarrow$ $\uparrow$ heart rate, $\uparrow$ systemic vascular resistance, $\uparrow$ BP $\rightarrow$ $\uparrow$ myocardial O_2 consumption = reason pain relief is a priority in the management of the patient with an acute coronary syndrome)
Indications	• Analgesic of choice for continuing ischemic chest discomfort unresponsive to nitrates • Pulmonary vascular congestion complicating acute coronary syndromes (SBP >90 mm Hg)
Dosing (Adult)	• 2 to 4 mg (give in 2-mg increments) slow IV push; give additional doses of 2 to 8 mg IV at 5- to 15-minute intervals*
Precautions	Watch closely for: • Bradycardia • CNS depression • Nausea/vomiting • Respiratory depression (most serious side effect—reversible with naloxone) • Hypotension
Contraindications	• Hypersensitivity to morphine or other opiates • Respiratory depression • CNS depression due to head injury, overdose, poisoning, etc. • Increased intracranial pressure • Asthma (relative) • Undiagnosed abdominal pain • Hypovolemia • Hypotension
Special Considerations	Make sure naloxone and airway equipment are within reach before giving
Onset of Action	IV: Immediate (peak 20 min)
Duration	IV: 2 to 4 hours

*2005 American Heart Association guidelines for cardiopulmonary resuscitation and emergency cardiovascular care, part 8: Stabilization of the patient with acute coronary syndromes. *Circulation* 2005;112(suppl IV):IV-98.

TABLE 5-10	Naloxone	
Generic Name	naloxone hydrochloride	
Trade Name	Narcan	
Classification	Narcotic (opioid) antagonist	
Mechanism of Action	Although the mechanism of action of naloxone is not fully understood, evidence suggests that naloxone antagonizes the effects of opiates by competing for the same receptor sites, thereby preventing or reversing the effects of narcotics including respiratory depression, sedation, and hypotension.	
Indications	• Complete or partial reversal of narcotic depression, including respiratory depression, induced by opioids including natural and synthetic narcotics, propoxyphene, methadone, and the narcotic-antagonist analgesics: nalbuphine, pentazocine, and butorphanol • Diagnosis of suspected acute opioid overdosage	
Dosing (Adult)	IV, IM, SubQ—known or suspected narcotic overdose • Initial dose 0.4 to 2 mg. If the desired degree of counteraction and improvement in respiratory function is not obtained, it may be repeated at 2 to 3 minute intervals.* • If no response is observed after 10 mg of naloxone have been given, reevaluate diagnosis. IM or SubQ administration may be necessary if IV route is not available.	
Precautions	Abrupt reversal of narcotic depression may result in: • Nausea, vomiting • Sweating • Tachycardia • Increased BP • Tremulousness • Seizures • Cardiac arrest	
Contraindications	Known hypersensitivity to the medication	
Special Considerations	• Ineffective if respiratory depression due to hypnotics, sedatives, anesthetics, or other nonnarcotic CNS depressants. • Effects of narcotics are usually longer than those of naloxone; thus, respiratory depression may return when naloxone has worn off. Monitor the patient closely • Naloxone can also be given by the intranasal or endotracheal routes. The IV, IM, or SubQ routes are preferred over the endotracheal route.[†]	
Onset of Action	IV: 2 minutes, SubQ/IM: <5 minutes	
Duration	IV: 45 minutes, SubQ/IM: 45 to 60 minutes	

* *Mosby's drug consult,* St. Louis: Mosby, 2006.

[†]2005 American Heart Association guidelines for cardiopulmonary resuscitation and emergency cardiovascular care, part 10.2: Toxicology in ECC. *Circulation* 2005;112(suppl IV):IV-129.

IM, Intramuscular; *SubQ,* subcutaneous.

TABLE 5-11	Aspirin
Generic Name	acetylsalicylic acid
Trade Names	Bufferin, Anacin, APC
Classification	Nonnarcotic analgesic; antipyretic; antiinflammatory; salicylate
How Supplied	81- and 325-mg tablets
Mechanism of Action	Blocks synthesis of thromboxane A2, inhibiting platelet aggregation
Indications	• Chest discomfort or other signs/symptoms suggestive of an acute coronary syndrome (unless hypersensitive-aspirin) • ECG changes suggestive of acute MI
Dosing (Adult)	160 to 325 mg (2 to 4 pediatric chewable tablets), chewed*
Precautions	• Asthma (relative contraindication) • Active ulcer disease (relative contraindication)
Contraindications	• Hypersensitivity to aspirin and/or nonsteroidal anti-inflammatory agents • Recent history of GI bleeding • Bleeding disorders (hemophilia)
Special Considerations	• Use with caution in the patient with a history of asthma, nasal polyps, or nasal allergies. Anaphylactic reactions in sensitive patients have occurred. • Consider ticlopidine, or clopidogrel if aspirin allergy, intolerant, or ineffective. • Rectal suppository may be used for patients who cannot take aspirin orally.
Onset of Action	20 to 30 minutes
Duration	4 to 6 hours

*2005 American Heart Association guidelines for cardiopulmonary resuscitation and emergency cardiovascular care, part 8: Stabilization of the patient with acute coronary syndromes. *Circulation* 2005;112(suppl IV):IV-98.

ECG, Electrocardiogram; *GI,* gastrointestinal.

QUICK REVIEW 5-3

1. In general, a patient experiencing an acute coronary syndrome should receive "MONA." Can you recall each medication and its dosage?

   M =

   O =

   N =

   A =

2. Name two indications for administration of morphine sulfate.

   1.

   2.

TABLE 5-12	Fibrinolytics
Generic Names (Trade Names)	alteplase recombinant; tissue plasminogen activator (Activase, tPA); reteplase (Retavase); tenecteplase (TNKase); anistreplase; anisoylated plasminogen streptokinase activator complex (APSAC; Eminase); streptokinase (Streptase, Kabikinase)
Classification	Fibrinolytic ("clot-buster")
Mechanism of Action	Fibrinolytics work by altering plasmin in the body, which then breaks down fibrinogen and fibrin clots
Indications	• Improvement of ventricular function following ST-elevation myocardial infarction with onset of symptoms of ≤12 hours and ECG findings consistent with ST-elevation myocardial infarction • tPA may be used in acute ischemic stroke, after intracranial hemorrhage has been excluded by computed tomography scan or other diagnostic imaging. • Acute pulmonary thromboembolism.
Contraindications	See Box 5-2
Special Considerations	• Pay careful attention to all potential bleeding sites (including catheter insertion sites, arterial and venous puncture sites, cutdown sites, and needle puncture sites). • Some fibrinolytics are associated with an increased risk of bleeding or hemorrhage if used with heparin, oral anticoagulants, vitamin K antagonists, aspirin, or dipyridamole. • Do not give heparin and reteplase simultaneously in the same IV line. If reteplase is to be injected through an IV line containing heparin, flush normal saline or a 5% dextrose solution through the line before and after the reteplase injection. • Tenecteplase is also known as TNK-tPA. "TNK" refers to the sites of the tPA molecule that have been modified.

BOX 5-2

Contraindications and Cautions for Fibrinolytic Use in ST-Elevation Myocardial Infarction

Absolute Contraindications
• Any prior intracranial hemorrhage
• Known structural cerebrovascular lesion (e.g., AVM)
• Known malignant intracranial neoplasm (primary or metastatic)
• Ischemic stroke within 3 months *except* acute ischemic stroke within 3 hours
• Suspected aortic dissection
• Active bleeding or bleeding diathesis (excluding menses)
• Significant closed head trauma or facial trauma within 3 months

Cautions/Relative Contraindications
• History of chronic, severe, poorly controlled hypertension
• Severe uncontrolled hypertension on presentation (SBP >180 mm Hg or DBP >110 mm Hg; could be an absolute contraindication in low-risk patients with myocardial infarction)
• History of prior ischemic stroke within 3 months, dementia, or known intracranial pathology not covered in contraindications
• Traumatic or prolonged (10 minutes) CPR or major surgery (<3 weeks)
• Recent (within 2 to 4 weeks) internal bleeding
• Noncompressible vascular punctures
• For streptokinase/anistreplase: prior exposure (5 days ago) or prior allergic reaction to these agents
• Pregnancy
• Active peptic ulcer
• Current use of anticoagulants: the higher the INR, the higher the risk of bleeding

*Viewed as advisory for clinical decision making and may not be all-inclusive or definitive.
AVM, Arteriovenous malformation; *CPR,* cardiopulmonary resuscitation; *DBP,* diastolic blood pressure; *INR,* International Normalized Ratio.
From Antman EM, Anbe DT, Armstrong PW, et al: www.acc.org/clinical/guidelines/stemi/index.pdf/

HEPARIN

TABLE 5-13	Unfractionated Heparin
Generic Name	heparin sodium
Trade Names	Calciparine, Liquaemin
Classification	Anticoagulant
Mechanism of Action	Indirectly inhibits thrombin, acting at multiple sites in the normal coagulation system. It is not a fibrinolytic; it does not dissolve existing clots.
Indications*	• Patients undergoing percutaneous or surgical revascularization • Patients undergoing reperfusion therapy with alteplase, reteplase, or tenecteplase • Patients treated with nonselective fibrinolytic agents (streptokinase, anistreplase, urokinase) who are at high risk for systemic emboli (large or anterior MI, AFib, previous embolus, or known LV thrombus)
Dosing (Adult)*	IV dosing in patients undergoing reperfusion therapy: • 60 U/kg (maximum 4000 U for patients weighing >70 kg) followed by an infusion of 12 U/kg/hr (maximum 1000 U/hr for patients weighing >70 kg) initially adjusted to maintain activated partial thromboplastin time at 1.5 to 2 times control (about 50 to 70 sec) for 48 hours or until angiography. • When given by continuous IV infusion, coagulation time should be determined about every 4 hours in the early stages of treatment.[†] Follow institutional heparin protocol.
Precautions	Discontinue promptly if a patient develops new thrombosis in association with a reduction in platelet count.
Contraindications	Should not be used in patients: • With severe thrombocytopenia. • In whom suitable blood coagulation tests (e.g., whole-blood clotting time, partial thromboplastin time) cannot be performed at appropriate intervals (this contraindication refers to full-dose heparin; there is usually no need to monitor coagulation parameters in patients receiving low-dose heparin). • With an uncontrollable active bleeding state, except when this is due to disseminated intravascular coagulation.
Special Considerations	Anticoagulants prevent new clots from forming, but do not dissolve previously formed clots.

*Antman EM, Anbe DT, Armstrong PW, et al: www.acc.org/clinical/guidelines/stemi/index.pdf/
[†]*Mosby's drug consult,* St. Louis: Mosby, 2006.

TABLE 5-14	Low Molecular Weight Heparin
Generic Name	enoxaparin sodium
Trade Name	Lovenox
Classification	Anticoagulant, low molecular weight heparin (LMWH)
Mechanism of Action	LMWH with antithrombotic properties
Indications*	Acceptable alternative to unfractionated heparin as ancillary therapy for patients younger than 75 years of age who are receiving fibrinolytic therapy, provided that significant renal dysfunction is not present
Precautions	• Should not be mixed with other injections or infusions • Periodic complete blood counts, including platelet count, and stool occult blood tests are recommended during the course of treatment
Contraindications	• Known hypersensitivity to heparin or pork products • Hypersensitivity to enoxaparin • Active major bleeding
Special Considerations	• Cannot be used interchangeably (unit for unit) with heparin or other LMWHs • Not intended for intramuscular administration

*2005 American Heart Association guidelines for cardiopulmonary resuscitation and emergency cardiovascular care, part 8: Stabilization of the patient with acute coronary syndromes. *Circulation* 2005;112(suppl IV):IV-101.

TABLE 5-15	Glycoprotein IIb/IIIa Inhibitors
Generic Names (Trade Names)	abciximab (ReoPro); eptifibatide (Integrilin); tirofiban (Aggrastat)
Mechanism of Action	Prevent fibrinogen binding and platelet clumping
Indications*	• In patients with high-risk stratification unstable angina/NSTEMI, treatment should begin as soon as possible in conjunction with aspirin, heparin, and clopidogrel and a strategy of early PCI. • Treatment with tirofiban or eptifibatide may be used in patients with high-risk stratification UA/NSTEMI in conjunction with standard therapy if PCI is not planned.
Precautions	Minimize arterial and venous punctures, IM injections, and use of urinary catheters, nasotracheal intubation, and nasogastric tubes. When establishing IV access, avoid noncompressible sites (e.g., subclavian or jugular veins).
Special Considerations	• High-risk features include persistent pain, hemodynamic or rhythm instability, diabetes, acute or dynamic ECG changes, and any elevation in cardiac troponins attributed to cardiac injury. • Abciximab should not be given unless PCI is planned.

*2005 American Heart Association guidelines for cardiopulmonary resuscitation and emergency cardiovascular care, part 8: Stabilization of the patient with acute coronary syndromes. *Circulation* 2005;112(suppl IV):IV-101-102.

NSTEMI, Non–ST-elevation myocardial infarction; *PCI,* percutaneous coronary intervention; *UA,* unstable angina.

TABLE 5-16	Clopidogrel
Generic Name	clopidogrel
Trade Name	Plavix
Classification	Antiplatelet agent, anticoagulant
Mechanism of Action	Clopidogrel is an antiplatelet agent that helps prevent platelets from sticking together and forming clots. Platelets exposed to clopidogrel are affected for the remainder of their lifespan.
Indications	An oral loading dose is recommended in the following situations:* • In addition to standard care (aspirin, UFH, or LMWH and GP IIb/IIIa inhibitors if indicated) to ED patients with ACS with elevated cardiac markers or new ECG changes consistent with ischemia (excluding STEMI) in whom a medical approach or PCI is planned • It is reasonable to give an oral dose of clopidogrel to ED patients with suspected ACS (without ECG or cardiac biomarker changes) who are unable to take aspirin because of hypersensitivity or major gastrointestinal intolerance • STEMI in patients up to 75 years of age receiving fibrinolysis, aspirin, and heparin.
Contraindications	Hypersensitivity to the drug substance or any component of the product. Active pathological bleeding such as peptic ulcer or intracranial hemorrhage.
Special Considerations	Platelet aggregation and bleeding time gradually return to baseline values after treatment is discontinued, generally in about 5 days.

*2005 American Heart Association guidelines for cardiopulmonary resuscitation and emergency cardiovascular care, part 8: Stabilization of the patient with acute coronary syndromes. *Circulation* 2005;112(suppl IV):IV-102.

LMWH, Low molecular weight heparin; *PCI,* percutaneous coronary intervention; *ACS,* acute coronary syndrome; *ED,* emergency Department; *GP IIb/IIIa,* glycoprotein IIb/IIIa inhibitor; *UFH,* unfractionated heparin.

TABLE 5-17	Angiotensin-Converting Enzyme Inhibitors
Generic Names (Trade Names)	captopril (Capoten); enalapril (Vasotec); lisinopril (Prinivil, Zestril); ramipril (Altace)
Classification	Antihypertensive, ACE inhibitor
Mechanism of Action	In the body, the hormone angiotensin I is converted to angiotensin II (the active form of angiotensin) by the action of ACE. Angiotensin II causes vasoconstriction (more potent than NE) and increased aldosterone secretion from the kidneys. Aldosterone causes the kidneys to retain salt and water and to excrete potassium, leading to an increase in blood volume and BP. ACE inhibitors prevent the conversion of angiotensin I to angiotensin II. As a result, blood vessels relax, reducing the pressure the heart must pump against, and decreasing myocardial workload. By increasing renal blood flow, ACE inhibitors help rid the body of excess sodium and fluid accumulation.
Indications*	• Recommended within the first 24 hours after onset of symptoms in STEMI patients with pulmonary congestion or LV ejection fraction <40%, in the absence of hypotension (SBP <100 mm Hg or more than 30 mm Hg below baseline) • Also recommended for all other patients with acute MI with or without early reperfusion therapy
Precautions	• Adjust dose in patients with renal impairment or renal failure • May cause a profound drop in BP following the first dose or if used with diuretics • Persistent nonproductive cough has been reported with all ACE inhibitors, resolving after discontinuation of therapy
Contraindications	• Hypersensitivity to ACE inhibitors (e.g., a patient who has experienced angioedema during therapy with an other ACE inhibitor) • SBP <100 mm Hg • Presence of clinically relevant renal failure • History of bilateral renal artery stenosis of the renal arteries
Special Considerations	• IV administration of ACE inhibitors is contraindicated in the first 24 hours because of risk of hypotension. • When used in pregnancy during the second and third trimesters, ACE inhibitors can cause injury and even death to the developing fetus.

*2005 American Heart Association guidelines for cardiopulmonary resuscitation and emergency cardiovascular care, part 8: Stabilization of the patient with acute coronary syndromes. *Circulation* 2005;112(suppl IV):IV-102.
ACE, Angiotensin-converting enzyme; *LV,* left ventricular; *MI,* myocardial infarction.

TABLE 5-18	3-Hydroxy-3-Methylglutaryl Coenzyme A Reductase Inhibitors (Statins)
Generic Names (Trade Names)	atorvastatin (Lipitor); fluvastatin (Lescol); lovastatin (Mevacor); pravastatin (Pravachol); rosuvastatin (Crestor); simvastatin (Zocor)
Mechanism of Action	Statins: • Slow cholesterol production • Lower LDL cholesterol and triglyceride levels • Increase HDL cholesterol • Increase the liver's ability to remove circulating LDL cholesterol
Indications	• Begin within 24 hours of an acute coronary syndrome • If the patient is already on statin therapy, continue the therapy
Precautions*	• Occasionally causes myopathy, which is manifested as muscle pain, tenderness, or weakness. • Muscle cell breakdown (rhabdomyolysis) can occur in severe cases. Myoglobin may be released into the bloodstream and can result in acute renal failure. Rare fatalities have occurred.
Special Considerations	• The risk of myopathy/rhabdomyolysis is increased by simultaneous administration of amiodarone or verapamil with simvastatin. • Grapefruit juice should be avoided when taking statins.

Mosby's drug consult, St. Louis: Mosby, 2006.
LDL, Low-density lipoprotein; *HDL,* high-density lipoprotein.

DRUGS USED FOR CONTROL OF HEART RHYTHM AND RATE

TABLE 5-19	Classification of Antiarrhythmics
Class	**Major Action**
IA	Block fast sodium channels in cardiac muscle, resulting in decreased excitability; prolong repolarization Examples: quinidine, procainamide, disopyramide
IB	Block fast sodium channels in cardiac muscle, resulting in decreased excitability; shorten repolarization or have little effect Examples: lidocaine, tocainide, mexiletine
IC	Profoundly slow conduction in normal tissues Examples: flecainide, propafenone
II	Beta-blockers; suppress automaticity and rate of impulse conduction, repolarization time unchanged Examples: propranolol, esmolol, atenolol
III	Markedly prolong repolarization time, usually by interfering with the outflow of potassium through potassium channels Examples: amiodarone, sotalol
IV	Calcium channel blockers; block inward movement of calcium to slow impulse conduction (particularly through the AV node) and vascular smooth muscle contraction Examples: verapamil, diltiazem

TABLE 5-20	Adenosine
Generic Name	adenosine
Trade Name	Adenocard
Classification	Endogenous nucleoside, antiarrhythmic
Mechanism of Action	• Found naturally in all body cells • Rapidly metabolized in the blood vessels • Slows sinus rate • Slows conduction time through AV node • Can interrupt reentry pathways through AV node • Can restore sinus rhythm in reentry SVT, including SVT associated with WPW syndrome
Indications*	• Stable, narrow-complex AV nodal or sinus nodal reentry tachycardias • For unstable reentry SVT while preparations are made for cardioversion • Undefined, stable, narrow-complex SVT as a combination therapeutic and diagnostic maneuver • Stable, wide-complex tachycardias in patients with a recurrence of a known reentry pathway that has been previously defined
Dosing (Adult)*	• 6-mg rapid IV push over 1 to 3 seconds. Decrease the dose to 3 mg in patients on dipyridamole (Persantine) or carbamazepine (Tegretol), those with transplanted hearts, or if given via a central IV line. Consider increasing the dose in patients on theophylline, caffeine, or theobromine. • If no response within 1 to 2 minutes, give 12 mg. May repeat 12-mg dose once in 1-2 minutes.
Precautions	• Side effects common but transient and usually resolve within 1-2 minutes • Cardiovascular: Facial flushing (common), chest pain (common), headache, sweating, palpitations, hypotension • Respiratory: Shortness of breath/dyspnea (common), chest pressure, hyperventilation • CNS: Lightheadedness, dizziness, tingling in arms, numbness, apprehension, blurred vision, burning sensation, heaviness in arms, neck and back pain • Gastrointestinal: Nausea, metallic taste, tightness in throat, pressure in groin • Use with caution in patients with obstructive lung disease not associated with bronchoconstriction (emphysema, bronchitis)
Contraindications	• Poison/drug-induced tachycardia • Bronchoconstriction or bronchospasm (asthma) • Second- or third-degree AV block • Sick sinus syndrome (except in patients with a functioning artificial pacemaker)
Special Considerations	• Recommended IV site is the antecubital fossa. Follow each dose immediately with a 20 mL normal saline flush and raise the arm for 10 to 20 seconds. Use the injection port nearest the hub of the IV catheter. *Constant ECG monitoring is essential.* • Must be injected into the IV tubing as fast as possible (over a period of seconds). Failure to do so may result in breakdown of the medication while still in the IV tubing. • Cases of prolonged asystole, VT, VF, transient increase in BP, bradycardia, AFib, and bronchospasm in association with adenosine use have been reported. • Discontinue in any patient who develops severe respiratory difficulty • Because adenosine works by decreasing conduction through the AV node, administration may result in first-, second-, or third-degree AV block. Because the half-life of adenosine is short, these effects are usually self-limiting.
Half-life	<10 seconds

*2005 American Heart Association guidelines for cardiopulmonary resuscitation and emergency cardiovascular care, part 7.3: Management of symptomatic bradycardia and tachycardia. *Circulation* 2005;112(suppl IV):IV-72-74.

AV, Atrioventricular; *SVT,* supraventricular tachycardia; *VT,* ventricular tachycardia; *VF,* ventricular fibrillation.

TABLE 5-21   Amiodarone

Generic Name	amiodarone hydrochloride
Trade Name	Cordarone
Classification	Class III antiarrhythmic. Although amiodarone is considered a class III antiarrhythmic, it possesses electrophysiologic characteristics of all four classes of antiarrhythmics. Amiodarone blocks sodium channels (class I action), inhibits sympathetic stimulation (class II action), and blocks potassium channels (class III action) as well as calcium channels (class IV action).
Mechanism of Action	• Slows conduction in the His-Purkinje system and in accessory pathway of patients with WPW syndrome • Inhibits alpha- and beta-receptors, and possesses both vagolytic and calcium-channel blocking properties • Lengthens the action potential duration and increases the refractory period in all cardiac tissues, including the SA node, AV node, atrial cells, Purkinje fibers, and ventricular myocardium Hemodynamic effects • Coronary and peripheral vasodilator • Mild decrease in myocardial contractility however, cardiac output may actually increase due to decreased afterload • Suppresses SA node function • Prolongs PR, QRS, and QT intervals • Slows conduction at the AV junction
Indications	• Pulseless VT/VF (after CPR, defibrillation, and a vasopressor) • Polymorphic VT • Wide-complex tachycardia of uncertain origin • Stable VT when cardioversion unsuccessful • Adjunct to electrical cardioversion of SVT/PSVT, atrial tachycardia • Pharmacological conversion of AFib • Rate control of AFib or flutter when other therapies ineffective
Dosing (Adult)	Cardiac arrest: Pulseless VT/VF. • Initial bolus: 300-mg IV/IO bolus. Consider repeat dose of 150-mg IV/IO bolus once in 5 minutes.* • If return of spontaneous circulation, consider continuous IV infusion† (1-mg/min infusion for 6 hours and then a 0.5-mg/min maintenance infusion over 18 hours). Maximum daily dose 2.2-g IV/24 hours. Other indications: • Loading dose: 150-mg IV bolus over 10 minutes (15 mg/min). May repeat every 10 minutes as needed. After conversion, follow with a 1-mg/min infusion for 6 hours and then a 0.5 mg/min maintenance infusion over 18 hours.‡ • Maximum cumulative dose 2.2-g IV/24 hr.
Precautions	Hypotension and bradycardia are most common side effects. Slow infusion rate or discontinue if seen.
Contraindications	• Known hypersensitivity • Severe sinus-node dysfunction causing marked sinus bradycardia • Second- and third-degree AV block • Syncope due to bradycardia (except when used in conjunction with a pacemaker) • Use with caution in patients with uncorrected electrolyte abnormalities, particularly hypokalemia and/or hypomagnesemia, because these conditions may predispose the patient to **proarrhythmias**
Special Considerations	• Additive effect with other medications that prolong the QT interval (e.g., Class Ia antiarrhythmics, phenothiazines, tricyclic antidepressants, thiazide diuretics, sotalol). • In therapeutic doses, amiodarone has only a mild negative effect on myocardial contractility. This is the reason it appears in multiple algorithms involving patients experiencing dysrhythmias, but who have signs of heart failure.

*2005 American Heart Association guidelines for cardiopulmonary resuscitation and emergency cardiovascular care, part 7.2: Management of cardiac arrest. *Circulation* 2005;112(suppl IV):IV-59–IV-63.

†2005 American Heart Association guidelines for cardiopulmonary resuscitation and emergency cardiovascular care, part 7.5: Postresuscitation support. *Circulation* 2005;112(suppl IV):IV-86.

‡2005 American Heart Association guidelines for cardiopulmonary resuscitation and emergency cardiovascular care, part 7.3: Management of symptomatic bradycardia and tachycardia. *Circulation* 2005;112(suppl IV):IV-74.

SA, Sinoatrial; *PSVT,* paroxysmal supraventricular tachycardia; *AFib,* atrial fibrillation.

TABLE 5-22	Atropine
Generic Name	atropine sulfate
Trade Name	Atropine
Classification	Parasympatholytic, antimuscarinic, muscarinic antagonist, anticholinergic, parasympathetic antagonist, parasympathetic blocker
How Supplied	0.5 mg/mL (prefilled syringe), 0.4 mg/mL (multidose vial)
Mechanism of Action	Cardiovascular • Increases heart rate (positive chronotropic effect) by accelerating SA node discharge rate and blocking vagus nerve • Increases conduction velocity (positive dromotropic effect) • Little or no effect on force of contraction (inotropic effect) • *May* restore cardiac rhythm in asystole or slow PEA Respiratory • Relaxes bronchial smooth muscle (bronchodilation); decreases body secretions (lungs, bronchi, GI tract, sweat, saliva) GI/GU • Decreased GI motility and secretions, urinary retention Other • Pupil dilation, decreased sweat production
Indications	• First-line drug for symptomatic narrow-QRS bradycardia • Asystole (after epinephrine) • Slow PEA (after epinephrine)
Dosing (Adult)	Symptomatic bradycardia • 0.5-mg IV push every 3 to 5 minutes to a total dose of 3 mg* Asystole/slow PEA • IV/IO: 1.0 mg every 3 to 5 minutes to a total dose of 3 mg • ET: 2 to 2.5 times IV/IO dose
Precautions	• Do not push slowly or in smaller than recommended doses. Small doses (<0.5 mg) produce modest paradoxical cardiac slowing that may last 2 minutes. • May result in tachycardia, palpitations, and ventricular ectopy. • May worsen ischemia or induce VT or VF. • Use with caution in acute MI. Excessive increases in heart rate may further worsen ischemia or increase size of infarction.
Special Considerations	• Although transplanted hearts do not usually respond to atropine because they lack vagal nerve innervation, atropine may be used with caution after heart transplantation.* Monitoring is essential. • Give oxygen before giving atropine. • Do not give unless solution is clear.
Onset of Action	IV: 1 minute (increased heart rate), 30 minutes (decreased secretions)
Duration	IV: 2 hours

*2005 American Heart Association guidelines for cardiopulmonary resuscitation and emergency cardiovascular care, part 7.3: Management of symptomatic bradycardia and tachycardia. *Circulation* 2005;112(suppl IV):IV-68-69.

PEA, Pulseless electrical activity; *ET,* endotracheal; *GU,* genitourinary.

TABLE 5-23	Beta-blockers	
Generic Names (Trade Names)	atenolol (Tenormin); esmolol (Brevibloc); labetalol (Normodyne, Trandate); metoprolol (Lopressor); propranolol (Inderal)	
Classification	Beta-blockers	
Mechanism of Action	• Slow sinus rate • Depress AV conduction • Reduce BP • Decrease myocardial oxygen consumption • Reduce the incidence of dysrhythmias by decreasing catecholamine levels • Reduce risk of sudden death in patients with an acute coronary syndrome	

Indications*†‡	• For rate control in:
	  • Narrow-complex tachycardias that originate from either a reentry mechanism (reentry SVT) or an automatic focus (junctional, ectopic, or multifocal tachycardia) uncontrolled by vagal maneuvers and adenosine in the patient with no signs of heart failure.
	  • AFib and atrial flutter in a patient who has no signs of heart failure.
	• Oral beta-blocker therapy should be given promptly for acute coronary syndromes of all types unless contraindications are present, regardless of the need for revascularization therapies.
	• Control of BP in hypertensive emergencies.
	• Use in the postresuscitation setting is reasonable if there are no contraindications.	

Precautions	Some beta-blockers should be used with caution in patients with impaired renal or liver function.	
Contraindications	• Moderate to severe LV failure and pulmonary edema • Heart rate <60 bpm • Hypotension (SBP <100 mm Hg) • Signs of poor peripheral perfusion • Second- or third-degree AV block • Reactive airway disease	
Special Considerations	• Use with caution in conjunction with medications that slow conduction (e.g., digitalis, calcium channel blockers) and in those that decrease myocardial contractility (e.g., calcium channel blockers). • In general, patients with reactive airway disease should not receive beta-blockers.	

*2005 American Heart Association guidelines for cardiopulmonary resuscitation and emergency cardiovascular care, part 7.3: Management of symptomatic bradycardia and tachycardia. *Circulation* 2005; 112(suppl IV):IV-74.

†2005 American Heart Association guidelines for cardiopulmonary resuscitation and emergency cardiovascular care, part 7.5: Postresuscitation support. *Circulation* 2005;112(suppl IV):IV-86.

‡2005 American Heart Association Guidelines for cardiopulmonary resuscitation and emergency cardiovascular care, part 8: Stabilization of the patient with acute coronary syndromes. *Circulation* 2005;112(suppl IV):IV-100.

TABLE 5-24	Digitalis
Note	Cardiac glycosides are a closely related group of medications that have common specific effects on the heart. "Digitalis" is a term that refers to the entire group of cardiac glycosides.
Generic Name	digoxin
Trade Name	Lanoxin
Classification	Cardiac glycoside
Mechanism of Action	• Slows conduction through AV node (prolonging PR interval) • In atrial flutter or atrial fibrillation, decreases number of atrial impulses reaching the ventricles; thus, decreasing the ventricular response (− chronotropic effect) • Increases force and velocity of myocardial contraction (+ inotropic effect) • Increases cardiac output
Indications	*Limited use in emergency cardiac care* • Control ventricular rate in patients with AFib or atrial flutter • PSVT • Heart failure due to poor left ventricular contractility
Precautions	• Toxic to therapeutic ratio is narrow • May result in toxicity in patients with hypokalemia or hypomagnesemia because potassium or magnesium depletion sensitizes the myocardium to digoxin • Hypercalcemia predisposes the patient to digitalis toxicity • May cause severe sinus bradycardia or SA block in patients with preexisting sinus node disease • May cause complete AV block in patients with preexisting incomplete AV block
Contraindications	• Known hypersensitivity • Digitalis toxicity
Special Considerations	• ACE inhibitors have largely replaced digoxin as first-line therapy for CHF due to systolic dysfunction. • In patients with AFib or atrial flutter, IV calcium channel blockers or beta-blockers are generally more effective than digoxin for initial control of ventricular rate.

CHF, Congestive heart failure.

QUICK REVIEW 5-5

1. How is adenosine given?

2. Name three indications for administration of atropine.
   1.
   2.
   3.
3. How is amiodarone given in pulseless ventricular tachycardia (VT)/ ventricular fibrillation (VF)?

TABLE 5-25	Diltiazem
Generic Name	diltiazem hydrochloride
Trade Name	Cardizem
Classification	Calcium channel blocker (calcium antagonist)
Mechanism of Action*	Inhibits movement of calcium ions across cell membranes in the heart and vascular smooth muscle, resulting in the following: • Relaxation of coronary vascular smooth muscle • Dilation of both large and small coronary arteries • Decreased sinoatrial and AV conduction • Decreased myocardial oxygen demand • Produces antihypertensive effects primarily by relaxation of vascular smooth muscle and a resultant decrease in peripheral vascular resistance
Indications†	• Stable narrow-QRS tachycardia due to reentry if the rhythm persists despite vagal maneuvers or adenosine • Stable narrow-QRS tachycardia due to automaticity (junctional, ectopic atrial, multifocal atrial tachycardia) if the rhythm persists despite vagal maneuvers or adenosine • To control the ventricular rate in patients with AFib or atrial flutter (Note: should *not* be given to patients with AFib or atrial flutter associated with known preexcitation [WPW syndrome])
Dosing (Adult)†	• Initial dose 0.25 mg/kg IV bolus over 2 minutes. • If needed, follow in 15 minutes with 0.35 mg/kg over 2 minutes. Subsequent IV bolus doses should be individualized for each patient.
Precautions	Avoid calcium channel blockers in patients with wide-QRS tachycardia unless it is **known with certainty** to be supraventricular in origin (may precipitate VF).
Contraindications	• Wide-QRS tachycardia of uncertain origin • Poison/drug-induced tachycardias • Digitalis toxicity (may worsen heart block) • AFib or atrial flutter with an accessory bypass tract (WPW) • Sick-sinus syndrome (bradycardia-tachycardia syndrome) except with a functioning ventricular pacemaker • Severe CHF • Second or third-degree AV block • Hypotension (SBP <90 mm Hg) • Cardiogenic shock
Special Considerations	• "Studies to date, primarily in patients with good ventricular function, have not revealed evidence of a negative inotropic effect; cardiac output, ejection fraction, and left ventricular end diastolic pressure have not been affected. Such data have no predictive value with respect to effects in patients with poor ventricular function, and increased heart failure has been reported in patients with preexisting impairment of ventricular function. There are as yet few data on the interaction of diltiazem and beta-blockers in patients with poor ventricular function."* • Monitor closely for hypotension and AV block. • Concurrent use of amiodarone and diltiazem can result in bradycardia and decreased cardiac output by an unknown mechanism. • IV calcium channel blockers and IV beta-blockers should not be given together or in close proximity (within a few hours)—may cause severe hypotension.
Onset of Action	IV: ½ to 1 hour
Duration	IV: 1 to 3 hours

*Mosby's drug consult, St. Louis: Mosby, 2006.
†2005 American Heart Association guidelines for cardiopulmonary resuscitation and emergency cardiovascular care, part 7.3: Management of symptomatic bradycardia and tachycardia. *Circulation* 2005;112(suppl IV):IV-74.

QUICK REVIEW 5-6

1. Name two indications for the use of diltiazem.
   1.
   2.
2. Describe the effects of digitalis on heart rate and myocardial contractility.

3. Name three situations in which the use of beta-blockers should generally be avoided.
   1.
   2.
   3.

TABLE 5-26	Epinephrine
Generic Name	epinephrine
Trade Name	Adrenalin
Classification	Natural catecholamine; sympathomimetic; adrenergic agonist
Mechanism of Action	• Stimulates alpha, beta$_1$, and beta$_2$ receptors • Alpha-agonist: constricts arterioles in skin, mucosa, kidneys, and viscera → increased systemic vascular resistance • Beta$_1$ agonist: increases force of contraction (+ inotropic effect), increases heart rate (+ chronotropic effect) → increased myocardial workload and oxygen requirements • Beta$_2$ agonist: relaxation of bronchial smooth muscle, dilation of vessels in skeletal muscle; dilation of cerebral, pulmonary, coronary, and hepatic vessels
Indications	• Cardiac arrest: VF, pulseless VT, asystole, PEA • Symptomatic bradycardia
Dosing (Adult)	Cardiac arrest • IV/IO: 1 mg (10 mL) of 1:10,000 solution, follow with 20-mL fluid flush. May repeat 1-mg dose every 3 to 5 minutes. • Endotracheal: 2 to 2.5 mg. Symptomatic bradycardia or hypotension* • Continuous infusion at 2 to 10 mcg/min. • To mix, add 1 mg epinephrine to 500 mL NS or D$_5$W for a resulting concentration of 4 mcg/mL. Begin at 1 mcg/min and titrate to desired hemodynamic response.
Precautions	• Increases myocardial oxygen demand • Avoid mixing with sodium bicarbonate Epinephrine infusion • Administer via infusion pump • Check IV site frequently for evidence of tissue sloughing
Special Considerations	Should not be administered in the same IV line as alkaline solutions—inactivates epinephrine
Onset of Action	IV: 1 to 2 minutes
Duration	IV: 5 to 10 minutes

*2005 American Heart Association guidelines for cardiopulmonary resuscitation and emergency cardiovascular care, part 7.4: Monitoring and medications. *Circulation* 2005;112(suppl IV):IV-79.

TABLE 5-27	Lidocaine Hydrochloride
Generic Name	lidocaine hydrochloride
Trade Name	Xylocaine
Classification	Class Ib antiarrhythmic
Mechanism of Action	Lidocaine inhibits the influx of sodium through the fast channels of the myocardial cell membrane and decreases conduction in ischemic cardiac tissue without adversely affecting normal conduction. Clinical studies with lidocaine have demonstrated no change in sinus node recovery time or SA conduction time. AV nodal conduction time is unchanged or shortened. In therapeutic doses, lidocaine does not affect BP, cardiac output, or myocardial contractility. No significant interactions between lidocaine and the ANS have been described; consequently, lidocaine has little or no effect on autonomic tone.
Indications	Pulseless VT/VF that persists after defibrillation and vasopressor administration
Dosing (Adult)	• Initial dose: 1- to 1.5-mg/kg IV/IO bolus. Consider repeat dose (0.5 to 0.75 mg/kg) in 5 to 10 minutes. • Cumulative IV/IO bolus dose should not exceed 3 mg/kg. • *Only bolus therapy is used in cardiac arrest.* It may be reasonable to continue an infusion of an antiarrhythmic drug that was associated with a return of spontaneous circulation.* • Maintenance infusion: 1 to 4 mg/min. • Endotracheal dose: 2 to 3 mg/kg (2 to 2.5 times IV dose).
Precautions	• The maintenance infusion of lidocaine is 1 to 4 mg/min. This should be reduced after 24 hours (to 1 to 2 mg/min) or in the setting of altered metabolism (CHF, hepatic dysfunction, acute MI with hypotension or shock, patients older than 70 years of age, poor peripheral perfusion) and as guided by blood level monitoring. • The elimination half-life of lidocaine following an IV bolus injection is typically 1.5 to 2 hours. Because of the rapid rate at which lidocaine is metabolized, any condition that affects liver function may alter lidocaine kinetics. The half-life may be prolonged twofold or more in patients with liver dysfunction. Renal dysfunction does not affect lidocaine kinetics but may increase the buildup of metabolites. • Signs and symptoms of lidocaine toxicity are primarily CNS related: dizziness, drowsiness, mild agitation, tinnitus, slurred speech, hearing impairment, disorientation and confusion, muscle twitching, seizures, and respiratory arrest.
Contraindications	• Hypersensitivity to lidocaine or amide-type local anesthetics • Severe degrees of sinoatrial, AV, or intraventricular block in the absence of an artificial pacemaker • Stokes-Adams syndrome (sudden recurring episodes of loss of consciousness caused by transient interruption of cardiac output by incomplete or complete heart block) • WPW syndrome
Special Considerations	Lidocaine may be *lethal* in a bradycardia with a ventricular escape rhythm.
Onset of Action	IV: 45 to 90 seconds
Duration	IV: 10 to 20 minutes

*2005 American Heart Association guidelines for cardiopulmonary resuscitation and emergency cardiovascular care, part 7.5: Postresuscitation support. *Circulation* 2005;112(suppl IV):IV-86.

TABLE 5-28	Magnesium Sulfate
Generic Name	magnesium sulfate
Classification	Antiarrhythmic, electrolyte
Mechanism of Action	• Second most plentiful intracellular cation. Essential for the activity of many enzyme systems and plays an important role with regard to neurochemical transmission and muscular excitability. • Some of the effects of magnesium on the nervous system are similar to those of calcium. An increased concentration of magnesium in the extracellular fluid causes depression of the CNS. Magnesium has a direct depressant effect on skeletal muscle. • Abnormally low concentrations of magnesium in the extracellular fluid result in increased acetylcholine release and increased muscle excitability that can produce tetany. • Magnesium slows the rate of SA nodal impulse formation. Higher concentrations of magnesium (>15 mEq/L) produce cardiac arrest in diastole. • Excess magnesium causes vasodilation by both a direct action on blood vessels and ganglionic blockade.
Indications	• Polymorphic VT with prolonged QT interval (TdP) • For rhythm control of AFib ≤48 hours duration
Dosing (Adult)*	• TdP (pulseless): 1 to 2 g (2 to 4 mL of 50% solution) IV push diluted in 10 mL. • TdP (with pulse) or AFib with a rapid ventricular response: 1 to 2 g IV in 50 to 100 mL D_5W over 5 to 60 minutes. Give the infusion slowly if the patient is stable and more rapidly if the patient is unstable.
Precautions	• Caution should be used in patients receiving digitalis • Use with caution in patients with impaired renal function • Use with caution in patients with preexisting heart blocks
Contraindications	• Respiratory depression • Hypocalcemia • Hypermagnesemia
Special Considerations	Signs and symptoms of magnesium overdose include: • Hypotension • Flushing, sweating • Bradycardia, AV block • Respiratory depression • Drowsiness, decreasing level of consciousness • Diminished reflexes or muscle weakness, flaccid paralysis Antidote = calcium

*2005 American Heart Association Guidelines for Cardiopulmonary Resuscitation and Emergency Cardiovascular Care, Part 7.3: Management of Symptomatic Bradycardia and Tachycardia. *Circulation* 2005;112(suppl IV):IV-73–IV-75.
TdP, Torsades de pointes.

QUICK REVIEW 5-7

1. Name the adrenergic-receptor sites stimulated by epinephrine.

2. Name four dysrhythmias for which epinephrine may be used.
   1.
   2.
   3.
   4.

3. What is the endotracheal dose of epinephrine in cardiac arrest?

4. What is the dose of epinephrine when given for bradycardia and hypotension?

5. What is the maximum IV bolus dose of lidocaine?

TABLE 5-29	Procainamide
Generic Name	procainamide
Trade Names	Pronestyl, Procan SR
Classification	Class Ia antiarrhythmic
Mechanism of Action	• In therapeutic doses, decreases conduction velocity in the atria, ventricles, and His-Purkinje system • Prolongs the effective refractory period of the atria • Shortens the effective refractory period of the AV node • Decreases automaticity in the His-Purkinje system and ectopic pacemakers • Prolongs the PR and QT intervals • Exerts a peripheral vasodilatory effect • In therapeutic doses, myocardial contractility of the undamaged heart is usually not affected
Indications	• Stable monomorphic VT in patients with no signs of heart failure • Control of rapid ventricular rate in AFib or atrial flutter in patients with no signs of heart failure • Control of rapid ventricular rate in AFib or atrial flutter in patients with known WPW syndrome and no signs of heart failure • AV reentrant narrow-complex tachycardias such as reentry SVT if no response to vagal maneuvers and adenosine and if no signs of heart failure
Dosing (Adult)*	20-mg/min IV infusion until one of the following occurs: • Dysrhythmia resolves • Hypotension • QRS widens by >50% of original width • Total dose of 17 mg/kg administered Maintenance infusion 1 to 4 mg/min
Precautions	• Use with caution with other medications that prolong the QT interval (e.g., phenothiazines, tricyclic antidepressants, thiazide diuretics, sotalol). • During administration, carefully monitor the patient's ECG and BP. If the BP falls 15 mm Hg or more, procainamide administration should be temporarily discontinued. Watch the ECG closely for increasing PR and QT intervals, widening of the QRS complex, heart block, and/or onset of TdP. • Reduce maintenance infusion rate in liver dysfunction (procainamide is metabolized by the liver), renal failure (procainamide is eliminated by the kidneys).
Contraindications	• Complete AV block in the absence of an artificial pacemaker • Patients sensitive to procaine or other ester-type local anesthetics • Lupus erythematosus • Patients with a prolonged QRS duration or QT interval because of the potential for heart block • Preexisting QT prolongation/TdP • Digitalis toxicity (procainamide may further depress conduction)
Special Considerations	Pharmacological effects of procainamide may be increased if amiodarone is also given.

*2005 American Heart Association guidelines for cardiopulmonary resuscitation and emergency cardiovascular care, part 7.3: Management of symptomatic bradycardia and tachycardia. *Circulation* 2005;112(suppl IV):IV-75-76.

TABLE 5-30	Sotalol
Generic Name	sotalol
Trade Name	Betapace
Classification	Class III antiarrhythmic
Mechanism of Action	• Class III antiarrhythmic with nonselective beta-blockade activity • Slows heart rate • Decreases AV nodal conduction • Increases AV nodal refractoriness • Prolongs the effective refractory period of atrial muscle, ventricular muscle, and AV accessory pathways (where present) in both anterograde and retrograde directions • Increases force of contraction
Indications*	• Monomorphic VT • For rhythm control of AFib or atrial flutter in patients with WPW syndrome if the rhythm has been present ≤48 hours and no signs of heart failure are present
Precautions	• Because of its effect on cardiac repolarization (QT interval prolongation), TdP is the most common dysrhythmia associated with sotalol administration. The risk of TdP progressively increases with prolongation of the QT interval, and is worsened by reduction in heart rate and reduction in serum potassium. Patients with sustained VT and a history of CHF appear to have the highest risk for serious proarrhythmia. • Should not be used in patients with hypokalemia or hypomagnesemia (these conditions can exaggerate the degree of QT prolongation, and increase the potential for TdP). • Bradycardia • Hypotension
Contraindications	• Bronchial asthma • Sinus bradycardia • Second- and third-degree AV block (unless a functioning pacemaker is present) • Congenital or acquired long QT syndromes • Cardiogenic shock • Uncontrolled CHF • Previous evidence of hypersensitivity to sotalol

*2005 American Heart Association Guidelines for cardiopulmonary resuscitation and emergency cardiovascular care, part 7.3: Management of symptomatic bradycardia and tachycardia. *Circulation* 2005;112(suppl IV):IV-76.

TABLE 5-31	Verapamil
Generic Name	verapamil
Trade Names	Calan, Isoptin, Verelan
Classification	Calcium channel blocker (calcium antagonist)
Mechanism of Action	Inhibits movement of calcium ions across cell membranes in the heart and vascular smooth muscle, resulting in: • Relaxation of coronary vascular smooth muscle • Dilation of both large and small coronary arteries • Decreased SA and AV conduction • Decreased myocardial oxygen demand
Indications*	• Stable narrow-QRS tachycardia due to reentry if the rhythm persists despite vagal maneuvers or adenosine • Stable narrow-QRS tachycardia due to automaticity (junctional, ectopic atrial, multifocal atrial tachycardia) if the rhythm persists despite vagal maneuvers or adenosine • To control the ventricular rate in patients with AFib or atrial flutter (Note: should *not* be given to patients with AFib or atrial flutter associated with known preexcitation [WPW syndrome])
Dosing (Adult)*	• 2.5- to 5-mg slow IV push over 2 minutes (give over 3 to 4 min in the elderly or when BP is within the lower range of normal). May repeat with 5 to 10 mg in 15 to 30 minutes (if no response and BP remains normal or elevated). Maximum total dose 20 mg. • Alternative dosing may include 5 mg IV push every 15 minutes to a total dose of 30 mg.
Precautions	• Avoid calcium channel blockers in patients with wide-QRS tachycardia unless it is *known with certainty* to be supraventricular in origin (may precipitate VF). • Calcium channel blockers decrease peripheral resistance and can worsen hypotension. These medications should not be given to patients with an SBP of <90 mm Hg and should be used with caution in patients with mild to moderate hypotension. Monitor BP, heart rate, and ECG closely. • IV calcium channel blockers and IV beta-blockers should not be given together or in close proximity (within a few hours); may cause severe hypotension.
Contraindications	• Wide-QRS tachycardia of uncertain origin • Poison/drug-induced tachycardias • Digitalis toxicity (may worsen heart block) • AFib or atrial flutter with an accessory bypass tract (WPW syndrome) • Sick-sinus syndrome (bradycardia-tachycardia syndrome) except with a functioning ventricular pacemaker • Severe CHF • Second- or third-degree AV block • Hypotension (SBP <90 mm Hg) • Cardiogenic shock
Special Considerations	• During administration, monitor closely for hypotension and AV block. • Verapamil has been found to significantly inhibit elimination of alcohol, resulting in elevated blood alcohol concentrations that may prolong alcohol's intoxicating effects.
Onset of Action	IV: 2 to 5 minutes
Duration	IV: 2 hours

*2005 American Heart Association guidelines for cardiopulmonary resuscitation and emergency cardiovascular care, part 7.3: Management of symptomatic bradycardia and tachycardia. *Circulation* 2005;112(suppl IV):IV-74.

DRUGS USED TO IMPROVE CARDIAC OUTPUT AND BLOOD PRESSURE

TABLE 5-32	Calcium Chloride
Generic Name	calcium chloride
Trade Name	N/A
Classification	Electrolyte, calcium salt
Mechanism of Action	• Fifth most abundant element in the body • Essential for functional integrity of nervous and muscular systems • Necessary for normal cardiac contractility and coagulation of blood • Increases force of cardiac contraction (positive inotropic effect) • Antidote for magnesium sulfate
Indications	• Known or suspected acute hyperkalemia • Hypocalcemia • Calcium channel blocker toxicity/overdose • Pretreatment for calcium channel blocker administration • Magnesium toxicity
Dosing (Adult)*	Hyperkalemia: 500 to 1000 mg (5 to 10 mL) IV of a 10% solution (100 mg/mL) over 2 to 5 minutes.[†] Dosage should be titrated by constant monitoring of ECG changes during administration.
Precautions	• Do not give calcium intramuscularly or subcutaneously—can cause severe tissue necrosis, sloughing, or abscess formation. • Irritating to veins. Monitor IV site closely. Ensure patency of IV line before giving. Patient may experience pain, burning at the IV site, severe venous thrombosis, and severe tissue necrosis if solution extravasates. Patient may complain of "heat waves," tingling, and/or a metallic taste if given too rapidly. • Calcium chloride administration may be accompanied by peripheral vasodilation, with a moderate fall in BP. • Use with caution in patients taking digitalis—increases ventricular irritability and can precipitate digitalis toxicity.
Contraindications	Hypercalcemia, concurrent digitalis therapy (relative contraindication), kidney stones, VF
Special Considerations	• Calcium chloride is preferred over calcium gluceptate or calcium gluconate because calcium chloride produces consistently higher and more predictable levels of ionized calcium in the plasma. A 10% solution of calcium chloride contains 1.36 mEq of calcium per 100 mg of salt per mL. • Incompatible with all medications. Flush line before and after giving. • Concurrent administration of sodium bicarbonate and calcium chloride will produce a precipitate, calcium carbonate (chalk).
Onset of Action	5 to 15 minutes
Duration	Depends on dose and total body stores of calcium

*2005 American Heart Association guidelines for cardiopulmonary resuscitation and emergency cardiovascular care, part 7.4: Monitoring and medications. *Circulation* 2005;112(suppl IV):IV-80.

[†]2005 American Heart Association guidelines for cardiopulmonary resuscitation and emergency cardiovascular care, part 10.1: Life-threatening electrolyte abnormalities. *Circulation* 2005;112(suppl IV):IV-122.

TABLE 5-33	Dobutamine
Generic Name	dobutamine
Trade Name	Dobutrex
Classification	Direct-acting sympathomimetic, cardiac stimulant, adrenergic agonist agent
Mechanism of Action	• Stimulates alpha, beta$_1$, and beta$_2$ receptors • Potent inotropic effect (i.e., increased myocardial contractility, increased stroke volume, increased cardiac output) • Less chronotropic effect (heart rate) • Minimal alpha effect (vasoconstriction)
Indications	Short-term management of patients with cardiac decompensation due to depressed contractility (CHF, pulmonary congestion)
Dosing (Adult)*	Continuous IV infusion. Usual dose is 2 to 20 mcg/kg/min IV, but patient response varies.
Precautions	• Tachycardia may occur with high doses, but this occurs less commonly than with dopamine. • Continuously monitor ECG and BP.
Contraindications	• Hypersensitivity to sulfites or dobutamine • Tachydysrhythmias • Severe hypotension • Hypertrophic aortic stenosis
Special Considerations	• May cause a marked increase in heart rate or BP, especially systolic pressure • Correct hypovolemia before treatment with dobutamine • Use with tricyclic antidepressants can cause an increased adrenergic effect and possibly result in severe hypertensive crisis or cardiac dysrhythmias
Onset of Action	1 to 2 minutes
Duration	10 to 15 minutes (half-life 2 min)

*2005 American Heart Association guidelines for cardiopulmonary resuscitation and emergency cardiovascular care, part 7.4: Monitoring and medications. *Circulation* 2005;112(suppl IV):IV-80.

QUICK REVIEW 5-8

1. Does verapamil affect myocardial contractility?

2. What is the typical dosage range for IV verapamil?

3. Name four signs and symptoms of lidocaine toxicity.
   1.
   2.
   3.
   4.

4. What is the recommended dose of atropine in the treatment of asystole?

TABLE 5-34	Dopamine
Generic Name	dopamine
Trade Names	Intropin, Dopastat
Classification	Direct- and indirect-acting sympathomimetic; cardiac stimulant and vasopressor; natural catecholamine
Mechanism of Action	• Naturally occurring immediate precursor of NE in the body • Pharmacologic effects change with increasing dosage • Stimulates dopaminergic, beta, and alpha-adrenergic receptor sites The effects of dopamine are dose related (there is some "overlap" of effects).
Low dose = dopaminergic	**Low dose (dopaminergic effects)** 0.5 to 2 mcg/kg/min • At this dose range, dopaminergic receptors are stimulated, resulting in dilation of the renal, mesenteric, coronary, and intracerebral vascular beds. • Diuresis usually occurs in this dose range and renal blood flow increases.
Medium dose = beta	**Medium dose (beta effects)** 2 to 10 mcg/kg/min ("cardiac dose") • At this dose range, dopamine acts directly on the beta$_1$ receptors on the myocardium resulting in resulting in improved myocardial contractility, increased SA rate, and enhanced impulse conduction in the heart.
High dose = alpha	**High dose (alpha effects) ("pressor dose")** 10 to 20 mcg/kg/min • At this dose range, alpha$_1$, and alpha$_2$ receptors are stimulated; BP and systemic vascular resistance increase. • Vasoconstrictor effects are first seen in the vascular beds of skeletal muscle; but with increasing doses, they are also evident in the renal and mesenteric vessels. >20 mcg/kg/min • Produces effects similar to NE. • Vasoconstriction may compromise the circulation of the limbs. • May increase heart rate and oxygen demand to undesirable limits.
Indications	• Symptomatic bradycardias that have not responded to atropine and/or when external pacing is unavailable or ineffective • Hypotension that occurs after return of spontaneous circulation • Hemodynamically significant hypotension in the absence of hypovolemia
Dosing (Adult)*†	• Dopamine is given as a continuous IV infusion of 2 to 10 mcg/kg/min. • Increase infusion rate according to BP and other clinical responses.
Precautions	Correct hypovolemia before beginning dopamine therapy for the treatment of hypotension and shock
Contraindications	• Hypersensitivity to sulfites or dopamine • Hypovolemia • Pheochromocytoma • Uncorrected tachydysrhythmias or VF • MAOIs
Special Considerations	• Extravasation into surrounding tissue may cause necrosis and sloughing. • Gradually taper drug before discontinuing the infusion. Monitor BP, ECG, and drip rate closely. • Dilute before giving (or used premixed bag of IV solution). Do not give as an IV bolus. Should only be infused via an infusion pump.
Onset of Action	2 to 5 minutes
Duration	5 to 10 minutes (half-life 2 min); duration may increase to 1 hour if MAOIs are present

*2005 American Heart Association guidelines for cardiopulmonary resuscitation and emergency cardiovascular care, part 7.3: Management of symptomatic bradycardia and tachycardia. *Circulation* 2005;112(suppl IV):IV-69.

†2005 American Heart Association guidelines for cardiopulmonary resuscitation and emergency cardiovascular care, part 7.4: Monitoring and medications. *Circulation* 2005;112(suppl IV):IV-79–IV-80.

MAOI, Monoamine oxidase inhibitor.

TABLE 5-35	Norepinephrine
Generic Name	norepinephrine
Trade Names	Levophed, Levarterenol
Classification	Direct-acting adrenergic agent
Mechanism of Action	• NE functions as a peripheral vasoconstrictor (alpha-adrenergic action) and as an inotropic stimulator of the heart and dilator of coronary arteries (beta-adrenergic action) • Alpha activity dominant • Increases myocardial oxygen demand
Indications	• Cardiogenic shock • Severe hypotension (SBP <70 mm Hg) not due to hypovolemia
Dosing (Adult)*	• 0.5 to 1.0 mcg/min by continuous IV infusion titrated to improve BP ((30 mcg/min); usual dose range is 8 to 12 mcg/min • When discontinuing infusion, taper off gradually
Precautions	Use with extreme caution in patients receiving MAOIs or antidepressants of the triptyline or imipramine types, because severe, prolonged hypertension may result.
Contraindications	• Hypersensitivity to sulfites or NE • Hypotension due to hypovolemia (except in emergencies) • Mesenteric or peripheral vascular thrombosis • Halothane or cyclopropane anesthesia (possibility of fatal dysrhythmias) • Pregnancy (may cause fetal anoxia or hypoxia)
Special Considerations	• Should be administered via an infusion pump into a central vein or a large peripheral vein (e.g., antecubital vein) to reduce the risk of necrosis of the overlying skin from prolonged vasoconstriction. Gangrene of the lower extremity has occurred when infusions of NE were administered via an ankle vein. • Extravasation into surrounding tissue may cause necrosis and sloughing. Antidote for extravasation = phentolamine (Regitine). • Monitor BP every 2 to 3 minutes until stabilized, then every 5 minutes. Monitor the patient's ECG continuously.
Onset of Action	Immediate
Duration	1 to 2 minutes

*2005 American Heart Association guidelines for cardiopulmonary resuscitation and emergency cardiovascular care, part 7.4: Monitoring and medications. *Circulation* 2005;112(suppl IV):IV-79.

TABLE 5-36	Vasopressin
Generic Name	vasopressin
Trade Name	Pitressin
Classification	Pituitary hormone, antidiuretic
Mechanism of Action	Causes constriction of peripheral, cerebral, pulmonary, and coronary vessels
Indications	Cardiac arrest
Dosing (Adult)*	One-time dose of 40 units IV/IO push; may be used in place of first or second dose of epinephrine in cardiac arrest (see Special Considerations below).
Precautions	• Can increase peripheral vascular resistance and provoke cardiac ischemia and angina pectoris • Nausea and vomiting • Tremors • Tissue necrosis if extravasation occurs
Contraindications	• Hypersensitivity • Responsive patient with coronary artery disease or peripheral vascular disease
Special Considerations	• Half-life approximately 10 to 20 minutes • Insufficient evidence to recommend for or against vasopressin use in PEA*

*2005 American Heart Association guidelines for cardiopulmonary resuscitation and emergency cardiovascular care, part 7.2: Management of pulseless arrest. *Circulation* 2005;112(suppl IV):IV-61-62.

QUICK REVIEW 5-9

1. When is norepinephrine indicated?

2. What is the usual dosage range for dobutamine administration?

3. True or False. Vasopressin should be given every 10 to 20 minutes in cardiac arrest.

4. True or False. Dopamine is given slow IV push at a rate of 0.5 to 2 mcg/kg/min.

VASODILATORS

TABLE 5-37	Sodium Nitroprusside
Generic Name	sodium nitroprusside
Trade Names	Nipride, Nitropress
Classification	Vasodilator, antihypertensive
Mechanism of Action	• Direct-acting arterial and venous vasodilator. • Relaxes vascular smooth muscle with consequent dilation of peripheral arteries and veins; other smooth muscle (e.g., uterus, duodenum) is not affected. • Nitroprusside is more active on veins than on arteries. • Venodilation promotes peripheral pooling of blood and decreases venous return to the heart, thereby reducing preload. • Arteriolar relaxation reduces systemic vascular resistance (afterload). • Dilates coronary arteries.
Indications	Immediate reduction of BP in a hypertensive emergency or hypertensive urgency
Precautions	• Nitroprusside can cause precipitous decreases in BP. In patients not properly monitored, these decreases can lead to irreversible ischemic injuries or death. • Monitor for signs of cyanide toxicity. • Solution is sensitive to certain wavelengths of light, and must be protected from light during clinical use.
Contraindications	Hypotension, severe refractory CHF
Onset of Action	1 to 2 minutes
Duration	Effects stop quickly upon discontinuation of infusion

OTHER DRUGS

TABLE 5-38	Furosemide	
Generic Name	furosemide	
Trade Name	Lasix	
Classification	Loop diuretic	
Mechanism of Action	• Inhibits the reabsorption of sodium and chloride in the ascending limb of the loop of Henle, resulting in an increase in the urinary excretion of sodium, chloride, and water → profound diuresis.	
	• Furosemide increases excretion of potassium, hydrogen, calcium, magnesium, bicarbonate, ammonium, and phosphate.	
	• Venodilation increases venous capacitance and decreases preload (venous return).	
Indications	Adjunctive therapy in acute pulmonary edema (SBP >90 to 100 mm Hg without signs and symptoms of shock)	
Dosing (Adult)*	The initial dose is 0.5- to 1-mg/kg IV push given at a rate no faster than 20 mg/min.	
Precautions	• Ototoxicity and resulting transient deafness can occur with rapid administration.	
	• Do not exceed the recommended rate of administration.	
	• Furosemide should be administered cautiously in patients with the following:	
	• Diabetes mellitus.	
	• Dehydration.	
	• Severe renal disease.	
	• Patients with sulfonamide hypersensitivity or thiazide diuretic hypersensitivity may also be hypersensitive to furosemide.	
Contraindications	• Hypersensitivity to furosemide or sulfonamides	
	• Hypovolemia	
	• Severe electrolyte depletion	
	• Hypotension	
	• Anuria	
Special Considerations	• Can cause excessive fluid loss and dehydration, resulting in hypovolemia and electrolyte imbalance.	
	• Use less than 0.5 mg/kg for new onset acute pulmonary edema without hypovolemia. Use 1 mg/kg for acute or chronic volume overload, renal insufficiency.[†]	
Onset of Action	• Venodilation: <5 minutes; diuresis: within 5 minutes	
	• Peak effect within ½ hour. Half-life about ½ to 1 hour	
Duration	Venodilation: <2 hours; diuretic effect: about 2 hours	

*2005 American Heart Association guidelines for cardiopulmonary resuscitation and emergency cardiovascular care, part 7.4: Monitoring and medications. *Circulation* 2005;112(suppl IV):IV-82.

[†]Antman EM, Anbe DT, Armstrong PW, et al: www.acc.org/clinical/guidelines/stemi/index.pdf/

TABLE 5-39	Sodium Bicarbonate
Generic Name	sodium bicarbonate
Trade Name	N/A
Classification	Alkalinizing agent, antacid, electrolyte
Mechanism of Action	• Increases plasma bicarbonate • Buffers excess hydrogen ion concentration • Raises blood pH • Reverses clinical manifestations of acidosis
Indications	• Known preexisting hyperkalemia • Preexisting metabolic acidosis • Overdose: tricyclic antidepressants, procainamide
Dosing (Adult)	• Initial dose 1 mEq/kg IV bolus. ½ the initial dose may be repeated every 10 minutes thereafter.* • Repeated IV boluses of 1 to 2 mEq/kg may be needed when sodium bicarbonate is used to treat drug-induced arrhythmias and hypotension.†
Precautions	Extravasation may lead to tissue inflammation and necrosis.
Contraindications	Significant metabolic or respiratory alkalosis Severe pulmonary edema
Special Considerations	• Do not mix with parenteral drugs because of the possibility of drug inactivation or precipitation. • Hyperkalemia produces ECG changes including tall, peaked (tented) T waves; widened QRS complexes, prolonged PR intervals, flattened ST segments, and flattened or absent P waves. Hyperkalemia may lead to ventricular dysrhythmias and asystole if not reversed. • Sodium bicarbonate is used in hyperkalemia to decrease serum potassium (K^+) levels by temporarily shifting K^+ into the intracellular fluid. • Sodium bicarbonate may be administered in tricyclic antidepressant overdose with QRS prolongation or hypotension. The drug is given as needed to maintain the arterial pH between 7.45 and 7.55.
Onset of Action	2 to 10 minutes
Duration	30 to 60 minutes

*2005 American Heart Association guidelines for cardiopulmonary resuscitation and emergency cardiovascular care, part 7.4: Monitoring and medications. *Circulation* 2005;112(suppl IV):IV-82.

†2005 American Heart Association guidelines for cardiopulmonary resuscitation and emergency cardiovascular care, part 10.2: Toxicology in emergency cardiovascular care. *Circulation* 2005;112(suppl IV):IV-130.

QUICK REVIEW ANSWERS

Quick Review Number	Answers
5-1	1. Maintain hydration; restore fluid and electrolyte balance; provide fluids for resuscitation; administration of medications, blood and blood components, and nutrient solutions; obtain venous blood specimens for laboratory analysis. 2. During circulatory collapse or cardiac arrest, the preferred vascular access site is the largest, most accessible vein that does not require the interruption of resuscitation efforts. If no IV is in place before the arrest, establish IV access using a peripheral vein—preferably the antecubital or external jugular vein. 3. Does not require interruption of cardiopulmonary resuscitation (CPR); easier to learn than central venous access; if IV attempt unsuccessful, site easily compressible to reduce bleeding; results in fewer complications. 4. The external jugular vein lies superficially along the lateral portion of the neck. It extends from behind the angle of the jaw and passes downward across the sternocleidomastoid muscle and then under the middle of the clavicle to join the subclavian vein.
5-2	1. Alpha$_1$ receptor sites are located in vascular smooth muscle, beta$_1$ receptor sites are located in the heart and kidneys, beta$_2$ receptor sites are located in the smooth muscle of the bronchi and skeletal blood vessels. 2. Increase, myocardial contractility 3. Decrease, heart rate
5-3	MONA is a memory aid that may be used to recall medications used in the management of acute coronary syndromes (although not in the order they are given). M = *M*orphine, O = *O*xygen, N = *N*itroglycerin, A = *A*spirin. 1. Oxygen 4 L/min, aspirin 160 to 325 mg (chewed), nitroglycerin 0.4 mg SL tablets or spray (3 (5 minutes apart), morphine 2 to 4 mg every 5 minutes 2. Analgesic of choice for continuing ischemic chest discomfort unresponsive to nitrates; pulmonary vascular congestion complicating acute coronary syndromes (systolic blood pressure [SBP] >90 mm Hg)
5-4	1. Prevent fibrinogen binding and platelet clumping. 2. In general, prevent conversion of angiotensin I to angiotensin II (a potent vasoconstrictor). As a result, blood vessels relax, reducing the pressure the heart must pump against, and decreasing myocardial workload. By increasing renal blood flow, help rid the body of excess sodium and fluid build up.
5-5	1. Due to its extremely short half-life, adenosine should be given via a large-gauge IV started as close to the heart as possible (such as the antecubital vein). When given via a peripheral vein, the initial bolus is 6-mg rapid IV bolus over 1 to 3 seconds followed by a 20-mL saline flush and elevation of the extremity. If no response, may repeat with 12 mg in 1 to 2 minutes. The 12-mg dose may be repeated once in 1 to 2 minutes. 2. First-line drug for symptomatic narrow-QRS bradycardia, asystole (after epinephrine), slow PEA (after epinephrine). 3. Initial bolus—300 mg IV/IO bolus. Consider repeat dose of 150-mg IV/IO bolus once in 5 minutes. If return of spontaneous

circulation, consider continuous IV infusion (1 mg/min infusion for 6 hours and then a 0.5 mg/min maintenance infusion over 18 hours). Maximum daily dose is 2.2 g IV/24 hours.

5-6   1. Stable narrow-QRS tachycardia due to reentry if the rhythm persists despite vagal maneuvers or adenosine; stable narrow-QRS tachycardia due to automaticity (junctional, ectopic atrial, multifocal atrial tachycardia) if the rhythm persists despite vagal maneuvers or adenosine; to control the ventricular rate in patients with atrial fibrillation or atrial flutter. 2. Slows heart rate (negative chronotrope), increases myocardial contractility (positive inotrope). 3. Beta-blockers should generally not be given to patients with hypotension, bradycardia, congestive heart failure (CHF), second- or third-degree AV block, or a history of reactive airway disease.

5-7   1. Alpha and beta-adrenergic (beta$_1$ and beta$_2$) receptor sites 2. Pulseless VT, VF, asystole, PEA, symptomatic bradycardia 3. 2 to 2.5 mg 4. 2 to 10 mcg/min IV infusion (not IV bolus) 5. 3 mg/kg

5-8   1. Yes. Verapamil is a calcium channel blocker and is a negative inotrope (decreases the force of myocardial contraction). 2. 2.5 to 5 mg slow IV push over 2 minutes. If no response to the initial dose (and the patient's BP normal or elevated), repeat with 5 to 10 mg as needed every 15 to 30 minutes to a maximum dose of 20 mg. 3. Dizziness, drowsiness, mild agitation, hearing impairment, disorientation and confusion, muscle twitching, seizures, respiratory arrest 4. IV dose 1 mg every 3 to 5 minutes to a maximum dose of 3 mg

5-9   1. Cardiogenic shock, severe hypotension (SBP <70 mm Hg) not due to hypovolemia 2. 2 to 20 mcg/kg/min 3. False 4. False

STOP & REVIEW

1. Which of the following is considered a peripheral vein?
   a. Femoral
   b. Subclavian
   c. Internal jugular
   d. External jugular

2. What is the usual IV dosage of furosemide?
   a. 0.5 to 1.0 mg rapid IV push
   b. 0.5 to 1.0 mg/kg slow IV push
   c. 1 to 2 g rapid IV push
   d. 1 to 2 mg/kg/min continuous IV infusion

3. Which of the following is used in the management of severe hypotension (SBP <70 mm Hg) that is not due to hypovolemia?
   a. Dobutamine
   b. Nitroglycerin
   c. Dopamine
   d. Norepinephrine

4. Diltiazem may be used to:
   a. Control the ventricular rate in atrial fibrillation and atrial flutter.
   b. Convert wide-QRS tachycardia of uncertain origin to a sinus rhythm.
   c. Control the ventricular rate in Wolff-Parkinson-White (WPW) syndrome.
   d. Increase the ventricular rate in second- or third-degree AV block.

5. The initial dose of diltiazem is:
   a. 0.25 mg/kg IV push over 2 minutes
   b. 0.5 mg every 5 minutes to a maximum of 3 mg
   c. 0.35 mg/kg IV push over 2 minutes
   d. 1 to 1.5 mg/kg IV push over 1 to 2 minutes

6. When given in a cardiac arrest, the correct IV/IO dose of epinephrine is:
   a. 0.5 mg every 3 to 5 minutes to a maximum dose of 3 mg
   b. 0.5 mg every 5 minutes to a maximum dose of 3 mg/kg
   c. 1.0 mg every 3 to 5 minutes
   d. 1.0 mg every 5 minutes to a maximum dose of 3 mg/kg

7. Atropine may be useful in treating which of the following?
   a. Sinus tachycardia, AFib, and asystole
   b. Slow PEA, narrow-QRS tachycardias, and wide-QRS tachycardias
   c. Wide-QRS tachycardias, symptomatic bradycardia, and sinus tachycardia
   d. Symptomatic bradycardia, asystole, and slow PEA

8. Dopamine:
   a. Is useful in relieving chest discomfort associated with acute coronary syndromes
   b. Suppresses ventricular ectopy
   c. Is used to increase heart rate and blood pressure
   d. Should be given until the QRS increases to more than 50% of its original width

9. During cardiac arrest, IV medications given via a peripheral IV should be given rapidly by bolus injection and followed with a ____ bolus of IV fluid.
   a. 5-mL
   b. 10-mL
   c. 20-mL
   d. 50- to 100-mL

10. Leg veins are generally avoided for IV therapy due to:
    a. Discomfort
    b. Increased likelihood of venous thrombosis
    c. Inadequate flow rates
    d. Increased likelihood of extravasation due to downward position

11. Which of the following decrease myocardial oxygen requirements?
    a. Atropine, morphine
    b. Epinephrine, atropine
    c. Nitroglycerin, morphine
    d. Norepinephrine, nitroglycerin

12. The recommended IV dose of atropine when used to treat asystole is:
    a. 0.5 mg every 3 to 5 minutes to a maximum dose of 3 mg
    b. 1.0 mg every 3 to 5 minutes to a maximum dose of 3 mg
    c. 0.5 to 1.0 mg every 3 to 5 minutes to a maximum dose of 3 mg
    d. 1 to 1.5 mg/kg every 3 to 5 minutes to a maximum dose of 3 mg/kg

13. A drug that is a positive inotrope will:
    a. Increase myocardial contractility
    b. Decrease the heart rate
    c. Increase the heart rate
    d. Decrease myocardial contractility

14. Atropine should not be pushed in doses below 0.5 mg because:
    a. It may cause transient deafness
    b. It will cause a rapid increase in blood pressure
    c. It will result in excessively fast heart rates
    d. It may result in slowing of the heart rate

15. List three rhythms for which vasopressin may be given.
    1.
    2.
    3.

16. Which of the following is not an endpoint for procainamide administration?
    a. Hypotension develops
    b. The dysrhythmia is suppressed
    c. A total of 3 mg/kg has been given
    d. The QRS widens by 50% of its original width

17. Which of the following statements is not true about giving calcium chloride?
    a. Calcium chloride should be routinely given in cardiac arrest
    b. Severe tissue necrosis may occur if the calcium solution extravasates
    c. Calcium chloride may be helpful in the treatment of acute hyperkalemia
    d. Constant ECG monitoring is essential when giving calcium

18. Digitalis:
    a. Increases heart rate
    b. Is contraindicated in asthmatics
    c. Is a calcium channel blocker
    d. Increases the force of myocardial contraction

19. Which of the following statements about sotalol is not true?
    a. Side effects of giving sotalol include bradycardia and hypotension
    b. Sotalol increases heart rate and decreases the force of contraction
    c. Sotalol may be used in the treatment of monomorphic VT
    d. Torsades de pointes is the most common dysrhythmia associated with giving so-talol

20. Drugs used in the treatment of a symptomatic bradycardia include:
    a. Atropine, dopamine, and epinephrine
    b. Adenosine, epinephrine, and verapamil
    c. Dopamine, dobutamine, and norepinephrine
    d. Lidocaine, amiodarone, and vasopressin

Questions 21-40. Match each of the drugs below with its correct description.

a) Sodium bicarbonate	k) Digitalis
b) Epinephrine	l) Glycoprotein
c) Sodium nitroprusside	m) Dopamine
d) Atropine	n) Lidocaine
e) Heparin	o) Furosemide
f) Magnesium sulfate	p) Sotalol
g) Dobutamine	q) Fibrinolytic
h) Nitroglycerin	r) ACE inhibitor
i) Calcium chloride	s) Vasopressin
j) Diltiazem	t) Adenosine

_____21. Diuretic

_____22. May be used to treat torsades de pointes

_____23. Prevents the conversion of angiotensin I to angiotensin II

_____24. Can be used in place of the first or second dose of epinephrine in cardiac arrest

_____25. __ IIb/IIIa inhibitors prevent fibrinogen binding and platelet clumping

_____26. May be used as an alternative to amiodarone in pulseless VT/VF arrest

_____27. Although given IV bolus in cardiac arrest, this drug is given by IV infusion in symp-tomatic bradycardia

_____28. Calcium channel blocker

_____29. Drug of choice for most narrow-QRS tachycardias

_____30. May be used in tricyclic antidepressant overdose

_____31. Used in the treatment of acute pulmonary edema if no signs/symptoms of shock and SBP 70 to 100 mm Hg

_____32. Potent vasodilator

____33. _____ therapy is one reperfusion therapy option for patients with ST-segment elevation MI

____34. Used to treat symptomatic narrow-QRS bradycardia and slow PEA

____35. Used in the treatment of AFib or atrial flutter with WPW

____36. Indirect inhibitor of thrombin

____37. Vasodilator used in normotensive patients with ischemic chest discomfort

____38. Slows heart rate and increases force of contraction, but has limited use in emergency cardiac care

____39. Used to treat hyperkalemia and calcium channel blocker overdose

____40. Used to treat hypotension, especially that associated with symptomatic bradycardia

Questions 41-56. Match each of the drug dosages below with its correct description.
a) 6 mg rapid IV push over 1 to 3 seconds
b) 0.4 mg every 5 minutes up to 3 doses
c) 1 mg (1:10,000 solution) every 3 to 5 minutes
d) Initial dose 2 to 4 mg slow IV push; additional doses of 2 to 8 mg IV at 5- to 15-minute intervals
e) 40 units
f) 1 mg every 3 to 5 minutes, maximum total dose 3 mg
g) 150 mg over 10 minutes
h) 20 mg/min; maximum total dose 17 mg/kg
i) 5 mcg/min
j) 0.25 mg/kg IV bolus over 2 minutes
k) 0.5 mg every 3 to 5 min, maximum total dose 3 mg
l) 160 to 325 mg
m) 300 mg
n) 1 to 2 g
o) 2.5 to 5 mg slow IV push
p) 1 to 1.5 mg/kg

____41. Atropine dose in symptomatic bradycardia

____42. Recommended dosage of aspirin

____43. Initial dosage of verapamil

____44. Initial IV/IO dosage of amiodarone in cardiac arrest

____45. Dosage of nitroglycerin sublingual tablet or spray

____46. Dosage of magnesium sulfate for torsades de pointes

____47. Initial dose of diltiazem IV

____48. Atropine dose in asystole or slow PEA

____49. Initial IV/IO dosage of lidocaine

____50. Initial dosage of adenosine

____51. Initial IV dosage of nitroglycerin

____52. Dosage of vasopressin IV in cardiac arrest

_____53. Dosage of morphine sulfate to relieve ischemic chest discomfort

_____54. Loading dose of IV amiodarone for indications other than cardiac arrest

_____55. Dosage of procainamide

_____56. IV/IO dosage of epinephrine in cardiac arrest

STOP & REVIEW ANSWERS

1. d. The external jugular is considered a peripheral vein. The femoral, subclavian, and internal jugular veins are central veins.

2. b. The usual IV dosage of furosemide (Lasix) is 0.5 to 1.0 mg/kg slow IV push.

3. d. For a SBP <70 mm Hg with signs/symptoms of shock use an NE IV infusion 0.5 to 30 mcg/min. For a SBP 70 to 100 mm Hg with signs/symptoms of shock use a dopamine IV infusion 5 to 15 mcg/kg/min. For a SBP 70 to 100 mm Hg and no sign/symptoms of shock, use a dobutamine IV infusion 2 to 20 mcg/kg/min. (This is discussed in more detail in Chapter 6.) Because nitroglycerin is a vasodilator, it is not used in the management of a patient with hypotension.

4. Diltiazem is a calcium channel blocker that may be used to control the ventricular rate in stable narrow-QRS tachycardias or atrial fibrillation or atrial flutter with a rapid ventricular response if the rhythm persists despite vagal maneuvers or adenosine in patients with an adequate BP. Calcium channel blockers should be avoided in patients with wide-QRS tachycardia—unless it is *known with certainty* to be supraventricular in origin—may precipitate VF! Calcium channel blockers should be avoided in patients with WPW and are contraindicated in second- or third-degree AV block.

5. a. The initial dose of diltiazem is 0.25 mg/kg IV push over 2 min. If needed, follow in 15 min with 0.35 mg/kg over 2 min. Subsequent IV bolus doses should be individualized for each patient.

6. c. The IV/IO dose of epinephrine in cardiac arrest is 1 mg every 3 to 5 minutes. There is no maximum dose.

7. d. Because atropine increases heart rate, it is not indicated in the treatment of rhythms that have a fast ventricular rate. Atropine may be useful in the treatment of symptomatic bradycardia, asystole, and slow PEA.

8. c. Dopamine increases heart rate and cardiac contractility directly by stimulating beta-1 receptors on the myocardium and indirectly by causing the release of NE from storage sites in sympathetic nerve endings. Dopamine is not an analgesic; therefore it is not useful in relieving pain or discomfort. Dopamine is not an antiarrhythmic; therefore it does not suppress ventricular ectopy. Dopamine does not affect the width of the QRS complex.

9. c. In cardiac arrest, drugs given from a peripheral vein require 1 to 2 minutes to reach the central circulation. Following the drug with a 20 mL bolus of IV fluid and raising the extremity for 10 to 20 seconds helps speed delivery of the drug to the central circulation.

10. b. Leg veins are generally avoided because of their distance from the central circulation and because blood flow from the distal extremities is markedly decreased, increasing the likelihood and severity of venous thrombosis.

11. c. Nitroglycerin and morphine decrease myocardial oxygen requirements. Epinephrine, NE, and atropine increase myocardial oxygen requirements.

12. b. The recommended IV/IO dose of atropine when used to treat asystole is 1 mg every 3 to 5 minutes to a maximum dose of 3 mg.

13. a. The term "inotrope" refers to a drug's effect on myocardial contractility. A drug that is a positive inotrope increases the heart's force of contraction. Digitalis, dopamine, and epinephrine are examples of drugs that are positive inotropes. Negative inotropes decrease the heart's force of contraction. Calcium channel blockers and beta-blockers are examples of negative inotropes.

14. d. Atropine should not be pushed slowly or in smaller than recommended doses. Small doses (<0.5 mg) produce modest paradoxical cardiac slowing that may last 2 minutes.

15. Vasopressin may be used to replace the first or second dose of epinephrine in cardiac arrest. The four cardiac arrest rhythms are asystole, PEA, pulseless VT, and VF.

16. c. Endpoints for procainamide administration include the onset of hypotension, suppression of the dysrhythmia, widening of the QRS by more than 50% of its original width, and administration of a maximum total dose of 17 mg/kg.

17. a. Because high serum calcium levels due to calcium administration may be detrimental, calcium chloride should not be routinely given in cardiac arrest. Calcium chloride may helpful in the treatment of acute hyperkalemia, hypocalcemia, magnesium overdose, and calcium channel blocker toxicity. Severe tissue necrosis may occur if the calcium solution extravasates.

18. d. Digitalis is a cardiac glycoside that slows conduction through the AV node (prolonging the PR interval), increases the force and velocity of myocardial contraction (positive inotropic effect), and increases cardiac output.

19. b. Sotalol decreases heart rate and increases the force of contraction. It may be used in the treatment of monomorphic VT and for rhythm control of atrial fibrillation or atrial flutter in patients with WPW syndrome if the rhythm has been present ≤48 hours and no signs of heart failure are present. Side effects include bradycardia, hypotension, and dysrhythmias. The most common dysrhythmia associated with giving sotalol is torsades de pointes.

20. a. Drugs used in the treatment of a symptomatic narrow-QRS bradycardia include atropine, dopamine, and epinephrine.

21. o	31. g
22. f	32. c
23. r	33. q
24. s	34. d
25. l	35. p
26. n	36. e
27. b	37. h
28. j	38. k
29. t	39. i
30. a	40. m

41. k   49. p

42. l   50. a

43. o   51. i

44. m   52. e

45. b   53. d

46. n   54. g

47. j   55. h

48. f   56. c

REFERENCES

1. Iwama H, Katsumi A, Shinohara K, et al: Clavicular approach to intraosseous infusion in adults. *Fukushima J Med Sci* Jun 1994;40(1):1-8.
2. Glaeser PW, Hellmich TR, Szewczuga D, et al: Five-year experience in prehospital intraosseous infusions in children and adults. *Ann Emerg Med* Jul 1993;22(7):1119-1124.
3. Iserson KV, Criss E: Intraosseous infusions: A usable technique. *Am J Emerg Med* Nov 1986;4(6):540-542.
4. Macnab A, Christenson J, Findlay J, et al: A new system for sternal intraosseous infusion in adults. *Prehosp Emerg Care* Apr-Jun 2000;4(2):173-177.
5. Efrati O, Ben-Abraham R, Barak A, et al: Endobronchial adrenaline: Should it be reconsidered? Dose response and hæmodynamic effect in dogs. *Resuscitation* Oct 2003;59(1):117-122.
6. Manisterski Y, Vaknin Z, Ben-Abraham R, et al: Endotracheal epinephrine: A call for larger doses. *Anesth Analg* Oct 2002;95(4):1037-1041, table of contents.
7. Vaknin Z, Manisterski Y, Ben-Abraham R, et al: Is endotracheal adrenaline deleterious because of the beta adrenergic effect? *Anesth Analg* Jun 2001;92(6):1408-1412.
8. Efrati O, Barak A, Ben-Abraham R, et al: Should vasopressin replace adrenaline for endotracheal drug administration? *Crit Care Med* Feb 2003;31(2):572-576.
9. Antman EM, Anbe DT, Armstrong PW, et al: ACC/AHA guidelines for the management of patients with ST-elevation myocardial infarction: A report of the American College of Cardiology/American Heart Association Task Force on Practice Guidelines (Committee to Revise the 1999 Guidelines for the Management of Patients with Acute Myocardial Infarction). 2004. Available at www.acc.org/clinical/guidelines/stemi/index.pdf/

Acute Coronary Syndromes

OBJECTIVES

Upon completion of this chapter, you will be able to:

1. Define acute coronary syndromes (ACS).
2. Describe the pathophysiology of coronary artery disease and the process of atherosclerosis.
3. Differentiate the characteristics of stable (classic) angina, unstable angina, and acute myocardial infarction (MI).
4. Explain atypical presentation and its significance in ACS.
5. Identify the electrocardiogram (ECG) changes associated with myocardial ischemia, injury, and infarction.
6. Explain the ECG criteria for significant ST-segment changes.
7. Describe the initial assessment and immediate general treatment of acute coronary syndromes.
8. Describe the initial management of a patient experiencing ST-elevation MI (STEMI), non–ST-elevation MI (NSTEMI), and unstable angina.
9. Explain the importance of the 12-lead ECG in ACS.
10. Identify the ECG leads that view the anterior wall, inferior wall, lateral wall, and septum.
11. Explain the clinical and ECG features of right ventricular infarction (RVI).
12. Identify the most common complications of an acute MI.

INTRODUCTION

Each year, about 1.1 million Americans experience a heart attack. About 460,000 of these events are fatal, and about half of these deaths occur within 1 hour of the onset of symptoms and before the person reaches the hospital.[1]

    When a temporary or permanent blockage occurs in a coronary artery, the blood supply to the heart muscle is impaired. An impaired blood supply results in a decreased supply of oxygen to the myocardium. When the heart's demand for oxygen exceeds its supply from the coronary circulation, chest discomfort or related symptoms often occur. A decreased supply of oxygenated blood to a body part or organ is called **ischemia.** This chapter discusses the pathophysiology of coronary artery disease and the process of atherosclerosis. Conditions ranging from myocardial ischemia or injury to death (necrosis) of the heart muscle are presented, including strategies to use when providing initial emergency care to patients who present with these conditions.

ACUTE CORONARY SYNDROMES

- Recognition of an acute coronary syndrome and giving appropriate and timely emergency care can have a big impact on patient outcome. **Acute coronary syndromes** (ACSs) are conditions caused by a similar sequence of pathologic events—a temporary or permanent blockage of a coronary artery. This sequence of events results in conditions ranging from myocardial ischemia or injury to death (necrosis) of heart muscle.
- ACSs include unstable angina, NSTEMI, and STEMI. Sudden cardiac death (SCD) can occur with any of these conditions.

 ACSs are also called acute ischemic coronary syndromes (AICSs).

PATHOLOGY

The usual cause of an ACS is the rupture of an atherosclerotic plaque. To understand this process, a quick review of some relevant anatomy follows.

- Arteries consist of three layers (Figure 6-1).
  - The outermost layer is the tunica adventitia. It consists of flexible connective tissue and helps hold the vessel open.
  - The middle layer is the tunica media. It consists of smooth muscle tissue and elastic connective tissue. This layer is encircled by smooth muscle and innervated by fibers of the autonomic nervous system that allows constriction and dilation of the vessel. Smooth muscle cells function to maintain vascular tone and regulate local blood flow depending on the body's metabolic needs. These cells are also capable of producing collagen, elastin, and other substances that are important in the formation of atherosclerotic plaques.
  - The innermost layer of an artery is the tunica intima. It is made up of endothelium that lines the vascular system. Endothelium is a single layer of cells in direct contact with the blood. The intima is at risk of damage from conditions such as hypertension, high cholesterol, smoking, and diabetes.
- **Arteriosclerosis** is a chronic disease of the arterial system characterized by abnormal thickening and hardening of the vessel walls. **Atherosclerosis** (athero = gruel or paste, sclerosis = hardness) is a form of arteriosclerosis in which the thickening and hardening of the vessel walls are caused by a build up of fat-like deposits in the inner lining of large and middle-sized muscular arteries. As the fatty deposits build up, the opening of the artery slowly narrows and blood flow to the muscle decreases (Figure 6-2).

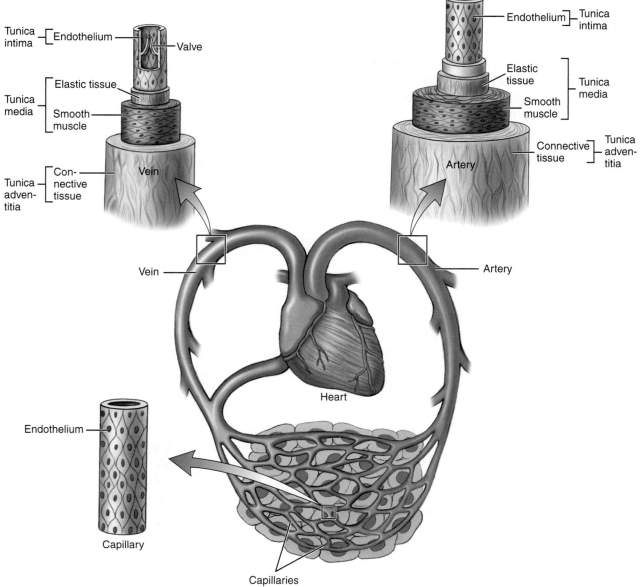

Figure 6-1 • Blood vessel wall layers.

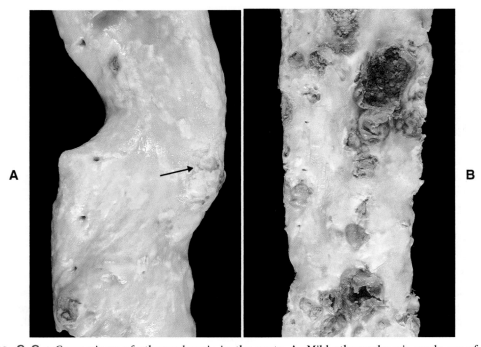

Figure 6-2 • Gross views of atherosclerosis in the aorta. **A,** Mild atherosclerosis made up of fibrous plaques *(arrow).* **B,** Severe disease with scattered and complicated lesions.

■ Any artery in the body can develop atherosclerosis.
  ▶ If the coronary arteries are involved (coronary artery disease [CAD]) and blood flow to the heart is decreased, angina or more serious signs and symptoms may result.
  ▶ If the arteries in the leg are involved (peripheral vascular disease), leg pain (claudication) may result.
  ▶ If the arteries supplying the brain are involved (carotid artery disease), a stroke or transient ischemic attack (TIA) may result.

■ Research has shown that oxidation and the body's inflammatory response contribute to atherosclerosis and heart disease. Oxidation is a normal chemical process in the body that is caused by the release of free radicals. Free radicals are oxygen atoms created during normal cell metabolism. Too many free radicals can seriously damage cells and impair the body's ability to fight against illness. Examples of conditions that can cause an overproduction of free radicals include stress and exposure to cigarette smoke, pesticides, air pollution, ultraviolet light, and radiation. Antioxidants, such as Vitamins C and E, work by binding to free radicals and transforming them into nondamaging substances or repairing cellular damage.

■ Oxidation causes injury to the inner lining of arteries. Low-density lipoproteins (LDLs) become damaged when they react with free radicals. LDL may be responsible for a buildup fat-like material on the artery walls. Injury to the inner lining of the arteries starts the body's inflammatory response. White blood cells are released at the site and oxidize LDL. Cytokines are also released. Cytokines trigger the inflammatory response, attracting even more white blood cells to the site. They also raise blood pressure (BP) and increase the tendency for blood to clot. Oxidation converts LDL to a foamy material. The foamy material sticks to the smooth muscle cells of the arteries. Over time, the foamy material builds up on artery walls and forms a hard plaque.

■ Atherosclerotic plaques differ in their makeup, vulnerability to rupture, and tendency to make a blood clot. "Stable" plaques are unlikely to rupture. They are made up mainly of collagen-rich tissue that has hardened. They have a thick fibrous cap over the lipid core that separates it from contact with the blood, making them less likely to rupture (Figure 6-3). As these plaques increase in size, the artery can become severely narrowed.

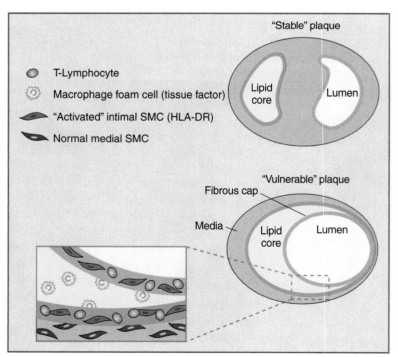

Figure 6-3 • Comparison of "stable" and "vulnerable" plaques. A stable plaque has a relatively thick fibrous cap separating the lipid core from contact with the blood. A vulnerable plaque typically has a large lipid core and a thin cap of fibrous tissue that separates it from the vessel lumen. *SMC*, Smooth muscle cell.

■ The walls of an artery outwardly expand (remodel) as plaque builds up inside it. This occurs so that the size of the vessel stays relatively constant, despite the increased size of the plaque.

  ▶ When the plaque fills about 40% of the inside of the artery, remodeling stops because the artery can no longer expand to make room for the increase in plaque size.

  ▶ Complete blockage of the artery may cause a heart attack (myocardial infarction [MI]). However, because the plaque usually increases in size over months and years, other vascular pathways may enlarge as portions of a coronary artery become blocked. These vascular pathways (collateral circulation) serve as an alternative route for blood flow around the blocked artery to the heart muscle. Thus, the presence of collateral arteries may prevent infarction despite complete blockage of the artery.

■ Plaques that are prone to rupture are called "vulnerable" plaques. They are soft and have a thin cap of fibrous tissue over the fatty center that separates it from the opening of the artery (Figure 6-4).

  ▶ If the fibrous cap tears or ruptures, the contents of the plaque are exposed to flowing blood. Platelets stick to the damaged lining of the vessel and to each other within 1 to 5 seconds and form a plug.

  ▶ "Sticky platelets" secrete several chemicals, including thromboxane A_2. These substances stimulate vasoconstriction, reducing blood flow at the site.

  ▶ Aspirin (an antiplatelet agent) blocks the production of thromboxane A_2, slowing down the clumping (aggregation) of platelets and lowering the risk of complete blockage of the vessel.

■ Once platelets are activated, glycoprotein IIb/IIIa receptors that are needed for platelet clumping appear on the surface of the platelet. Fibrinogen molecules bind to these receptors to form bridges ("cross-links") between nearby platelets, allowing them to clump. Glycoprotein IIb/IIIa receptor inhibitors prevent fibrinogen binding and platelet clumping.

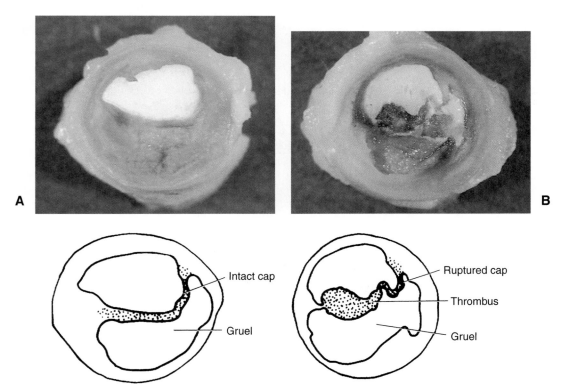

Figure 6-4 • View of a vulnerable plaque. **A,** The yellow, soft fatty material ("gruel") is separated from the opening of the vessel by a thin fibrous cap. White radiographic contrast medium is visible in the vessel opening. **B,** This specimen was just a few millimeters distal to the one shown in **A.** In this specimen, the thin fibrous cap is ruptured. A mural thrombus has developed where the fatty gruel has been exposed. White contrast medium has penetrated the gruel through the ruptured fibrous cap.

■ As the process continues, fibrinogen cross-links platelets, thrombin is made, and fibrin is formed, ultimately producing a clot (Figure 6-5). Clots can be dissolved by a process called **fibrinolysis.** Fibrinolytics ("clot-busters") are drugs that stimulate the conversion of plasminogen to plasmin, which dissolves the clot (Figure 6-6).

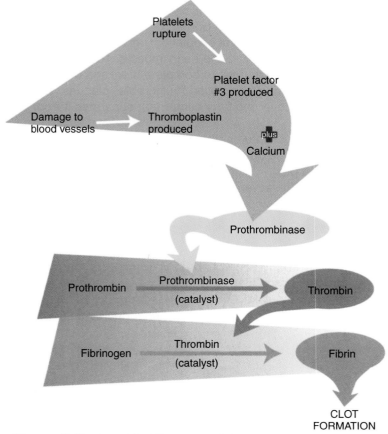

Figure 6-5 • Simplified illustration of the process of clot formation.

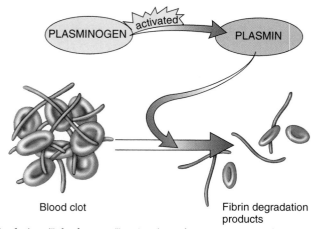

Figure 6-6 • Fibrinolytics ("clot-busters") stimulate the conversion of plasminogen to plasmin, which dissolves the clot.

■ Rupture of a vulnerable plaque may follow extreme physical activity (especially in some-one unaccustomed to regular exercise), severe emotional trauma, sexual activity, expo-sure to illicit drugs (cocaine, marijuana, or amphetamines), exposure to cold, or acute in-fection.[2] Contributing factors to plaque rupture may include the frictional force from blood flow; coronary spasm at the site of the plaque; internal plaque changes; and the effects of risk factors, such as high BP and high cholesterol.

■ Blockage of a coronary artery by a clot may be complete or incomplete.

   ▶ Complete blockage of a coronary artery may result in STEMI or sudden death.
   ▶ Partial (incomplete) blockage of a coronary artery by a clot may result in no clinical signs and symptoms (silent MI), unstable angina, NSTEMI or, possibly, sudden death.

■ The patient's signs, symptoms, and outcome depend on factors including the following:

   ▶ Amount of heart muscle supplied by the affected artery
   ▶ Severity and duration of myocardial ischemia
   ▶ Electrical instability of the ischemic myocardium
   ▶ Degree and duration of coronary vessel blockage
   ▶ Presence (and extent) or absence of collateral coronary circulation

---

QUICK REVIEW 6-1

1. The innermost layer of the vessel walls is made up of _____.
2. "Sticky platelets" secrete several chemicals, including thromboxane A_2. Name a common drug used to block the synthesis of thromboxane A_2, inhibiting platelet clumping.

3. Once platelets are activated, _____ receptors that are essential for platelet aggregation appear on the surface of the platelet. Fibrinogen molecules bind to these receptors to form bridges ("cross-links") between adjacent platelets, allowing them to clump.
4. _____ stimulate the conversion of plasminogen to plasmin, which dis-solves a clot.

Answers can be found at the end of this chapter.

ANGINA PECTORIS

■ **Angina pectoris** is chest discomfort that occurs when the heart muscle does not receive enough oxygen (myocardial ischemia). Angina is not a disease. It is a symptom of myocar-dial ischemia. Angina most often occurs in patients with coronary artery disease involving at least one coronary artery. However, it can be present in patients with normal coronary arter-ies. Angina also occurs in persons with uncontrolled high BP or valvular heart disease.

■ Angina means squeezing or tightening, not pain. The discomfort associated with angina occurs because of the stimulation of nerve endings by lactic acid and carbon dioxide that builds up in ischemic tissue. Common words used by patients experiencing angina to describe the sensation they are feeling are shown in Box 6-1. Some patients have diffi-culty describing their discomfort.

■ Chest discomfort associated with myocardial ischemia usually begins in the central or left chest and then radiates to the arm (especially the little finger [ulnar] side of the left arm), wrist, jaw, epigastrium, left shoulder, or between the shoulder blades (Figure 6-7). Isch-emic chest discomfort is usually not sharp, worsened by deep inspiration, affected by moving muscles in the area where the discomfort is localized, or positional in nature.

■ Ischemia can occur because of increased myocardial oxygen demand (demand ischemia), reduced myocardial oxygen supply (supply ischemia), or both. If the cause of the ischemia is not reversed and blood flow restored to the affected area of the heart muscle, ischemia may lead to cellular injury and, ultimately, infarction.

■ Ischemia can quickly resolve by reducing the heart's oxygen demand (by resting or slow-ing the heart rate with medications such as beta-blockers) or increasing blood flow by dilating the coronary arteries with drugs such as nitroglycerin (NTG).

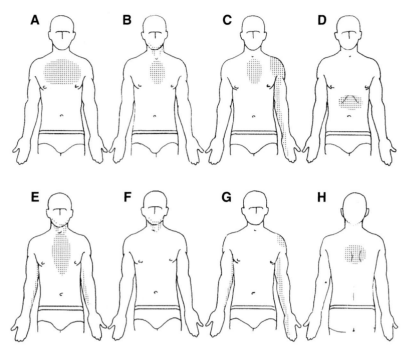

Figure 6-7 • Common sites for anginal pain. **A,** Upper part of chest. **B,** Beneath sternum radiating to neck and jaw. **C,** Beneath sternum radiating down left arm. **D,** Epigastric. **E,** Epigastric radiating to neck, jaw, and arms. **F,** Neck and jaw. **G,** Left shoulder. **H,** Interscapular.

BOX 6-1

Common Terms Patients Use To Describe Angina

- Heaviness
- Pressing
- Suffocating
- Squeezing
- Strangling
- Constricting
- Bursting
- Burning
- Grip-like
- "A band across my chest"
- "A weight in the center of my chest"
- "A vise tightening around my chest"

■ Early assessment, including a focused history, and emergency care are essential to prevent worsening ischemia. Serial ECGs and continuous ECG monitoring should be performed.

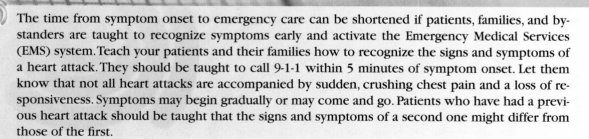

The time from symptom onset to emergency care can be shortened if patients, families, and bystanders are taught to recognize symptoms early and activate the Emergency Medical Services (EMS) system. Teach your patients and their families how to recognize the signs and symptoms of a heart attack. They should be taught to call 9-1-1 within 5 minutes of symptom onset. Let them know that not all heart attacks are accompanied by sudden, crushing chest pain and a loss of responsiveness. Symptoms may begin gradually or may come and go. Patients who have had a previous heart attack should be taught that the signs and symptoms of a second one might differ from those of the first.

Stable Angina

■ Stable (classic) angina remains relatively constant and predictable in terms of severity, signs and symptoms, precipitating events, and response to treatment. It is characterized by brief episodes of chest discomfort related to activities that increase the heart's need for oxygen such as emotional upset, exercise/exertion, and exposure to cold weather. Possible related signs and symptoms are shown in Box 6-2.

■ Symptoms typically last 2 to 5 minutes and occasionally 5 to 15 minutes. Prolonged discomfort (>30 minutes) is uncommon in stable angina.

BOX 6-2

Stable Angina

Common Precipitating Events	Related Signs and Symptoms
• Emotional upset	• Shortness of breath
• Exercise/exertion	• Palpitations
• Exposure to cold weather	• Sweating
	• Nausea or vomiting

Unstable Angina

■ Unstable angina (also known as preinfarction angina) is a condition of intermediate severity between stable angina and acute MI. It occurs most often in men and women 60 to 80 years of age who have one or more of the major risk factors for coronary artery disease.

■ Unstable angina is characterized by one or more of the following:
  ▶ Symptoms that occur at rest (or minimal exertion) and usually lasting >20 minutes
  ▶ Symptoms that are severe and/or of new onset (i.e., within the previous 4-6 weeks)
  ▶ Symptoms that are more severe, prolonged, or frequent in a patient with a history of stable angina

■ Unlike stable angina, the discomfort associated with unstable angina may be described as painful.

■ Patients with untreated unstable angina are at high risk of a heart attack or death. Early assessment and emergency care are essential to prevent worsening ischemia.

QUICK REVIEW 6-2

1. _____ is a decreased supply of oxygenated blood to a body part or organ.
2. Can you describe the typical pain pattern associated with chronic stable angina?

3. Name the "3 I's" of an acute coronary event.
    1.
    2.
    3.
4. Describe the characteristics of unstable angina.

Prinzmetal's Angina

▨ Prinzmetal's angina (also called Prinzmetal's variant angina or variant angina) is an uncommon form of angina. It is the result of intense spasm of a segment of a coronary artery.

▨ This variant angina may occur in otherwise healthy individuals (usually between 40 and 50 years of age) with no demonstrable coronary heart disease. The episode of coronary artery spasm occurs almost exclusively at rest, often occurs in the early morning hours, and may awaken the patient from sleep. It is not usually brought on by physical exertion or emotional stress.

▨ Episodes usually last only a few minutes, but this may be long enough to produce serious dysrhythmias including ventricular tachycardia and fibrillation, as well as sudden death. If the spasm persists, infarction may result.

 Myocardial ischemia, injury, and infarction are referred to as "The 3 I's" of an acute coronary event.

MYOCARDIAL INFARCTION

▨ Ischemia prolonged more than just a few minutes results in myocardial *injury*. Myocardial injury refers to myocardial tissue that has been cut off from or experienced a severe reduction in its blood and oxygen supply.

▨ Injured myocardial cells are still alive but will die (infarct) if the ischemia is not quickly corrected. If the blocked vessel can be quickly opened, restoring blood flow and oxygen to the injured area, no tissue death occurs.

  ▶ Methods to restore blood flow include giving fibrinolytics, coronary angioplasty, and a coronary artery bypass graft (CABG), among others.

▨ A **myocardial infarction (MI)** occurs when blood flow to the heart muscle stops or is suddenly decreased long enough to cause cell death. Possible locations of infarctions in the ventricular wall are shown in Figure 6-8.

  ▶ In the strictest sense, the term MI relates to dead heart muscle tissue. In a practical sense, the term MI is applied to the *process* that results in the death of myocardial tissue. Think of the "process" of MI as a continuum rather than the presence of dead heart

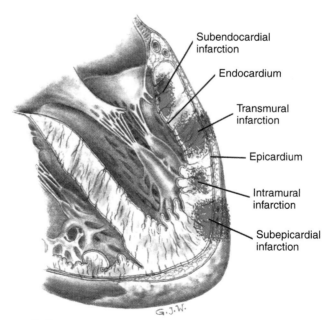

Figure 6-8 • Possible locations of infarctions in the ventricular wall.

tissue. If efforts are made to recognize the process of MI, patients may be identified earlier. If they are promptly treated, the loss of heart tissue may be avoided.[3]

■ An acute MI usually results from a thrombus. Less commonly, acute MI may occur because of coronary spasm (as in cocaine abuse) or coronary embolism (rare).

■ Nearly 10% of MIs occur in people younger than age 40 years, and 45% occur in people younger than age 65 years.[4] Between the ages of 40 and 60 years, the incidence of MI increases fivefold.[5]

■ Infarcted cells cannot respond to an electrical stimulus or provide any mechanical function.

It has been estimated that there are 30 patients with stable angina for every patient with infarction who is hospitalized.[6]

HISTORY AND PHYSICAL FINDINGS

Precipitating Factors

■ A precipitating factor is present in about 50% of patients experiencing MI. Examples include unusually vigorous exercise, severe emotional stress, or serious illness. Cocaine use may be a factor, particularly in patients younger than 40 years of age.

■ Patients at risk for SCD may have signs and symptoms such as chest discomfort, dyspnea, weakness or fatigue, palpitations, syncope, or nonspecific complaints before an MI or SCD.

  ▶ Among patients interviewed after successful resuscitation following out-of-hospital cardiac arrest, 28% said that they had had new or changing angina pectoris or dyspnea in the 4 weeks before arrest. During this time 31% had seen a physician, but only 12% had seen the physician because of these symptoms.[7]

■ Not all chest discomfort is cardiac-related. Obtaining an accurate history is important to help determine if a patient's signs and symptoms are most likely related to ischemia due to coronary artery disease. The five most important factors, ranked in the order of importance, are as follows:[8]
  1. The nature of the anginal symptoms
  2. Previous history of coronary artery disease
  3. Gender
  4. Age
  5. The number of risk factors present

■ Because time is muscle when caring for patients with an ACS, it is important to ask targeted questions to determine the patient's probability of an ACS and not delay reperfusion therapy (if indicated). Important information to obtain when eliciting a targeted history is shown in Table 6-1.

  ▶ If the patient has STEMI, the goals of reperfusion therapy are to give fibrinolytics within 30 minutes of arrival in the emergency department (ED) ("door-to-drug") or to provide percutaneous coronary intervention (PCI) within 90 minutes of arrival ("door-to-balloon inflation").[9]

■ Chest discomfort is the most common symptom of infarction. It is present in 75% to 80% of patients with acute MI. Patients experiencing a heart attack may describe the sensation they are feeling as similar to angina, or use words such as *heartburn, indigestion, dull, squeezing, gnawing, aching, tightness,* or *pressure.*

■ The patient may describe his discomfort with a clenched fist held against his sternum (Levine's sign). The discomfort typically lasts longer than 30 minutes. It may be constant or come and go, and occasionally may be relieved with belching.[10]

■ Patients with possible symptoms of ischemic chest discomfort should be taught the importance of calling 9-1-1 rather than arranging for their own transport to the hospital.

  ▶ In 2000, a follow-up survey of chest pain patients who presented to EDs in 20 U.S. communities was done. The patients in the survey were either released or admitted to the

TABLE 6-1	Acute Coronary Syndromes—Targeted History
Historical Information to Obtain	**Notes**
Patient age, gender	Important risk factors
SAMPLE History	
Signs/Symptoms	"What prompted you to seek medical assistance today?"
Allergies	Medications, food, environmental causes (pollen), and products (latex)
Medications	• Prescription and over-the-counter medications (including herbal supplements), recreational substance use • History of Viagra (or similar medication) use in the past 24 to 48 hours?
Past medical history	• History of coronary artery disease, stable or unstable angina, MI, coronary bypass surgery, or PCI? • History of high BP or diabetes? • Risk factors present? How many? • History of bleeding problems, ulcer disease, TIA, or stroke?
Last oral intake	Time of most recent meal and fluid intake
Events prior	"What were you doing when it began?"
OPQRST (Pain Presentation)	
Onset	• "When did your symptoms begin?" • "Did your symptoms begin suddenly or gradually?"
Provocation/Palliative	• "Did anything bring on your discomfort?" • "Does anything make it better or worse?" (Associated with respiration, movement)
Quality	"How would you describe your discomfort?"
Region/Radiation/Referral	• "Where is your discomfort?" (Ask the patient to point to it.) • "Does it go anywhere else?"
Severity	"On a scale of 0 to 10, with 0 being the least and 10 being the worst, what number would you assign your pain or discomfort?"
Timing	"Does your discomfort come and go, or is it constant?"
Presence of associated symptoms?	Nausea, vomiting, sweating, weakness, fatigue
Special considerations	Consider possibility of potentially lethal conditions that mimic acute MI such as aortic dissection, acute pericarditis, acute myocarditis, and pulmonary embolism.

hospital with a confirmed coronary event. The survey revealed that about 23% of the patients used EMS. Most of them were driven by someone else (60%) or drove themselves to the hospital (16%).[11]

▶ Teach your patients that EMS professionals can provide life-saving care if they develop complications en route to the hospital.

 "Although typical characteristics substantially raise the probability of CAD, features not characteristic of chest pain, such as sharp stabbing pain or reproduction of pain on palpation, *do not exclude* the possibility of acute coronary syndrome."[12]

Atypical Presentation

▦ Chest discomfort is absent in about 20% of patients experiencing an infarction. In a 2000 study, 33% of patients admitted to a hospital with an MI did not have chest pain on presentation to the hospital. MI patients without chest pain had a longer delay before hospital presentation, were less likely to be diagnosed as having confirmed MI at the time of hospital admission, and were less likely to receive fibrinolytics, angioplasty, aspirin, beta-blockers, or heparin.[13]

▦ Atypical chest discomfort is localized to the chest area but has musculoskeletal, positional, or pleuritic features. Atypical presentation refers to the uncharacteristic signs and symptoms experienced by some patients. Patients experiencing an ACS who are most likely to present atypically include the elderly, diabetic individuals, and women.

QUICK REVIEW 6-3

1. What is meant by the phrase, "myocardial injury"?

2. How does myocardial injury differ from MI?

3. A 62-year-old man is complaining of chest discomfort. When taking this patient's history, list three important factors that may help determine if his signs and symptoms are most likely related to ischemia due to coronary artery disease.
    1.
    2.
    3.

- Older adults may present with atypical symptoms such as a change in mental status, generalized weakness, syncope, shortness of breath, fatigue, unexplained nausea, and abdominal or epigastric discomfort. They are also more likely to present with more severe preexisting conditions, such as hypertension, heart failure, or a previous acute MI, than a younger patient.
- Diabetic individuals may present atypically with generalized weakness, syncope, lightheadedness, or a change in mental status.
- Women who experience an ACS often describe their discomfort as aching, tightness, pressure, sharpness, burning, fullness, or tingling. The location of the discomfort is often in the back, shoulder, or neck.
  - Some women have vague chest discomfort that tends to come and go with no known aggravating factors. Frequent acute symptoms include shortness of breath, weakness, unusual fatigue, cold sweats, dizziness, and nausea or vomiting.
  - Women are twice as likely as men to die in the early weeks after an acute MI and experience reinfarction more frequently.

Anginal Equivalents

- **Anginal equivalent** symptoms are symptoms of myocardial ischemia other than chest pain or discomfort. Examples of anginal equivalents include the following:
  - Generalized weakness
  - Difficulty breathing
  - Excessive sweating
  - Unexplained nausea or vomiting
  - Dizziness
  - Syncope or near-syncope
  - Palpitations
  - Isolated arm or jaw pain
  - Fatigue
  - Dysrhythmias

Delays in Seeking Medical Care

- After the onset of ischemic chest pain symptoms, most patients do not seek medical care for 2 hours or more. Women often delay seeking medical help longer than men. Common reasons for the delay in seeking medical care are shown in Box 6-3.

- The likelihood of death from acute MI decreases as the interval between symptom onset and initiation of treatment decreases. According to the National Heart Attack Alert Program, each hour of delay equals a 1% increase in the likelihood of death.

- In the past, patients with known CAD who were prescribed NTG were often advised to take one NTG dose sublingually, 5 minutes apart, for up to 3 doses before calling for help. Because this practice has been associated with delays in seeking medical care, this recommendation has been changed. Physicians are now advising their patients to take *1* NTG dose sublingually promptly for chest discomfort. If symptoms are unimproved or worsening 5 minutes after 1 NTG dose has been taken, patients are advised to call 9-1-1 immediately.[10]

- Delays in calling 9-1-1 have also occurred because patients take an aspirin in response to their symptoms. Teach your patients to call 9-1-1 first. If there are no contraindications, emergency medical dispatchers may advise the patient to chew aspirin while EMS personnel are en route, aspirin may be given during EMS care or on arrival at the hospital if it was not given in the prehospital setting.

About 1 in every 300 patients with chest pain or discomfort transported to the ED by private vehicle goes into cardiac arrest en route.[14]

BOX 6-3

Common Reasons for Delays in Seeking Medical Care for Ischemic-Type Chest Discomfort[10]

- Unaware of the importance of calling EMS/9-1-1 for symptoms
- Unaware of the need for rapid treatment
- Mild discomfort began slowly, not abruptly and with severe pain as depicted on television or in the movies ("Hollywood heart attack")
- Believed symptoms would go away or were not serious
- Believed symptoms were due to another chronic condition, such as arthritis, muscle strain, or "the flu"
- Did not want to "bother" EMS personnel or their physician
- Afraid of embarrassment if symptoms turned out to be a false alarm
- Wanted family approval before seeking medical care
- Felt they were not at risk for a heart attack (especially women or young, healthy men)

From Antman EM, Anbe DT, Armstrong PW, et al: www.acc.org/clinical/guidelines/stemi/index.pdf.

Qᴜɪᴄᴋ Rᴇᴠɪᴇᴡ 6-4

1. What is the most common symptom associated with MI?

2. What types of patients are more likely to present atypically when experiencing an ACS?

3. What is meant by the phrase, "anginal equivalent" symptoms?

4. List two examples of anginal equivalents.
   1.
   2.

ELECTROCARDIOGRAM FINDINGS

The sudden blockage of a coronary artery may result in ischemia, injury, and/or death of the area of the myocardium supplied by the affected artery. The area supplied by the blocked artery goes through a characteristic sequence of events that have been identified as "zones" of ischemia, injury, and infarction. Each zone is associated with characteristic ECG changes (Figure 6-9). The ECG changes described below are not seen in every lead. They appear only in leads looking at the area fed by the blocked vessel.[3]

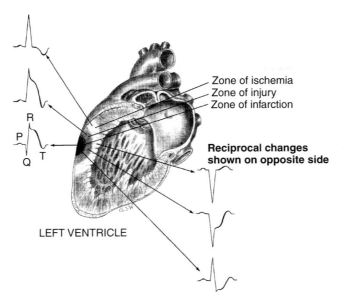

Figure 6-9 • Zones of ischemia, injury, and infarction showing ECG waveforms and reciprocal waveform changes corresponding to each zone.

Because most infarctions occur in the left ventricle (LV) and a standard 12-lead ECG views the surfaces of the LV from 12 different angles, obtain a 12-lead ECG as quickly as possible in a patient experiencing a possible ACS.

Myocardial Ischemia

■ Ischemia affects the heart's cells responsible for contraction as well as those responsible for the generation and conduction of electrical impulses. Because ischemia affects repolarization, its effects can be viewed on the ECG as brief changes in ST-segments and T waves in the leads facing the affected area of the ventricle.

■ ST-segment *depression* is suggestive of myocardial ischemia.

  ▶ Remember that the ST-segment represents the early part of repolarization of the RV and LV. The normal ST-segment begins at the isoelectric line, extends from the end of the S wave, and curves gradually upward to the beginning of the T wave.

  ▶ When looking for ST-segment displacement on an ECG, find the junction—or J-point— the connection between the end of the QRS complex and the beginning of the ST-segment. Locate a QRS complex on the 12-lead ECG, and follow that QRS complex to the end. Look to see where the end of the QRS complex makes a sudden sharp change in direction. That point identifies the J-point (Figure 6-10).

  ▶ Compare the ST-segment deviation to the isoelectric line. The TP-segment is best used for this comparison however, some authorities prefer to use the PR-segment as the baseline (Figure 6-11). If the ST-segment is below the baseline, ST-segment depression is present. This ECG finding is considered significant if the ST-segment is ≥0.5 mm below the baseline.

  ▶ ECG changes are significant when they are seen in two *contiguous* leads. Two leads are contiguous if they look at the same area of the heart or if they are numerically consecutive chest leads. This is explained in more detail later in this chapter.

There is some difference of opinion as to where ST-segment deviation should be measured. Some authorities simply measure deviation at the J-point while others look for displacement 0.04 second after the J-point. Still others measure ST-segment deviation 0.06 second after the J-point.[3]

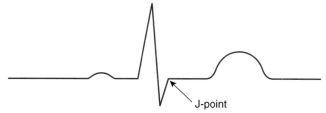

J-point

Figure 6-10 • The point where the QRS complex and the ST-segment meet is called the "junction" or "J" point.

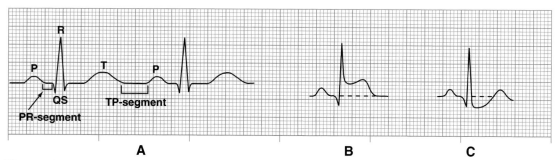

A   B   C

Figure 6-11 • The PR-segment and TP-segment. **A,** The TP-segment is best used to determine the presence of ST-segment displacement from the baseline. However, some authorities prefer to use the PR-segment as the baseline. **B,** ST-segment elevation. **C,** ST-segment depression.

- Negative (inverted) T waves may also be present. T-wave inversion is significant if it is new and the T waves are ≥3 mm.
- These ECG changes, and the chest discomfort that accompanies myocardial ischemia, usually resolve when:
  - The demand for oxygen is reduced (by resting or slowing the heart rate with drugs such as beta-blockers) to a level that can be supplied by the coronary artery.
  - Blood flow is increased by dilating the coronary arteries with drugs such as NTG.
- After the episode of chest discomfort is resolved, ST-segments usually return to the baseline.

 Although typical angina produces ST-segment *depression,* Prinzmetal's angina produces ST-segment *elevation.* Because NTG is effective at relieving coronary artery spasm, the ECG evidence of Prinzmetal's angina may be lost if no baseline (pretreatment) ECG is obtained.[3]

Myocardial Injury

- Injured myocardium does not function normally because depolarization is incomplete and repolarization is impaired. Myocardial injury can be extensive enough to produce a decrease in pump function or electrical conductivity in the affected cells.
- ECG evidence of myocardial injury in progress can be seen on the ECG as ST-segment elevation in the leads facing the affected area. In leads opposite the affected area, ST-segment depression (reciprocal changes) may be seen.
- Remember that ST-segment elevation in the shape of a "smiley" face is usually benign, particularly when it occurs in an otherwise healthy, asymptomatic patient. However, the appearance of coved ST-segment elevation is called an *acute injury pattern*.
- ST-segment elevation is considered significant when it is >1 mm in two or more contiguous leads.

Throughout this text, ST-segment elevation of more than 1 mm in two contiguous leads is used as the primary criterion for infarct recognition. However, some cardiologists use a more stringent requirement for ST-segment elevation. In this alternate means of infarct recognition, at least 2 mm of ST-segment elevation is required in the chest leads before infarction is suspected. Each method has its advantage: The 1-mm threshold for ST-segment elevation favors sensitivity, and the 2-mm criteria favors specificity. Sensitivity refers to a test's ability to identify true disease. Specificity refers to a test that is correctly negative in the absence of disease. A test with high specificity has few false-positives.[3]

Myocardial Infarction

Recognition of infarction on the ECG relies on the detection of changes in the shape of the QRS complex, the T wave, and the ST-segment. These changes occur in relation to certain events during the infarction.

Non–ST-Elevation Myocardial Infarction

■ As its name implies, patients experiencing NSTEMI do not show signs of myocardial injury (ST-segment elevation) on their ECG.

■ The diagnosis of NSTEMI is made based on the patient's signs and symptoms, history, and blood test results (cardiac biomarkers) that confirm the presence of an infarction.

▶ ST-segment depression, transient ST-segment elevation, and/or T-wave inversion occur in 30% to 50% of patients with unstable angina, depending on the severity of the patient's clinical presentation.[15] Cardiac biomarkers should be obtained on initial patient presentation to rule out infarction and again in 6 hours. If biomarkers reveal evidence of myocardial necrosis, the diagnosis is NSTEMI.

■ Patients with NSTEMI are known to be at higher risk for death and reinfarction than are those with unstable angina. NSTEMIs tend to be smaller and have a better short-term prognosis than ST-elevation infarctions. However, the overall prognosis is similar to that for STEMIs.

▶ Recurrence of the infarction is common in the days to weeks after the patient has been sent home. This is referred to as "completion" of the infarction. Studies suggest that the incidence of NSTEMI is increasing as the population of older patients with more advanced disease increases.

ST-Elevation Myocardial Infarction

In the past, an MI was classified according to its location (anterior, inferior, etc.), and whether or not it produced Q waves on the ECG (Q wave versus non-Q wave MI). However, because a pathologic Q wave may take hours to develop (and in some cases, never develops), the patient's signs and symptoms, laboratory results, and the presence of ST-segment elevation provide the strongest evidence for the early recognition of MI.

Most patients with ST-segment elevation will develop Q-wave MI. Only a minority of patients with ischemic chest discomfort at rest who do not have ST-segment elevation will develop Q-wave MI.

One third of patients who experience STEMI will die within 24 hours of the onset of ischemia.[10]

ECG changes due to STEMI often occur in a predictable pattern. The ECG changes described below appear in leads looking at the area fed by the blocked vessel.[3]

■ *Hyperacute phase.* The first change you might notice in the ECG is the development of a tall T wave. Hyperacute T waves are sometimes called "tombstone" T waves. Because of their size, it is often possible to inscribe "RIP" (rest in peace) in the waveform on the ECG. Hyperacute T waves typically measure more than 50% of the preceding R wave. In addition to an increase in height, the T wave becomes more symmetric and may become pointed (Figure 6-12A). These changes are often not recorded on the ECG because they have typically resolved by the time the patient seeks medical assistance.

■ *Early acute phase.* As time progresses, ST-segment elevation may develop, indicating myocardial injury in progress (Figure 6-12B). ST-segment elevation may occur within the first hour or first few hours of infarction.

■ *Later acute phase.* In the later acute phase of the infarction, you may see the presence of T-wave inversion, suggesting the presence of ischemia (Figure 6-12C). In fact, T-wave inversion may precede the development of ST-segment elevation, or they may occur at the same time.

■ *Fully evolved phase.* A few hours later, the ECG may show the first signs that tissue death has occurred. That evidence comes with the development of abnormal (pathologic) Q waves (Figure 6-12D).

   ▶ Remember that a Q wave that is 0.04 second or more wide (one small box or more) or more than ⅓ of the amplitude of the R wave in that lead is suggestive of infarction.

   ▶ An abnormal Q wave indicates the presence of dead myocardial tissue and subsequently, a loss of electrical activity. They can appear within hours after blockage of a coronary artery but more commonly appear several hours or days after the onset of signs and symptoms of an acute MI. However, when combined with ST-segment or T-wave changes, the presence of abnormal Q waves suggests an acute MI.

■ *Healed phase.* In time, the T wave regains its normal shape and the ST-segment returns to the baseline. The Q wave, however, often remains as evidence that an infarction has occurred (Figure 6-12E). When this pattern is seen, establishing the time of the infarction is impossible. It is only possible to recognize the presence of a previous MI.

KEEPING IT SIMPLE

Q waves occur normally in some leads. To figure out whether a Q wave is physiologic or pathologic, take an imaginary cup of water and pour it over the Q wave. Physiologic Q waves are narrow and do not hold water. Pathologic Q waves are 0.04 second or more wide or more than ⅓ of the amplitude of the following R wave in that lead. Pathologic Q waves do hold water. If the Q wave looks like it would hold even a drop of water, assume that it is probably pathologic, and if you see a QS complex (a QRS complex with no R wave), think of it as a huge pathologic Q wave.[3]

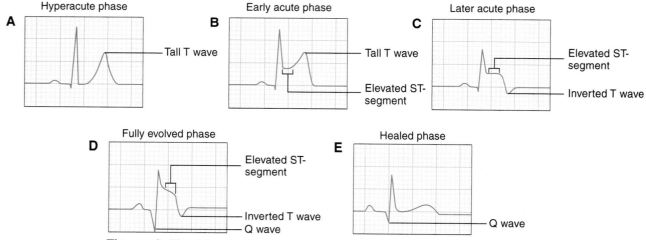

Figure 6-12 • The evolving pattern of ST-elevation myocardial infarction on the ECG.

Contiguous Leads[3]

- The ECG changes just described are called *indicative changes* of myocardial ischemia, injury, and infarction.
  - ▶ Indicative changes are significant when they are seen in at least two *contiguous* leads.
  - ▶ Two leads are contiguous if they look at the same area of the heart or if they are numerically consecutive chest leads.
- To better understand this, look at Figure 6-13 and Table 6-2. The colors in the table were added to highlight the areas of the heart viewed by the same leads. For example, leads II, III, and aVF appear the same color in the table because they view the inferior wall of the LV. Because these leads "see" the same part of the heart, they are considered contiguous leads.
  - ▶ Leads I, aVL, V_5, and V_6 are contiguous because they all look at adjoining tissue in the lateral wall of the LV.
  - ▶ Leads V_1 and V_2 are contiguous because both leads look at the septum.
  - ▶ Leads V_3 and V_4 are contiguous because both leads look at the anterior wall of the LV.
  - ▶ If right chest leads such as V_4R, V_5R, and V_6R are used, they are contiguous because they view the RV. Leads V_7, V_8, and V_9 are contiguous because they look at the posterior surface of the heart.
  - ▶ Are leads II and V_2 contiguous? No. Leads II and V_2 are not contiguous. Remember: Two leads are contiguous if they look at the same area of the heart or they are numerically consecutive *chest* leads. Lead II is a *limb* lead that looks at the inferior wall. V_2 is a *chest* lead that looks at the septum.

TABLE 6-2		Localizing ECG Changes						
I	Lateral	aVR	------------	V_1	Septum	V_4	Anterior	V_4R	Right Ventricle
II	Inferior	aVL	Lateral	V_2	Septum	V_5	Lateral	V_5R	Right Ventricle
III	Inferior	aVF	Inferior	V_3	Anterior	V_6	Lateral	V_6R	Right Ventricle

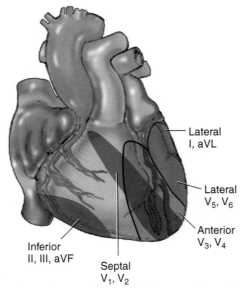

Figure 6-13 • The surfaces of the heart. The posterior surface is not shown.

■ Now look at Figure 6-14. We have already determined that V_1 and V_2 are contiguous leads. Are leads V_2 and V_3 contiguous? Yes. V_2 and V_3 are right next to each other on the patient's chest. When each of these positive electrodes "looks in" at tissue, they see adjoining tissue in the heart as well.

■ Leads V_3, V_4, and V_5 are contiguous, as well as V_4, V_5, and V_6.

 A completely normal ECG in a patient with chest pain or discomfort does not exclude the possibility of an ACS. Between 1% and 6% of such patients eventually are proved to have had an acute MI. At least 4% will be found to have unstable angina.[8]

Localization of a Myocardial Infarction

■ To recognize ECG signs of ischemia, injury, and infarction, you need to be able to recognize changes in the shape of the QRS complex, ST-segment, and T wave. To localize the site of infarction, note which leads are displaying that evidence, and consider which part of the heart those leads "see." Because an MI is the result of a blocked coronary artery, it is useful to know which arteries supply the heart. Once the infarction has been recognized and localized, an understanding of coronary artery anatomy makes it possible to predict which coronary artery is affected.[3]

■ The main coronary arteries lie on the epicardial surface of the heart. They branch into progressively smaller vessels, eventually becoming arterioles, and then capillaries. Thus, the epicardium has a rich blood supply to draw from. Branches of the main coronary arteries penetrate into the heart's muscle mass and supply the subendocardium with blood. The diameter of these "feeder branches" is much narrower. An MI often begins in the subendocardial part of the LV because this area has a high demand for oxygen and a relatively weak blood supply.[3]

▶ Another way to think about the coronary arteries that lie on the epicardial surface of the heart is to compare them with the high-pressure fire hose used by firefighters (Figure 6-15). The hose used by firefighters has multiple internal layers that can delaminate and

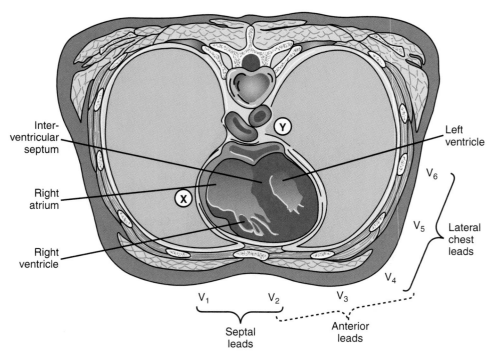

Figure 6-14 • This drawing shows the areas of the heart as seen by the chest leads. Note that neither the right ventricular wall (X) nor the posterior wall of the LV (Y) is well visualized by any of the usual six chest leads.

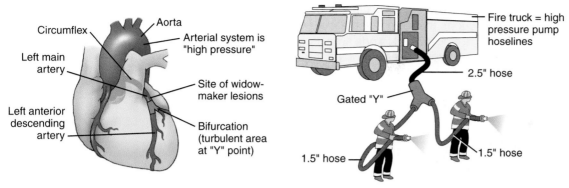

Figure 6-15 • The epicardial coronary arteries can be compared with a high-pressure hose used by firefighters.

fail, causing the fire hose to become obstructed by its own internal sheeting. This obstruction then causes the fire hose to lose water flow and pressure distal to the obstruction. This places the firefighters at the end of that hose line at great risk of injury and even death. Hence the firefighters have lost their protective hose line because of the lack of water flow.

▶ Much like coronary artery disease, the fire hose can be in the delaminating process for some time before the subsequent failure or occlusion occurs. It can fail with or without warning signs and indications, much like the setting of an ACS.[3]

KEEPING IT SIMPLE

In the standard 12-lead ECG, leads II, III, and aVF "look" at tissue supplied by the right coronary artery (RCA). Eight leads "look" at tissue supplied by the left coronary artery (LCA): leads I, aVL, $V_1, V_2, V_3, V_4, V_5,$ and V_6. When evaluating the extent of infarction produced by an LCA occlusion, decide how many of these leads are showing indicative changes. The more of these eight leads that show indicative changes, the larger the infarction is presumed to be.[3]

■ The LV has been divided into regions where an MI may occur—septal, anterior, lateral, inferior, and posterior.

■ If an ECG shows changes in leads II, III, and aVF, the inferior wall is affected. Because the inferior wall of the LV is supplied by the right coronary artery (RCA) in most people, it is reasonable to suppose that these ECG changes are due to partial or complete blockage of the RCA.

■ When indicative changes are seen in the leads viewing the septal, anterior, and/or lateral walls of the LV (V_1-V_6, I, and aVL), it is reasonable to suspect that these ECG changes are due to partial or complete blockage of the left coronary artery (LCA).[3]

▶ One way to gauge the relative extent or size of an infarction is to evaluate how many leads are showing indicative changes. An ECG showing changes in only a few leads suggests a smaller infarction than one that produces changes in many leads. In general, the more proximal the blockage in the vessel, the larger the infarction and the greater the number of leads showing indicative changes.[3]

■ Although ECG localization of the infarct site is possible, it is not perfect.

▶ For example, what appears to be a lateral wall infarction on the ECG may actually be an anterior wall infarction. This can occur with any location of infarction and is due to the fact that the ECG is simply a measurement of current flow on the patient's skin. Factors including anatomic variations, patient position, and other underlying conditions may affect the perceived infarct location versus the actual location. The patient's unique pattern of coronary artery distribution can also affect the location of infarct and so can the presence of collateral circulation. For these reasons, you may occasionally encounter infarctions that are difficult to localize into the previously mentioned areas.[3]

◾ An MI may not be limited to one area. For example, if the chest leads indicate ECG changes in leads V_3 and V_4 (suggestive of an anterior wall MI) and indicative changes are also present in V_5 and V_6, the infarction would be called an anterolateral infarction or an anterior infarction with lateral extension.[3] Table 6-3 summarizes the pattern in which coronary arteries most commonly supply the myocardium.

TABLE 6-3	Localization of a Myocardial Infarction		
Location of Myocardial Infarction	Indicative Changes (Leads Facing Affected Area)	Reciprocal Changes (Leads Opposite Affected Area)	Affected Coronary Artery
Anterior	V_3, V_4	V_7, V_8, V_9	LCA • LAD: diagonal branch
Anteroseptal	V_1, V_2, V_3, V_4	V_7, V_8, V_9	LCA • LAD: diagonal branch • LAD: septal branch
Anterolateral	I, aVL, V_3, V_4, V_5, V_6	II, III, aVF, V_7, V_8, V_9	LCA • LAD: diagonal branch and/or • Circumflex branch
Inferior	II, III, aVF	I, aVL	RCA (most common) posterior descending branch or LCA—circumflex branch
Lateral	I, aVL, V_5, V_6	II, III, aVF	LCA • LAD: diagonal branch and/or • Circumflex branch RCA
Septum	V_1, V_2	V_7, V_8, V_9	LCA • LAD: septal branch
Posterior	V_7, V_8, V_9	V_1, V_2, V_3	RCA or left circumflex artery
RV	V_1R-V_6R	I, aVL	RCA • Proximal branches

LAD, Left anterior descending.

Quick Review 6-5

1. ST-segment depression is considered significant if the ST-segment is _____ mm below the baseline.
2. When are two ECG leads considered contiguous?

3. ECG evidence of myocardial injury in progress can be seen on the ECG as ST-segment _____ in the leads facing the affected area.
4. In a standard 12-lead ECG, how many leads look at tissue supplied by the RCA?

Anterior Wall

◾ Leads V_3 and V_4 face the anterior wall of the LV. The left main coronary artery supplies the left anterior descending (LAD) artery and the circumflex artery. A blockage in the left main coronary artery (the "widow maker") often leads to cardiogenic shock and death without prompt reperfusion.
◾ Blockage of the midportion of the LAD results in an anterior infarction (Figure 6-16). However, an infarction involving the anterior wall is usually not localized only to this area. For example, proximal occlusion of the LAD may become an anteroseptal infarction if the septal branch is involved or an anterolateral infarction if the marginal branch is involved.

■ If the blockage occurs proximal to both the septal and diagonal branches, an extensive anterior infarction (anteroseptal-lateral MI) will result. An example of an infarction involving the anterior wall is shown in Figure 6-17.

■ Because the LAD artery supplies about 40% of the heart's blood and a critical section of the LV, blockage of this vessel can lead to complications including heart failure and cardiogenic shock. Sympathetic hyperactivity is common, with resulting sinus tachycardia and/or hypertension. An anterior wall MI may cause other dysrhythmias including premature ventricular complexes (PVCs), atrial flutter, or atrial fibrillation (AFib). Because the bundle branches travel through this area, bundle branch blocks (BBBs) may also result from injury in this area.

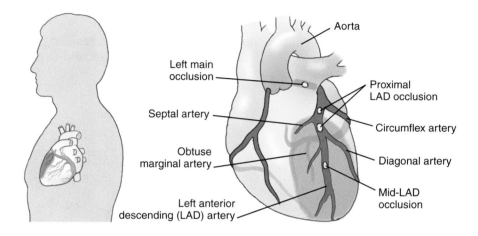

I Lateral	aVR	V₁ Septum	V₄ Anterior
II Inferior	aVL Lateral	V₂ Septum	V₅ Lateral
III Inferior	aVF Inferior	V₃ Anterior	V₆ Lateral

Figure 6-16 • Anterior wall infarction. Blockage of the middle area of the LAD artery results in an anterior infarction. Proximal blockage of the LAD may become an anteroseptal infarction if the septal branch is involved or an anterolateral infarction if the marginal branch is involved. If the blockage occurs proximal to both the septal and diagonal branches, an extensive anterior infarction (anteroseptal-lateral MI) will result.

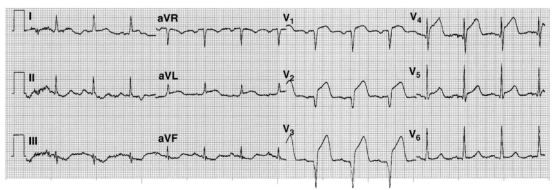

Figure 6-17 • Extensive anterior infarction.

Inferior Wall

- ■ Leads II, III, and aVF view the inferior surface of the LV. In most individuals, the inferior wall of the LV is supplied by the posterior descending branch of the RCA (Figure 6-18). In most individuals, the inferior wall of the LV is supplied by the posterior descending branch of the RCA ("right dominant system"). Blockage of the RCA proximal to the marginal branch will result in an inferior wall MI and RVI. Blockage of the RCA distal to the marginal branch will result in an inferior infarction, sparing the RV.

- ■ In some individuals, the circumflex artery supplies the inferior wall through the posterior descending artery ("left dominant system") (Figure 6-19). Blockage of the posterior descending artery will result in an inferior infarction; however, a proximal occlusion of the circumflex may result in infarction in the lateral and posterior walls. An example of an inferior wall infarction is shown in Figure 6-20.

- ■ Parasympathetic hyperactivity is common with inferior wall MIs, resulting in bradydysrhythmias. Conduction delays such as first-degree AV block and second-degree AV block type I are common and usually transient.

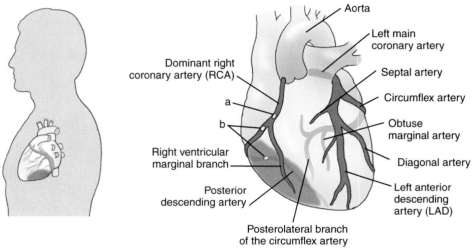

Figure 6-18 • Inferior wall infarction. Coronary anatomy shows a dominant RCA. A blockage at point "A" results in an inferior infarction and an RVI. A blockage at point "B" involves only the inferior wall.

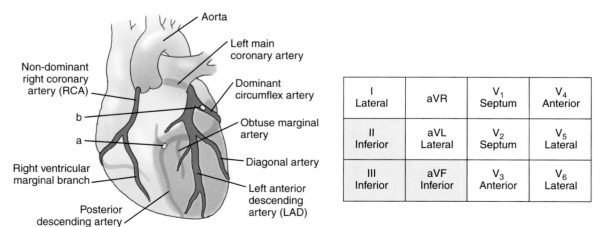

I Lateral	aVR	V$_1$ Septum	V$_4$ Anterior
II Inferior	aVL Lateral	V$_2$ Septum	V$_5$ Lateral
III Inferior	aVF Inferior	V$_3$ Anterior	V$_6$ Lateral

Figure 6-19 • Inferior wall infarction. Coronary anatomy shows a dominant left circumflex artery. Blockage at point "A" results in an inferior infarction. A blockage at "B" may result in a lateral and posterior wall infarction.

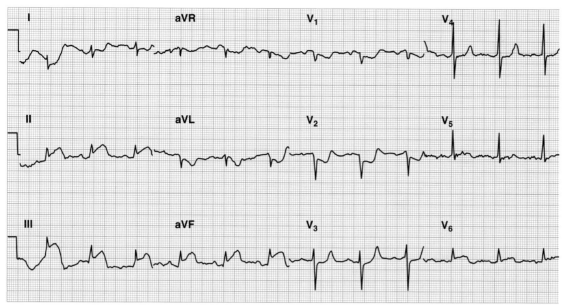

Figure 6-20 • Inferior wall infarction. Reciprocal changes are present in leads I and aVL.

Lateral Wall

■ Leads I, aVL, V$_5$, and V$_6$ view the lateral wall of the LV. The lateral wall of the LV may be supplied by the left circumflex artery, the LAD artery, or a branch of the RCA (Figure 6-21).

■ Lateral wall infarctions often occur as extensions of anterior or inferior infarctions. Isolated lateral wall infarctions usually involve occlusion of the circumflex artery and are frequently missed. More commonly, the lateral wall is involved with proximal occlusion of the LAD artery (anterolateral MI) or a branch of the RCA (inferolateral MI).

■ Blockage of the marginal branches of the circumflex artery may cause a posterolateral MI. An example of an infarction involving the lateral wall is shown in Figure 6-22.

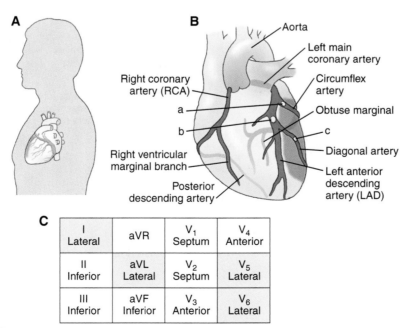

I Lateral	aVR	V$_1$ Septum	V$_4$ Anterior
II Inferior	aVL Lateral	V$_2$ Septum	V$_5$ Lateral
III Inferior	aVF Inferior	V$_3$ Anterior	V$_6$ Lateral

Figure 6-21 • Lateral wall infarction. Coronary artery anatomy shows the following: **A,** Blockage of the circumflex artery, **B,** Blockage of the proximal LAD artery, and **C,** Blockage of the diagonal artery.

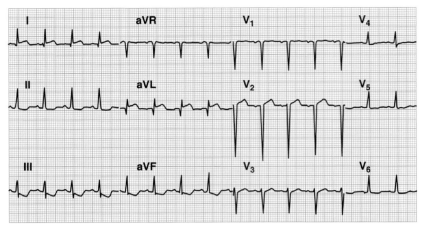

Figure 6-22 • Lateral wall infarction. Lead I shows a small Q wave with ST-segment elevation. A larger Q wave with ST-segment elevation can be seen in lead aVL. This patient had an anterior NSTEMI 4 days earlier with ST-segment elevation and T-wave inversion in leads V_2 through V_6. A coronary arteriogram at that time showed a blocked LAD artery distal to its first large septal perforator. The ST-segment elevation evolved and the T waves in all of the chest leads had become upright the day before this tracing was recorded. The patient then had another episode of chest pain associated with the appearance of signs of acute lateral infarction as shown in this tracing. A repeat coronary arteriogram showed new blockage of the obtuse marginal branch of the left circumflex artery.

Septum

▣ Leads V_1 and V_2 face the septal area of the LV. The septum, which contains the bundle of His and bundle branches, is normally supplied by the LAD artery (Figure 6-23). A blockage in this area may result in right BBB, left BBB (more common), second-degree AV block type II, and third-degree AV block.

▣ If the site of infarction is limited to the septum, ECG changes are seen in V_1 and V_2. If the entire anterior wall is involved, ECG changes will be visible in V_1, V_2, V_3, and V_4. An example of a septal infarction is shown in Figure 6-24.

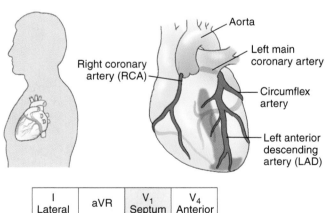

I Lateral	aVR	V_1 Septum	V_4 Anterior
II Inferior	aVL Lateral	V_2 Septum	V_5 Lateral
III Inferior	aVF Inferior	V_3 Anterior	V_6 Lateral

Figure 6-23 • Septal infarction.

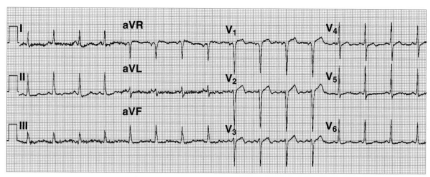

Figure 6-24 • Septal infarction.

Posterior Wall

■ Posterior wall MIs usually occur in conjunction with an inferior or lateral infarction. The posterior wall of the LV is supplied by the left circumflex coronary artery in most patients; however, in some patients it is supplied by the RCA (Figure 6-25). If the posterior wall is supplied by the RCA, complications may include dysrhythmias involving the sinoatrial (SA) node, AV node, and bundle of His.

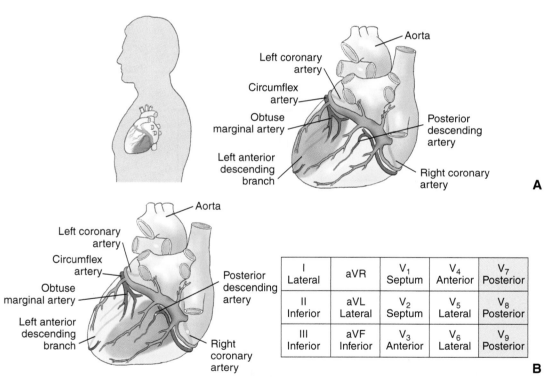

I Lateral	aVR	V₁ Septum	V₄ Anterior	V₇ Posterior
II Inferior	aVL Lateral	V₂ Septum	V₅ Lateral	V₈ Posterior
III Inferior	aVF Inferior	V₃ Anterior	V₆ Lateral	V₉ Posterior

Figure 6-25 • Posterior infarction. **A,** Coronary anatomy shows a dominant RCA. Blockage of the RCA commonly results in an inferior and posterior infarction. **B,** Coronary anatomy shows a dominant left circumflex artery. Blockage of a marginal branch is the cause of most isolated posterior infarctions.

- Because no leads of a standard 12-lead ECG directly view the posterior wall of the LV, additional chest leads should be used to view the heart's posterior surface. Changes indicative of a posterior wall infarction include ST-segment elevation in these leads.
- If placement of posterior chest leads is not feasible, changes in the opposite (anterior) wall of the heart can be viewed as reciprocal changes. A posterior wall MI usually produces tall R waves and ST-segment depression in leads V_1, V_2, and to a lesser extent in lead V_3. To assist in the recognition of ECG changes suggesting a posterior wall MI, the "mirror test" is helpful (Figure 6-26). Flip over the ECG to the blank side and turn it upside down. When held up to the light, the tall R waves become deep Q waves and ST-segment depression becomes ST-segment elevation—the "classic" indicative changes associated with MI.

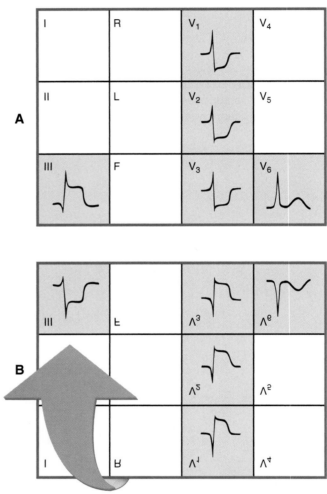

Figure 6-26 • The "mirror test." This test is helpful when assessing the ECG of a patient with an acute inferior infarction in whom you suspect an acute posterior infarction. **A,** This schematic 12-lead ECG shows changes indicative of inferior infarction in lead III. Note the tall R wave in lead V_1 and the ST-segment depression in leads V_1, V_2, and V_3. **B,** To check for a possible posterior infarction, flip the tracing over. Looking through the paper (as it is held up to the light), you now see Q waves and ST-segment elevation in leads V_1, V_2, and V_3. This is a positive mirror test and suggests that the lead changes observed in A may reflect an associated acute posterior infarction.

Right Ventricle

■ Suspect an RVI when ECG changes suggesting an inferior infarction (ST-segment elevation in leads II, III, and/or aVF) are seen. About 50% of patients with inferior infarction have some involvement of the RV.

■ The RV is supplied by the right ventricular marginal branch of the RCA (Figure 6-27). A blockage of the right ventricular marginal branch results in an isolated RVI. Blockage of the RCA proximal to the right ventricular marginal branch results in an inferior infarction and an RVI.

■ To view the RV, right chest leads are used. Placement of right chest leads is identical to placement of the standard chest leads except on the right side of the chest. These leads then "look" directly at the RV and can show the ST-segment elevation created by the infarct. If time does not permit obtaining all six right-sided chest leads, the lead of choice is V₄R. An example of an infarction involving the RV is shown in Figure 6-28.

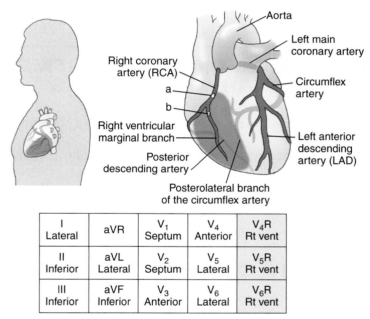

I Lateral	aVR	V₁ Septum	V₄ Anterior	V₄R Rt vent
II Inferior	aVL Lateral	V₂ Septum	V₅ Lateral	V₅R Rt vent
III Inferior	aVF Inferior	V₃ Anterior	V₆ Lateral	V₆R Rt vent

Figure 6-27 • RVI. At a, blockage of the RCA proximal to the right ventricular marginal branch results in an inferior and RVI. At b, blockage of the right ventricular marginal branch results in an isolated RVI.

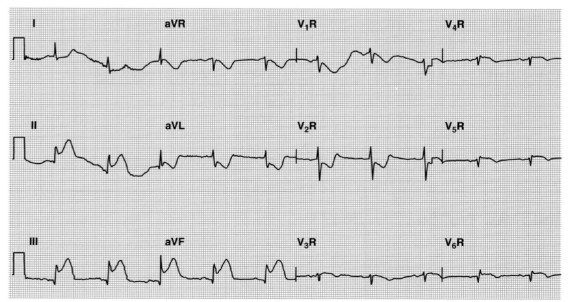

Figure 6-28 • Inferior wall MI and RVI.

▶ Complications associated with RVI include hypotension, cardiogenic shock, AV blocks, atrial flutter or fibrillation, and premature atrial complexes. AV blocks are particularly common, occurring in about ½ of patients with RVI.

QUICK REVIEW 6-6

1. ST-segment elevation is considered significant when the ST-segment is more than ___ mm above the baseline to the right of the J-point.
2. How is death of myocardial tissue recognized on the ECG?

3. True or False. Myocardial ischemia prolonged more than just a few minutes often results in myocardial injury.

INITIAL MANAGEMENT OF ACUTE CORONARY SYNDROMES

GOALS IN THE IMMEDIATE MANAGEMENT OF ACUTE CORONARY SYNDROMES

According to the American Heart Association, the primary goals of therapy for patients with ACS include the following:[16]

■ Reduce the amount of myocardial necrosis that occurs in patients with MI, preserving left ventricular function and preventing heart failure

■ Prevent major adverse cardiac events (MACEs): death, nonfatal MI, and need for urgent revascularization

■ Treat acute, life-threatening complications of ACS, such as ventricular fibrillation (VF)/pulseless ventricular tachycardia (VT), symptomatic bradycardias, and unstable tachycardias

POSSIBLE ACUTE CORONARY SYNDROME

■ A *possible* acute coronary syndrome has been defined as the following:[12]
  ▶ Recent episode of chest discomfort at rest not entirely typical of ischemia but pain free at time of initial evaluation
  ▶ Normal or unchanged ECG
  ▶ No cardiac biomarker elevation
■ Patients experiencing a possible ACS are managed by either observation in the ED chest pain unit or admittance to a monitored hospital bed.

DEFINITE ACUTE CORONARY SYNDROME

■ A *definite* ACS is a recent episode of typical ischemic discomfort that is either of new onset or severe or exhibits an accelerating pattern of previous stable angina (especially if it occurred at rest or within 2 weeks of a previously documented MI).
■ Triage of these patients is based on their 12-lead ECG.
   The diagnosis of an ACS is made based on the patient's history, signs and symptoms, risk factors, 12-lead ECG, cardiac biomarkers, and other diagnostic tests.

INITIAL MANAGEMENT

Although only a physician can make a final diagnosis of an ACS, an ACLS provider must take responsibility for recognizing infarction and take steps to speed the process of data collection, physician evaluation, and, when appropriate, reperfusion therapy. The reality of this expectation is that nurses, paramedics, and all other cardiac care providers must be able to develop a "working diagnosis" of infarction. Although this working diagnosis must be confirmed by a physician before definitive treatment may begin, it has been clearly demonstrated that early recognition of infarction by a nonphysician can greatly reduce the time to treatment.[3]

Once a working diagnosis of infarction has been made, strategies for reducing time to treatment vary with the setting. Paramedics should obtain a 12-lead ECG in all situations involving a patient with a possible ACS. The 12-lead should be transmitted (or the paramedic's interpretation of it should be relayed) to the receiving facility as soon as possible to reduce time to reperfusion. Paramedics should routinely use a focused checklist (developed in conjunction with the receiving facility) to assist in the identification of patients eligible for reperfusion therapy. Prehospital identification of such patients has been shown to be accurate.[17] The preferences of the receiving facility and system protocols determine which preparatory steps are appropriate. In general, aspirin is given, additional intravenous (IV) lines are established, and medications are given for pain control.

In the ED, nurses should have immediate access to a 12-lead ECG monitor. When the 12-lead shows evidence of infarction or causes the nurse to suspect infarction, the tracing should be brought to the attention of a physician immediately. Much of the routine laboratory work should be made a standing order so that the nursing staff can begin to collect data for physician review. This process allows the nurse to identify patients with a high likelihood of infarction and quickly gather the data necessary for physician review.[3]

The initial management of all ACSs is generally the same, and management of the patient must be done efficiently. If the patient has an STEMI, time targets for reperfusion are to give fibrinolytics within 30 minutes of arrival ("door-to-drug") or provide primary angioplasty within 90 minutes of arrival ("door-to-balloon inflation").[18]

If patient findings are consistent with a possible or definite ACS, the following interventions (including obtaining and reviewing a 12-lead ECG) should be performed within 10 minutes of patient contact (prehospital) or arrival in the ED. The American Heart Association's recommendations for the initial treatment of ACSs are summarized in Figure 6-29.[19]

Targeted History and Physical Exam

Obtain a targeted history and physical exam. This can be done at the same time as other procedures. For example, questions can be asked of the patient while obtaining vital signs and attaching the pulse oximeter and ECG. The reperfusion checklist begun in the prehospital setting should be continued and completed on the patient's arrival in the ED.

Determine the patient's age, gender, signs and symptoms (including location of pain, duration, quality, relation to effort, and time of symptom onset), history of CAD, and presence of CAD risk factors. Assess the degree of the patient's pain/discomfort using a 0 to 10 scale. Consider the possibility of other potentially lethal conditions that mimic acute MI such as aortic dissection, acute pericarditis, acute myocarditis, and pulmonary embolism.

Several factors contribute to the efficacy of reperfusion therapy, but probably the most significant is the duration from symptom onset to treatment. The benefits of reperfusion therapy are often time dependent. Remember: *time is muscle*. Time of symptom onset is defined as the beginning of continuous, persistent discomfort that prompted the patient to seek medical attention. In canine studies, it has been estimated that 50% of tissue loss occurs within 2 hours of coronary occlusion. Tissue death may be noted as early as the first 20 minutes of infarction, and studies estimate that about 90% of tissue loss occurs within the first 6 hours. Therefore, if myocardium is to be saved, the blockage must be eliminated before irreversible tissue death occurs. The results from fibrinolytic trials suggest that a similar pattern occurs in humans. Very early treatment provides the greatest reduction in mortality.[3]

Assess the patient's vital signs and determine oxygen saturation. Give oxygen, establish IV access, and place the patient on a cardiac monitor if not already done. Give aspirin 160 to 325 mg (chewed) if there are no contraindications.

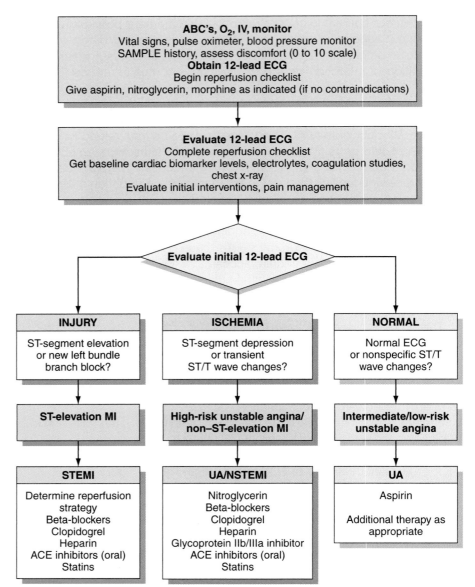

Figure 6-29 • Ischemic chest discomfort algorithm.

12-Lead Electrocardiogram

Obtaining and reviewing a 12-lead ECG is an important component of the initial assessment of the patient presenting with ischemic chest discomfort. Obtain the first 12-lead ECG with 10 minutes of patient contact or the patient's arrival in the ED. Repeat with each set of vital signs, when the patient's symptoms change, and as often as necessary.

When prehospital care professionals have the ability to perform 12-lead ECGs, the door-to-drug or door-to-primary angioplasty, time begins on arrival of the EMS providers. This can decrease the door-to-reperfusion therapy time on arrival at the ED. Prehospital use of a 12-lead ECG has led to substantially higher use of reperfusion therapy with either fibrinolysis or primary angioplasty.[20] Unfortunately, the prehospital 12-lead ECG is underused nationally. It should be incorporated into any EMS system where feasible.[21]

 BBB, left ventricular hypertrophy, an idioventricular rhythm, or a paced rhythm may make the ECG signs of ischemia or injury difficult or impossible to interpret.

Once the 12-lead has been obtained, it should be reviewed carefully. Look at each lead for the presence of ST-segment displacement (elevation or depression). If ST-segment elevation is present, note its elevation in millimeters. Examine the T waves for any changes in orientation, shape, and size. Examine each lead for the presence of a Q wave. If a Q wave is present, measure its duration. Assess the areas of ischemia or injury by assessing lead groupings. Remember: ECG evidence must be found in at least two contiguous leads. Based on the 12-lead ECG findings, categorize the patient into one of three groups:

1. *ST-segment elevation.* ST-segment elevation >1 mm in two or more contiguous leads or new-onset left BBB suggests myocardial injury. This patient is classified as ST-elevation MI. Patients with obvious ST-segment elevation in leads II, III, and/or aVF should also be evaluated for possible right ventricular MI.

2. *ST-segment depression.* ST-segment depression ≥0.5 mm or transient ST-segment/ T-wave changes that occur with pain or discomfort suggest myocardial ischemia. This patient is classified as high-risk unstable angina/non-ST-elevation MI. Patients with obvious ST-segment depression should be evaluated for possible posterior MI.

3. *Normal/nondiagnostic ECG.* A normal ECG or nonspecific ST- and T-wave changes are nondiagnostic and require further evaluation. This patient is classified as intermediate/ low-risk unstable angina. Patients with normal ECGs, nonspecific ST- and T-wave changes, or ST-segment depression have a much lower likelihood of total coronary occlusion and do not benefit from, and may in fact be harmed by, fibrinolysis. Obtain serial ECGs (ECGs every 5 to 10 minutes) in patients with a history suggesting an ACS and a nondiagnostic ECG.[10]

An absence of signs of ischemia, injury, or infarction on an ECG or in early laboratory data does not exclude the possibility of an ACS.

QUICK REVIEW 6-7

1. What are the goals in the management of an ACS?

2. True or False. A 56-year-old man presents with chest discomfort that has been present for 90 minutes. The 12-lead ECG shows nonspecific ST-segment and T-wave changes. Based on this information, this patient is a candidate for reperfusion therapy.
3. The 12-lead ECG plays a central role in the management of a patient with an ACS. When the patient's initial 12-lead is obtained, the ECG should be carefully reviewed and then the patient should be categorized into one of three groups, based on the 12-lead findings. What are the three groups?
    1.
    2.
    3.

Cardiac Biomarkers

▪ Obtain baseline cardiac biomarker levels, other laboratory studies including a CBC, lipid profile, coagulation studies, and electrolytes. Obtain a portable chest x-ray, preferably upright.

- ▶ As myocardial cells die, intracellular substances pass through broken cell membranes and leak substances into the bloodstream. The presence of these substances in the blood can subsequently be measured by means of blood tests to verify the presence of an infarction. These substances (called cardiac biomarkers, serum cardiac markers, or inflammatory markers) include creatine kinase (CK), creatine kinase myocardial band (CK-MB), myoglobin, troponin I (TnI), and troponin T (TnT).
- ▶ Cardiac biomarkers are useful for confirming the diagnosis of MI when patients present without ST-segment elevation, when the diagnosis may be unclear, and to distinguish patients with unstable angina from those with NSTEMI. Cardiac biomarkers are also useful for confirming the diagnosis of MI for patients with STEMI. Because there is no tissue death, there is no cardiac biomarker release in stable or unstable angina.
- ▶ Treatment decisions and reperfusion therapy for patients with STEMI should not be delayed pending cardiac biomarker test results. Studies have shown that the delay in release of biomarkers from damaged myocardium makes these tests insensitive for ruling out the diagnosis of STEMI or NSTEMI in the first 4 to 6 hours of onset of symptoms.[22]

"As many as 2-10% of patients sent home after an initial evaluation in the ED or urgent care for suspected cardiac ischemia will have an unexpected MI. Misinterpretation of the ECG is the main reason for an incorrect discharge in approximately 25% of such cases, although automatic ECG interpretation has improved this process. Among patients who are discharged home with an unrecognized MI, as many as 25% subsequently die."[21]

Routine Measures

- ▪ Oxygen
  - ▶ Give oxygen to all patients with obvious pulmonary congestion or arterial oxygen saturation <90% (Class I).
  - ▶ Reasonable to give supplemental oxygen to all patients with ACS for the first 6 hours of therapy (Class IIa).
- ▪ Aspirin
  - ▶ Give 160 to 325 mg of nonenteric aspirin as soon as possible after symptom onset, if there are no contraindications.
    - • Chewable aspirin allows for quicker absorption.
    - • Aspirin can rival fibrinolytic therapy in its impact on mortality reduction. It is effective, inexpensive, available, and produces few side effects.
    - • Flavored chewable aspirin may be better accepted by the patient over standard aspirin tablets.
- ▪ Nitroglycerin
  - ▶ NTG relaxes vascular smooth muscle, including dilation of the coronary arteries (particularly in the area of plaque disruption). It also decreases myocardial oxygen consumption.
  - ▶ Before giving NTG, make sure an IV is in place, the patient's systolic blood pressure (SBP) is >90 mm Hg, the patient's heart rate is >50 and <100 beats per min (bpm), there are no signs of RVI, and the patient has not used Viagra, Cialis, or similar medication in the previous 24 to 48 hours.
  - ▶ NTG sublingual (SL) tablets or spray may be given at 5-minute intervals to a maximum of 3 doses.
  - ▶ Consider the presence of RVI if the patient with an inferior wall infarction becomes hypotensive after administration of nitrates.
- ▪ Morphine
  - ▶ Morphine is the drug of choice to relieve pain associated with ACSs. It decreases anxiety, pain, and myocardial oxygen requirements.
  - ▶ Give morphine 2 to 4 mg (give in 2 mg increments) slow IV push. Give additional doses of 2 to 8 mg IV at 5- to 15-minute intervals.[23]
  - ▶ Several doses may be required for adequate pain relief.

KEEPING IT SIMPLE

MONA

MONA is a memory aid that may be used to recall medications used in the management of ACSs (but not in the order they are given).

M = Morphine
O = Oxygen
N = Nitroglycerin
A = Aspirin

Relief of pain is a priority in the management of a patient experiencing an ACS. Relief of pain decreases anxiety, myocardial oxygen demand, and the risk of cardiac dysrhythmias. When treating a patient with an ACS, it is not enough to simply reduce the patient's degree of pain or discomfort. The goal is to ensure that the patient is pain free, while closely monitoring his or her vital signs.

Initial Management of ST-Elevation Myocardial Infarction

■ Reperfusion therapy is the mainstay of treatment for STEMI. Because STEMI is usually the result of a blocked coronary artery, the blockage may be removed by giving fibrinolytics (pharmacologic reperfusion) or primary PCI (mechanical reperfusion) (Box 6-4).

  ▸ Fibrinolytic therapy is considered a Class I intervention for patients who have an onset of symptoms ≤12 hours, ST-segment elevation >1 mm in two or more contiguous leads (or BBB [obscuring ST-segment analysis]) and a history suggesting acute MI.

  ▸ If no contraindications exist, fibrinolytics may also be given to patients who have an onset of symptoms within 12 hours and findings of a true posterior MI on their ECG.

  ▸ Fibrinolytics are generally not recommended for patients presenting more than 12 hours after symptom onset. They should not be given to patients who present >24 hours after the onset of symptoms or to patients who show ST-segment depression (unless a true posterior MI is suspected).[23]

Patients routinely taking nonsteroidal anti-inflammatory drugs (except for aspirin), before STEMI should have those agents discontinued at the time of presentation with STEMI because of the increased risk of mortality, reinfarction, hypertension, heart failure, and myocardial rupture associated with their use.[24]

BOX 6-4

Reperfusion Therapy—Fibrinolytics or Percutaneous Coronary Intervention?

Fibrinolysis is generally preferred if
- Patient presents ≤3 hours from symptom onset.
- Invasive strategy is not an option (catheterization lab occupied/not available, vascular access difficulties, lack of access to skilled PCI facility).
- Invasive strategy would be delayed (prolonged transport, medical contact-to-balloon or door-balloon >90 min, [door-to-balloon] minus [door-to-needle] is >1 hr).
- No contraindications to fibrinolysis.

An invasive strategy is generally preferred if
- Patient presents >3 hours from symptom onset.
- Diagnosis of STEMI is in doubt.
- Skilled PCI facility available with surgical backup (medical contact-to-balloon or door-balloon <90 min, (door-to-balloon) minus (door-to-needle) is <1 hour.
- Contraindications to fibrinolysis, including increased risk of bleeding and intracranial hemorrhage.
- High risk from STEMI (such as congestive heart failure [CHF]).

If presentation <3 hours and no delay for PCI, then no preference for either strategy.
From Antman EM, Anbe DT, Armstrong PW, et al: www.acc.org/clinical/guidelines/stemi/index.pdf; 2005 American Heart Association Guidelines for cardiopulmonary resuscitation and emergency cardiovascular care, part 8. *Circulation* 2005;112(suppl IV):IV-95.

▶ According to the American Heart Association, prehospital "administration of fibrinolytics to patients with STEMI with no contraindications is safe, feasible, and reasonable. This intervention may be performed by trained paramedics, nurses, and physicians for patients with symptom duration of 30 minutes to 6 hours. System requirements include protocols with fibrinolytic checklists, ECG acquisition and interpretation, experience in ACLS, the ability to communicate with the receiving institution, and a medical director with training/experience in management of STEMI. A process of continuous quality improvement is required. Given the operational challenges required to provide out-of-hospital fibrinolytics, most EMS systems should focus on early diagnosis with 12-lead ECGs, rapid transport, and advance notification of the ED (verbal interpretation or direct transmission of ECG) instead of out-of-hospital delivery of fibrinolysis."[25]

▶ A primary PCI refers to angioplasty that is performed as a primary reperfusion strategy without prior fibrinolytic therapy. By removing the blockage, perfusion should be restored and myocardial tissue salvaged.

   • PCI is recommended as an alternative to fibrinolysis for STEMI if balloon inflation can be performed within 90 minutes in centers with experience and an appropriate laboratory environment. PCI is preferred for patients with a symptom duration of >3 and ≤12 hours. It may also be performed in patients who have an acute MI complicated by cardiogenic shock or heart failure. PCI should be considered as a reperfusion strategy in candidates for reperfusion who have a contraindication to fibrinolytic therapy.

▶ Reperfusion goals: door-to-drug time within 30 minutes or door-to-balloon inflation time within 90 minutes. Use a reperfusion checklist to evaluate the patient's candidacy for reperfusion therapy.

 During fibrinolytic therapy, monitor the ECG and the patient's vital signs closely. Watch for reperfusion dysrhythmias as blood flow is reestablished through the infarct-related artery. Reocclusion may occur. Watch for ST-segment changes, dysrhythmias, and hypotension, and question the patient about chest discomfort.

■ Patients with STEMI should receive:

   ▶ Aspirin 160 to 325 mg (chewed and swallowed) if not already taken by the patient (and no contraindications).

   ▶ Beta-blockers (if no contraindications).

      • Oral beta-blocker therapy should be started in the first 24 hours for patients who do not have any of the following: 1) signs of heart failure, 2) evidence of a low output state, 3) increased risk for cardiogenic shock (age greater than 70 years, systolic blood pressure less than 120 mm Hg, sinus tachycardia greater than 110 bpm or heart rate less than 60 bpm, and increased time since onset of symptoms of STEMI), or 4) other relative contraindications to beta blockade (PR interval greater than 0.24 seconds, second- or third-degree AV block, active asthma, or reactive airway disease).[24]

   ▶ Heparin[26]

      • Unfractionated heparin (UFH) recommended for patients 75 years of age or older as additional therapy to fibrinolysis (Class IIa) and for any STEMI patient who is undergoing revascularization.

      • In STEMI patients who are not receiving fibrinolytic therapy or revascularization, low molecular weight heparin (LMWH) (specifically enoxaparin) may be considered an acceptable alternative to UFH in the ED setting.

   ▶ Glycoprotein IIb/IIIa inhibitors—insufficient evidence to recommend for or against use in STEMI.

   ▶ Oral angiotensin-converting enzyme (ACE) inhibitor therapy is recommended within first 24 hours after onset of symptoms in STEMI patients with pulmonary congestion or left ventricular ejection fraction <40%, in the absence of hypotension (SBP <100 mm Hg or more than 30 mm Hg below baseline) (Class I). Oral ACE inhibitor therapy can also be recommended for all other patients with acute MI with or without early reperfusion therapy (Class IIa).[27]

▶ Early therapy (within 24 hours of patient presentation) with HMG Coenzyme A reductase inhibitors (statins) is feasible in patients with an ACS or acute MI (Class I).[27] If the patient is already on statin therapy, therapy should be continued.

▶ Clopidogrel 75 mg per day orally should be added to aspirin in patients with STEMI regardless of whether they undergo reperfusion with fibrinolytic therapy or do not receive reperfusion therapy. Treatment with clopidogrel should continue for at least 14 days. In patients taking clopidogrel in whom CABG is planned, the drug should be withheld for at least 5 days and preferably for 7 days unless the urgency for revascularization outweighs the risks of excess bleeding.

Because of the risk of hypotension, IV administration of ACE inhibitors is contraindicated in the first 24 hours of STEMI.

Initial Management of Unstable Angina/Non–ST-Segment Elevation Myocardial Infarction

■ Patients with unstable angina/NSTEMI (and no contraindications) should receive:
  ▶ Oxygen, IV access, continuous ECG monitoring.
  ▶ Aspirin 160 to 325 mg (chewed and swallowed) if not already taken by the patient (and no contraindications).
  ▶ Beta-blockers if the patient is not already taking beta-blockers or is inadequately treated on current dose of beta-blocker (if no contraindications).
  ▶ NTG SL tablet or spray, followed by IV NTG if symptoms persist despite SL NTG therapy and beta-blocker therapy, and if SBP is >90 mm Hg.
  ▶ Morphine 2 to 4 mg IV if discomfort is not relieved or symptoms recur despite NTG therapy. Make sure the patient's SBP is >90 mm Hg.
  ▶ Clopidogrel, heparin, glycoprotein IIb/IIIa inhibitors.
■ Patients who present with a high or intermediate likelihood of ischemia are admitted to the hospital and treated for unstable angina/NSTEMI.

Initial Management of Patients with a Suspected Acute Coronary Syndrome and a Nondiagnostic/Normal Electrocardiogram

■ The ECG is nondiagnostic in about 50% of patients with chest discomfort. A normal ECG does not rule out an acute MI, particularly in the early hours of a coronary artery occlusion.
■ Nondiagnostic ECGs are more common in the elderly and patients with previous MI.
■ Give aspirin and other therapy as appropriate (such as beta-blockers and NTG).
■ Patients who present with a low likelihood of ischemia are initially managed in the ED chest pain unit and then managed as outpatients with detailed evaluation within 72 hours.

QUICK REVIEW 6-8

1. Why is pain relief a high priority in the management of an ACS?

2. Fibrinolytic therapy is recommended for patients who have ST-segment _____ in two or more contiguous leads, a history suggesting acute MI, and time from symptom onset to therapy that is _____ hours.

3. Which leads on a standard 12-lead ECG should be viewed for changes when identifying an inferior wall MI?

4. Patients who experience a(n) _____ MI have a greater incidence of heart failure and cardiogenic shock than those who have MIs affecting other areas of the LV.

COMPLICATIONS OF ACUTE MYOCARDIAL INFARCTION

HYPOTENSION AND SHOCK

- ▨ Shock
  - ▶ **Shock** is inadequate tissue perfusion that results from the failure of the cardiovascular system to deliver enough oxygen and nutrients to sustain vital organ function.
    - The underlying cause must be recognized and treated promptly, or cell and organ dysfunction and death may result.
    - Signs and symptoms differ according to underlying cause and compensatory mechanisms.
  - ▶ Adequate tissue perfusion requires an intact cardiovascular system.
    - This includes an adequate fluid volume (the blood), a container to regulate the distribution of the fluid (the blood vessels), and a pump (the heart) with sufficient force to move the fluid throughout the container.
    - A problem with any of these components can affect perfusion.
- ▨ Cardiovascular triad
  - ▶ Conduction system (rate)
  - ▶ Tank/vascular system (volume)
  - ▶ Myocardium (pump)

 If a patient is hypotensive or has signs of shock, ask yourself, "Is there a rate problem, a pump problem, or a volume/vascular resistance problem?"

- ▨ Hypotension
  - ▶ Hypotension occurs as a result of a problem with one part of the cardiovascular triad.
  - ▶ Conduction system (rate)
    - Too slow—sinus bradycardia, second- and third-degree AV blocks, pacemaker failure
    - Too fast—sinus tachycardia, atrial flutter or AFib with a rapid ventricular response, supraventricular tachycardias, ventricular tachycardia
  - ▶ Tank/vascular system (volume)
    - Empty tank (absolute hypovolemia)—hemorrhage, gastrointestinal tract loss, renal losses, insensible losses, adrenal insufficiency (aldosterone)
    - Change in tank size (relative hypovolemia)—central nervous system (CNS) injury, spinal injury, third-space loss, sepsis, anaphylaxis, drugs that alter vascular tone, adrenal insufficiency (cortisol)
  - ▶ Myocardium (pump)
    - Primary causes—MI, papillary muscle dysfunction, myocarditis, cardiomyopathies, acute aortic insufficiency, prosthetic valve dysfunction, septal rupture
    - Secondary causes—cardiac tamponade, pulmonary embolism, drugs that alter function, superior vena cava syndrome

Hypotension and Rate Problems

- ▨ A rate problem is *not* synonymous with a "conduction problem."
  - ▶ An adequate rate may be present although a conduction defect exists.
  - ▶ Assess the patient for possible pump, volume, or vascular resistance problem if the patient is hypotensive but his or her rate is within normal limits.
- ▨ If a rate problem exists and you are unclear if a significant pump, volume, or vascular resistance problem coexists, correct the rate problem first. For example, correct the heart rate of a hypotensive, bradycardic patient before giving a fluid challenge, vasopressor, or inotrope.
- ▨ If a rate problem coexists with a suspected pump, volume, or vascular resistance problem, treat simultaneously.

- Management
  - ▶ Primary and secondary surveys, O$_2$, IV, cardiac monitor, pulse oximetry, assess vital signs, review history, physical examination, 12-lead ECG, portable chest x-ray.
  - ▶ If the patient is hypotensive (and symptomatic) and the heart rate is too slow, speed it up (use bradycardia algorithm).
  - ▶ If the patient is hypotensive (and symptomatic) and the heart rate is too fast, slow it down (determine width of QRS, then use appropriate tachycardia algorithm).

Hypotension and Volume Problems

- Consider possible causes of volume deficit.
  - ▶ Empty tank (absolute hypovolemia = actual fluid deficit)
    - Hemorrhage
    - Gastrointestinal loss (vomiting, diarrhea)
    - Renal losses (polyuria)
    - Insensible losses (perspiration, respiration)
    - Adrenal insufficiency (aldosterone)
    - Phlebotomy
    - Reduced fluid intake due to pain, nausea/vomiting
  - ▶ Change in tank size (relative hypovolemia = vasodilation from any cause or redistribution of fluid to third spaces)
    - CNS injury
    - Spinal injury
    - Third-space loss
    - Adrenal insufficiency (cortisol)
    - Sepsis
    - Drugs that alter vascular tone
    - Anaphylaxis
- Initial management
  - ▶ Primary and secondary surveys, O$_2$, IV, cardiac monitor, pulse oximetry, assess vital signs, review history, physical examination, 12-lead ECG, portable chest x-ray.
  - ▶ Generally, first priority = fluid replacement to increase volume.
    - Fluid challenge (250- to 500-mL IV boluses—reassess)
    - Blood transfusion (if appropriate)
  - ▶ If cause known, institute appropriate intervention (such as for septic shock, anaphylaxis).
  - ▶ Consider vasopressors, if indicated, to improve vascular tone if no response to fluid challenge(s).

Hypotension and Pump Problems

- **Cardiac output** is the amount of blood pumped into the aorta each minute by the heart.
  - ▶ Defined as the stroke volume (amount of blood ejected from a ventricle with each heart beat) times the heart rate.
  - ▶ Cardiac output may be affected by an increase or decrease in heart rate *or* stroke volume.
- Stroke volume is affected by preload, afterload, and contractility.
  - ▶ **Preload** is the force exerted on the walls of the ventricles at the end of diastole. The volume of blood returning to the heart influences preload. More blood returning to the right atrium increases preload; less blood returning decreases preload. If the ventricle is stretched beyond its physiological limit, cardiac output may fall due to volume overload and overstretching of the muscle fibers.
  - ▶ **Afterload** is the pressure or resistance against which the ventricles must pump to eject blood. Afterload is influenced by arterial BP, arterial distensibility (ability to become stretched), and arterial resistance. The less the resistance (lower afterload), the more

easily blood can be ejected. Increased afterload (increased resistance) results in increased cardiac workload.

▶ **Ejection fraction** is the percentage of total ventricular volume ejected during each myocardial contraction. It is used as a measure of ventricular function.
  • Normally, the heart empties (ejects) slightly more than ½ the blood that it contains with each beat; thus, a normal ejection fraction is >50%. Impaired ventricular function = ejection fraction <40%.

▨ Pump failure due to acute MI may result in decreased cardiac output and may produce signs and symptoms of tissue hypoperfusion or pulmonary congestion.
  ▶ May be primary or secondary.
    • Causes of primary pump problems—MI, drug overdose/poisoning.
    • Causes of secondary pump problems—as oxygen, glucose, and adenosine triphosphate (ATP) are depleted, essentially all patients in shock will eventually develop a secondary pump problem.

▨ Signs and symptoms of hypoperfusion include hypotension, weak pulse, weakness, skin findings (pallor, sweating), fatigue.

▨ Signs and symptoms of pulmonary congestion include tachypnea, labored respirations, jugular venous distention, frothy sputum, cyanosis, and dyspnea.

▨ Patients in pump failure may require the following:
  ▶ Treatment of a coexisting rate or volume problem
  ▶ Correction of underlying problems (hypoglycemia, hypoxia, drug overdose, poisoning)
  ▶ Support for failing pump
    • Drugs to increase contractility (dopamine, dobutamine, etc.)
    • Vasodilators to decrease afterload
    • Vasodilators, diuretics to decrease preload
    • Mechanical assistance (intra-aortic balloon pump)
    • Surgery (CABG, valve, heart transplant)

KEEPING IT SIMPLE

Cardiac dysrhythmias are the primary *electrical* complication of acute MI. The primary *mechanical* complications of acute MI are CHF and cardiogenic shock.[28]

Left Ventricular Failure

▨ MI may result in left ventricular dysfunction/CHF.

▨ As the heart begins to fail, compensatory mechanisms attempt to maintain adequate perfusion pressure and improve cardiac output by manipulating one or more of the following—heart rate, stroke volume, preload, contractility, and/or afterload.

▨ Compensatory mechanisms may, over time, worsen the degree of failure.
  ▶ Tachycardia—increases myocardial oxygen demand, decreases time for coronary artery perfusion.
  ▶ Sodium and water retention lead to overdistention of ventricles and, ultimately, decreased force of ventricular contraction.

▨ Left ventricular failure is manifested as pulmonary venous congestion and pulmonary edema.
  ▶ As the LV fails, blood backs up into the pulmonary veins and capillaries (Figure 6-30). As the pulmonary capillaries become congested, fluid is pushed from the pulmonary capillaries across the alveolar wall into the alveoli, resulting in pulmonary edema.
  ▶ Pulmonary edema inhibits gas exchange by impairing diffusion between the alveoli and capillary membrane (Figure 6-31).
    • Results in excessive accumulation of fluid in the interstitial spaces and alveoli of the lungs.
  ▶ Hypotension develops as cardiac output decreases.

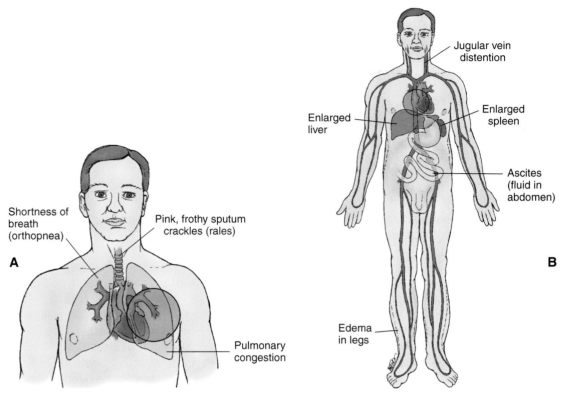

Figure 6-30 • Heart failure. **A,** Left ventricular failure results in a backup of fluid in the lungs. **B,** Right ventricular failure results in a backup of blood in the vascular system.

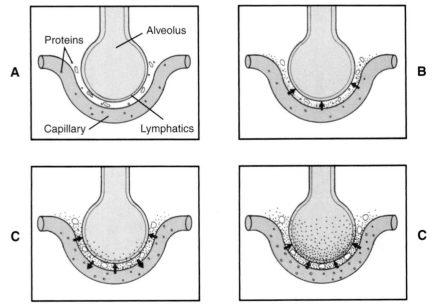

Figure 6-31 • As pulmonary edema progresses, it inhibits the exchange of oxygen and carbon dioxide between the alveoli/capillary membrane. **A,** Normal relationship. **B,** Increased pulmonary capillary hydrostatic pressure causes fluid to move from the vascular space into the pulmonary interstitial space. **C,** Lymphatic flow increases in an attempt to pull fluid back into the vascular or lymphatic space. **D,** Failure of lymphatic flow and worsening of left ventricular failure result in further movement of fluid into the interstitial space and the alveoli.

> ❯ Other signs of LV failure include anxiety, orthopnea, cough with frothy sputum, tachypnea, diaphoresis, dyspnea.

 Heart failure can be defined based on symptom onset, the primary ventricle involved, and overall cardiac output.

Right Ventricular Failure

- The most common cause of right ventricular failure (RVF) is left ventricular failure.
- RVF is manifested as systemic venous congestion and peripheral edema.
- Other signs of RVF include diaphoresis, tachycardia, dyspnea, jugular venous distention (Figure 6-32), fatigue, dependent edema, weakness, weight gain.

Initial Management of Acute Pulmonary Edema

- Primary and secondary surveys, O_2 (intubation may be needed), IV, cardiac monitor, pulse oximetry, assess vital signs, review history, physical examination, 12-lead ECG, portable chest x-ray.
- If feasible and BP permits, place patient in sitting position with feet dependent. This increases lung volume and vital capacity, decreases work of respiration, and decreases venous return to the heart.
- First-line actions[10] (unless SBP <100 mm Hg or more than 30 mm Hg below baseline):
  - ❯ NTG SL or spray (maximum of 3 doses) to reduce preload and afterload.
  - ❯ Furosemide IV 0.5 to 1 mg/kg for venodilation, then diuresis; mobilizes fluid from the lungs into the circulation. Use less than 0.5 mg/kg for new onset acute pulmonary edema without hypovolemia. Use 1 mg/kg for acute or chronic volume overload, renal insufficiency.[10]
  - ❯ Morphine IV 2 to 4 mg to reduce preload and afterload, decrease anxiety/tachypnea.
  - ❯ Dopamine 5 to 15 mcg/kg/min if signs/symptoms of shock present and SBP 70 to 100 mm Hg.
  - ❯ Dobutamine 2 to 20 mcg/kg/min if *no* signs/symptoms of shock and SBP 70 to 100 mm Hg.

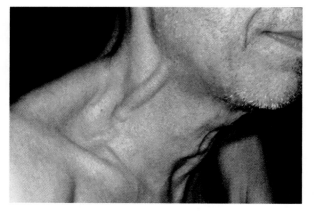
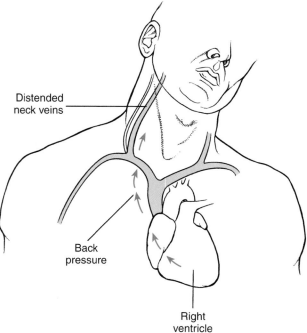

Distended neck veins

Back pressure

Right ventricle

Figure 6-32 • Neck vein distention because of right ventricular failure.

Cardiogenic Shock

▨ Cardiogenic shock occurs because of impaired cardiac muscle function that leads to decreased cardiac output. It may occur as a complication of shock of any cause.
▨ Causes
  ▶ MI
    • Large left ventricular infarction (usually >40% of LV) in 80% of shock patients. Remember that dead tissue does not contribute to contractility. Therefore, extensive muscle damage due to a large infarction is likely to result in cardiogenic shock.
    • RVI in 10% of shock patients.
  ▶ Mechanical complications (e.g., ventricular septal defect, acute mitral regurgitation, cardiac tamponade) in 10% of shock patients
▨ Assessment findings
  ▶ Compensated shock—anxiety, pale skin, cool extremities; diaphoresis, weak, thready peripheral pulses; mild tachycardia, jugular venous distention (indicating right ventricular failure), narrowed pulse pressure (rise in diastolic pressure with normal SBP), mild basilar crackles, normal or mild decrease in urine output, orthopnea
  ▶ Decompensated shock—lethargy; pale, mottled, or cyanotic skin; diaphoresis, weak, thready central pulses; peripheral pulses may be absent; hypotension, tachypnea with decreased tidal volume, increasing pulmonary congestion and crackles, oliguria
▨ If pulmonary edema is associated with hypotension, cardiogenic shock exists.[10]
▨ Initial management[10]
  ▶ Primary and secondary surveys, O_2, IV, cardiac monitor, pulse oximetry, assess vital signs, review history, physical examination, 12-lead ECG, portable chest x-ray
  ▶ SBP <70 mm Hg with signs/symptoms of shock—Norepinephrine IV infusion 0.5 to 30 mcg/min
  ▶ SBP 70 to 100 mm Hg with signs/symptoms of shock—Dopamine IV infusion 5 to 15 mcg/kg/min
  ▶ SBP 70 to 100 mm Hg and *no* sign/symptoms of shock—Dobutamine IV infusion 2 to 20 mcg/kg/min
  ▶ SBP >100 mm Hg—NTG IV infusion 10 to 20 mcg/min, titrate to effect every 5 to 10 minutes

Cardiogenic shock is the leading cause of death for patients hospitalized with acute MI.[29] The treatment of cardiogenic shock is generally based on increasing contractility, altering preload and afterload, and controlling dysrhythmias if they are present and contributing to shock.

RIGHT VENTRICULAR INFARCTION[3]

When an inferior wall MI is suspected (indicative changes in leads II, III, and aVF), obtain right-sided chest leads to screen for a RVI. At a minimum, obtain lead V_4R and look for ST-segment elevation. The ST-segment elevation seen with RVI is transient, disappearing in less than 10 hours following the onset of symptoms in about ½ of patients.[30]

A quick review of related physiology helps us to better understand what happens in the setting of RVI. As blood leaves the right atrium, it enters the RV and is then pumped from the RV into the lungs. While circulating through the pulmonary circuit, the blood is oxygenated and delivered into the left atrium. From the left atrium, blood fills the LV and is then forcefully sent into the systemic circulation. In the setting of RVI, the RV may lose some of its ability to pump blood into the pulmonary circuit. When this happens blood "stalls" in the RV and may begin to "back up." (Technically, the blood does not back up; the venous return exceeds ventricular output and blood begins to accumulate.) This stalling and backing up produce the hypotension (of varying degrees), jugular venous distention, and absence of pulmonary edema (clear lung sounds) that are considered the clinical triad of RVI. This triad is present in only about 10% to 15% of patients with RVI.

As blood backs up from the RV, the jugular veins become enlarged. Hypotension results from the decrease in blood volume moving into the lungs and LV. The LV can only pump as much blood as it receives, and if less blood reaches the LV, less blood is pumped into the systemic circulation. The net effect of this reduction in left ventricular output is a decrease in BP.

In the setting of MI, hypotension is often accompanied by pulmonary edema. However, this is not the case with RVI. In the setting of RVI, blood does not back up from the LV into the lungs, so pulmonary edema is not expected. Shortness of breath may occur but not as a result of pulmonary edema. Instead, it occurs in response to the decrease in perfusion (hypotension and/or hypoxia).

If the patient is hypotensive with a known or suspected RVI, repeat IV fluid challenges of 250 to 500 mL may be necessary every 15 minutes, up to 1 to 2 L. The patient's breath sounds and BP must be reassessed after *each* fluid challenge. Discontinue fluid therapy if pulmonary edema develops. It is important to remember that although vigilant fluid administration often resolves the hypotension that accompanies an RVI and improves cardiac output, there also is a simultaneous infarction occurring in the inferior wall of the LV. This coexistent infarction may reduce the LV's pump function and the possibility of provoking pulmonary edema is a very real concern.

Pain Management Considerations[3]

Routine measures used in the initial management of the normotensive patient experiencing an ACS include giving oxygen, aspirin, and NTG followed by morphine if chest discomfort persists (and there are no contraindications). This approach is effective and indicated in most patients experiencing an ACS. However, the patient experiencing an RVI may require an altered approach to the management of chest discomfort.

Morphine and NTG are vasodilators, and thus they reduce preload. This reduction in preload, although usually beneficial, can be undesirable in the setting of RVI and may cause profound hypotension. Therefore, caution must be exercised when giving NTG and morphine to patients experiencing RVI. If hypotension does occur, it will bring with it the serious consequence of a decrease in coronary artery perfusion.

Because the coronary arteries are supplied from the aorta, a decrease in BP will reduce blood flow through the coronary arteries. When this occurs in an already infarcting heart, it can reduce collateral circulation to the infarcting areas or create ischemia in previously unaffected areas of the heart. Therefore, hypotension is more than just an inconvenience; it can reduce coronary artery perfusion and worsen the area of injury. Hypotension secondary to pain management is a complication that should be anticipated when treating RVI.

When does the risk of hypotension outweigh the benefits of pain management? In most cases, it is best to have physician input. If the decision is made to give vasodilators, there are a few methods of administration that may lessen the patient's hypotensive response. First, establish an IV before giving a vasodilator. This should be routinely done for all patients; however, it is particularly important in RVI. Second, give an IV fluid challenge of 250 to 500 mL (usually with normal saline) if the patient's breath sounds are clear, and reassess the patient's response. This approach attempts to increase preload and offset the anticipated decrease in preload.

It is important to recognize that not every patient experiencing RVI will experience significant hypotension after nitrate administration. Just as there are varying degrees of severity in left ventricular infarctions, RVI is not always so extensive as to manifest great hemodynamic significance.

KEEPING IT SIMPLE

Because of the risk of severe hypotension, nitrates, diuretics, and other vasodilators (such as ACE inhibitors) should be avoided in RVI.

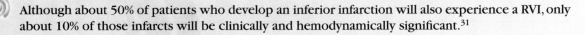

Although about 50% of patients who develop an inferior infarction will also experience a RVI, only about 10% of those infarcts will be clinically and hemodynamically significant.[31]

Complications Associated with Myocardial Infarction
- Dysrhythmias (most common)
- Heart failure, pulmonary edema
- Cardiogenic shock
- Systemic or pulmonary thromboembolism
- Papillary muscle rupture, mitral insufficiency
- Dressler's syndrome (pericarditis occurring 2 to 4 weeks after MI)
- Ventricular aneurysm/rupture
- Ventricular septal defect

DYSRHYTHMIAS ASSOCIATED WITH ISCHEMIA, INJURY, AND INFARCTION

- Dysrhythmias are the most common complication in the first few hours following MI.
- For many years, PVCs observed in patients experiencing an acute MI were thought to be "warning" dysrhythmias of impending VF, particularly multiform PVCs, R-on-T PVCs, couplets, and frequent (>6/min) PVCs. It is considered prudent clinical practice to observe these premature beats closely, consider the reason for their occurrence (such as hypoxemia, acid-base disturbance, electrolyte imbalance, or heart failure), and correct the underlying cause. Routine administration of lidocaine to prevent VF is no longer recommended.
- Beta-blockers have been shown to decrease the incidence of VF and decrease the incidence of sudden death associated with acute MI when given to patients without contraindications.
- Primary VF is VF that occurs during the acute phase of a MI. The incidence of VF is highest during the first 4 hours after onset of symptoms and remains an important contributing factor to death in the first 24 hours. VF as a result of heart failure or cardiogenic shock can also contribute to death from acute MI.[27]
  - ◗ If VF occurs, there is no conclusive data to support the use of lidocaine or any particular strategy for preventing the recurrence of VF. The use of beta-blockers is preferred if they were not begun before the episode of VF. If a maintenance infusion of lidocaine is used, current recommendations are to continue the infusion for no more than 24 hours (unless symptomatic VT persists) and discontinue it to assess the patient's ongoing need for antiarrhythmic treatment.[32]

QUICK REVIEW 6-9

1. Cardiogenic shock is most often due to extensive MI, involving approximately ____% or more of the LV.
2. What drug is usually used in the management of a suspected pump problem with an SBP of 70 to 90 mm Hg?
3. True or False. Norepinephrine is the drug of choice for a suspected volume problem accompanied by hypertension.
4. Why is tachycardia often associated with RVF?

5. Why is nitroglycerin given to patients with acute pulmonary edema who have an SBP >100 mm Hg?

6. When is an RVI suspected?

QUICK REVIEW ANSWERS

Quick Review Number	Answers
6-1	1. Endothelium 2. Aspirin 3. Glycoprotein IIb/IIIa 4. Fibrinolytics
6-2	1. Ischemia 2. Chronic stable angina is predictable and consistent. Duration of symptoms typically 2 to 5 minutes, occasionally 5 to 15 minutes; prolonged discomfort (>30 min) uncommon and usually relieved with rest or within 45 seconds to 5 minutes of NTG administration. 3. (Myocardial) ischemia, injury, and infarction 4. Unstable angina is characterized by one or more of the following: • Symptoms of angina at rest (usually >20 minutes) • Progressively worsening of preexisting stable angina • New onset (<2 months) angina that is severe and brought on by minimal exertion
6-3	1. Myocardial injury refers to myocardial tissue that has been cut off from or experienced a severe reduction in its blood and oxygen supply. 2. Injured myocardial cells are still alive but will die (infarct) if the ischemia is not quickly corrected. If the blocked vessel can be quickly opened, restoring blood flow and oxygen to the injured area, no tissue death occurs. An MI occurs when blood flow to the heart muscle stops or is suddenly decreased long enough to cause cell death. 3. The five most important factors, ranked in the order of importance, are as follows: • The nature of the anginal symptoms • Previous history of coronary artery disease • Gender • Age • The number of risk factors present
6-4	1. Chest discomfort 2. Older adults (elderly), women, and diabetic individuals 3. Anginal equivalent symptoms are symptoms of myocardial ischemia other than chest pain or discomfort. 4. Examples of anginal equivalents include generalized weakness, difficulty breathing, excessive sweating, unexplained nausea or vomiting, dizziness, syncope or near-syncope, palpitations, isolated arm or jaw pain, fatigue, and dysrhythmias.
6-5	1. ST-segment depression is considered significant if the ST-segment is ≥0.5 mm below the baseline. 2. Two leads are contiguous if they look at the same area of the heart or if they are numerically consecutive chest leads. 3. ECG evidence of myocardial injury in progress can be seen on the ECG as ST-segment elevation in the leads facing the affected area. 4. In the standard 12-lead ECG, three leads (II, III, and aVF) "look" at tissue supplied by the RCA.
6-6	1. 1 mm 2. Abnormal (pathologic) Q waves 3. True

6-7

1. The primary goals of therapy for patients with ACS include the following:
- Reduce the amount of myocardial necrosis that occurs in patients with MI, preserving (LV function and preventing heart failure
- Prevent MACE: death, nonfatal MI, and need for urgent re-vascularization
- Treat acute, life-threatening complications of ACS, such as VF/pulseless VT, symptomatic bradycardias, and unstable tachycardias

2. False 3. 1) ST-segment elevation (or new left BBB), 2) ST-segment depression or transient ST-segment/T-wave changes, 3) normal/nondiagnostic ECG

6-8

1. Relief of pain decreases anxiety, myocardial oxygen demand, and the risk of cardiac dysrhythmias. 2. Fibrinolytic therapy is recommended for patients who have ST-segment elevation in two or more contiguous leads, a history suggesting acute MI, and time from symptom onset to therapy that is ≤12 hours. 3. Leads II, III, aVF 4. Anterior

6-9

1. 40% 2. Dopamine IV infusion 3. False 4. The body attempts to maintain cardiac output by increasing heart rate. The increased heart rate, however, results in decreased ventricular filling time and decreased coronary artery perfusion. 5. To increase venous capacitance (promote venous pooling), thereby reducing preload and afterload 6. When the patient has experienced an inferior wall MI of the LV (ST-segment elevation in leads II, III, aVF)

STOP & REVIEW

Questions 1-22. Match the term or phrase with its corresponding description.

a) Contiguous
b) Tombstone
c) Dysrhythmias
d) Viagra
e) Claudication
f) Biomarkers
g) Left
h) MACE
i) Elevation
j) Morphine
k) MONA
l) Absolute
m) Plaque
n) Depression
o) Reperfusion
p) Right
q) Prinzmetal's
r) Dead
s) Volume
t) Endothelium
u) Reciprocal
v) Infarction

_____ 1. Acronym for major adverse cardiac events

_____ 2. Most myocardial infarctions occur in the __ ventricle

_____ 3. This type of angina is the result of intense spasm of a segment of a coronary artery

_____ 4. Leads V_4R, V_5R, and V_6R view the __ ventricle

_____ 5. Memory aid used to recall the medications typically given in the management of ACS

_____ 6. This lines the vascular system

_____ 7. The presence of a pathologic Q wave on an ECG indicates the presence of __ myocardial tissue

_____ 8. Leg pain due to peripheral vascular disease

_____ 9. ECG changes seen in leads opposite the affected area are called __ changes

_____10. Hyperacute T waves are sometimes called __ T waves

_____11. Most common complication of MI

_____12. The usual cause of an ACS

_____13. ST-segment __ is suggestive of myocardial ischemia

_____14. One part of the cardiovascular triad

_____15. Narcotic analgesic of choice to relieve ACS pain/discomfort

_____16. Cardiac __ are blood tests used to help verify the presence of an MI

_____17. ST-segment __ is suggestive of myocardial injury

_____18. ECG changes are significant when they are seen in two __ leads

____19. Before giving NTG, make sure the patient has not used this medication (or a similar medication) within 24 to 48 hours

____20. An actual fluid deficit is also called a(n) __ hypovolemia

____21. One of "the 3 I's" of an acute coronary event

____22. This therapy is the mainstay of treatment for STEMI

A 62-year-old man is complaining of chest discomfort. The patient states his discomfort is located in the center of his chest and radiates to his left arm. He was reading the newspaper when his discomfort began about 1½ hours ago. On a 0 to 10 scale, the patient rates his discomfort a "9." He has no significant past medical history, takes no medications regularly, and states he has "never had anything like this before." His father died of a heart attack at the age of 66 years. The patient is an investment banker and states he is under considerable daily stress. Questions 23 to 34 pertain to the initial assessment and management of this patient.

23. Initial management of this patient should include ABCs, O_2, IV, monitor, and
   a. Aspirin and a 12-lead ECG
   b. Preparations for immediate defibrillation
   c. Preparations for transcutaneous pacing
   d. A 500 mL fluid challenge of normal saline

24. The patient's vital signs are as follows: BP 146/74, pulse 128 (regular), respirations 18, oxygen saturation 97% on oxygen at 4 L/min. Breath sounds are clear bilaterally. The patient's skin is warm and moist. The cardiac monitor shows a sinus tachycardia. This rhythm
   a. Requires immediate treatment with synchronized cardioversion
   b. Is most likely associated with the discomfort and ACS the patient is experiencing
   c. Requires immediate treatment with vagal maneuvers and adenosine
   d. Is common and no reason for concern in a patient experiencing an ACS

25. An IV has been established. The cardiac monitor now reveals sinus tachycardia with occasional uniform PVCs. Which of the following statements is true regarding obtaining a 12-lead ECG in this situation?
   a. A 12-lead ECG should be obtained within 10 minutes of patient contact (prehospital) or arrival in the ED
   b. A 12-lead ECG is necessary only if the patient's symptoms persist for more than 30 minutes
   c. A 12-lead ECG is an unnecessary expense and should be reserved for those situations in which you are unsure if the patient is experiencing an ACS
   d. A 12-lead ECG is essential to decision-making in the emergency care of a patient with an acute coronary syndrome and should be obtained with 30 minutes of patient contact (prehospital) or arrival in the ED

26. Sublingual nitroglycerin (NTG) is ordered for this patient. What is the rationale for giving NTG in this situation?
   a. NTG is a potent narcotic analgesic
   b. NTG increases myocardial oxygen consumption
   c. NTG relaxes vascular smooth muscle, including dilation of the coronary arteries
   d. NTG blocks the formation of thromboxane A_2, which causes platelets to clump and arteries to constrict

27. What precautions should be taken before giving NTG?
    a. Make sure the patient's heart rate is at least 70 bpm
    b. Make sure there is no evidence of an RVI
    c. Make sure the patient's SBP is >110 mm Hg
    d. Make sure the patient has not used a diuretic or antihypertensive medication in the past 24 hours

28. NTG SL tablets or spray may be given:
    a. Only once. If no relief of discomfort after one dose, give morphine
    b. At 15-minute intervals to a maximum of 2 doses. If no relief of discomfort after 2 doses, give midazolam (Versed) or meperidine (Demerol)
    c. Every 5 minutes until discomfort is relieved
    d. At 5-minute intervals to a maximum of 3 doses

29. A beta-blocker has been ordered for this patient. What is the rationale for giving a beta-blocker in this situation?
    a. Increase heart rate
    b. Improve ventilation through bronchodilation
    c. Decrease myocardial oxygen consumption
    d. Increase myocardial contractility

30. A 12-lead ECG has been obtained. Which of the following components of the ECG should be carefully examined to determine the most appropriate treatment course for this patient?
    a. P waves and PR intervals
    b. ST-segments, Q waves, and T waves
    c. P waves and QRS complexes
    d. ST-segments and PR intervals

31. When viewing the ECG of a patient experiencing an ACS, the presence of ST-segment elevation suggests myocardial __.
    a. Ischemia
    b. Injury
    c. Infarction
    d. Necrosis

32. The patient's 12-lead ECG reveals 3-mm ST-segment elevation in leads V_1, V_2, V_3, and V_4. What portion of the heart do these leads "see?"
    a. The septum and anterior surface of the LV
    b. The right ventricle and the lateral surface of the LV
    c. The anterior and inferior surfaces of the LV
    d. The posterior and lateral surfaces of the LV

33. The patient rates his chest discomfort a "9" despite SL NTG therapy. His BP is 140/70, pulse 96, and respirations 18. Assuming the patient's vital signs remain stable, which of the following statements is true about relieving this patient's chest discomfort?
    a. Morphine 2 to 4 mg IV should be given and repeated every 5 minutes until the patient determines his discomfort is tolerable
    b. Give 2 mg of morphine IV and then reassess the degree of the patient's discomfort every 30 minutes
    c. Give an initial dose of 8 mg of morphine IV and repeat every 30 minutes until the patient is pain free
    d. Morphine 2 to 4 mg should be given slow IV push and additional doses given at 5- to 15-minute intervals until the patient is pain free

34. The patient has been diagnosed with an anteroseptal MI. Which of the following complications should be reasonably anticipated with this type of infarction?
    a. Bradycardias and pulmonary embolism
    b. Tension pneumothorax and BBBs
    c. Heart failure and cardiogenic shock
    d. AFib and stroke

35. An MI is
    a. A thin-walled bulge in a dead area of the LV that balloons out when the ventricle contracts
    b. Death of myocardial cells due to myocardial ischemia
    c. The inability of the heart to maintain cardiac output adequate to meet the metabolic demands of the body
    d. A gradual process involving obstruction and hardening of the arterial wall

36. Drugs given in the initial management of acute pulmonary edema without hypotension include
    a. Oxygen, NTG, morphine, and furosemide
    b. Oxygen, NTG, aspirin, and dopamine
    c. Oxygen, furosemide, and amiodarone
    d. Oxygen, morphine, and atropine

37. What is the most common complication in the first few hours of MI?
    a. Ventricular aneurysm
    b. Dysrhythmias
    c. CHF
    d. Papillary muscle dysfunction

STOP & REVIEW ANSWERS

1. h	12. m
2. g	13. n
3. q	14. s
4. p	15. j
5. k	16. f
6. t	17. i
7. r	18. a
8. e	19. d
9. u	20. l
10. b	21. v
11. c	22. o

23. a. Initial management of a patient experiencing an ACS should include primary and secondary surveys, O_2, IV, monitor, vital signs, aspirin if not already taken by the patient (and no contraindications), and a 12-lead ECG within 10 minutes of patient contact or patient arrival in the ED. Thus far, we have no idea what the patient's cardiac rhythm is, so preparations for defibrillation and transcutaneous pacing are not warranted. A fluid challenge is not routinely given to a patient experiencing an ACS. Furthermore, we do not yet know the patient's vital signs or the status of his lung sounds.

24. b. The sinus tachycardia seen on the cardiac monitor is most likely associated with the discomfort and ACS the patient is experiencing. The treatment for a sinus tachycardia is treatment of the underlying cause. In this case, the patient should be given medications to relieve his discomfort as soon as possible. A tachycardia is a concern in a patient experiencing an ACS because it results in decreased ventricular filling time and decreased coronary artery perfusion. Vagal maneuvers and adenosine are not appropriate interventions for a sinus tachycardia. These interventions are used for stable patients who are symptomatic because of a narrow-QRS tachycardia such as AV nodal reentrant tachycardia. Synchronized cardioversion is not appropriate for a sinus tachycardia. It is used to treat unstable patients who have a rhythm with a clearly identifiable QRS complex and a rapid ventricular rate (such as some narrow-QRS tachycardias and VT).

25. a. A 12-lead ECG is essential to decision making in the emergency care of a patient with an ACS and should be obtained with 10 minutes of patient contact (prehospital) or arrival in the ED.

26. c. NTG relaxes vascular smooth muscle, including dilation of the coronary arteries (particularly in the area of plaque disruption). It also decreases myocardial oxygen consumption. Aspirin (not nitroglycerin) blocks the formation of thromboxane A_2 (thromboxane A_2 causes platelets to clump and arteries to constrict).

27. b. Before giving NTG, make sure an IV is in place, the patient's SBP is >90 mm Hg, his heart rate is >50 and <100 bpm, there are no signs of RVI (absence of ST-segment elevation in leads II, III, and aVF), and the patient has not used Viagra, Cialis, or similar medication in the previous 24 to 48 hours.

28. d. NTG SL tablets or spray may be given at 5-minute intervals to a maximum of 3 doses, assuming that the patient's vital signs remain stable.

29. c. Beta-blockers are used in ACSs to reduce myocardial oxygen consumption, decrease the incidence of dysrhythmias, lower BP, block catecholamine stimulation, decrease myocardial contractility, and decrease the incidence of VF.

30. b. Once the 12-lead has been obtained, it should be reviewed carefully. Look at each lead for the presence of ST-segment displacement (elevation or depression). If ST-segment elevation is present, note its elevation in millimeters. Examine the T waves for any changes in orientation, shape, and size. Examine each lead for the presence of a Q wave. If a Q wave is present, measure its duration. Assess the areas of ischemia or injury by assessing lead groupings. Remember: ECG evidence must be found in at least two contiguous leads.

31. b. When viewing the ECG of a patient experiencing an ACS, the presence of ST-segment elevation suggests myocardial *injury*.

32. a. Leads V$_1$ and V$_2$ view the septum. Leads V$_3$ and V$_4$ view the anterior surface of the LV. ST-segment elevation in these leads suggests an anteroseptal MI.

33. d. Give morphine 2- to 4-mg (give in 2-mg increments) slow IV push. Give additional doses of 2 to 8 mg IV at 5- to 15-minute intervals. Relief of pain is a priority in the management of a patient experiencing an ACS. Relief of pain decreases anxiety, myocardial oxygen demand, and the risk of cardiac dysrhythmias. When treating a patient with an ACS, it is not enough to simply reduce the patient's degree of pain or discomfort. The goal is to ensure that the patient is pain-free, while closely monitoring his or her vital signs.

34. c. Blockage of the midportion of the LAD artery results in an anterior infarction. Proximal occlusion of the LAD may become an anteroseptal infarction if the septal branch is involved or an anterolateral infarction if the marginal branch is involved. Because the LAD artery supplies about 40% of the heart's blood and a critical section of the LV, blockage of this vessel can lead to complications including heart failure and cardiogenic shock. Sympathetic hyperactivity is common with resulting sinus tachycardia and/or hypertension. An anterior wall MI may cause other dysrhythmias including PVCs, atrial flutter, or AFib. Because the bundle branches travel through this area, BBBs may also result from injury in this area.

35. b. MI is death of myocardial cells due to myocardial ischemia. MI occurs when there is a sudden decrease or total cessation of blood flow through a coronary artery to an area of the myocardium. A thin-walled bulge in a dead area of the LV that balloons out when the ventricle contracts describes a ventricular aneurysm. The inability of the heart to maintain cardiac output adequate to meet the metabolic demands of the body describes heart failure. Arteriosclerosis is a gradual process involving obstruction and hardening of the arterial wall.

36. a. Venodilators such as NTG and morphine and diuretics such as furosemide are used to reduce preload in the initial management of the normotensive patient with congestive heart failure/acute pulmonary edema. Atropine and amiodarone are antiarrhythmics and are not indicated in the management of acute pulmonary edema. Dopamine may be used in the initial management of acute pulmonary edema if signs/symptoms of shock are present and the patient has a SBP of 70 to 100 mm Hg.

37. b. Dysrhythmias are the most common complication in the first few hours of MI. Other complications of MI include CHF, pulmonary edema, cardiogenic shock, systemic or pulmonary thromboembolism, papillary muscle rupture, mitral insufficiency, Dressler's syndrome (pericarditis occurring 2 to 4 weeks after MI), ventricular aneurysm/rupture, and ventricular septal defect.

REFERENCES

1. Greenlund KJ, Keenan NL, Giles WH, et al: Public recognition of major signs and symptoms of heart attack: Seventeen states and the US Virgin Islands, 2001. *Am Heart J* Jun 2004;147(6):1010-1016.
2. Shah PK: Mechanisms of plaque vulnerability and rupture. *J Am Coll Cardiol* Feb 19, 2003;41(4 Suppl S):15S-22S.
3. Phalen T, Aehlert B: *The 12-lead ECG in acute coronary syndromes.* St. Louis: Mosby, 2006.
4. Schoen FJ: The heart. In Kumar V, Abbas AK, Fausto N (Eds.): *Robbins and Cotran pathologic basis of disease* (7th ed.) Philadelphia: Elsevier, 2005.
5. Schoen FJ: Blood vessels. In Kumar V, Abbas AK, Fausto N (Eds.): *Robbins and Cotran pathologic basis of disease* (7th ed.) Philadelphia: Elsevier, 2005.
6. Gibbons RJ, Abrams J, Chatterjee K, et al: ACC/AHA 2002 guideline update for the management of patients with chronic stable angina: A report of the American College of Cardiology/American Heart Association Task Force on Practice Guidelines (Committee to Update the 1999 Guidelines for the Management of Patients with Chronic Stable Angina). 2002. Available at www.acc.org/clinical/guidelines/stable/stable.pdf/
7. Liberthson RR, Nagel EL, Hirschman JC, Nussenfeld SR: Prehospital ventricular defibrillation: Prognosis and follow-up course. *N Engl J Med* Aug 15, 1974;291(7):317-321.
8. Braunwald E, Antman EM, Beasley JW, et al: ACC/AHA 2002 guideline update for the management of patients with unstable angina and non–ST-segment elevation myocardial infarction: A report of the American College of Cardiology/American Heart Association Task Force on Practice Guidelines (Committee on the Management of Patients with Unstable Angina). 2002. Available at: http://www.acc.org/clinical/guidelines/unstable/unstable.pdf/
9. American Heart Association guidelines for cardiopulmonary resuscitation and emergency cardiovascular care, part 8: Stabilization of the patient with acute coronary syndromes. *Circulation* 2005;112(suppl IV):IV-93.
10. Antman EM, Anbe DT, Armstrong PW, et al: ACC/AHA guidelines for the management of patients with ST-elevation myocardial infarction: A report of the American College of Cardiology/American Heart Association Task Force on Practice Guidelines (Committee to Revise the 1999 Guidelines for the Management of Patients with Acute Myocardial Infarction). 2004. Available at www.acc.org/clinical/guidelines/stemi/index.pdf/
11. Brown AL, Mann NC, Daya M, et al: Demographic, belief, and situational factors influencing the decision to utilize emergency medical services among chest pain patients. Rapid Early Action for Coronary Treatment (REACT) study. *Circulation* Jul 11, 2000;102(2):173-178.
12. Braunwald E, Antman EM, Beasley JW, et al: ACC/AHA guidelines for the management of patients with unstable angina and non–ST-segment elevation myocardial infarction: A report of the American College of Cardiology/American Heart Association Task Force on Practice Guidelines (Committee on the Management of Patients with Unstable Angina). *J Am Coll Cardiol* 2000;36:970-1062.
13. Canto JG, Shlipak MG, Rogers WJ, et al: Prevalence, clinical characteristics, and mortality among patients with myocardial infarction presenting without chest pain. *JAMA* Jun 28, 2000;283(24):3223-3229.
14. Becker L, Larsen MP, Eisenberg MS: Incidence of cardiac arrest during self-transport for chest pain. *Ann Emerg Med* 1996;28:612-616.
15. Savonitto S, Ardissino D, Granger CB, et al: Prognostic value of the admission electrocardiogram in acute coronary syndromes. *JAMA* 1999;281:707-713.

16. 2005 American Heart Association guidelines for cardiopulmonary resuscitation and emergency cardiovascular care, part 8: Stabilization of the patient with acute coronary syndromes. *Circulation* 2005;112(suppl IV):IV-89.

17. Aufderheide TP, Keelan MH, Hendley GE, et al: Milwaukee Prehospital Chest Pain Project—phase I: Feasibility and accuracy of prehospital thrombolytic candidate selection. *Am J Cardiol* 1992;69:991-996.

18. 2005 American Heart Association guidelines for cardiopulmonary resuscitation and emergency cardiovascular care, part 8: Stabilization of the patient with acute coronary syndromes. *Circulation* 2005;112(suppl IV):IV-93.

19. 2005 American Heart Association guidelines for cardiopulmonary resuscitation and emergency cardiovascular care, part 8: Stabilization of the patient with acute coronary syndromes. *Circulation* 2005;112(suppl IV):IV-90.

20. Canto JG, Rogers WJ, Bowlby LJ, et al: The prehospital electrocardiogram in acute myocardial infarction: is its full potential being realized? National Registry of Myocardial Infarction 2 Investigators. *J Am Coll Cardiol* 1997;29:498-505.

21. Ohman EM, Hudson MP: Acute ST Elevation Myocardial Infarction: Early Assessment and Stratification. In Weaver WD, Hudson MP (Eds.): *Focus on acute coronary syndromes*, American College of Cardiology Foundation, 2003.

22. Schuchert A, Hamm C, Scholz J, et al: Prehospital testing for troponin T in patients with suspected acute myocardial infarction. *Am Heart J* 1999;138:45-48.

23. 2005 American Heart Association guidelines for cardiopulmonary resuscitation and emergency cardiovascular care, part 8: Stabilization of the patient with acute coronary syndromes. *Circulation* 2005;112(suppl IV):IV-98.

24. Antman EM, Hand M, Armstrong PW, Bates ER, Green LA, Halasyamani LK, Hochman JS, Krumholz HM, Lamas GA, Mullany CJ, Pearle DL, Sloan MA, Smith SC Jr. 2007 focused update of the ACC/AHA 2004 Guidelines for the Management of Patients with ST-Elevation Myocardial Infarction: a report of the American College of Cardiology/American Heart Association Task Force on Practice Guidelines (Writing Group to Review New Evidence and Update the ACC AHA 2004 Guidelines for the Management of Patients with ST-Elevation Myocardial Infarction). *J Am Coll Cardiol* 2008;51:210-247.

25. 2005 American Heart Association guidelines for cardiopulmonary resuscitation and emergency cardiovascular care, part 8: Stabilization of the patient with acute coronary syndromes. *Circulation* 2005;112(suppl IV):IV-91-92.

26. 2005 American Heart Association guidelines for cardiopulmonary resuscitation and emergency cardiovascular care, part 8: Stabilization of the patient with acute coronary syndromes. *Circulation* 2005;112(suppl IV):IV-101.

27. 2005 American Heart Association guidelines for cardiopulmonary resuscitation and emergency cardiovascular care, part 8: Stabilization of the patient with acute coronary syndromes. *Circulation* 2005;112(suppl IV):IV-102.

28. Crawford MV, Spence MI: *Common sense approach to coronary care* (6th ed.) St. Louis: Mosby-Year Book, 1995, p. 129.

29. Braat SH, Brugada P, De Zwaan C, et al: Value of electrocardiogram in diagnosing right ventricular involvement in patients with an acute inferior wall myocardial infarction. *Br Heart J* 1983;49:368-372.

30. Goldberg RJ, Gore JM, Thompson CA, Gurwitz JH: Recent magnitude of and temporal trends (1994-1997) in the incidence and hospital death rates of cardiogenic shock complicating acute myocardial infarction: The second national registry of myocardial infarction. *Am Heart J* 2001;141:65-72.

31. Stewart S, Haste M: Prediction of right ventricular and posterior wall ST-elevation by coronary care nurses: The 12-lead electrocardiograph versus the 18-lead electrocardiograph. *Heart Lung* 1996;25:14-23.

32. 2005 American Heart Association guidelines for cardiopulmonary resuscitation and emergency cardiovascular care, part 8: Stabilization of the patient with acute coronary syndromes. *Circulation* 2005;112(suppl IV):IV-103.

Stroke and Special Resuscitation Situations

OBJECTIVES

Upon completion of this chapter, you will be able to:

1. Describe the two major types of stroke.
2. Describe the sequence of events that occurs during a stroke.
3. Discuss why stroke must be treated within the early hours of symptom onset.
4. Identify the signs and symptoms of stroke.
5. Understand the significance of a transient ischemic attack (TIA).
6. Describe the initial emergency care for each of the following situations:
   - Stroke
   - Drowning
   - Near-fatal asthma
   - Anaphylaxis
   - Hypothermia
   - Traumatic cardiac arrest
   - Cardiac arrest and pregnancy
   - Electric shock and lightning strike

INTRODUCTION

ACLS algorithms are guidelines to use when caring for patients who are experiencing a cardiac-related emergency. The most common ACLS algorithms are discussed in Chapter 8. Some situations require modification of the ACLS algorithms to increase the likelihood of a positive outcome. In this chapter, the initial emergency care for stroke and special resuscitation situations (such as drowning, near-fatal asthma, anaphylaxis, traumatic cardiac arrest, and hypothermia) is discussed. Stroke is discussed in most ACLS courses; however, the special resuscitation situations mentioned in this chapter are not routinely discussed in an ACLS course. A detailed discussion of these topics is typical in an advanced ACLS course.

ADULT STROKE

A **stroke** is a sudden change in neurologic function caused by a change in cerebral blood flow. A stroke is also called a "brain attack." The public is familiar with the phrase "heart attack." Because a stroke happens in the brain rather than the heart, the phrase "brain attack" may convey the events involved in a stroke more clearly to the public than the word "stroke." The term "brain attack" and its application to stroke are credited to Vladimir C. Hachinski and John Norris, neurologists from Canada. The National Stroke Association (NSA) began using the term in 1990.

STROKE FACTS

- Stroke is the third leading cause of death in the United States, after heart disease and cancer.
- Every minute in the United States, someone experiences a stroke; and every 3.3 minutes, someone dies of one.
- Stroke kills more than twice as many American women every year as breast cancer.
- About one third of all stroke survivors will have another stroke within 5 years.
- About 700,000 people suffer a stroke each year. Of these, about 500,000 are first attacks, and 200,000 are recurrent attacks.
- About 50% of stroke deaths occur before the person reaches the hospital.

"STROKE BELT"

The Centers for Disease Control and Prevention has identified a "Stroke Belt" in the United States. Twelve contiguous states and the District of Columbia have stroke death rates consistently more than 10% higher than the rest of the country: Virginia, North Carolina, South Carolina, Georgia, Florida, Alabama, Mississippi, Louisiana, Arkansas, Tennessee, Kentucky, Indiana, and Washington, DC. The higher incidence and mortality may be linked to a number of factors, including a higher-than-average population of African Americans, higher-than-average population of older adults, and dietary factors.

RISK FACTORS

- Deaths from stroke can be reduced or delayed by preventing and controlling risk factors.
  - Important nonmodifiable risk factors for strokes include older age, family history of stroke and/or cardiovascular disease, gender, and ethnicity (higher rates in African Americans than in whites).
  - Modifiable risk factors include high blood pressure (BP), cigarette smoking, transient ischemic attacks (TIAs), heart disease (particularly atrial fibrillation), diabetes mellitus, carotid artery disease, hypercoagulopathy, and hyperlipidemia.

■ Other factors may affect the risk of stroke. Because stroke deaths tend to occur more often during extremely hot or cold temperatures, season and climate may increase the risk of stroke. People of lower income and educational levels may be at increased risk for stroke.

CLASSIFICATION OF STROKE BY ANATOMIC LOCATION

■ The carotid arteries supply 80% of blood flow to the brain; 20% is supplied through the vertebrobasilar system (Figure 7-1).

■ Strokes involving the carotid arteries are called *anterior circulation strokes* or *carotid territory strokes*. They usually involve the cerebral hemispheres.

■ Strokes affecting the vertebrobasilar arteries are called *posterior circulation strokes* or *vertebrobasilar territory strokes*. They usually affect the brain stem or cerebellum.

Signs and symptoms of stroke are shown in Table 7-1. The lobes of the brain are shown in Figure 7-2. The functional subdivisions of the cerebral cortex are shown in Figure 7-3.

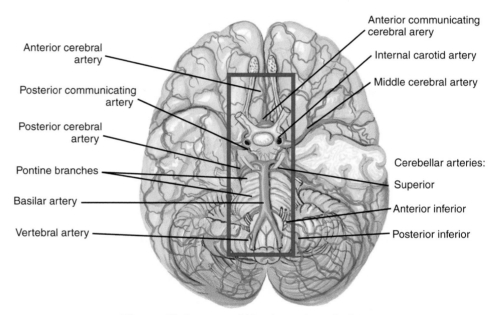

Figure 7-1 • Arterial blood supply to the brain.

TABLE 7-1	Signs and Symptoms of Stroke	
Affected Artery	**Structures Supplied by Affected Vessel**	**Signs and Symptoms of Blockage**
Anterior cerebral	Supplies medial surfaces and upper portions of frontal and parietal lobes	• Emotional lability • Confusion • Weakness, numbness on affected side • Paralysis of contralateral foot and leg • Impaired mobility, with sensation greater in lower extremities than in upper • Urinary incontinence • Loss of coordination • Personality changes • Impaired sensory function
Middle cerebral (Most commonly blocked vessel in stroke; largest branch of the internal carotid artery)	Supplies a portion of the frontal lobe, lateral surface of the temporal and parietal lobes, including the primary motor and sensory areas of the face, throat, hand, and arm and in the dominant hemisphere, the areas for speech	Changes in communication, cognition, mobility, and sensation including: • Aphasia • Dysphasia • Reading difficulty (dyslexia) • Inability to write (dysgraphia) • Visual field deficits • Contralateral sensory deficit • Contralateral hemiparesis (more severe in the face and hand than in the leg) • Altered level of responsiveness
Posterior cerebral	Supplies medial and inferior temporal lobes, medial occipital lobe, thalamus, posterior hypothalamus, visual receptive area	• Hemiplegia • Receptive aphasia • Sensory impairment • Dyslexia • Coma • Visual field deficits • Cortical blindness from ischemia
Internal carotid	Supplies cerebral hemispheres and diencephalon	• Headaches • Altered level of responsiveness • Bruits over the carotid artery • Profound aphasia • Ptosis • Weakness, paralysis, numbness, sensory changes, and visual deficits (blurring) on the affected side • Unilateral blindness
Vertebral or basilar	Supplies brainstem and cerebellum	Incomplete blockage • TIAs • Unilateral and bilateral weakness of extremities • Visual deficits on affected side (diplopia, color blindness, lack of depth perception) • Nausea, vertigo, tinnitus • Headache • Dysarthria • Numbness • Dysphagia • "Locked-in" syndrome: no movement except eyelids; sensation and consciousness preserved Complete blockage • Coma • Extension (decerebrate) posturing • Respiratory and circulatory abnormalities

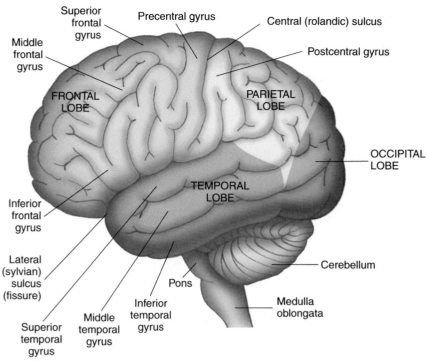

Figure 7-2 • Lobes and principal fissures of the cerebral cortex, cerebellum, and brainstem.

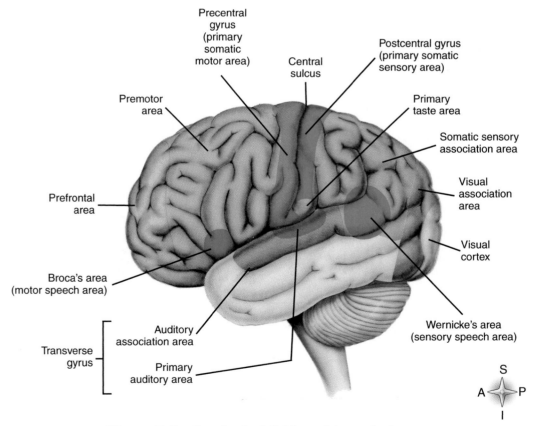

Figure 7-3 • Functional subdivisions of the cerebral cortex.

ISCHEMIC AND HEMORRHAGIC STROKE

There are two major types of stroke—ischemic and hemorrhagic. An ischemic stroke occurs when a blood vessel supplying the brain is blocked. It can be life-threatening but rarely leads to death within the first hour. A hemorrhagic stroke occurs when a cerebral artery bursts. It can be fatal at onset.

Ischemic Stroke

Ischemic strokes account for more than 80% of strokes. There are two types of ischemic strokes—thrombotic and embolic.

Thrombotic Stroke

■ A thrombotic stroke is the most common cause of stroke (Figure 7-4).
■ In a thrombotic stroke, atherosclerosis of large vessels in the brain causes progressive narrowing and platelet clumping. Platelet clumping results in the development of blood clots within the brain artery itself (cerebral thrombosis). When the blood clots are of sufficient size to block blood flow through the artery, the area previously supplied by that artery becomes ischemic.
■ Ischemia occurs because the tissue supplied by the blocked artery does not receive oxygen (O_2) and the essential nutrients needed for normal brain function. The patient's signs and symptoms depend on the location of the artery affected and the areas of brain ischemia.

About 5% of patients with acute ischemic stroke present with a seizure, and up to 30% have a headache.[1]

Embolic Stroke

■ In an embolic stroke, material from an area outside the brain (such as the heart, aorta, or other major artery) becomes dislodged and travels through the bloodstream to the brain (cerebral embolism).
■ Embolic material may consist of fragments of valves, tumors, or plaques; air, fat, amniotic fluid, a foreign body, or a blood clot.
■ An embolus tends to become lodged where arteries branch because blood flow is most turbulent in these areas. Fragments of the embolus may become lodged in smaller vessels.

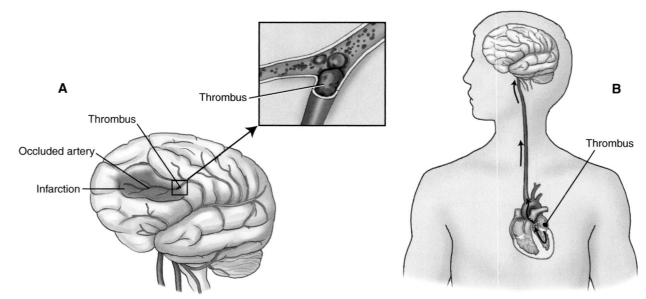

Figure 7-4 • An ischemic stroke may occur because of a thrombus or embolus. **A,** Thrombotic stroke. **B,** Embolic stroke.

■ As with thrombotic strokes, the patient's signs and symptoms depend on the location of the artery affected and the areas of brain ischemia.

Interesting Stroke Facts[2]

- Patients who have atrial fibrillation are 5 to 17 times more likely to develop a stroke than those who do not have atrial fibrillation.
- Almost 20% of stroke patients have atrial fibrillation on their admission electrocardiogram (ECG).
- About 1% to 2% of patients who have an acute myocardial infarction (MI) have a subsequent stroke within the first month after their cardiac event. Half of these occur within the first 5 days of the MI.
- Independent predictors of who will develop a stroke after an acute MI include a history of atrial fibrillation (new-onset or chronic), prior stroke, and ST-segment elevation.
- Aspirin use reduces the incidence of post-MI stroke by 42%.
- Ischemic stroke is associated with changes in the autonomic function of the heart that may lead to sudden death in 6% to 11% of patients.

Evolution of an Ischemic Stroke

Complete blockage of an artery may lead to death of an area of cells in the brain because blood flow is obstructed (ischemic infarction). The evolution of the thrombosis may take place in a few minutes, hours, or even days. Large blood vessels, such as the carotid, middle cerebral, and basilar arteries, can take longer to become blocked than smaller vessels.

Warning signs of impending stroke may be present. A TIA is one of the most important warning signs. A **transient ischemic attack** has been traditionally defined as a neurologic deficit caused by focal brain ischemia that completely resolves within 24 hours. This definition has been changed to "a brief episode of neurologic dysfunction caused by focal brain or retinal ischemia, with clinical symptoms typically lasting less than 1 hour, and without evidence of acute infarction."[3] This definition is tissue-based rather than time-based because some patients with traditionally defined TIAs have, in fact, had a stroke.[3] Some studies have shown positive magnetic resonance imaging (MRI) findings of stroke in up to two thirds of patients with a clinical TIA diagnosis. The longer the duration of symptoms, the more likely that the MRI result is positive.[3]

Most TIAs last only about 2 to 20 minutes.

A TIA is a significant indicator of stroke risk. About one quarter of patients presenting with stroke have had a previous TIA. About 5% of patients with a TIA will develop a completed stroke within 1 month if untreated.

A TIA should be treated with the same urgency as a completed stroke. When obtaining the patient's medical history, be sure to ask about previous TIAs and their frequency.

A **reversible ischemic neurologic deficit (RIND)** is a neurologic deficit that lasts more than 24 hours but leaves little or no neurologic deficit. However, full resolution may take weeks.

Brain damage may occur because of the infarction as well as an excessive buildup of fluid in the brain (cerebral edema). As brain tissue dies, fluid begins to build up, resulting in swelling. Because the skull is a rigid container, as swelling increases, nearby brain tissue is compressed (nerve cells, nerve tracts, and cerebral arteries), and intracranial pressure (ICP) increases. A sustained increase in pressure causes continued ischemia, irreparable damage to brain cells, and potentially death.

Cerebral edema usually peaks 2 to 5 days after the onset of the stroke. The fluid buildup then stabilizes and may begin to decrease.

Ischemic Penumbra. In an ischemic stroke, there are two main areas of injury (Figure 7-5). The first area is the zone of ischemia. Because of the blockage in the artery, there is little blood flow through this area. As a result, brain tissue previously supplied by the blocked vessel is deprived of O_2, glucose, and other essential nutrients. Unless blood flow is quickly restored, nerve cells and other supporting nervous system cells will be irreversibly damaged or die (infarct) within a few minutes of the blockage.

The second area of injury is called the ischemic penumbra ("transitional zone"). The penumbra is a rim of brain tissue that surrounds the zone of ischemia. It is supplied with blood by collateral arteries that connect with branches of the blocked vessel. The size of the penumbra depends on the number and patency of the collateral arteries. Blood flow to brain tissue in this area is decreased (between 20% and 50% of normal), but not absent. Brain tissue in the penumbra is "stunned" but not yet irreversibly damaged. Because the collateral blood supply is not enough to maintain the brain's demand for O_2 and glucose indefinitely, brain cells in the penumbra may live or die depending on how quickly blood flow is restored in the early hours of a stroke.

The time from onset of stroke symptoms until treatment is a key factor for success of any therapy. The earlier the treatment for stroke, the more favorable the results are likely to be. Blood flow needs to be restored to the affected area as quickly as possible. To date, only intravenous (IV) administration of a recombinant form of TPA (tissue plasminogen activator) (rtPA) has been proven to be effective. Intra-arterial fibrinolysis has been studied for treatment of selected patients with major stroke of less than 6 hours duration due to blockage of the middle cerebral artery.[4] Studies have shown that intraarterial administration of fibrinolytics is associated with a reduction in mortality and an improvement in favorable outcomes after a stroke. However, it is also associated with an increased risk of hemorrhagic complications. At present, no evidence is available to show that intraarterial fibrinolytic therapy is better than IV treatment.[5]

The window of opportunity to use IV rtPA to treat ischemic stroke patients is 3 hours. To be evaluated and receive treatment, patients need to be at a hospital within 60 minutes of symptom onset. Unfortunately, some stroke victims and their family members usually either cannot seek or fail to seek medical attention fast enough, precluding the use of rtPA.

KEEPING IT SIMPLE

- Trauma: "Golden Hour"
- Heart attack: "Time Is Muscle"
- Stroke: "Time Is Neurons" "Time Is Brain"

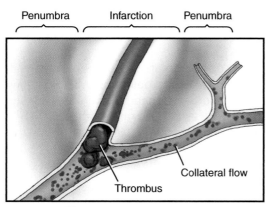
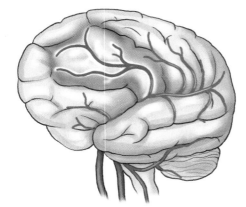

Figure 7-5 • Ischemic stroke. Zone of ischemia and the ischemic penumbra.

Hemorrhagic Stroke

A hemorrhagic stroke is caused by either rupture of an artery with bleeding onto the surface of the brain (subarachnoid hemorrhage [SAH]) or bleeding into the brain (intracerebral hemorrhage [IH]) (Figure 7-6).

Subarachnoid Hemorrhage

An aneurysm is the most common cause of SAH. A sudden onset of "the worst headache of my life" is a classic description of SAH. Arteriovenous (AV) malformations account for about 5% of all SAHs.

Initial mortality is high and rebleeding is common. Mortality from rebleeding is also high. Rebleeding most commonly occurs during the first day, usually within 12 hours after the initial hemorrhage.

Intracerebral Hemorrhage

Most IHs are associated with chronic hypertension. Small vessels within the brain are damaged by long-standing hypertension and eventually rupture and bleed. This type of stroke may require neurosurgery.

When we think of stroke, we usually associate it with older adults. But stroke can occur in persons of any age. Strokes can occur in utero, in infants, and in children. In infants and children, strokes are usually associated with:

- Birth defects
- Infections, such as meningitis, encephalitis
- Trauma
- Blood disorders, such as sickle cell disease

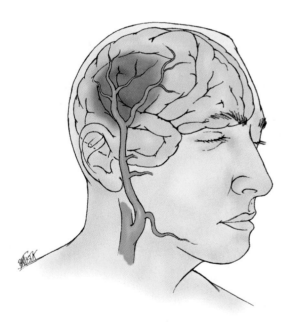

Figure 7-6 • Hemorrhagic stroke.

STROKE: CHAIN OF RECOVERY

Like the Chain of Survival used to describe the sequence of events needed to survive sudden cardiac death, the Chain of Recovery is a metaphor for the series of events that must occur in the emergency care of the possible stroke patient to improve his or her chances of full recovery (Figure 7-7). The critical links in the chain include the following[6]:

- Identification of stroke signs and symptoms by the patient or bystanders
- Immediate emergency medical services (EMS) system activation and appropriate dispatch with prearrival instructions
- Rapid EMS response, assessment, evacuation, and appropriate prehospital care
- Forewarning of the receiving stroke center for resource preparation and immobilization
- Rapid definitive diagnosis by experienced specialists at the stroke center

The Chain of Recovery has been modified in American Heart Association publications and is called the "The Stroke Chain of Survival and Recovery."[7,8] The chain consists of seven links:

1. *Detection* of the onset of stroke signs and symptoms

2. *Dispatch* through activation of the EMS system and prompt EMS response

3. *Delivery* of the patient to the receiving hospital while providing appropriate prehospital assessment and care and prearrival notification

4. *Door* (emergency department [ED] triage)

5. *Data* (ED evaluation, including computed tomography [CT])

6. *Decision* about potential therapies

7. *Drug* therapy

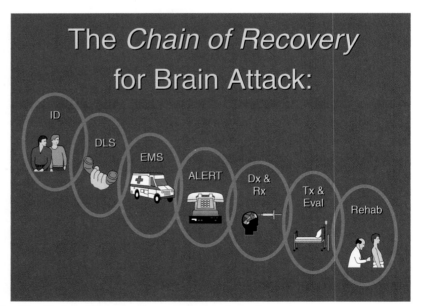

Figure 7-7 • The Chain of Recovery for acute ischemic stroke patients.
ID, identification of symptoms by the patient or bystanders; *DLS,* dispatch life support; *EMS,* Emergency Medical Services; *ALERT,* forewarning of receiving facility of impending arrival of stroke patient; *Dx & Rx,* diagnosis and medication; *Tx & Eval,* treatment and evaluation; *Rehab,* rehabilitation.

Components of the Stroke Chain of Survival and Recovery

Detection

In 1996, the Gallup Organization conducted a survey regarding stroke awareness for the National Stroke Association. In a survey of adults age 50 years or older

- 38% did not know where in the body a stroke occurs.
- 19% were unaware that there are things you can do to help prevent a stroke.
- Only 40% would call 9-1-1 immediately if they were having a stroke.
- Two thirds were unaware of the short time frame in which a person must seek treatment.
- 91% of older Americans could not identify sudden blurred or decreased vision in one or both eyes as a symptom of stroke.
- 85% could not identify loss of balance or coordination (a major sign when accompanied by another symptom) as a symptom of stroke.
- 68% could not identify difficulty in speaking or understanding simple statements as a stroke symptom.
- 42% could not identify weakness, numbness, or paralysis in face, arm, or leg as a stroke symptom.
- 17% were unable to name any symptoms at all.

Recognition of stroke signs and symptoms by the patient, family, or bystanders is critical. Although the Gallup Survey results listed here are more than 10 years old, they clearly reflect a need for public and patient education. This need is still present today.

Dispatch

Stroke victims and their families must be taught to activate the EMS system immediately on recognition of brain attack signs and symptoms. Currently, only half of stroke victims use the EMS system. Teach your patients and their family members the three Rs of stroke:

- Reduce risk.
- Recognize symptoms.
- Respond by calling 9-1-1.

Delivery

- Prehospital professionals should quickly perform a primary survey (initial assessment). If the patient's signs and symptoms suggest an acute stroke, begin transport and notify the receiving facility that the patient is en route. Consider transporting to a designated stroke center if time and protocols permit. Perform a focused or detailed physical examination en route as dictated by the patient's condition.
- Make sure the patient's airway remains open. Monitor the patient's breathing effort and be prepared to assist ventilations. If inadequate breathing is present, consider intubation. Apply a pulse oximeter and cardiac monitor. Give O_2 as needed and per physician instructions.
- Check the patient's serum glucose level. This helps to differentiate stroke from other common causes of stroke symptoms, such as hypoglycemia. Give dextrose if the patient is hypoglycemic. Give thiamine to alcoholic or malnourished individuals.
- Establish IV access with a saline lock or an IV line containing normal saline or lactated Ringer's solution and run at a keep-open rate (30 mL/hr). Obtain a 12-lead ECG. Do not delay transport to definitive care to perform these procedures.
- Perform a neurologic evaluation using the Cincinnati Prehospital Stroke Scale or other validated evaluation tool.
- Assess and support the patient's vital signs. In general, hypertension should not be treated in the prehospital setting. Hypotension should be treated aggressively in accordance with the underlying cause of the hypotension.
- Obtain an accurate history. Find out the patient's normal baseline mental status. Use a Prehospital Stroke Alert Checklist to screen patients for stroke signs and symptoms, time of onset, and contraindications to fibrinolytic therapy or other therapies that may become

available. Obtaining this information should not delay patient transport. Any information obtained should be relayed to the receiving facility.

- ▨ Encourage family members or bystanders to accompany the patient to the hospital so they can provide historical information to the treating team and provide support to the patient. If they cannot go to the hospital, obtain a telephone number where they can be contacted.
- ▨ Collect and/or document all medications. Medications that are particularly important include aspirin, warfarin (Coumadin), insulin, vand antihypertensives.
- ▨ Be familiar with the categorization/designation of hospitals in your area. Ideally, patients showing signs and symptoms of an acute stroke should be transported to a designated stroke center if the patient can be delivered to the center in 2 hours or less from the onset of stroke symptoms. The center should be notified of the patient's impending arrival.

Cincinnati Prehospital Stroke Scale

Facial droop/weakness: Ask patient, "Show me your teeth," or "Smile for me."
- Normal: Both sides of face move equally well
- Abnormal: One side of face does not move at all

Motor weakness (arm drift): With eyes closed, ask patient to extend arms out in front of him or her 90 degrees (if sitting) or 45 degrees (if supine). Drift is scored if the arm falls before 10 seconds.
- Normal: Both arms move the same *or* both arms do not move at all
- Abnormal: One arm either does not move or one arm drifts down compared to the other

Aphasia (speech): Ask the patient to say "A rolling stone gathers no moss," "You can't teach an old dog new tricks," "The sky is blue in Cincinnati," or a similar phrase.
- Normal: Phrase is repeated clearly and correctly
- Abnormal: Patient uses inappropriate words, words are slurred (dysarthria), or the patient is unable to talk

If any one of these signs is abnormal, stroke probability = 72%.

Modified from Kothari RU, Pancioli A, Liu T, Brott T, Broderick J. "Cincinnati Prehospital Stroke Scale: reproducibility and validity." *Ann Emerg Med* 1999 Apr;33(4):373-8.

Determining the time of symptom onset is critical. "For the purposes of treatment, the onset is assumed as the time that the patient was last known to be symptom-free. Because ischemic stroke is often painless, most patients are not awakened by its occurrence. Thus, for a patient with symptoms of stroke on awakening, the time of onset is assumed to be the time the patient was last known to be symptom-free before retiring. If a patient had mild impairments but then had worsening over the subsequent hours, the time the first symptom began is assumed to be the time of onset. In contrast, if a patient has symptoms that completely resolved (TIA) and then has a second event, the time of onset of the new symptoms is used."[4]

Door

Hospital EDs that accept stroke patients from EMS professionals should have the necessary personnel and procedures in place (such as a stroke team) to rapidly assess and treat stroke patients. The National Institute of Neurological Disorders and Stroke (NINDS) has established recommended target times for in-hospital evaluation and treatment of potential fibrinolytic candidates (Table 7-2).

Within 10 minutes of the patient's arrival:
- ▨ Reassess the patient's airway, breathing, circulation (ABCs) and take the patient's vital signs. Check the patient's BP in both upper extremities. BP elevation is common in the acute phase of stroke and may be a compensatory mechanism for reduced blood flow in the ischemic penumbra. Any treatment given should be based on multiple measurements taken 10 to 20 minutes apart, *never* on a single BP reading. Aggressive BP control may be provided if hemorrhagic stroke is present or if fibrinolytic therapy has been given.
- ▨ Check the patient's O_2 saturation and give O_2 as indicated.
- ▨ Make sure that an IV has been established. Avoid dextrose-containing solutions because they can increase swelling of the brain.

TABLE 7-2	NINDS-Recommended Stroke Evaluation Targets for Potential Fibrinolytic Candidates
Activity	**Target**
Door-to-physician evaluation	10 minutes
Door to access to neurological expertise (in person or by phone)	15 minutes
Door to computed tomography completion	25 minutes
Door to computed tomography read	45 minutes
Door to drug/intervention	60 minutes
Door to neurosurgical availability (on-site or by transport)	2 hours
Door to admission to monitored bed	3 hours

■ Check the patient's blood sugar and treat if indicated. Give dextrose if the patient is hypoglycemic. Give insulin if the patient's serum glucose is more than 300. Give thiamine if the patient is an alcoholic or malnourished.

■ Obtain a 12-lead ECG and assess for dysrhythmias.

■ Perform a general neurologic screening assessment and alert the stroke team: neurologist, radiologist, CT technician.

Within 25 minutes of the patient's arrival:

■ Review the patient's history.

■ Establish the time of symptom onset (<3 hours required for IV fibrinolytics). When was the last time the patient was known to be without symptoms? What was the patient doing when the symptoms began? Did the patient complain of a headache? Did he or she have a seizure? Has there been a change in his or her level of responsiveness? Is there a history of any recent trauma?

■ Review the patient's past medical history. Determine the presence of stroke risk factors. Find out the medications the patient is currently taking and the patient's allergies to medications.

■ Perform a physical exam.

■ Perform a neurologic exam. Scales are used in order to give quantifiable information to other members of the stroke team.

  ▶ Use the Glasgow Coma Scale (GCS) to determine level of responsiveness (Table 7-3). The GCS measures impairment but is of limited use in an intubated patient, a patient with orbital trauma, or a patient with previous neurologic impairment.

  ▶ Use the National Institutes of Health Stroke Scale (NIHSS) to determine the severity of the stroke (Table 7-4). The NIHSS is used to assess neurologic outcome and degree of recovery. Use of this scale allows a standardized way to assess outcome and compare outcomes with other centers. The scale consists of an 11-item, 42-point standardized scale. The NIHSS is usually performed by a neurologist and takes roughly 7 minutes to perform. Treatment should not be delayed by using this scale.

  • Scores of 0 or 1 indicate a normal or near-normal examination.

  • Scores of 1 to 4 indicate minor strokes, a score of 5 to 15 a moderate stroke, 15 to 20 a moderately severe stroke, and a score of more than 20 a severe stroke.

  • About 60% to 70% of patients with an acute ischemic stroke and a baseline NIHSS score <10 will have a favorable outcome after 1 year as compared with only 4% to 16% of those with a score >20.[4]

■ Diagnostic studies that should be obtained in all patients with suspected acute ischemic stroke include the following[4]:

  ▶ Urgent noncontrast CT scan of the brain. The purpose of the scan is to rule out other potential mimics of an ischemic event such as an intracranial tumor, abscess, or hemorrhage.[9] A CT scan may not detect an ischemic stroke for 6 to 72 hours after the initial infarction.[10] Brain MRI could be considered at qualified centers because it provides much more detailed infarct localization (which can be used to determine eligibility for localized fibrinolytic administration versus generalized administration) and more specificity in detecting ischemia in cases presenting in less than 6 hours.

  ▶ ECG, serum glucose, serum electrolytes, renal function tests.

  ▶ Complete blood count, including platelet count.

TABLE 7-3	Glasgow Coma Scale	
Eye Opening	**E-Score**	
Spontaneous	4	
To speech	3	
To pain	2	
No response	1	
Best Verbal Response	**V-Score**	
Oriented	5	
Confused	4	
Inappropriate	3	
Incomprehensible	2	
No response	1	
Best Motor Response	**M-Score**	
Obeys commands	6	
Localizes pain	5	
Withdrawal	4	
Abnormal flexion	3	
Extension	2	
No response	1	
No response	1	
Score: E+V+M	**15**	

> Prothrombin time/international normalized ratio (INR), activated partial thromboplastin time.

■ Diagnostic studies that should be obtained in selected patients with suspected acute ischemic stroke include the following[4]:

> Hepatic function tests
> Toxicology screen
> Blood alcohol determination
> Pregnancy test
> O_2 saturation or arterial blood gas tests (if hypoxia is suspected)
> Chest radiography (if lung disease is suspected)
> Lumbar puncture (if SAH is suspected and CT is negative for blood)
> Electroencephalogram (if seizures are suspected)
> Lateral cervical spine x-ray if the patient is comatose or has a history of trauma

Differential Diagnosis of Acute Stroke
- Hypoglycemia
- Trauma (such as a subdural hematoma)
- Hemorrhagic stroke (SAH, intracranial hemorrhage)
- Transient ischemic events that have not resolved at presentation
- Meningitis/encephalitis
- Hypertensive encephalopathy
- Intracranial mass
- Spinal cord, peripheral nerve disease
- Brain abscess
- Seizures/Todd's paralysis
- Infections
- Complex migraines
- Metabolic abnormalities (hypoglycemia/hyperglycemia, drug overdose)
- Bell's palsy

Item #	Category	Description	Score
TABLE 7-4	**National Institutes of Health Stroke Scale**		
1A	Level of consciousness (LOC)	Alert	0
		Drowsy	1
		Stuporous	2
		Coma/unresponsive	3
1B	Orientation questions (two): Ask patient month and age	Answers both correctly	0
		Answers one correctly	1
		Answers neither correctly	2
1C	Response to commands (two): Ask patient to open/close eyes, make fist, let go	Obeys both correctly	0
		Obeys one correctly	1
		Obeys neither correctly	2
2	Gaze: Look at position of eyes at rest, then ask patient to look to the left or right	Normal horizontal movements	0
		Partial gaze palsy	1
		Complete gaze palsy	2
3	Visual fields: Test by asking patient to count fingers in all four quadrants	No visual field defect	0
		Partial hemianopia	1
		Complete hemianopia	2
		Bilateral hemianopia	3
4	Facial movement: Ask patient to grimace or smile, puff out cheeks, pucker, and squeeze eyes shut	Normal	0
		Minor facial weakness	1
		Partial facial weakness	2
		Complete unilateral palsy	3
5	Motor function: Raise arm palm down to 90 degrees (sitting) or 45 degrees (supine) and score drift/movement a. Left arm b. Right arm	No drift: holds for full 10 seconds	0
		Drifts before 5 seconds	1
		Falls before 10 seconds	2
		No effort against gravity	3
		No movement	4
		Not tested (amputation, joint fusion)	9
6	Motor function: Raise leg to 30 degrees and score drift/movement a. Left leg b. Right leg	No drift: holds for full 5 seconds	0
		Drifts before 5 seconds	1
		Falls before 5 seconds	2
		No effort against gravity	3
		No movement	4
		Not tested (amputation, joint fusion)	9
7	Limb ataxia: Finger-to-nose and heel-to-shin tests	No ataxia	0
		Ataxia in one limb	1
		Ataxia in two limbs	2
8	Sensory: Pinprick to face, arm, trunk, leg, comparing side to side	No sensory loss	0
		Mild sensory loss	1
		Severe sensory loss	2
9	Language: Name groups of objects, read short sentences, describe a picture	Normal	0
		Mild aphasia	1
		Severe aphasia	2
		Mute or global aphasia	3
10	Articulation (speech clarity): Ask patient to read words or repeat a phrase	Normal	0
		Mild dysarthria	1
		Severe dysarthria	2
11	Extinction and inattention (neglect): Ask patient to describe features on right and left sides of a picture	Absent/no neglect	0
		Partial neglect	1
		Complete neglect	2
			Total:

Data

Data from the history and physical examination, laboratory studies, and imaging studies are used to help determine the patient's treatment plan.

Decision

A decision about potential therapies is made based on the data gathered and the type (hemorrhagic versus nonhemorrhagic), location (carotid/vertebrobasilar), and severity of the stroke.

Drug

If the patient meets the inclusion criteria, fibrinolytic therapy may be ordered for the treatment of acute ischemic stroke. Characteristics of patients with ischemic stroke who could be treated with rtPA are shown in Box 7-1. If the decision is made to use fibrinolytic therapy (rtPA), close monitoring of the patient is critical.

■ Monitor for bleeding and neurologic deterioration. Monitor the patient's BP every 15 minutes for 2 hours after the start of the infusion; then every 30 minutes for 6 hours; then every hour, from the 8th hour until 24 hours after the start of rtPA; then per routine.

■ Do not give antiplatelet or anticoagulant therapies for 24 hours.

■ Do not perform invasive procedures, intramuscular (IM) injections, or arterial punctures on noncompressible sites for 24 hours.

■ Obtain a brain CT scan 24 hours postinfusion or sooner if neurologic deterioration occurs.

BOX 7-1

Characteristics of Patients with Ischemic Stroke Who Could Be Treated with Recombinant Tissue Plasminogen Activator

- Diagnosis of ischemic stroke causing measurable neurologic deficit
- The neurological signs should not be clearing spontaneously
- The neurological signs should not be minor and isolated
- Caution should be exercised in treating a patient with major deficits
- The symptoms of stroke should not be suggestive of SAH
- Onset of symptoms <3 hours before beginning treatment
- No head trauma or prior stroke in previous 3 months
- No myocardial infarction in the previous 3 months
- No gastrointestinal or urinary tract hemorrhage in previous 21 days
- No major surgery in the previous 14 days
- No arterial puncture at a noncompressible site in the previous 7 days
- No history of previous intracranial hemorrhage
- BP not elevated (systolic BP <185 mm Hg and diastolic <110 mm Hg)
- No evidence of active bleeding or acute trauma (fracture) on examination
- Not taking an oral anticoagulant or if anticoagulant being taken, INR ≤1.7
- If receiving heparin in previous 48 hours, activated partial thromboplastin time must be in normal range
- Platelet count ≥100,000 mm^3
- Serum glucose concentration ≥50 mg/dL (2.7 mmol/L)
- No seizure with postictal residual neurologic impairments
- CT does not show a multilobar infarction (hypodensity >⅓ cerebral hemisphere)
- The patient or family understand the potential risks and benefits from treatment

From Adams H, Adams R, Del Zoppo G, Goldstein LB: *Stroke* Apr 2005;36(4):916-923.

QUICK REVIEW 7-1

1. The brain receives most of its blood via the _____ arteries.
2. True or False. Breast cancer affects more American women every year than stroke.
3. Briefly explain the difference between the two types of stroke.

4. What are the two main areas of injury in an ischemic stroke?
   1.
   2.
5. List the three areas evaluated when using the Cincinnati Prehospital Stroke Scale.
   1.
   2.
   3.

Answers can be found at the end of this chapter.

ELECTROLYTE ABNORMALITIES

Electrolyte disturbances are a common cause of dysrhythmias. If not corrected, electrolyte abnormalities can lead to cardiac arrest and complicate resuscitation and postresuscitation care. Knowing the possible causes and recognizing the signs and symptoms of electrolyte disorders can help prevent cardiac arrest.

POTASSIUM

Normal values: 3.5 to 5 mEq/L.

Hyperkalemia

Possible Causes

- Potassium supplements (oral and parenteral)
- Dietary—salt substitutes
- Stored blood
- Potassium-containing medications
- Acute and chronic renal failure
- Sickle cell disease
- Potassium-sparing diuretics
- Drug-induced (nonsteroidal anti-inflammatory drugs, angiotensin-converting enzyme [ACE] inhibitors, heparin)
- Transcellular shifts due to acidosis, hypertonicity, insulin deficiency; drugs such as beta-blockers and succinylcholine; digitalistoxicity; or exercise
- Rhabdomyolysis
- Burns and crush injuries

Clinical Features

Signs and symptoms of hyperkalemia are primarily seen as cardiovascular and neurologic changes.
- ECG changes correlate with the degree of hyperkalemia (Figure 7-8).

Serum Potassium Level	ECG Change
5.6-6 mEq/L	Tall, peaked (tented) T waves
6-6.5 mEq/L	Prolonged PR and QT intervals
6.5-7 mEq/L	P wave amplitude decreases, flattened ST-segments
7-8 mEq/L	P waves eventually disappear, QRS widens
8-12 mEq/L	Wide QRS complexes
>15 mEq/L	Ventricular fibrillation (VF), asystole

- Dysrhythmias may include second- and third-degree atrioventricular (AV) block, wide-complex tachycardia, VF, and asystole.
- Neuromuscular signs and symptoms include muscle cramps, weakness, paralysis, paresthesias, tetany, and focal neurologic deficits.

Initial Emergency Care

- ABCs, O$_2$, IV, monitor.
- Stop potassium intake (oral and IV).

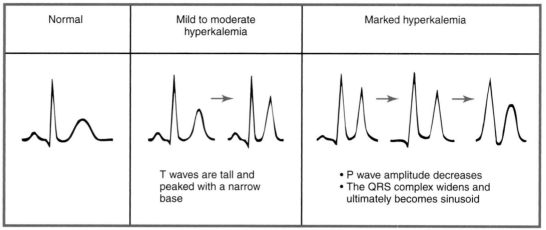

Normal	Mild to moderate hyperkalemia	Marked hyperkalemia
	T waves are tall and peaked with a narrow base	• P wave amplitude decreases • The QRS complex widens and ultimately becomes sinusoid

Figure 7-8 • ECG signs of hyperkalemia.

- Stop all medications that might be associated with hyperkalemia (ACE inhibitors, potassium-sparing diuretics).
- Mild hyperkalemia (5-6 mEq/L): Remove potassium from the body with furosemide, Kayexalate.
- Moderate hyperkalemia (6-7 mEq/L): Shift potassium into the cells with glucose plus insulin, sodium bicarbonate, or nebulized albuterol.
- Severe hyperkalemia (>7 mEq/L)
  - Shift potassium into the cells with calcium chloride, glucose plus insulin, sodium bicarbonate, or nebulized albuterol.
  - Remove potassium from the body with furosemide, Kayexalate, or dialysis.

Hypokalemia

Possible Causes

- Decreased intake of dietary potassium
- Impaired absorption of potassium
- Clay ingestion
- Increased loss due to hyperaldosteronism, glycyrrhizic acid (licorice, chewing tobacco), excessive adrenocorticosteroids, Cushing's syndrome, steroid therapy
- Drugs such as diuretics, aminoglycosides, and mannitol
- Gastrointestinal (GI) losses due to vomiting, nasogastric suction, diarrhea, malabsorption, ileostomy, laxative abuse
- Increased losses from the skin due to excessive sweating or burns
- Transcellular shifts due to vomiting, diuretics, bicarbonate therapy, insulin, $beta_2$ agonists (albuterol, terbutaline, epinephrine)
- IV hyperalimentation
- Acute mountain sickness

Clinical Features

- Lethargy, depression, irritability, and confusion
- Paresthesias, depressed deep tendon reflexes, fasciculations, and muscle pain and weakness
- Abdominal distention, cramping, nausea, and vomiting
- Severe deficiency results in death due to respiratory paralysis
- ECG changes correlate with the degree of hypokalemia (Figure 7-9).
  - T wave amplitude decreases.
  - T waves flatten, U waves appear.

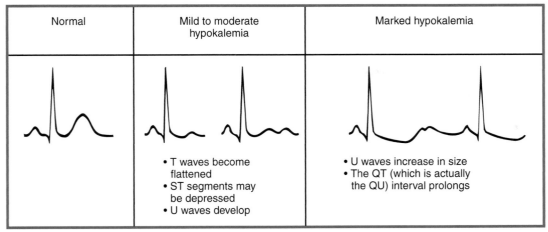

Normal	Mild to moderate hypokalemia	Marked hypokalemia
	• T waves become flattened • ST segments may be depressed • U waves develop	• U waves increase in size • The QT (which is actually the QU) interval prolongs

Figure 7-9 • ECG signs of hypokalemia.

▶ ST-segment becomes depressed.
▶ U waves increase in size; PR, QRS, and QT intervals lengthen.
▪ Bradydysrhythmias, AV blocks, AV dissociation, and ventricular tachycardia (VT) can occur.

Initial Emergency Care

▪ ABCs, O$_2$, IV, monitor
▪ Oral potassium preferred for mild hypokalemia, IV if unable to tolerate oral therapy
▪ Moderate hypokalemia (2.5-3 mEq/L): Oral potassium preferred, IV if unable to tolerate oral therapy
▪ Severe hypokalemia (<2.5 mEq/L): IV potassium replacement

SODIUM

Normal values: 135-145 mEq/L.

Hypernatremia

Hypernatremia most often occurs in very young, elderly, debilitated, or altered patients.

Possible Causes

Excessive sweating, burns, diarrhea, nasogastric suctioning, vomiting, and third-space fluid loss (ileus, pancreatitis, or bowel obstruction).

Clinical Features

▪ Clinical features typically result in central nervous system (CNS) changes such as altered mental status, agitation, irritability, focal neurologic deficits, seizures, and coma.
▪ Weakness, tremor, rigidity, and increased deep tendon reflexes may be present.
▪ Hypernatremia is not associated with any characteristic ECG changes.

Initial Emergency Care

▪ ABCs, O$_2$, IV, monitor.
▪ Treat the underlying cause.
▪ Replace fluid orally or via nasogastric tube if patient is stable and asymptomatic.
▪ IV normal saline or a 5% dextrose in half-normal saline solution is used to restore extracellular fluid volume in hypovolemic patients.

Hyponatremia

Possible Causes

- Hyperglycemia
- Sodium deficit due to hypovolemia: renal losses, GI losses, third-space losses, excessive sweating, Addison's disease
- Sodium deficit in the presence of normal volume: adrenal insufficiency, hypothyroidism, syndrome of inappropriate antidiuretic hormone secretion (SIADH), psychogenic polydipsia
- Sodium deficit due to hypervolemia: congestive heart failure, hepatic cirrhosis, nephrotic syndrome, renal failure

Clinical Features

- Signs and symptoms are dependent on the rate at which sodium is lost and the actual serum sodium level.
- Lethargy, confusion, disorientation, agitation, depression, psychosis, seizures, coma, and death.
- Hyponatremia is not associated with any characteristic ECG changes.

Initial Emergency Care

- ABCs, O_2, IV, monitor.
- Treatment depends on the patient's volume status.
- Hypovolemic patients need oral or IV sodium. Isotonic saline is usually used initially and then changed to a hypotonic fluid, such as 0.45% saline, once hypovolemia is corrected.
- Patients who have a normal volume or are hypervolemic are usually treated by restricting water. If significant fluid overload is present, a loop diuretic may be necessary.

MAGNESIUM

Normal values: 1.2 to 2.6 mEq/L.

Hypermagnesemia

Possible Causes

- Renal failure
- Lithium therapy
- Excessive use of magnesium-containing substances such as antacids, laxatives, cathartics, or excessive parenteral magnesium
- Impaired magnesium elimination due to anticholinergics, narcotics, chronic constipation, bowel obstruction
- Rhabdomyolysis
- Adrenal insufficiency
- Hyperparathyroidism
- Hypothyroidism

Clinical Features

- Early signs including nausea, vomiting, weakness, and flushing of the skin.
- Decreased and eventual loss of deep tendon reflexes.
- Hypotension, respiratory depression, coma.
- ECG changes include a prolonged PR interval, widening of the QRS complex, and elevated T waves. Dysrhythmias may include third-degree AV block and asystole.

Initial Emergency Care

- ABCs, O_2, IV, monitor.
- Stop magnesium intake (oral and IV).

■ Calcium chloride may be given IV if severe hypermagnesemia is present to reverse respiratory depression, hypotension, and cardiac dysrhythmias.
■ Dialysis, if severe.

Hypomagnesemia

Possible Causes

■ Diuretic therapy
■ Alcohol abuse
■ Excessive calcium or vitamin D intake
■ Giving IV fluids or total parenteral nutrition without magnesium replacement
■ GI losses such as chronic diarrhea, nasogastric suctioning, bowel fistula, and acute pancreatitis
■ Endocrine disorders such as diabetes mellitus, hyperaldosteronism, hyperthyroidism, and hyperparathyroidism
■ Pregnancy
■ Drugs such as diuretics, beta-agonists, aminoglycosides, cancer chemotherapy, and theophylline

Clinical Features

■ Altered mental status, muscle weakness, tremor, hyperreflexia, tetany, ataxia, dizziness, seizures, and dysphagia
■ Positive Chvostek's or Trousseau's sign
■ Supraventricular dysrhythmias: atrial fibrillation, multifocal atrial tachycardia, paroxysmal supraventricular tachycardia
■ Ventricular dysrhythmias: premature ventricular complexes (PVCs), VT, torsades de pointes, VF
■ ECG changes include diminished voltage of P waves and QRS complexes, prolongation of the PR, QRS, and QT intervals; ST-segment changes; flattening and widening of T waves; and presence of U waves

Initial Emergency Care

■ ABCs, O_2, IV, monitor
■ For severe or symptomatic hypomagnesemia, give magnesium sulfate IV

CALCIUM

Normal values: 4.5 to 5.5 mEq/L or 9 to 11 mg/dL.

Hypercalcemia

Possible Causes

Primary hyperparathyroidism and malignancy are the cause of most cases of hypercalcemia.

Clinical Features

■ Neurologic symptoms include depression, weakness, fatigue, and confusion that may progress to hallucinations, disorientation, seizures, and coma.
■ ECG changes include shortening of the QT interval, prolongation of the PR and QRS intervals, and flattening of T waves (Figure 7-10). Cardiac dysrhythmias may occur, particularly AV blocks. Bundle branch blocks may occur.
■ Other symptoms include nausea and vomiting, abdominal pain, dysphagia, constipation, peptic ulcers, and pancreatitis.

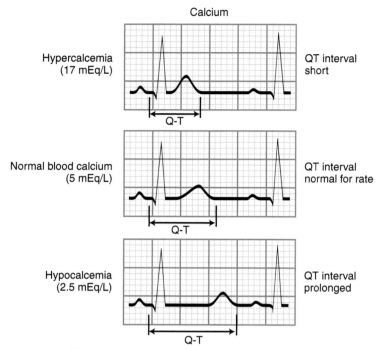

Figure 7-10 • ECG changes due to calcium.

Initial Emergency Care

- ABCs, O$_2$, IV, monitor.
- Give 0.9% saline IV to restore intravascular volume and induce diuresis.
- Watch potassium and magnesium levels closely.
- Patients with heart failure or renal insufficiency may need hemodialysis to rapidly decrease serum calcium.

Hypocalcemia

Possible Causes

- Hypoalbuminemia due to cirrhosis, nephrosis, malnutrition, burns, chronic illness, and sepsis
- Toxic shock syndrome, serum magnesium abnormalities, after thyroid surgery

Clinical Features

Paresthesias of the extremities and face, muscle cramping, shortness of breath due to bronchospasm, stridor, tetanic contractions, hyperreflexia, positive Chvostek's and Trousseau's signs, distal extremity numbness, angina, syncope, and heart failure due to decreased contractility.

Initial Emergency Care

- ABCs, O$_2$, IV, monitor.
- Calcium chloride or calcium gluconate IV.
- Watch magnesium, potassium, and pH closely.

TOXICOLOGY

■ A **poison** is a substance that, on ingestion, inhalation, absorption, application, injection, or development within the body in relatively small amounts, may cause structural damage or functional disturbance.

■ Poisons can be found in four forms: solid, liquid, spray, or gas.

  ▶ Solid poisons include medicines, plants, powders (e.g., laundry detergent, automatic dishwasher detergent), granular pesticides, and fertilizers.

  ▶ Liquid poisons include lotions, liquid laundry soap, furniture polish, lighter fluid, and syrup medicines.

  ▶ Poisons in spray form include insecticides, spray paint, and some cleaning products.

  ▶ Gases or vapors that are poisonous (invisible poisons) include carbon monoxide from hot water heaters and furnaces, exhaust fumes from automobiles, and fumes from gas or oil burning stoves.

POISON CONTROL CENTERS

■ Poison control centers (PCCs) provide free, 24-hour emergency telephone service for the public and medical professionals. 1-800-222-1222 is the telephone number for every poison center in the United States. Call this number 24 hours a day, 7 days a week to talk to a poison expert.

■ The telephone is staffed by medical personnel highly trained in the recognition and assessment of poisonings, first aid treatment, and drug information, reducing the time required to diagnose and establish definitive care for the poisoned patient.

■ The PCC is often contacted from the scene by EMS personnel requesting information and advice regarding the management of a poisoned patient. The ability to accept treatment orders/instructions from a PCC is based on local medical direction and local protocols.

ASSESSMENT OF THE PATIENT WITH A POSSIBLE TOXIC EXPOSURE

History

The history provides critical information in the assessment of the patient with a suspected toxic exposure. In addition to a SAMPLE history, critical questions to ask in a toxic exposure situation include what, when, where, why, and how.

■ What is the poison?

  ▶ Determine the exact name of the product, if possible.

  ▶ Obtain histories from different family members to help confirm the type and dose of exposure.

  ▶ Are there any pill bottles, commercial products, or plants to support the history?

■ How was it taken (i.e., ingested, inhaled, absorbed, or injected)?

■ When was it taken?

  ▶ Knowing the time of ingestion is critical when considering gastric emptying and antidote administration.

■ Where was the patient found? Any witnesses? Any others around?

■ How much was taken?

  ▶ Number of pills, amount of liquid.

  ▶ How many/amount available before ingestion?

  ▶ How many/much now in the container?

  ▶ Where is the substance stored?

  ▶ What is the patient's age? Weight?

  ▶ Has the patient vomited? How many times?

  ▶ What home remedies have been attempted? (Ask specifically about herbal or folk remedies.)

▶ Has a PCC been contacted? If so, what instructions were received? What treatment has already been given?

▶ Has the patient been depressed or experienced recent emotional stress?

Focused Physical Examination

When performing a physical examination on a patient with a known or suspected toxic exposure, be alert in your search for information regarding the severity and cause of the exposure. Changes in the patient's mental status, vital signs, skin temperature and moisture, and pupil size may provide a collection of physical findings that are typical of a specific toxin. Characteristic findings that are useful in recognizing a specific class of poisoning are called a *toxidrome* (Tables 7-5 and 7-6). Your physical examination findings may provide the only clues to the presence of a toxin if the patient is unresponsive. Familiarity with common toxidromes will enable you to recognize the diagnostic significance of your history and physical examination findings and implement an appropriate treatment plan.

TABLE 7-5	Clinical Presentations of Specific Toxidromes		
Toxidrome			
Anticholinergic	Signs/symptoms		Agitation or reduced responsiveness; tachypnea; tachycardia; slightly elevated temperature; blurred vision; dilated pupils; urinary retention; decreased bowel sounds; dry, flushed skin
	Typical agents		Atropine, diphenhydramine, scopolamine
	Primary antidote		Physostigmine
Cholinergic	Signs/symptoms		Altered mental status, tachypnea, bronchospasm, bradycardia or tachycardia, salivation, constricted pupils, polyuria, defecation, emesis, fever, lacrimation, seizures, diaphoresis
	Typical agents		Organophosphate insecticides (malathion), carbamate insecticides (carbaryl), some mushrooms, nerve agents
	Primary antidote		Atropine
Opioid	Signs/symptoms		Altered mental status, bradypnea or apnea, bradycardia, hypotension, pinpoint pupils, hypothermia
	Typical agents		Codeine, fentanyl, heroin, meperidine, methadone, oxycodone, dextromethorphan, propoxyphene
	Primary antidote		Naloxone
Sedative/Hypnotic	Signs/symptoms		Slurred speech, confusion, hypotension, tachycardia, pupil dilation or constriction, dry mouth, respiratory depression, decreased temperature, delirium, hallucinations, coma, paresthesias, blurred vision, ataxia, nystagmus
	Typical agents		Ethanol, anticonvulsants, barbiturates, benzodiazepines
	Primary antidote		Benzodiazepines: flumazenil
Sympathomimetic	Signs/symptoms		Agitation, tachypnea, tachycardia, hypertension, excessive speech and motor activity, tremor, dilated pupils, disorientation, insomnia, psychosis, fever, seizures, diaphoresis
	Typical agents		Albuterol, amphetamines (e.g., "ecstasy"), caffeine, cocaine, epinephrine, ephedrine, methamphetamine, phencyclidine, pseudoephedrine
	Primary antidote		Benzodiazepines

TABLE 7-6	Toxicology Memory Aids
Anticholinergic Syndrome (antihistamines, tricyclic antidepressants)	• Mad as a hatter: confused, delirium • Red as a beet: flushed skin • Dry as a bone: dry mouth • Hot as Hades: hyperthermia • Blind as a bat: dilated pupils
Cholinergic Syndrome	SLUDGE • **S**alivation, **L**acrimation, **U**rination, **D**efecation, **G**astrointestinal distress, **E**mesis DUMBELS • **D**iarrhea, **U**rination, **M**iosis (pinpoint pupils), **B**ronchospasm/**B**ronchorrhea/**B**radycardia, **E**mesis, **L**acrimation, **S**alivation

Mental Status

▓ Mental status is often affected by drugs and toxins.

▓ Anticholinergic agents, cocaine, amphetamines, ethanol, sedative-hypnotic withdrawal, and hypoglycemic agents frequently cause CNS stimulation, which is manifested as agitation and delirium.

▓ Benzodiazepines, sedative-hypnotics, barbiturates, and alcohols cause CNS depression. Agents such as ethanol and salicylates induce hypoglycemia, which may contribute to CNS depression. Some drugs, such as tricyclic antidepressants, cause dose-related CNS excitation and depression.

Toxins that Commonly Cause Seizures

• Camphor
• Cocaine
• Lithium
• Tricyclic antidepressants
• Isoniazid
• Lead
• Lidocaine
• Phenothiazines
• Salicylates
• Theophylline
• Beta-blockers
• Amphetamines

Airway

▓ Look for signs of airway edema, burns, excessive crying, stridor, and drooling. If the patient has any of these signs, suspect a significant airway injury.

▓ As you assess the patient's airway, note the presence of any odors that may help determine the cause of the patient's condition (Table 7-7).

▓ Use positioning or airway adjuncts as necessary to maintain an open airway and suction as needed.

▓ Perform endotracheal intubation if the airway cannot be maintained by positioning or if prolonged assisted ventilation is anticipated. Consider the use of pharmacologic adjuncts to aid in intubation.
  ▶ Severe upper airway injury following a caustic ingestion may prevent routine endotracheal intubation.
  ▶ The use of succinylcholine for rapid sequence intubation can result in prolonged paralysis in patients with organophosphate toxicity.

The effects of toxins may result in altered mental status, vomiting, or seizures, increasing the patient's risk of airway obstruction, aspiration, and lung damage. Be alert to potential airway problems and make sure suction is within reach.

TABLE 7-7	Odors and Toxins
Odor	**Toxin**
Acetone	Acetone, isopropyl alcohol, salicylates
Alcohol	Ethanol, isopropyl alcohol
Bitter almonds	Cyanide
Carrots	Water hemlock
Fishy	Zinc or aluminum phosphide
Fruity	Isopropyl alcohol, chlorinated hydrocarbons (e.g., chloroform)
Garlic	Arsenic, organophosphates, phosphorus, thallium
Glue	Toluene
Mothballs	Camphor
Pears	Chloral hydrate, paraldehyde
Rotten eggs	Sulfur dioxide, hydrogen sulfide
Shoe polish	Nitrobenzene
Vinyl	Ethchlorvynol
Wintergreen	Methyl salicylates

Breathing

- An increased respiratory rate may result from theophylline or hydrocarbon ingestion or from agents that cause metabolic acidosis such as ethylene glycol, methanol, and salicylates (the increased respiratory rate is a compensatory mechanism for acidosis).
- Noncardiogenic pulmonary edema is possible with any overdose that has led to apnea and has been associated with the following:
    - Heroin, meperidine, methadone, barbiturates, cocaine, or salicylates
    - Aspiration of chemicals such as kerosene and gasoline
    - Exposure to toxic gases such as chlorine, phosgene, and carbon monoxide
- Bradypnea may result from exposure to sedative/hypnotics, barbiturates, opioids, clonidine, alcohol, organophosphates, carbamates, strychnine, venom from the Mojave rattlesnake, and botulinum toxin.
- If ventilation is adequate, give 100% supplemental O_2 as necessary. If breathing is inadequate, assist ventilation using a bag-valve-mask device with 100% O_2. If abdominal distention occurs, consider placing a nasogastric tube (if not contraindicated) to release air from the stomach.

 Consider the possibility of a toxic exposure in an otherwise healthy patient with pulmonary edema.

Circulation

- Place the patient on a cardiac monitor.
- Sedative/hypnotics, opioids, beta-blockers, calcium channel blockers, digoxin, clonidine, organophosphates, and carbamate insecticides cause bradycardia.
- Examples of substances associated with an increased heart rate include amphetamines, caffeine, cocaine, ephedrine, phencyclidine, and theophylline.

 Remember, toxic exposures may include one or more toxidromes, especially in the case of intentional ingestion.

Vital Signs

Many toxins can produce changes in the patient's BP, heart rate, respiratory rate, and temperature (Table 7-8). The patient's mental status, skin temperature and moisture, and pupil size should also be assessed and documented. Frequent reassessment is important to note any trends or changes in the patient's condition.

Vital Sign	Increased	Decreased
Temperature	Amphetamines, anticholinergics, antihistamines, antipsychotic agents, cocaine, monoamine oxidase inhibitors, nicotine, phenothiazines, salicylates, sympathomimetics, theophylline, tricyclic antidepressants, serotonin reuptake inhibitors	Barbiturates, carbon monoxide, clonidine, ethanol, insulin, opiates, oral hypoglycemic agents, phenothiazines, sedative/hypnotics
Pulse	Amphetamines, anticholinergics, antihistamines, cocaine, phencyclidine, sympathomimetics, theophylline	Alcohol, beta-blockers, calcium channel blockers, carbamates, clonidine, cardiac glycosides, opiates, organophosphates
Respirations	Amphetamines, barbiturates (early), caffeine, cocaine, ethylene glycol, methanol, salicylates	Alcohols and ethanol, barbiturates (late), clonidine, opiates, sedative/hypnotics
BP	Amphetamines, anticholinergics, antihistamines, caffeine, clonidine, cocaine, marijuana, phencyclidine, sympathomimetics, theophylline	Antihypertensives, barbiturates, beta-blockers, calcium channel blockers, clonidine, cyanide, opiates, phenothiazines, sedative/hypnotics, tricyclic antidepressants (late)

TABLE 7-8 Toxins and Vital Sign Changes

■ When assessing the patient's O_2 saturation, remember the following:
  ▶ Any condition that reduces the strength of the arterial pulse may interfere with the measurement of the arterial oxyhemoglobin saturation (SpO_2). This includes hypotension, hypothermia, vasoconstrictive drugs, or placement of the oximeter sensor distal to a BP cuff.
  ▶ Pulse oximeters may record falsely elevated amounts of oxyhemoglobin in patients with abnormal forms of hemoglobin, such as carboxyhemoglobin or methemoglobin. Be alert for signs of adequate ventilation but poor perfusion (frequently seen in significant cyanide exposures).

Pupils

Assessment of pupil size is important in the evaluation of a toxic patient. Pupil dilation is a less specific physical finding than pupil constriction.
■ Substances such as opioids, clonidine, phencyclidine, and some sedative/hypnotics may cause constricted pupils. Meperidine (Demerol) is an opioid that may cause pupil dilation.
■ Pupil dilation may result from sympathomimetics, anticholinergics, antihistamines, and hypoxia.
■ Nystagmus (rapid, jerky eye movement) may be seen with exposure to anticonvulsants (especially carbamazepine and phenytoin), lithium, ethanol, barbiturates, sedative/hypnotics, monoamine oxidase inhibitors, isoniazid, and phencyclidine.

GENERAL GUIDELINES FOR MANAGING THE POISONED PATIENT

Most poisoned patients require only supportive therapy. General guidelines for management of the poisoned patient include the following:
■ Use personal protective equipment. Ensure adequate airway, ventilation, and circulation. If cervical spine trauma is suspected, manually stabilize the spine until the patient has been fully stabilized to a backboard or the cervical spine has been cleared.
■ Obtain a thorough history and perform a focused physical examination.
■ Consider hypoglycemia in an unresponsive or seizing patient. Check blood sugar.
■ Initiate cardiac monitoring and obtain vascular access as indicated.
■ Frequently monitor vital signs and ECG.

- In the prehospital setting, safely obtain any substance or substance container of a suspected poison and transport it with the patient.
- Consult with a clinical toxicologist/PCC as needed for specific treatment to prevent further absorption of the toxin (or antidotal therapy).

Tables 7-9 through 7-20 provide a list of commonly ingested substances, associated signs and symptoms, and possible treatment.

 The poisoned patient may require treatment that differs from standard ACLS guidelines. It is important to recognize the signs and symptoms of poisoning and consult a clinical toxicologist/PCC for assistance in determining an appropriate patient treatment plan.

TABLE 7-9	Anticholinergics
Description	Common products: diphenhydramine, doxylamine
Signs/Symptoms	• Tachycardia, supraventricular and ventricular dysrhythmias
	• Impaired conduction, shock, cardiac arrest
Treatment	• ABCs, O$_2$, IV, monitor
	• Physostigmine

TABLE 7-10	Beta-Blockers
Description	• Slow-release forms may lead to delayed and prolonged toxicity
	• Common products: propranolol, metoprolol , atenolol, sotalol
Signs/Symptoms	• Bradycardia, heart blocks, and hypotension are the hallmarks of significant beta-blocker toxicity*
	• Possible altered mental status; dyspnea due to bronchospasm or heart failure
	• Possible bronchospasm in asthmatic individuals
	• Seizures, coma, shock, cardiac arrest
Treatment	• ABCs, O$_2$, IV, monitor
	• Have pacemaker at bedside
	• Atropine has shown inconsistent effects in reversing bradycardia and hypotension*
	• Fluid challenges of normal saline and vasopressors may be needed to maintain BP
	• Possible calcium infusion
	• Possible glucose plus insulin infusion or glucagon
	• CBC, electrolytes, glucose

*Holstege CP, Dobmeier S: Cardiovascular challenges in toxicology. *Emerg Med Clin North Am* Nov 2005;23(4):1195-1217.
CBC, Complete blood (cell) count.

TABLE 7-11	Calcium Channel Blockers

Description	• Calcium channel blockers consist of four structural classes:
	  1. Dihydropyridines (nicardipine, nifedipine, isradipine, amlodipine, felodipine, and nimodipine)
	  2. Phenylalkylamines (verapamil)
	  3. Benzothiazepines (diltiazem)
	  4. Diarylaminopropylamine ethers (bepridil)
	• Slow-release forms may lead to delayed and prolonged toxicity

Signs/Symptoms	• Bradycardia with variable degrees of AV block and hypotension • Lightheadedness or dizziness, especially upon standing • Possible altered mental status • Hyperglycemia (secondary to blockage of insulin release); seizures, coma • Symptomatic patients are prone to development of pulmonary edema
Treatment	• ABCs, O_2, IV, monitor • Treat bradycardia per resuscitation guidelines; have pacer at bedside; atropine may be ineffective at reversing the bradycardia • Possible calcium chloride or calcium gluconate • Possible glucose plus insulin infusion or glucagon • Fluid challenges of normal saline and vasopressors may be needed to maintain BP • Pacemakers, intra-aortic balloon pump, extracorporeal membrane oxygenation, and cardiopulmonary bypass may all be considered in cases not responding to drug therapy* • CBC, electrolytes, glucose

*Holstege CP, Dobmeier S: Cardiovascular challenges in toxicology. *Emerg Med Clin North Am* Nov 2005;23(4):1195-1217.

TABLE 7-12	Carbamate Insecticides
Description	• Less toxic than organophosphates, but effects are similar • Toxicity is usually limited to muscarinic effects; nicotinic effects uncommon • Common products: flea and tick powders, ant killers
Signs/Symptoms	Muscarinic effects: vomiting, diarrhea, abdominal cramping, bradycardia, excessive salivation, and sweating
Treatment	• Protective equipment, remove contaminated clothing • ABCs, O_2, IV, monitor • Atropine is given until signs of muscarinic toxicity (e.g., symptomatic bradycardia, bronchorrhea, or wheezing) are reversed • Treat coma and seizures if they occur

TABLE 7-13	Cardiac Glycosides
Description	• Used for treatment of congestive heart failure and supraventricular dysrhythmias • Several plants contain cardiac glycosides (digoxin-like substances), including foxglove, oleander, and lily of the valley
Signs/Symptoms	• Altered mental status, nausea and vomiting, abdominal pain, headache • Almost any cardiac dysrhythmia may occur
Treatment	• ABCs, O_2, IV, monitor • Restore potassium, magnesium, intravascular volume • Treat symptomatic or unstable dysrhythmias per resuscitation guidelines; pacemaker should be used with caution • Monitor for ventricular dysrhythmias • Give antidote (digoxin immune Fab [Digibind]) for life-threatening dysrhythmias caused by digoxin overdose • Gastric aspiration or lavage may increase vagal tone and precipitate bradydysrhythmias • Avoid calcium when treating digoxin toxicity • Serum digoxin level, electrolytes (especially potassium, calcium, magnesium), renal panel, liver function tests, continuous ECG

TABLE 7-14	Clonidine
Description	• Used for the treatment of hypertension and sometimes used to alleviate opioid and nicotine withdrawal symptoms • Available in pills and sustained-release transdermal patches
Signs/Symptoms	• Altered mental status, pupil constriction, respiratory depression (Note: these symptoms can appear exactly like opiate toxicity, making it difficult to distinguish clonidine ingestion from opiate overdose). • Hypotension, bradycardia, (may be initially hypertensive)
Treatment	• ABCs, O_2, IV, monitor • Treat coma, hypotension, bradycardia and hypothermia (usually resolve with supportive measures such as fluids, atropine, dopamine, and warming) • Naloxone may be helpful in reversing effects (conflicting evidence) • Gastric decontamination (lavage preferred)

TABLE 7-15	Isoniazid
Description	• Used in the treatment of tuberculosis; depletes vitamin B_6, which is required for synthesis of GABA, an inhibitory neurotransmitter. Reduced GABA concentration can lead to seizures. • Initial signs of poisoning typically appear within 30 minutes to 2½ hours of ingestion.
Signs/Symptoms	• Altered mental status, tachypnea, hypotension, slurred speech, dizziness, ataxia, vomiting, bradycardia or tachycardia. • Lactic acidosis with or without seizures. • May progress to coma, shock, cardiac arrest.
Treatment	• ABCs, O_2, IV, monitor. • Treat coma, seizures, and metabolic acidosis if they occur. • Pyridoxine (vitamin B_6) is specific antidote and usually stops diazepam-resistant seizures; large doses of pyridoxine may be needed.

GABA, Gamma-aminobutyric acid.

"Coma Cocktail"
- **D**$_{50}$W
- **O**xygen
- **N**aloxone
- **T**hiamine

TABLE 7-16	Opiates
Description	Common products: codeine, fentanyl, heroin, meperidine, methadone, oxycodone, dextromethorphan, propoxyphene.
Signs/Symptoms	• Altered mental status, slow and shallow respirations or apnea, bradycardia, hypotension, pinpoint pupils. • Suspect opioid toxicity when the triad of CNS depression, respiratory depression, and miosis (pinpoint pupils) is present.
Treatment	• ABCs, O_2, IV, monitor. • Endotracheal intubation is indicated in patients who cannot protect their airway. • Obtain serum glucose level; give dextrose if indicated. • Give Naloxone for significant CNS and/or respiratory depression. Assist respirations with a bag-valve mask as necessary. If an IV cannot be established, naloxone can be given by the IM, SubQ, intranasal, or endotracheal routes. • Larger than usual doses of naloxone may be required for diphenoxylate/atropine (Lomotil), methadone, propoxyphene, pentazocine, and the fentanyl derivatives.

SubQ, Subcutaneous

TABLE 7-17	Organophosphates
Description	• Widely used pesticides; signs and symptoms usually occur within 30 minutes to 2 hours of exposure but may be delayed up to several hours • Chemical pneumonitis may occur if a product containing a hydrocarbon solvent is aspirated • In the acute phase, there is no test that can identify organophosphate toxicity; initial management based on clinical findings • Common products: No-Pest Strips, roach killers, diazinon, malathion, parathion
Signs/Symptoms	• Early signs are muscarinic: nausea, vomiting, abdominal cramps, urinary and fecal incontinence, increased bronchial secretions, cough, wheezing, dyspnea, sweating, salivation, miosis, blurred vision, lacrimation • Nicotinic effects include twitching, fasciculations, weakness, hypertension, tachycardia, and in severe cases paralysis and respiratory failure; death is usually caused by respiratory muscle paralysis • There is often a solvent odor and some describe a garlic-like odor of the organophosphate • Pay careful attention to respiratory muscle weakness; sudden respiratory arrest may occur
Treatment	• Protective equipment, remove contaminated clothing, decontamination procedures; ABCs, O_2, IV, monitor • Atropine is antidote for muscarinic effects; goal is drying of airway secretions to maintain oxygenation and ventilation—tachycardia is *not* a contraindication to its use—treatment must usually continue for at least 24 hours • Pralidoxime is antidote for nicotinic effects; treatment is generally necessary for at least 48 hours • If intubation is required, note potential interactions between neuromuscular blockers and organophosphates

TABLE 7-18	Sodium Channel Blockers
Description	Common substances: carbamazepine, Class I antiarrhythmics (disopyramide, quinidine, procainamide, lidocaine, encainide, flecainide, propafenone), cocaine
Signs/Symptoms	Bradycardia, ventricular dysrhythmias, widening of the QRS complex, seizures, shock, cardiac arrest
Treatment	• ABCs, O_2, IV, monitor • Sodium bicarbonate if QRS >0.10 second, persistent hypotension despite adequate hydration, or dysrhythmias* • Pacing may be needed • Lidocaine for treatment of ventricular dysrhythmias (except in lidocaine overdose) • Closely monitor electrolytes, pH, and fluid balance

*Holstege CP, Dobmeier S: Cardiovascular challenges in toxicology. *Emerg Med Clin North Am* Nov 2005;23(4):1195-1217.

TABLE 7-19	Stimulants (Sympathomimetics)
Description	Common substances: Amphetamines, methamphetamines, cocaine, PCP, ephedrine
Signs/Symptoms	• Tachycardia, supraventricular and ventricular dysrhythmias
	• Hypertensive crises, acute coronary syndromes, shock, cardiac arrest
Treatment	• ABCs, O$_2$, IV, monitor
	• Watch for and treat seizures
	• Assess temperature to rule out hyperthermia
	• Interventions may include benzodiazepines, lidocaine, sodium bicarbonate (for cocaine-related ventricular dysrhythmias), nitroglycerin, nitroprusside, phentolamine
	• Beta-blockers are relatively contraindicated

PCP, Phencyclidine.

TABLE 7-20	Tricyclic Antidepressants
Description	• Cause intraventricular conduction delays and serious dysrhythmias; also have anticholinergic effects
	• Progression from early to late symptoms may be rapid
	• Common products: amitriptyline, desipramine, imipramine, nortriptyline
Signs/Symptoms	• Early signs: tachycardia, restlessness, anxiety, increased temperature
	• Late signs (4 Cs): coma, convulsions, conduction defects (PR lengthening, widening of QRS complex, prolonging of QT interval), decreased contractility
	• Hypertension initially, then hypotension, dilated pupils, slurred speech, blurred vision, dry mouth, urinary retention
	• Supraventricular and ventricular dysrhythmias
Treatment	• ABCs, O$_2$, IV, monitor
	• Watch for and treat seizures, prevent injury
	• Continuous ECG monitoring, even in the patient who is asymptomatic at presentation
	• Treat symptomatic or unstable dysrhythmias per resuscitation guidelines; sodium bicarbonate for ventricular dysrhythmias
	• If hypotension present, IV fluid bolus; monitor for pulmonary edema; vasopressors for persistent hypotension
	• Other interventions may include hyperventilation and the use of magnesium sulfate, lidocaine, epinephrine IV
	• Serum/urine toxicology screen, cardiac enzymes, electrolytes; serum drug levels do not necessarily predict outcome and are not helpful in acute management

The "4 Cs" of Tricyclic Antidepressant Overdose
- **C**oma
- **C**onvulsions
- **C**onduction defects
- Decreased **c**ontractility

Prolonged resuscitation may be warranted for victims of poisoning or overdose.

DROWNING

Drowning is "a process resulting in primary respiratory impairment from submersion/immersion in a liquid medium. Implicit in this definition is that a liquid/air interface is present at the entrance of the victim's airway, preventing the victim from breathing air. The victim may live or die after this process, but whatever the outcome, he or she has been involved in a drowning incident"[11] (Figure 7-11).

■ "Immersion means to be covered in water or other fluid. For drowning to occur, usually at least the face and airway must be immersed. Submersion implies that the entire body, including the airway, is under the water or other fluid."[12]

■ The term "near-drowning" should no longer be used. The International Liaison Committee on Resuscitation (ILCOR) also recommends that the following terms should no longer be used: dry and wet drowning, active and passive drowning, silent drowning, secondary drowning, and drowned versus near-drowned.[13]

■ The major physiologic consequences of submersion are hypoxia, acidosis, and pulmonary edema. Of these, hypoxia is the most important.

■ Factors affecting patient outcome include water temperature, duration and degree of hypothermia, the diving reflex, the victim's age, water contamination, duration of cardiac arrest, the promptness and effectiveness of initial treatment, and cerebral resuscitation.[14]

■ Hypothermia may be associated with drowning.

■ Begin efforts to restore oxygenation, ventilation, and perfusion as quickly as possible.
  ❯ Bystander CPR
  ❯ Immediate EMS activation

■ If *any* type of resuscitation is required for a drowning victim, the patient should be transported to the hospital for evaluation.
  ❯ The most important factors that determine patient outcome are the duration and severity of hypoxia.

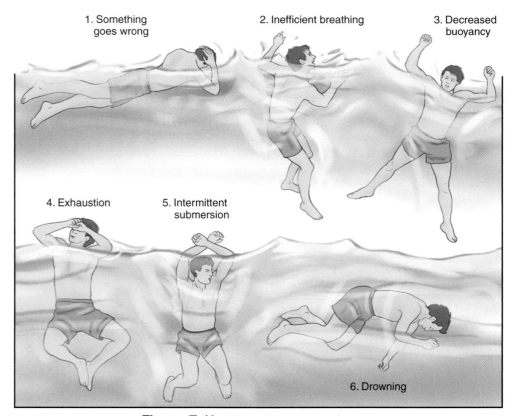

1. Something goes wrong
2. Inefficient breathing
3. Decreased buoyancy
4. Exhaustion
5. Intermittent submersion
6. Drowning

Figure 7-11 • Drowning events and stages.

▶ Resuscitation should begin at the scene and the patient should be transported unless there are signs of obvious death.

 When providing emergency care for a drowning victim, always remember personal safety.

 In situations involving a drowning victim, it is important to find out how long the victim was submersed, the fluid in which the victim was submersed, and the events surrounding the incident.

BASIC LIFE SUPPORT FOR DROWNING

■ Remove the victim from the water as quickly as possible.
■ Ventilation is the most important treatment for a drowning victim. Rescue breathing should be started as soon as the victim's airway can be opened and the rescuer's safety can be assured (usually when the victim is in shallow water or out of the water) (Figure 7-12).
■ Cervical spine stabilization is unnecessary unless there is a history of diving, use of a water slide, signs of injury, or signs of alcohol intoxication.[11] If the incident was not witnessed, assume cervical spine injury and provide in-line stabilization.
■ There is no need to clear the airway of aspirated water; however, debris, gastric contents, or other foreign material may need to be removed. Routine use of abdominal thrusts or the Heimlich maneuver is not recommended. These procedures can cause injury, vomiting, and aspiration, and delay CPR.
■ After removal from the water, begin CPR at once if a pulse cannot be felt. It may be difficult to feel a pulse because of peripheral vasoconstriction and decreased cardiac output. If the rescuer is alone, give 5 cycles (about 2 minutes) of CPR before leaving the victim to activate the EMS system.
■ Attach an automated external defibrillator (AED) and attempt defibrillation if a shockable rhythm is identified.

See Box 7-2 for interesting facts about drowning.

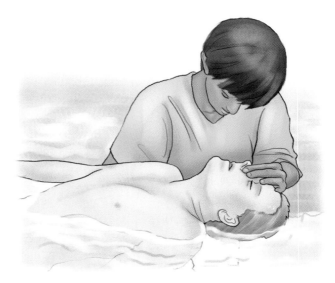

Figure 7-12 • Rescue breathing for a drowning victim in shallow water.

BOX 7-2

Interesting Drowning Facts

- Drowning is the fourth most common cause of all accidental deaths in the United States.
- Drowning is one of the leading causes of injury deaths among children and adolescents.
- Toddlers (younger than 2 years old) and teenage boys (aged 10 to 19 years) at greatest risk of drowning.
- Drowning occurs in freshwater lakes and rivers, saltwater bodies, swimming pools, bathtubs, and buckets.
- The residential swimming pool is the number one site of drowning for victims younger than 5 years of age; the bathtub is the second most common home site.
- Lakes, rivers, and saltwater bodies are common sites of adolescent and adult drowning.
- Inadequate supervision appears to be the most common factor predisposing a toddler to a submersion event. For adults and adolescents, alcohol is a significant risk factor.
- "The use of a solar blanket on a residential pool is also identified as a risk for submersion injuries. The solar blanket is a double layer of heavy plastic—with small air spaces that float on the surface of the pool—but that is not secured at the edge of the pool. The blanket will support a small or lightweight toy, but not the weight of a child. If a toddler attempts to retrieve an object from the blanket, it will slip and allow the child to submerge in the pool. Often, the blanket slides back over the child, trapping him or her in the pool, while obscuring view of the submerged child."

From Feldhaus KM: Submersion. In Marx JA (Ed.): *Rosen's emergency medicine: concepts and clinical practice* (5th ed.), Mosby, 2002.

ADVANCED LIFE SUPPORT FOR DROWNING

■ Give high flow O_2. Continuous positive airway pressure may be necessary to improve oxygenation.

■ Early endotracheal intubation may be necessary. "The decision to intubate a spontaneously breathing patient should be based on the degree of respiratory distress, the presence or absence of protective airway reflexes, the ability to maintain adequate tissue oxygenation based on pulse oximetry, and the presence of associated head or chest injuries. Patients with a PaO_2 level less than 50 mm Hg or a partial pressure of carbon dioxide (CO_2) more than 50 mm Hg on 100% O_2 require intubation."[14]

■ If the patient is in cardiac arrest, consider endotracheal intubation early in the resuscitation effort. Treat cardiac arrest rhythms according to the appropriate ACLS algorithm.

■ Suspect hypothermia in any drowning incident. Hypothermia is discussed later in this chapter.

■ Avoid excessive fluid administration, which may cause pulmonary edema.

NEAR-FATAL ASTHMA

Asthma is a reversible obstructive airway disease characterized by three important abnormalities: chronic airway inflammation, episodes of bronchoconstriction, and mucus plugging (Figure 7-13). Wheezing is an unreliable sign when evaluating the degree of distress in an asthmatic patient. An absence of wheezing may represent severe obstruction. With improvement, wheezing may become more prominent. Causes of wheezing other than asthma are shown in Box 7-3.

A

B

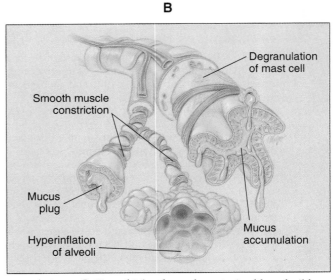

Figure 7-13 • Airway obstruction caused by asthma. **A,** The normal airway. **B,** Bronchial asthma characterized by a build up of mucus, swelling of the mucosa, and smooth muscle spasm, which causes obstruction of small airways.

BOX 7-3

Causes of Wheezing Other Than Asthma

- Pulmonary edema
- Chronic obstructive pulmonary disease
- Pneumonia
- Anaphylaxis
- Foreign bodies
- Pulmonary embolism
- Bronchiectasis
- Subglottic mass

INITIAL STABILIZATION

Assess the asthma patient's ability to complete a sentence (age dependent), presence of a cough, breathlessness, and chest tightness. Assess pulse rate, respiratory rate, breath sounds, use of accessory muscles, and presence of suprasternal retractions. Close monitoring is essential. Initial stabilization of the patient who has life-threatening asthma includes the use of O_2, bronchodilators, and steroids. A pulmonologist or intensivist should be consulted if the patient does not respond to treatment.

- Give O_2 to all patients to maintain O_2 saturation >92%.
- Give albuterol. Continuous administration may be more effective than intermittent administration.
- To reduce inflammation, all asthma patients should receive systemic corticosteroids as early as possible, although effects may not be evident for several hours. Because patients with near-fatal asthma may vomit or be unable to swallow, the IV route is preferred.[15] Prehospital administration of systemic corticosteroids should be considered.

ADJUNCTIVE THERAPY[16]

- Anticholinergics
  - Ipratropium bromide
    - Anticholinergic bronchodilator
    - Slow onset of action (about 20 minutes), peak effects at 60 to 90 minutes
    - Considered as an adjunct to albuterol

- ◗ Tiotropium
  - New, longer-acting anticholinergic
  - Currently undergoing clinical testing for use in acute asthma
- Magnesium sulfate
  - ◗ Causes bronchial smooth muscle relaxation
  - ◗ When given IV, can improve pulmonary function when combined with nebulized beta-agonists and corticosteroids
    - Usually given IV over 20 minutes
  - ◗ Nebulized magnesium sulfate may also improve pulmonary function during acute asthma when given with a beta$_2$-agonist
- Parenteral epinephrine or terbutaline
  - ◗ Can be given SubQ to patients with acute severe asthma
  - ◗ SubQ epinephrine is given in three divided doses about 20 minutes apart
    - Use 1:1000 epinephrine
    - May increase heart rate, myocardial irritability, and O_2 demand
  - ◗ Terbutaline is given SubQ and can be repeated in 30 to 60 minutes
- Ketamine
  - ◗ Dissociative anesthetic with bronchodilatory properties
  - ◗ Stimulates copious bronchial secretions
- Heliox
  - ◗ Mixture of helium and O_2 (usually a 70:30 helium to O_2 ratio mix)
  - ◗ Has been shown to improve delivery and deposition of nebulized albuterol
  - ◗ May be useful for asthma that is refractory to conventional therapy
  - ◗ If more than 30% O_2 needed by patient, cannot be used
  - ◗ Inadequate evidence to recommend for or against use of heliox during cardiac arrest
- Methylxanthines
  - ◗ Infrequently used due to erratic pharmacokinetics and side effects
- Leukotriene antagonists
  - ◗ Effectiveness during acute asthma exacerbations unproven
- Inhaled anesthetics
  - ◗ May work as bronchodilators
  - ◗ May reduce O_2 demand and CO_2 production
  - ◗ Requires an intensive care unit (ICU)
  - ◗ No studies to evaluate effectiveness

ASSISTED VENTILATION[17]

- Intubation and positive-pressure ventilation can trigger further bronchoconstriction and complications such as breath stacking and barotrauma.
  - ◗ Breath stacking can lead to hyperinflation, tension pneumothorax, and hypotension.
  - ◗ Manual and mechanical ventilation differs from that provided to nonasthmatic patients.
    - Use slower respiratory rate (6 to 10 breaths/min).
    - Use smaller tidal volumes (6 to 8 mL/kg).
    - Use shorter inspiratory time (adult inspiratory flow rate 80-100 mL/min).
    - Use longer expiratory time (inspiratory to expiratory ratio 1:4 or 1:5).
- Perform elective intubation if the asthmatic patient deteriorates despite aggressive therapy.
  - ◗ Rapid sequence intubation is technique of choice.
  - ◗ To decrease airway resistance, use the largest endotracheal tube available.
  - ◗ Confirm tube placement after insertion.
  - ◗ Sedation may be needed after intubation.
- If the patient deteriorates or becomes difficult to ventilate after intubation, use the DOPE memory aid to troubleshoot (Box 7-4).

> **BOX 7-4**
>
> **Troubleshooting Inadequate Ventilation or Oxygenation (DOPE)**
>
> - **D**isplaced tube (right mainstem or esophageal intubation)—Reassess tube position
> - **O**bstructed tube (secretions obstructing air flow)—Suction
> - **P**neumothorax (tension)—Needle thoracostomy
> - **E**quipment problem/failure—Check equipment and O_2 source

ANAPHYLAXIS

Anaphylaxis occurs when the body is exposed to a substance that produces a severe allergic reaction that usually occurs within minutes of the exposure. Type I hypersensitivity occurs when an individual is exposed to a specific allergen and develops immunoglobulin E (IgE) antibodies. These antibodies attach to mast cells in specific body locations, creating sensitized mast cells. On reexposure to the same allergen, histamine and other substances are released. These substances cause widespread arterial and venous vasodilation and increase capillary permeability (Figure 7-14).

Intravascular fluid leaks into the interstitial space, resulting in a decrease in intravascular volume (relative hypovolemia). The decrease in intravascular volume results in decreased cardiac preload and worsens hypotension. Increased blood vessel permeability causes swelling that is noticeable in the mucous membranes of the larynx (stridor), trachea, and bronchial tree, increasing the potential for complete airway obstruction due to severe edema.

CAUSES

- Latex
- Medications including antibiotics (especially penicillins, sulfa), aspirin, nonsteroidal anti-inflammatory drugs, muscle relaxants, antiserum, and IV radiocontrast agents
- Insect stings (ants, bees, hornets, wasps, yellow jackets)
- Foods such as peanuts, tree nuts, shellfish, wheat, and strawberries
- Unidentified cause (idiopathic)

ASSESSMENT FINDINGS

- Anxiety, restlessness
- Stridor, wheezing, coughing, hoarseness, intercostal and suprasternal retractions
- Tachycardia, hypotension, dysrhythmias
- Abdominal pain, vomiting, diarrhea
- Facial swelling and angioedema
- Urticaria (hives)
- Abdominal pain, cramping
- Pruritus (itching)

INITIAL EMERGENCY CARE

- ABCs, O_2, IV, cardiac monitor, pulse oximeter.
- Remove/discontinue the causative agent.
  - If a stinger is present, remove it by scraping it away or brushing it off.
- Give epinephrine 0.3 to 0.5 mg IM (use 1:1000 solution) early to all patients who have signs of a systemic reaction, especially hypotension, airway swelling, or definite difficulty breathing.[18] This dose can be repeated in 15 to 20 minutes if there is no improvement.
  - Give epinephrine 0.1 mg IV if anaphylaxis appears severe. Use 1:10,000 solution and give it slowly over 5 minutes.[18]

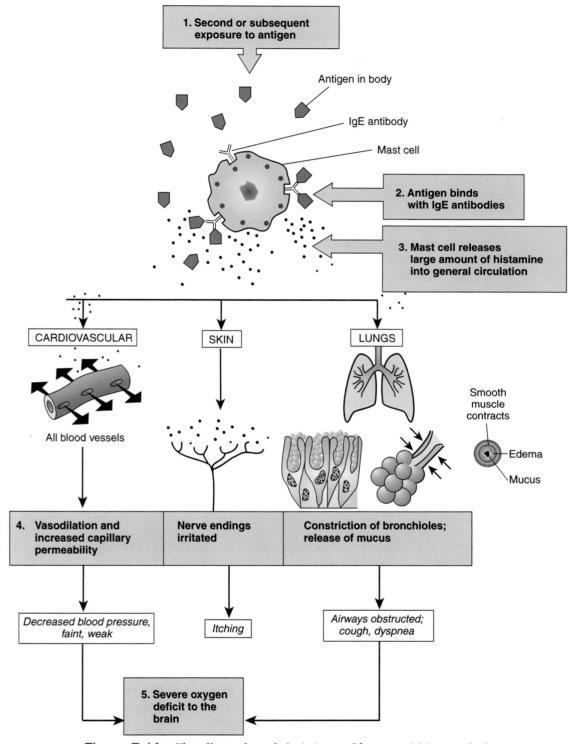

Figure 7-14 • The effects of anaphylaxis (a type I hypersensitivity reaction).

■ "Patients who are taking beta-blockers have increased incidence and severity of anaphylaxis and can develop a paradoxical response to epinephrine. Consider glucagon as well as ipratropium for these patients."[18]

■ If hypotension does not improve despite epinephrine therapy, give a fluid bolus of normal saline and assess the patient's response. If perfusion does not improve, repeat 1 or 2 fluid boluses and reassess response, repeating the primary survey after each fluid bolus. Monitor closely for increased work of breathing and the development of crackles.

- Give other drugs as needed to help stop the inflammatory reaction.
  - ▶ Diphenhydramine 25 to 50 mg IM or slowly IV
  - ▶ H$_2$ blockers such as cimetidine (orally, IM, or IV)
  - ▶ Inhaled bronchodilator therapy
    - Use albuterol if bronchospasm is present.
    - If the patient is on beta-blockers, use ipratropium to treat bronchospasm.
  - ▶ Use IV corticosteroids early in the course of treatment; effects may be delayed 4 to 6 hours.
- If cardiac arrest occurs[19]:
  - ▶ The arrest rhythm in anaphylaxis is often pulseless electrical activity (PEA) or asystole. Treat using the appropriate algorithm.
  - ▶ Volume expansion. Make sure at least two large-gauge IVs are in place. Rapidly infuse isotonic crystalloid solution. Between 4 and 8 liters may need to be given.
  - ▶ Give high-dose epinephrine IV. The American Heart Association says that a common dosing sequence is 1 to 3 mg IV (3 minutes), 3 to 5 mg IV (3 minutes), then a 4 to 10 mcg/min epinephrine infusion.
  - ▶ Consider an antihistamine IV.
  - ▶ Consider the use of steroids, which may be helpful in the postresuscitation period.
  - ▶ Prolonged CPR is appropriate because patients are often young with healthy hearts and cardiovascular systems.

HYPOTHERMIA

Hypothermia (core body temperature <95° F [35° C]) may result from a decrease in heat production, an increase in heat loss, or a combination of these factors. Hypothermia may be divided into three categories:

1. Mild (93.2° to 96.8° F [34° to 36° C])

2. Moderate (86° to 93° F [30° to 34° C])

3. Severe (<86° F [30° C])

Hypothermia is a result of exposure to conditions resulting in excessive heat loss. Exposure may include a body of water. It may also occur because of an abnormal control of body temperature as seen in conditions such as sepsis, metabolic disorders, ingestions, CNS disorders, and endocrine disorders. Neonates, trauma victims, intoxicated patients, the mentally ill, and the chronically disabled are particularly at risk for hypothermia. Hypothermia may be missed, especially in association with other injuries, such as multiple trauma.

ASSESSMENT FINDINGS

- The major areas of heat loss from the body are the head and the back of the neck.
- Shivering ceases below 86° F to 89.6° F (30° C to 32° C) as glycogen stores are depleted, or insulin is no longer available for glucose transfer.
- In severe hypothermia, the skin is pale or cyanotic, pupils may be fixed and dilated, muscles are rigid, and there may be no palpable pulses. Table 7-21 lists the signs and symptoms and initial emergency care for hypothermia.

INITIAL EMERGENCY CARE

- Emergency care depends on the degree of heat loss.
- Handle the patient gently; avoid jostling.
- Assess responsiveness, breathing (assess for 30 to 45 seconds), and pulse (assess for 30 to 45 seconds).

TABLE 7-21	Signs/Symptoms and Initial Management for Hypothermia		
Assessment	Mild Core Temp 93.2° to 96.8° F (34° to 36° C)	Moderate Core Temp 86° to 93° F (30° to 34° C)	Severe Core Temp <86° F (<30° C)
Airway Breathing	Open/patent Normal	Open/patent Decreased respiratory rate	Compromised Slow, shallow, or absent respirations; pulmonary edema may develop
Circulation	• Normal heart rate • Adequate BP • Pale, dry or wet skin	• Normal heart rate or bradycardia, atrial fibrillation, PVCs • Adequate BP or hypotension; difficult to obtain • Pale, cyanotic, or mottled skin	• Heart rate slows • Possible Osborne waves on ECG • Cyanotic or mottled skin • Body appears lifeless • Eventual VF or asystole
Mental Status	• AVPU = A • Slurred speech	• AVPU = V • Confusion to decreased responsiveness	• AVPU = P or U • Extreme disorientation
Other S/S	• Shivering • Uncoordinated movement	• Stiffening muscles • Shivering decreases and then stops below 86° F to 89.6° F (30° C to 32° C)	• Loss of deep tendon reflexes • Stiff, rigid muscles
Initial Care	• Move to warm environment • Remove wet clothing • Apply warm, dry clothing and blankets • Apply radiant heat, warm air, or heat packs • Protect from wind chill	• Move to warm environment • Remove wet clothing If perfusing rhythm: • Active external rewarming • Apply warm, dry clothing and blankets • Apply radiant heat, warm air, or heat packs If cardiac arrest: • Begin CPR and apply AED; if shockable rhythm present, shock once • Start IV and give IV drugs spaced at longer intervals • Active internal rewarming	• Move to warm environment • Remove wet clothing If perfusing rhythm: • Active internal rewarming If cardiac arrest: • Begin CPR and apply AED; if shockable rhythm present, shock once • Withhold drugs until temperature >86° F (30° C) • Active internal rewarming • Continue rewarming until core temperature >95° F (35° C), return of spontaneous circulation, or resuscitation efforts cease

AVPU, Alert, verbal stimulus response, painful stimulus response, unresponsive.

■ Give warmed and humidified 100% O_2. Perform endotracheal intubation if the hypothermic patient is unresponsive or if ventilation is inadequate.

■ Monitor core temperature, heart and respiratory rates, and BP continuously. Use low-reading thermometers to measure core temperature at 5-minute intervals.

■ Rewarming.
  ▶ Passive external rewarming is appropriate for all hypothermic patients. If sustained warmth can be ensured, provide active external rewarming for mildly hypothermic patients; active external rewarming for moderately hypothermic patients; and active internal rewarming for severely hypothermic patients.
  ▶ Begin CPR before internal rewarming for severely hypothermic patients who are not breathing and pulseless.

■ Warming methods.
  ▶ Passive external rewarming (appropriate for all types of hypothermia) includes moving the patient to a warm environment and application of warm, dry clothing and blankets.

- ▶ Active external rewarming includes application of radiant heat, warm air, or heat packs.
- ▶ Active internal rewarming includes warm IV fluids (normal saline); warm, humidified O_2; peritoneal lavage; esophageal rewarming tubes; or extracorporeal rewarming through partial cardiopulmonary bypass.
- ■ If the hypothermic patient is in cardiac arrest and VT or ventricular fibrillation (VF) is present, attempt defibrillation.
  - ▶ Deliver one shock. If there is no response, focus on CPR and rewarming. Postpone additional defibrillation attempts until the core temperature rises above 86° F (30° C).
  - ▶ IV medications are often withheld if the patient's core body temperature is lower than 86° F (30° C). If the core temperature is or rises above 86° F (30° C), IV drugs are given but spaced at longer than standard intervals.

TRAUMATIC CARDIAC ARREST

Traumatic prehospital cardiac arrests rarely survive. Cardiac arrests due to blunt trauma have a higher mortality rate than cardiac arrests due to penetrating trauma.

POSSIBLE CAUSES

- ■ Airway obstruction or chest injuries (large open pneumothorax, severe tracheobronchial injury [such as a laceration or crush injury], or thoracoabdominal injury) that lead to compromised ventilation and cardiac arrest due to hypoxia
- ■ Severe injury to vital structures (heart, aorta, pulmonary arteries)
- ■ Severe head injury leading to depressed respirations and cardiac arrest due to hypoxia
- ■ Underlying medical problems that led to the injury (such as sudden VF)
- ■ Decreased cardiac output or cardiac arrest caused by tension pneumothorax or cardiac tamponade
- ■ Hypovolemia and diminished delivery of O_2

Assume spinal injury if the patient is unresponsive or has an altered mental status, has experienced blunt trauma above the nipple line, has a significant mechanism of injury, complains of neck or back pain, numbness or tingling, loss of movement, or weakness, or if the patient has multiple injuries of any cause.

BASIC LIFE SUPPORT FOR TRAUMATIC CARDIAC ARREST

- ■ Rescuer safety is essential. Law enforcement personnel are needed to secure scenes involving potential violence, ensure safe traffic flow, and so forth.
- ■ Safe patient extrication.
- ■ Airway.
  - ▶ Use a jaw thrust without head-tilt maneuver to open the airway.
  - ▶ When possible, use a second rescuer to manually stabilize the head and neck until full spinal immobilization can be accomplished.
  - ▶ Clear the airway of secretions with suctioning as needed.
- ■ Breathing.
  - ▶ Assist breathing if respirations are absent, agonal, or slow and shallow.
  - ▶ Continued manual stabilization of the head and neck by a second rescuer is needed when ventilation is provided with a barrier device, a pocket mask, or a bag-valve-mask device.
  - ▶ Each ventilation should be delivered slowly with enough force to produce gentle chest rise.

▶ Consider the possibility of a flail chest, tension pneumothorax, or hemothorax if the chest does not rise during ventilation despite an open airway.

Deadly Chest Injuries

Life-threatening injuries that must be identified and treated in the primary survey:

- Airway obstruction
- Open pneumothorax
- Tension pneumothorax
- Massive hemothorax
- Flail chest
- Cardiac tamponade

■ Circulation.
  ▶ Stop any obvious major bleeding using direct pressure and dressings.
  ▶ Feel for a carotid pulse. If a carotid pulse cannot be felt within 10 seconds, begin chest compressions at a rate of about 100/min.
  ▶ Attach an AED/monitor/defibrillator if available. If a shockable rhythm is present, deliver one shock and then resume CPR.
■ Disability. Assess the patient's neurologic status (GCS).
■ Expose. Preserve body heat and maintain appropriate temperature. Respect the patient's modesty. Keep the patient covered if possible and replace clothing promptly after examining each body area.

Do *not* apply traction to the neck. In a patient with possible cervical spine trauma, applying traction can worsen an existing injury or convert a stable cervical fracture to an unstable fracture. If an attempt to move the head and neck into a neutral in-line position results in any of the following, *stop* any movement and stabilize the head in that position.

- Compromise of the airway or ventilation
- Neck muscle spasm
- Increased pain
- Onset or increase of a neurological deficit such as numbness, tingling, or loss of motor ability

ADVANCED CARDIAC LIFE SUPPORT FOR TRAUMATIC CARDIAC ARREST

(Advanced) Airway

■ Indications for immediate intubation of the injured patient include the following[20]:
  ▶ Respiratory arrest or apnea
  ▶ Respiratory failure, including severe hypoventilation or hypoxemia despite O_2 therapy
  ▶ Severe head injury (GCS score <8)
  ▶ Inability to protect the upper airway (loss of gag reflex, depressed level of consciousness)
  ▶ Chest injuries such as flail chest, pulmonary contusion, penetrating trauma
  ▶ Injuries associated with potential airway obstruction such as crushing facial or neck injuries
■ When intubation is indicated, maintain manual in-line stabilization of the head and neck during the procedure.
■ In the prehospital setting, intubation should be performed en route to definitive care (when possible).
■ Avoid nasotracheal intubation if severe maxillofacial injuries are present.
■ Confirm proper position of the tube by assessment techniques and use of a mechanical device, such as an exhaled CO_2 monitor. Check (and document) the centimeter markings at the patient's lips or teeth immediately after intubation, during transport, and any time the patient is moved.

■ Cricothyrotomy is indicated if endotracheal intubation is unsuccessful in a patient with massive facial injury and swelling. If cricothyrotomy is necessary, it should be performed by the most experienced person available.

Breathing

■ All injured patients should received supplemental O_2.

■ If breathing is absent, insert an oral airway to keep the airway open (if not already done and not contraindicated) and provide positive-pressure ventilation. Make sure the patient's chest wall rises with each ventilation.

■ If a sucking chest wound is present, promptly cover the wound with an airtight dressing (Figures 7-15 and 7-16). Examples of dressings that may be used include plastic wrap, petroleum gauze, or a defibrillation pad. Tape the dressing on three sides (flutter-valve effect—the dressing is sucked over the wound as the patient inhales, preventing air from entering; the open end of the dressing allows air to escape as the patient exhales).

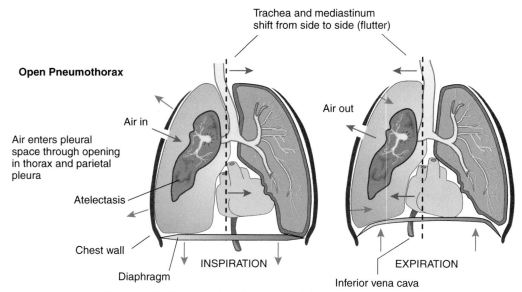

Figure 7-15 • Sucking chest wound (open pneumothorax).

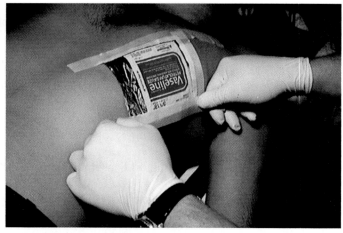

Figure 7-16 • If a sucking chest wound (open pneumothorax) is present, cover the wound with a sterile airtight dressing taped on three sides.

■ If breath sounds are decreased or absent on one side of the chest, consider the possibility of a tension pneumothorax or hemothorax.

▶ A tension pneumothorax is a life-threatening chest injury that can occur because of blunt or penetrating trauma or as a complication of treatment of an open pneumothorax (Figure 7-17). Signs and symptoms of a tension pneumothorax are shown in Box 7-5.

▶ If the patient has an open chest wound with signs of a tension pneumothorax, remove the dressing over the wound for a few seconds. If the wound in the chest wall has not sealed under the dressing, air will rush out of the wound. Reseal the wound with the airtight dressing once the pressure has been released. This procedure may need to be repeated periodically if pressure again builds up in the chest. If this procedure does not relieve the signs of a tension pneumothorax, needle decompression should be performed.

• Needle decompression (also called needle thoracostomy) is the insertion of an over-the-needle catheter into the chest to relieve a tension pneumothorax. The procedure converts a tension pneumothorax to a simple, open pneumothorax. In the hospital, this procedure is typically followed by insertion of a chest tube.

BOX 7-5

Signs and Symptoms of Tension Pneumothorax

- Cool, clammy skin
- Increased pulse rate
- Cyanosis (a late sign)
- Jugular venous distention (may be absent if hypovolemia present)
- Hypotension
- Severe respiratory distress
- Agitation, restlessness, anxiety
- Bulging of intercostal muscles on the affected side
- Decreased or absent breath sounds on the affected side
- Tracheal deviation toward the unaffected side (late sign)
- Possible subcutaneous emphysema in the face, neck, or chest wall
- Increased resistance felt during positive-pressure ventilation
- Falling O_2 saturation

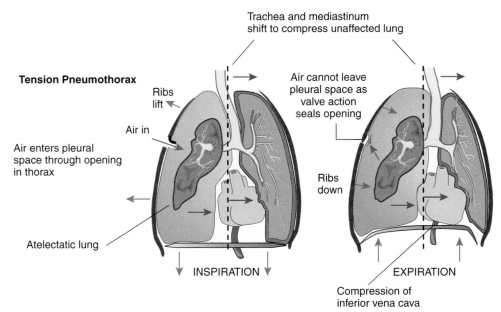

Figure 7-17 • Tension pneumothorax.

■ A hemothorax occurs as a result of blunt or penetrating chest trauma when large amounts of blood build up in the pleural space and compress the lung (Figure 7-18). Signs and symptoms of a hemothorax are listed in Box 7-6.

❱ Treat hypovolemia and shock with IV fluids and blood administration as indicated

❱ Tube thoracostomy—in-hospital management (make sure IV fluid resuscitation is begun before procedure)

Potentially Deadly Chest Injuries

Potentially life-threatening injuries that must be identified and for which treatment must begin in the secondary survey:

• Pulmonary contusion
• Myocardial contusion
• Aortic injury
• Traumatic diaphragmatic tear/rupture
• Tracheobronchial disruption
• Esophageal injury

BOX 7-6

Signs and Symptoms of a Hemothorax

• Tachypnea
• Tachycardia
• Dyspnea
• Respiratory distress
• Hypotension
• Narrowed pulse pressure
• Flat neck veins
• Pleuritic chest pain
• Pale, cool, moist skin
• Decreased breath sounds and dullness to percussion on affected side with or without obvious respiratory distress

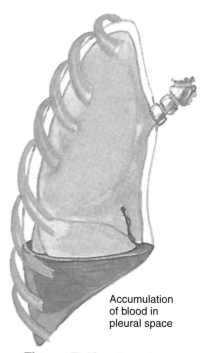

Accumulation
of blood in
pleural space

Figure 7-18 • Hemothorax.

Circulation

▦ Control major bleeding, if present. Apply direct pressure over the bleeding site with sterile dressings.

▦ Consider possible areas of major internal hemorrhage. Significant internal hemorrhage may occur in the chest, abdomen, pelvis, retroperitoneum, and femoral areas. Pain or swelling in any of these areas may be an indicator of possible internal hemorrhage.

▦ Establish IV access with normal saline or lactated Ringer's solution. If signs of shock are present, establish IV access in two sites using large-gauge catheters.

  ▶ In the field, the presence of shock in an injured patient indicates that rapid stabilization and transport are needed immediately. Obtain IV access quickly or (preferably) on the way to an appropriate receiving facility, such as a trauma center. Do not delay transport for multiple vascular access attempts at the scene.

▦ Volume replacement[21]

  ▶ Rapid infusion of IV fluids to maintain a systolic blood pressure (SBP) ≥100 mm Hg is now recommended only for patients with isolated blunt or penetrating head or extremity trauma.

  ▶ In urban settings, aggressive prehospital volume resuscitation for penetrating trauma is no longer recommended.
    • Increase in BP speeds rate of blood loss.
    • Delays arrival at a trauma center.
    • Delays surgical repair of bleeding vessels.

  ▶ Recommendations regarding volume resuscitation of trauma patients in a rural setting differ from those in an urban setting.
    • Transport times from rural areas to trauma centers are longer.
    • If in a rural setting, provide volume resuscitation during transport for blunt or penetrating trauma.
    • Goal: maintain SBP of 90 mm Hg.

▦ Cardiac arrest

  ▶ The most common terminal cardiac rhythms observed in injured victims are PEA, bradyasystolic rhythms, and occasionally VF/VT.[21]

  ▶ PEA
    • Consider reversible causes.
      • Severe hypovolemia. ECG signs usually include a narrow QRS complex at a rapid rate. Find source of volume loss and manage with volume replacement.
      • Hypothermia. ECG signs typically show an initial tachycardia, then progressive bradycardia. Osborne waves may be present on ECG. Emergency care depends on core temperature.
      • Cardiac tamponade (Figure 7-19). ECG signs of impending cardiac tamponade usually include a narrow QRS complex at a rapid rate. This deteriorates to sudden bradycardia as a terminal event. Pericardiocentesis is definitive treatment.
      • Tension pneumothorax. ECG signs usually include a narrow QRS complex at a slow rate (due to hypoxia). Definitive treatment includes needle decompression—second intercostal space, midclavicular line on affected side of the chest.

  ▶ Bradyasystolic rhythms
    • A bradyasystolic rhythm is a cardiac rhythm in which the ventricular rate is less than 60 bpm and/or there are periods of asystole.[22]
    • Presence suggests severe hypovolemia, severe hypoxemia, or cardiorespiratory failure.

  ▶ Pulseless VT/VF
    • Begin CPR and attempt defibrillation.
    • Epinephrine will probably be ineffective if uncorrected severe hypovolemia is present.

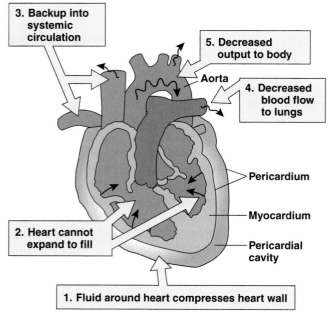

3. Backup into systemic circulation

5. Decreased output to body

Aorta

4. Decreased blood flow to lungs

Pericardium

Myocardium

Pericardial cavity

2. Heart cannot expand to fill

1. Fluid around heart compresses heart wall

Figure 7-19 • Cardiac tamponade.

Differential Diagnosis

■ Continue resuscitation
■ Consider insertion of urinary catheter, nasogastric tube if no contraindications

Evaluate

■ Reassess care provided

In the field, it is important to remember that definitive care for a trauma patient requires physician evaluation of the patient at an appropriate facility. With this in mind, limit scene time to 10 minutes or less if the patient's condition is critical. The patient should be rapidly packaged after starting essential field care and transported to the closest appropriate facility.

In an urgent care or hospital setting, the physician evaluating the patient should determine if the patient requires transfer to another facility for definitive care. If this decision is made, additional patient care and evaluation can be performed while preparations are made for the patient's transfer. Communication between the referring physician and receiving physician is essential.

CARDIAC ARREST AND PREGNANCY
BASIC LIFE SUPPORT MODIFICATIONS

■ The weight of the pregnant uterus on the inferior vena cava and aorta can hinder venous return and cardiac output (supine hypotension). To shift the weight of the uterus off of these major blood vessels, a patient who is 20 weeks pregnant or more should be placed 15 to 30 degrees back from the left lateral position. Maintain this position by placing a wedge, rolled blanket, or other object under the patient's right hip and lower back. If chest compressions are necessary, they should be performed with the patient in this position. Alternately, the uterus can be manually displaced to the left.
■ Chest compressions should be performed higher on the sternum (slightly above the center of the sternum).
■ It is not necessary to modify energy settings or pad/paddle position if defibrillation is required.
■ Before delivering a shock, remove fetal or uterine monitors (if present).

ADVANCED CARDIAC LIFE SUPPORT MODIFICATIONS

■ Because of the increased likelihood of regurgitation, use continuous cricoid pressure before and during attempted endotracheal intubation.

■ Because of possible airway narrowing due to swelling, it may be necessary to use an endotracheal tube 0.5 to 1 mm smaller in internal diameter than that used for a nonpregnant woman of similar size.

■ Support oxygenation and ventilation.

■ If an endotracheal tube is used, verify correct tube position using assessment techniques and an exhaled CO_2 detector. Esophageal detector devices may be less accurate in late pregnancy.

■ Because the pregnant patient's diaphragm is elevated during pregnancy, it may be necessary to ventilate using less volume.

■ The femoral vein or other lower extremity veins should not be used for venous access.

■ If pulseless VT/VF is present, defibrillate as recommended in the pulseless VT/VF algorithm.

■ Give ACLS drugs without modification during cardiac arrest.

■ Consider possible reversible causes of the cardiac arrest.

■ If the pregnant patient has an ST-elevation MI, percutaneous coronary intervention is the reperfusion strategy of choice.

EMERGENCY CESAREAN DELIVERY FOR THE PREGNANT PATIENT IN CARDIAC ARREST[23]

Consider the need for emergency cesarean delivery as soon as a pregnant patient develops cardiac arrest. The decision to perform emergency cesarean delivery should be made rapidly (within 4 to 5 minutes of the arrest) to maximize chances of maternal and infant survival. Factors to consider include the following:

■ Gestational age of fetus?
  ▶ <20 weeks—no cesarean delivery because the size of the fetus does not usually impact arrest
  ▶ 20 to 23 weeks—cesarean delivery if needed to successfully resuscitate mother; infant survival unlikely (if appropriately trained personnel, equipment, and facilities available)
  ▶ ≥24 to 25 weeks—cesarean delivery to save life of mother and infant (if appropriately trained personnel, equipment, and facilities available)

■ Availability of appropriate equipment?

■ Skilled personnel available to perform procedure?

■ Skilled personnel available to care for infant?

■ Skilled personnel (obstetric support) available for mother after the procedure?

ELECTRIC SHOCK AND LIGHTNING STRIKES

Factors that determine the site and severity of electrical injury include the following:

■ Voltage and amperage.

■ Type of current.
  ▶ Lightning acts as massive direct current shock, depolarizing the entire myocardium at once, and resulting in asystole.
  ▶ Alternating current (household and industrial current) is more damaging than direct current.
    • May cause tetanic muscle contractions.
    • May prevent the victim's self-release from the electrical source, increasing the duration of contact with the circuit.

- In the muscles, electric energy is converted to thermal energy. The heat produced can result in severe burns.
- Greater chance of current hitting during the relative refractory period (vulnerable period) of the cardiac cycle, resulting in VF.

▨ Duration of contact. The longer the contact with source, the greater the body exposure to current, the greater the damage.

▨ Resistance of tissues to current flow. Dry skin is resistant to current. However, resistance is greatly decreased when the skin is wet or the body is immersed in water. A low-voltage shock can become life-threatening if the skin is wet.

▨ Current pathway (Figure 7-20).
  ▶ In a horizontal (hand-to-hand or transthoracic) shock, current passes from one hand or arm across the chest and through the heart to the other hand or arm. Since the current passes through the heart, it is the most dangerous type of shock.
  ▶ In a vertical shock (hand-to-foot), the current passes from the hand and then down and out the lower leg or foot.
  ▶ In a straddle shock (foot-to-foot), current passes from one foot to the other. Because there are no major organs in the pathway of the current, this is the least dangerous type of shock.

An electric shock can produce respiratory arrest secondary to:

▨ Paralysis of the brain's respiratory center function

▨ Tetanic contraction of the diaphragm and muscles of the chest wall

▨ Prolonged paralysis of respiratory muscles, which may continue for minutes after the electric shock has terminated

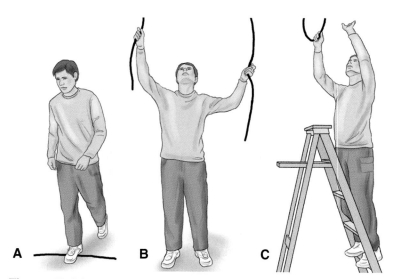

Figure 7-20 • Current pathways. **A,** Straddle; **B,** Horizontal; and **C,** Vertical.

LIGHTNING STRIKE FACTS[24]

■ According to American case reports since 1900, lightning strike carries a mortality of 30% and a morbidity of 70%. More recent studies have shown the mortality to be as low as 5% to 10%.

■ Only a small percentage of lightning strike victims actually sustain deep thermal burns.

■ The only immediate cause of death is from cardiac arrest.

■ The most dangerous time for a fatal lightning strike is the time preceding a storm. This is because lightning can travel horizontally as far as 10 miles or more in front of a thunderstorm.

BASIC LIFE SUPPORT MODIFICATIONS

■ Make sure the scene is safe to enter.

■ Turn off current.

■ Assess the patient's ABCs.

■ Begin CPR, attach an AED, and deliver a shock if indicated.

■ Assume cardiac arrest involving electricity is also associated with trauma until proven otherwise; protect the cervical spine and treat injuries.

■ Remove smoldering clothing.

ADVANCED CARDIAC LIFE SUPPORT MODIFICATIONS

■ Treat dysrhythmias per the ACLS guidelines for these rhythms.

■ Intubation may be difficult in patients with electrical burns of the face, mouth, or anterior neck due to soft tissue swelling.

■ If hypovolemic shock or significant tissue destruction is present, rapid IV fluid administration is indicated to counteract shock, correct ongoing fluid losses, and maintain a diuresis to avoid renal shutdown due to myoglobinuria.

■ If a lightning strike involves multiple victims, treat those who are unconscious or appear to be in cardiac arrest first ("reverse triage") (Figure 7-21). All victims of a lightning strike should be evaluated by a physician.

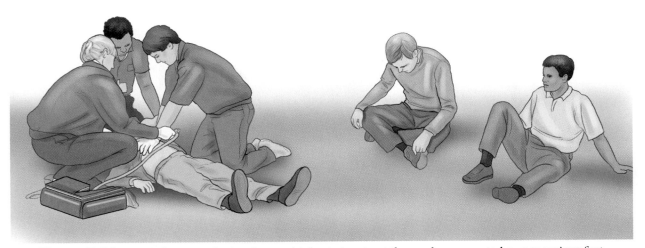

Figure 7-21 • If a lightning strike involves multiple victims, treat those who appear to be unconscious first.

QUICK REVIEW ANSWERS

Quick Review Number	Answers
7-1	1. Carotid. 2. False. Stroke kills more than twice as many American women every year as breast cancer. 3. There are two major types of stroke—ischemic and hemorrhagic. An ischemic stroke occurs when a blood vessel supplying the brain is blocked. It can be life-threatening but rarely leads to death within the first hour. A hemorrhagic stroke occurs when a cerebral artery bursts. It can be fatal at onset. 4. The two main areas of injury in an ischemic stroke are: 1) the zone of ischemia, and 2) the ischemic penumbra (transitional zone). 5. Facial droop/weakness, motor weakness (arm drift), and aphasia (speech).

STOP & REVIEW

Questions 1-20. Match each term with its correct description.

a) Ischemic
b) Jugular venous distention
c) Hypertension
d) Three
e) Peanuts
f) Embolic
g) Hypokalemia
h) Ventilation
i) Penetrating
j) Brain attack
k) Ipratropium
l) Heliox
m) Carotid
n) Straddle
o) Direct pressure
p) Alternating
q) Glucagon
r) Asystole
s) Tachycardia
t) Direct

_____ 1. Consider this drug in patients taking beta-blockers who develop anaphylaxis.

_____ 2. In urban settings, aggressive prehospital volume resuscitation for __ trauma is no longer recommended.

_____ 3. Least dangerous type of electrical current pathway.

_____ 4. Most of the blood flow to the brain is supplied by these arteries.

_____ 5. U waves may appear on the ECG with this electrolyte disorder.

_____ 6. Major bleeding should be controlled using __.

_____ 7. __ current may "freeze" a victim to the electrical source.

_____ 8. The most common type of stroke.

_____ 9. An open chest wound should be taped on __ sides.

_____10. A common arrest rhythm in anaphylaxis.

_____11. In this type of stroke, material from an area outside the brain becomes dislodged and travels through the bloodstream to the brain.

_____12. A sign of a tension pneumothorax that may be absent if hypovolemia is present.

_____13. Anticholinergic bronchodilator.

_____14. This is the cause of most intracerebral hemorrhages.

_____15. With this type of current, the victim is likely to be thrown from the electrical source.

_____16. The most important treatment for a drowning victim.

_____17. A possible cause of anaphylaxis.

_____18. A less "formal" name for stroke.

_____19. Side effect of epinephrine.

_____20. May be useful for asthma that is refractory to conventional therapy.

21. The most commonly blocked vessel in a stroke is the:
    a. Vertebral artery.
    b. Middle cerebral artery.
    c. Posterior cerebral artery.
    d. Anterior cerebral artery.

22. The most common cause of a subarachnoid hemorrhage is:
    a. Cerebral aneurysm.
    b. AV malformation.
    c. Chronic hypertension.
    d. Atrial fibrillation.

23. Which of the following dysrhythmias is most likely to precipitate a stroke?
    a. Sinus bradycardia
    b. Junctional rhythm
    c. Atrial fibrillation
    d. Idioventricular rhythm

24. Currently, the "window of opportunity" to use IV rtPA to treat ischemic stroke patients is within _____ of the onset of symptoms.
    a. 1 hour
    b. 3 hours
    c. 6 hours
    d. 12 hours

25. True or False. Strokes occur only in individuals older than 65 years of age.

26. Supine hypotension:
    a. Occurs as a result of prolonged labor.
    b. Occurs as a result of significant spinal injury.
    c. Occurs as a result of compression of the abdominal aorta and inferior vena cava by the pregnant uterus when the mother is supine.
    d. Is characterized by a tearing sensation in the abdomen and constant pain.

27. The greatest amount of body heat is lost from the:
    a. Head and feet.
    b. Feet and torso.
    c. Upper and lower extremities.
    d. Head and back of the neck.

28. Immediate treatment for an open pneumothorax should include:
    a. Needle decompression of the affected side of the chest.
    b. Starting two large-gauge peripheral IVs.
    c. Covering the wound with an airtight dressing.
    d. Insertion of a chest tube.

29. Why should the serum glucose level be determined during the initial management of a possible stroke patient?

    _____

    _____

30. Which one of the following is *not* one of the "4 Cs" of tricyclic antidepressant overdose?
    a. Conduction defects
    b. Cramping
    c. Decreased contractility
    d. Convulsions

31. A direct current shock is most likely to result in:
    a. Asystole.
    b. VF.
    c. VT.
    d. Third-degree AV block.

32. List four factors that determine the site and severity of an electrical injury.
    1.
    2.
    3.
    4.

33. Early ECG changes that are usually seen with hyperkalemia include:
    a. Development of U waves.
    b. ST-segment elevation and shortening of the QT interval.
    c. Widening of the QRS complex.
    d. Tall, peaked T waves.

34. Which of the following statements about providing care for a trauma patient is incorrect?
    a. When intubation is indicated, apply traction to the patient's head and neck during the procedure.
    b. If a carotid pulse cannot be felt within 10 seconds, begin chest compressions.
    c. A flail chest must be identified and treated during the primary survey.
    d. Consider the possibility of a tension pneumothorax if breath sounds are decreased or absent on one side of the chest.

STOP AND REVIEW ANSWERS

1. q	11. f
2. i	12. b
3. n	13. k
4. m	14. c
5. g	15. t
6. o	16. h
7. p	17. e
8. a	18. j
9. d	19. s
10. r	20. l

21. b. The middle cerebral artery is the most commonly blocked vessel in a stroke. It is the largest branch of the internal carotid artery.

22. a. A cerebral aneurysm is the most common cause of an SAH.

23. c. Patients experiencing atrial fibrillation may develop intra-atrial emboli because the atria are not contracting and blood stagnates in the atrial chambers. This predisposes the patient to systemic emboli, particularly stroke, if the clots dislodge spontaneously or because of conversion to a sinus rhythm.

24. b. Currently, the window of opportunity to use IV rtPA to treat ischemic stroke patients is 3 hours. To be evaluated and receive treatment, patients need to be at a hospital within 60 minutes of symptom onset.

25. False. Stroke can occur in persons of any age. Strokes can occur in utero, in infants, and in children.

26. c. Supine hypotension occurs as a result of compression of the abdominal aorta and inferior vena cava by the pregnant uterus when the mother is supine.

27. d. The greatest amount of body heat is lost from the head and back of the neck.

28. c. When a sucking chest wound (open pneumothorax) is present, the wound should be quickly covered with an airtight dressing. Examples of dressings that may be used include plastic wrap, petroleum gauze, or a defibrillation pad. Tape the dressing on three sides (flutter-valve effect—the dressing is sucked over the wound as the patient inhales, preventing air from entering; the open end of the dressing allows air to escape as the patient exhales).

29. The serum glucose level should be determined during the initial management of a possible stroke patient because hypoglycemia can mimic the signs and symptoms of a stroke. The glucose test is performed to rule out hypoglycemia before proceeding with stroke treatment.

30. b. The "4 Cs" of tricyclic antidepressant overdose are **c**oma, **c**onvulsions, **c**onduction defects (PR lengthening, widening of QRS complex, prolonging of QT interval), and decreased **c**ontractility.

31. a. Alternating current tends to cause ventricular fibrillation. Direct current tends to cause asystole.

32. Factors that determine the site and severity of electrical injury include voltage, amperage, type of current (alternating versus direct current), resistance of tissues, current pathway, and duration of contact.

33. d. ECG changes correlate with the degree of hyperkalemia. Early ECG changes include the appearance of tall, peaked T waves.

34. a. When intubation is indicated, maintain manual in-line stabilization of the head and neck (*without traction*) during the procedure. As with all patients, if a carotid pulse cannot be felt within 10 seconds, begin chest compressions. Life-threatening injuries that must be identified and treated in the primary survey include airway obstruction, open pneumothorax, tension pneumothorax, massive hemothorax, flail chest, and cardiac tamponade. If breath sounds are decreased or absent on one side of the chest, consider the possibility of a tension pneumothorax or hemothorax.

REFERENCES

1. Lewandowski CA, Libman R: Acute presentation of stroke. *J Stroke Cerebrovasc Dis* 1999;8: 117-126.
2. Kothari R, Barsan WG: Stroke. In Marx JA (Ed.), *Rosen's emergency medicine: Concepts and clinical practice* (5th ed.). St. Louis: Mosby, 2002.
3. Albers GW, Caplan LR, Coull BM: Transient ischemic attack: Proposal for a new definition. *N Engl J Med* 2002;347:1713-1716.
4. Adams HP Jr, Adams RJ, Brott T, et al: Stroke Council of the American Stroke Association. Guidelines for the early management of patients with ischemic stroke: A scientific statement from the Stroke Council of the American Stroke Association. *Stroke* Apr 2003;34(4):1056-1083.
5. Adams H, Adams R, Del Zoppo G, Goldstein LB: Stroke Council of the American Heart Association, American Stroke Association: Guidelines for the early management of patients with ischemic stroke: 2005 guidelines update a scientific statement from the Stroke Council of the American Heart Association/American Stroke Association. *Stroke* Apr 2005;36(4):916-923.
6. Pepe PE: Overview: Prehospital emergency medical care systems. The initial links in the chain of recovery for brain attack—access, prehospital care, notification, and transport. In Marler JR, Winters Jones P, Emr M (Eds.), *Proceedings of a National Symposium on Rapid Identification and Treatment of Acute Stroke.* Bethesda, MD: The National Institute of Neurological Disorders and Stroke, National Institutes of Health, 1997.
7. Hazinski MF: Demystifying recognition and management of stroke. *Curr Emerg Cardiac Care* 1996;7:8.
8. Cummins RO (Ed.): *Textbook of advanced cardiac life support,* Dallas: American Heart Association, 1997.
9. Schneck MJ: Acute Stroke: An aggressive approach to intervention and prevention. *Hospital Medicine* 1998;34(1):11-12, 17-20, 25-26, 28.
10. Plantz SH, Adler JN (Eds): *National medical series for independent study: Emergency medicine.* Baltimore: Williams & Wilkins, 1998.
11. 2005 American Heart Association guidelines for cardiopulmonary resuscitation and emergency cardiovascular care, part 10.3: Drowning. *Circulation* 2005;112(suppl IV):IV-133.
12. Soar J, Deakin CD, Nolan JP, et al: European Resuscitation Council guidelines for resuscitation 2005. section 7. Cardiac arrest in special circumstances. *Resuscitation* Dec 2005;67(Suppl 1): S135-170.
13. Idris AH, Berg RA, Bierens J, et al: Recommended guidelines for uniform reporting of data from drowning: The "Utstein style." *Resuscitation* 2003;59:45-57.
14. Feldhaus KM: Submersion. In Marx JA (Ed.): *Rosen's emergency medicine: Concepts and clinical practice* (5th ed.). St. Louis: Mosby, 2002.

15. 2005 American Heart Association guidelines for cardiopulmonary resuscitation and emergency cardiovascular care, part 10.5: Near-fatal asthma. *Circulation* 2005;112(suppl IV):IV-139.

16. 2005 American Heart Association guidelines for cardiopulmonary resuscitation and emergency cardiovascular care, part 10.5: Near-fatal asthma. *Circulation* 2005;112(suppl IV):IV-140.

17. 2005 American Heart Association guidelines for cardiopulmonary resuscitation and emergency cardiovascular care, part 10.5: Near-fatal asthma. *Circulation* 2005;112(suppl IV):IV-140-141.

18. 2005 American Heart Association guidelines for cardiopulmonary resuscitation and emergency cardiovascular care, part 10.6: Anaphylaxis. *Circulation* 2005;112(suppl IV):IV-144.

19. 2005 American Heart Association guidelines for cardiopulmonary resuscitation and emergency cardiovascular care, part 10.6: Anaphylaxis. *Circulation* 2005;112(suppl IV):IV-145.

20. 2005 American Heart Association guidelines for cardiopulmonary resuscitation and emergency cardiovascular care, part 10.7: Cardiac arrest associated with trauma. *Circulation* 2005;112(suppl IV):IV-147.

21. 2005 American Heart Association guidelines for cardiopulmonary resuscitation and emergency cardiovascular care, part 10.7: Cardiac arrest associated with trauma. *Circulation* 2005;112(suppl IV):IV-148.

22. Ornato JP, Peberdy MA: The mystery of bradyasystole during cardiac arrest. *Ann Emerg Med* May 1996;27:576-587.

23. 2005 American Heart Association guidelines for cardiopulmonary resuscitation and emergency cardiovascular care, part 10.8: Cardiac arrest associated with pregnancy. *Circulation* 2005;112(suppl IV):IV-152.

24. O'Keefe Gatewood M, Zane RD: Lightning injuries. *Emerg Med Clin North Am* May 2004;22(2): 369-403.

Putting It All Together

OBJECTIVES

Upon completion of this chapter, you will be able to:

1. Describe the role of each member of the resuscitation team.
2. Discuss the "phase response" of code organization.
3. Describe the critical actions necessary in caring for the adult patient in cardiac arrest.
4. Identify the immediate goals of postresuscitation care.
5. Given a patient situation, describe the initial emergency care (including mechanical, pharmacological, and electrical therapy where applicable) for each of the following situations:
   - Cardiac arrest rhythms—Pulseless ventricular tachycardia (VT)/ventricular fibrillation (VF), asystole, pulseless electrical activity (PEA)
   - Too slow rhythms—Symptomatic bradycardia
   - Too fast rhythms—Narrow-QRS tachycardia, wide-QRS tachycardia, irregular tachycardia
   - Acute coronary syndromes—ST-elevation myocardial infarction (STEMI), unstable angina/non–ST-elevation myocardial infarction (NSTEMI), nondiagnostic/normal electrocardiogram (ECG)

INTRODUCTION

Knowledge of the algorithms is essential to successful completion of an advanced cardiac life support (ACLS) course. The ACLS algorithms can be found on the following pages. During an ACLS course, your knowledge of the ACLS algorithms is evaluated in simulated situations and on the course posttest. The simulations (also called "cases") are evaluated by an ACLS instructor. The cardiac arrest algorithms are evaluated in the Cardiac Arrest Management (also called the Mega Code) station. In this station, you work in teams of four or five. Each person takes a turn as the team leader and as individual resuscitation team members, performing each of the critical tasks of resuscitation. Each team leader's knowledge is evaluated on the ACLS algorithms, ability to manage the resuscitation team, and decisions regarding patient management. Although the team leader is responsible for directing the overall actions of the team, a resuscitation effort requires *teamwork.* Each member of the team must know his or her responsibilities and be able to anticipate the team leader's instructions. This is true in real life, as well as in simulated situations.

To help you prepare for the ACLS course, each ACLS algorithm is presented on the following pages in a specific sequence:

- Examples of rhythms pertaining to the algorithm
- Brief explanation of the drugs used in the algorithm
- Flow chart of the algorithm
- Putting it all together

The putting it all together section for each algorithm is represented as simulated dialogue between the evaluator and team leader in an ACLS course. As you read the dialogue that pertains to each ACLS algorithm, assume you are the team leader. As the team leader, you are expected to assess a simulated patient and verbalize the treatment of all conditions you discover. You are also responsible for directing the actions of the team members that are present to assist you. Assume that each team member will correctly carry out your instructions; however, they will not do anything without your direction.

Please understand that it is difficult to demonstrate with text the actions and conversations that occur simultaneously between team members and the team leader (and the evaluator in a simulated situation). It is also impossible to predict all possible actions for a given situation. There may be alternative actions that are perfectly acceptable yet not presented in the dialogue.

THE RESUSCITATION TEAM

As a healthcare professional, it is important to know what to do if you encounter a patient who is in cardiac arrest. If you are off duty and encounter an unresponsive patient, activate the Emergency Medical Services (EMS) system by calling 9-1-1.

In the prehospital setting, Emergency Medical Technicians (EMTs) and paramedics often work in teams of two to four. The number varies depending on the environment in which the EMT or paramedic works. For example, a fire department crew that responds to an EMS call may be staffed with two EMTs and two paramedics on the vehicle. Although staffing may differ, the ambulance that arrives on the scene is typically staffed with two EMTs or an EMT and a paramedic.

Healthcare facilities have policies and procedures in place for activating the resuscitation team. Just as it is important to know how to use a piece of equipment before using it in an emergency, you must know your facility's procedure for activating the team. Members of the resuscitation team often carry pagers that are activated by the facility operator. For example, team activation procedures may include pressing a "code button" at the patient's bedside, calling a specific phone extension, or using a "quick dial button" located on telephones within the facility. When the operator is reached, the type of emergency and its location are stated. Once the operator is notified of the emergency, members of the team are usually activated via pagers and/or an overhead page.

How the team is activated may vary depending on the location and nature of the emergency. For example, a code/emergency response team is typically called for patients who are not in cardiac arrest but need emergency medical care as well as for patients who have experienced a respiratory or cardiac arrest. This team generally responds within the healthcare facility. Members of the team typically include a critical care or emergency department (ED) nurse (depending on the location of the emergency within the facility), respiratory therapist, administrative supervisor, nurse from the patient care area in which the emergency occurs, and at least one physician.

If the facility is a hospital, the code team may not be the same team to respond to an emergency that occurs within 250 yards of the hospital's main buildings. A response to an emergency within 250 yards of the facility usually involves an emergency response team from the hospital's ED (called an EMTALA Response Team in some facilities) and may also involve an EMS response. Because the emergency is located outside the main hospital, activation of this team may require procedures different from those used for an in-hospital emergency.

As you can see, it is important to know, learn, and practice your facility's code procedure. It is also important to learn what is expected of you as a member of the resuscitation team.

GOALS OF THE RESUSCITATION TEAM

Regardless of where a cardiac arrest occurs, the goals of the resuscitation team are to restore spontaneous breathing and circulation and preserve vital organ function throughout the resuscitation effort.

THE CRITICAL TASKS OF RESUSCITATION AND CONFIGURATION OF THE RESUSCITATION TEAM

Every resuscitation effort must have someone who assumes responsibility for overseeing the actions of the resuscitation team. If more than one person attempts to make decisions regarding the patient's care, confusion reigns and chaos will most likely result. The person in charge of the resuscitation effort is typically called the code director or team leader. The team leader directs the members of the team and oversees the resuscitation effort, making sure each team member performs tasks safely and correctly. Ideally, the team leader should be in a position to "stand back" to view and direct the resuscitation effort instead of performing specific tasks. However, the size of a resuscitation team and the skills of each team member vary. Some tasks can be performed by personnel with basic life support training, while others require advanced training.

A resuscitation effort requires coordination of four critical tasks:
1. Airway management
2. Chest compressions
3. ECG monitoring and defibrillation
4. Vascular access and drug administration

If the code team consists of five individuals, each of these critical tasks is assigned to a team member and the team leader oversees their actions (Figure 8-1). If the roles of each member of the code team have not already been preassigned, the team leader must quickly assign these tasks as the team members are assembled.

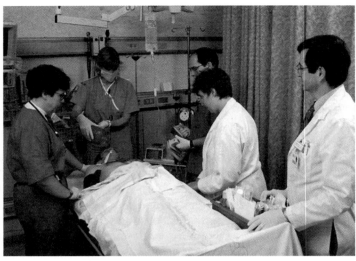

Figure 8-1 • The team leader assigns the four critical resuscitation tasks: airway management, chest compressions, ECG monitoring and defibrillation, and vascular access and drug administration.

Keeping It Simple

Four Critical Tasks of Resuscitation
Airway management
Chest compressions
ECG monitoring and defibrillation
Vascular access and medication administration

TEAM LEADER RESPONSIBILITIES

The team leader has many responsibilities during the resuscitation effort:
- Assesses the patient.
- Orders emergency care according to protocols.
- Considers reasons for the cardiac arrest and possible reversible causes.
- Supervises team members, ensuring that each member of the team performs tasks safely and correctly.
- Evaluates the adequacy of chest compressions including hand position, depth of cardiac compressions, proper rate, and ratio of compressions to ventilations.
- Ensures that the patient is receiving 100% O_2.
- Evaluates the adequacy of ventilation by assessing bilateral, symmetrical chest expansion with each ventilation.
- Ensures that defibrillation, when indicated, is performed safely and correctly.
- Ensures the correct choice and placement of vascular access.
- Confirms proper position of an advanced airway (if used).
- Ensures that drugs given are appropriate for the clinical situation/dysrhythmia and the correct dose, route, and concentration (if applicable).
- Ensures that IV bolus medications are followed with a 20-mL fluid flush and elevation of the extremity.
- Ensures the safety of all members of the resuscitation team, especially when procedures such as defibrillation are performed.
- Problem solves, including reevaluating possible causes of the arrest and recognizing malfunctioning equipment and/or misplaced or displaced tubes or lines.
- Decides when to terminate resuscitation efforts in consultation with team members.

TEAM MEMBER RESPONSIBILITIES

Airway Management Team Member

The ACLS team member responsible for airway management should do the following:
- Perform the head-tilt/chin-lift maneuver and jaw thrust without head-tilt maneuver.
- Correctly size and insert an oral airway and nasal airway.
- Correctly apply and understand the indications, contraindications, advantages, disadvantages, complications, liter flow range, and concentration of delivered O_2 for O_2 delivery devices including the nasal cannula, simple face mask, pocket mask, nonrebreathing mask, and bag-mask device.
- Suction the upper airway by selecting an appropriate suction device and catheter, and by using correct technique.
- Know how to correctly perform cricoid pressure.
- Know the indications, contraindications, advantages, disadvantages, complications, equipment, and technique for (if within his or her scope of practice) insertion of an advanced airway.
- Know how to confirm placement of an advanced airway.
- Know how to use an esophageal detector device and exhaled carbon dioxide detector.
- Know how to properly secure an advanced airway.

Cardiopulmonary Resuscitation Team Member

The ACLS or basic life support (BLS) team member responsible for cardiopulmonary resuscitation (CPR) must know how to properly perform CPR and provide chest compressions of adequate rate, force, and depth in the correct location.

Electrocardiographic Monitoring and Defibrillation Team Member

The ACLS team member responsible for ECG monitoring and defibrillation should know the following:
- How to operate an automated external defibrillator (AED) and manual defibrillator
- The difference between defibrillation and synchronized cardioversion, and the indications for and potential complications of these electrical procedures
- The proper placement of hand-held defibrillator paddles and combination adhesive pads
- The safety precautions that must be considered when performing electrical therapy
- The indications for and possible complications of transcutaneous pacing
- How to problem solve equipment failure

Vascular Access and Medications Team Member

The ACLS team member responsible for vascular access and medication administration should know the following:
- Site(s) of first choice for vascular access if no intravenous (IV) catheter is in place at the time of cardiac arrest
- Procedure for performing intraosseous (IO) access in an adult
- IV fluids of first choice in cardiac arrest
- Importance of following each drug given in a cardiac arrest with a 20-mL IV fluid bolus and elevation of the extremity
- Routes of administration and appropriate dosages for IV, IO, and endotracheal resuscitation medications

Support Roles

Support roles in a resuscitation effort include the following:
- Management of supplies
- Assistance with procedures
- Documentation of the resuscitation effort
- Liaison functions
- Crowd control

- ACLS algorithms are general guidelines for the management of specific dysrhythmias and clinical conditions.
- A change in the rhythm or a change in the pulse changes the algorithm.
- Continually reassess the patient—conditions change.

CODE ORGANIZATION: "PHASE RESPONSE"

Phase I: Anticipation

During the anticipation phase of a resuscitation effort, rescuers either respond to the scene of a possible cardiac arrest or await the patient's arrival from outside the hospital. Important steps to take at this time include the following:
- Analyzing initial information such as patient age, estimated time of arrest, circumstances surrounding the arrest, and presence of a do not attempt resuscitation (DNAR) order
- Assembling the resuscitation team
- Identifying the team leader
- Assigning critical resuscitation tasks
- Preparing advanced life support (ALS) equipment and positioning the code cart for easy access to defibrillator pads or paddles, O_2, suction equipment, drugs and supplies, and viewing the ECG monitor
- Positioning the team leader and resuscitation team members to begin (or continue) resuscitation efforts

Phase II: Entry

During the entry phase, the team leader identifies himself or herself and begins to obtain information as the resuscitation effort begins or continues.

In the field, care should begin where the patient is found unless EMS personnel do not have enough space to resuscitate the patient or conditions exist that may be hazardous to them or the patient. Quickly perform a primary survey. Check for signs of obvious death. If signs of obvious signs of death are present, do not begin CPR. If there are no signs of obvious death but the patient is unresponsive, not breathing, and has no central pulse, make sure the patient is on a firm surface while a team member quickly checks for documentation or other evidence of a DNAR order.
- If a properly completed DNAR form exists, do not begin CPR.
- If a DNAR order exists but its validity is questionable, place the patient on a cardiac monitor and consult with a physician immediately for direction about how to proceed. Follow your local protocol about what should be done on the scene in these situations while waiting to talk with medical direction.
- If a DNAR does not exist and there are no signs of obvious death, begin resuscitation.

In the hospital, the team leader ensures that a code board is placed under the patient. Most hospital beds have a "code" feature that quickly places the bed flat and deflates cushioning devices at the same time. If the patient is being transferred from another bed, the team leader ensures that the transfer occurs in a safe and orderly manner from the stretcher/gurney to the resuscitation bed.

The team leader:

■ Instructs team members to obtain baseline ABCD information and communicate this information to the team leader in the ABCD sequence. In the primary survey, ABCD stands for airway, breathing, circulation, and defibrillation. In the secondary survey, ABCD stands for advanced airway, breathing, circulation, and differential diagnosis.

■ When applicable, the team leader of the previous setting provides a concise history of the event and care given to the team leader accepting the patient. For example, a first responder relays information to arriving paramedics. Paramedics relay information to the ED nurse or physician.

■ Considers baseline laboratory values and other relevant data if necessary.

■ Evaluates the information at hand and acts on that information.

Although not always available, information related to the arrest should be sought including the following:

- When and where did the arrest occur?
- Was the arrest witnessed?
- Was CPR performed? If yes, how long was the patient down before CPR was started?
- What was the patient's initial cardiac rhythm? If VF or pulseless VT, when was the first shock delivered?
- Are there any special circumstances to consider such as hypothermia, trauma, drug overdose, DNAR orders?
- What treatment has been given?
- What information is available regarding the patient's past medical history?

Phase III: Resuscitation

This phase focuses on the ABCDs of resuscitation. The team leader directs the resuscitation team through the various resuscitation protocols. As the team leader, it is essential to act professionally throughout the resuscitation effort. Speak in a firm, confident tone to the members of your team. Be open to and actively seek suggestions from team members.

Ask your team members to tell you when there is any change in the patient's airway, breathing, or circulation (ABCs). Also, ask that they tell you when procedures are completed and drugs are given. For example, if you instructed a team member to establish an IV or give a drug, the response should be something like, "IV started—left antecubital vein," "1-mg 1:10,000 epinephrine given IV" when the task is completed. Team members should be instructed to ask you for clarification if your instructions are unclear.

Remember that during a cardiac arrest, your two most important priorities are CPR and, if a shockable rhythm is present, defibrillation. Vascular access, giving drugs, and inserting an advanced airway are of secondary importance. The rhythm present on the cardiac monitor will guide the sequence of procedures that need to be done next. For example, if the patient is in cardiac arrest and the cardiac monitor shows no electrical activity, asystole is present. If the monitor shows an organized rhythm despite no central pulse when you assess the patient, PEA is present. Defibrillation is not indicated for asystole or PEA. If the monitor shows VF or VT, defibrillation is indicated. Throughout the resuscitation effort, keep in mind that a change in the patient's cardiac rhythm usually results in a change in the recommended treatment sequence (algorithm). For instance, if defibrillation of VF results in a sinus rhythm, the algorithm changes because of the rhythm change. If the sinus rhythm on the monitor *does not* produce a pulse, the patient has PEA and treatment continues using that algorithm. If the sinus rhythm on the monitor *does* produce a pulse, supportive measures must be taken to maintain the perfusing rhythm. This is called postresuscitation support. The patient's breathing and blood pressure (BP) must be assessed with a return of a pulse. If defibrillation of VT results in VF (or vice versa), there is no change in the algorithm because pulseless VT and VF are treated in the same way.

In the field, if the patient's collapse is *witnessed* and the monitor shows VT or VF, defibrillation should be performed immediately. If there is a delay applying the cardiac monitor or preparing the defibrillator, begin CPR. If the patient's collapse was *not* witnessed and the monitor shows VT or VF, begin CPR. After five cycles of CPR (about 2 minutes), attempt defibrillation. In the hospital setting, there are insufficient data to support or refute CPR before defibrillation.[1]

When pulseless VT/VF is present, defibrillation is indicated. When the team leader indicates it is time to deliver a shock, all team members with the exception of the person performing chest compressions should *immediately* clear the patient. The airway team member must make sure that O_2 is not flowing near the patient's chest. Once the defibrillator is charged, the chest compressor should clear the patient and a shock should be delivered immediately to the patient. In this way, chest compressions are interrupted for the least amount of time possible during the resuscitation effort.

Once the shock is delivered, immediately resume CPR, starting with chest compressions. Perform five cycles of CPR (about 2 minutes), and then recheck the patient's rhythm. Continue emergency care according to the appropriate algorithm.

Establish vascular access. If no IV is in place at the time of the arrest, start a peripheral IV with a large-gauge catheter without interrupting CPR. The antecubital or external jugular veins are preferred. The preferred IV solution for use in cardiac arrest is normal saline or lactated Ringer's. Glucose-containing solutions should be avoided unless documented hypoglycemia exists. If peripheral IV attempts are unsuccessful, IO access should be attempted before trying a central line.

Give drugs using the correct algorithm. Drugs given during cardiac arrest should be given during brief pauses for rhythm checks and then followed with a 20-mL flush of IV fluid and elevation of the extremity. The drug is then circulated when CPR is resumed.

If the decision is made to insert an advanced airway, the procedure should be performed in less than 30 seconds. Make sure that the position of the tube is confirmed and then appropriately secured.

If a pulse returns, repeat the primary survey. If a pulse is present, assess the patient's breathing and BP. If there is no response to appropriately performed interventions, consider termination of efforts.

KEEPING IT SIMPLE

Remember to repeat the primary survey:
With any sudden change in the patient's condition.
When interventions do not appear to be working.
When vital signs are unstable.
Before any procedures.
When a change in rhythm is observed on the cardiac monitor.

Phase IV: Maintenance

In the maintenance phase of the resuscitation effort, a spontaneous pulse has returned or the patient's vital signs have stabilized. Efforts of the resuscitation team should be focused on the following:

- Anticipating and preventing deterioration of the patient's condition
- Repeated assessment of the patient's ABCs
- Stabilizing vital signs
- Securing tubes and lines
- Troubleshooting any problem areas
- Preparing the patient for transport/transfer
- Accurately documenting the events during the resuscitation effort
- Drawing blood for laboratory tests and treating as needed based on results

Phase V: Family Notification

Surveys have revealed that most relatives of patients requiring CPR would like to be offered the possibility of being in the resuscitation room.[2,3] In follow-up surveys with family members that had witnessed a resuscitation effort, most felt their adjustment to the death or grieving was facilitated by their witnessing the resuscitation and that their presence was beneficial to the dying family member.[4]

If family members are not present during the resuscitation effort, they should be told that resuscitation efforts have begun and should be periodically updated. The result of the resuscitation effort, whether successful or unsuccessful, should be relayed to the family promptly with honesty and compassion.

When speaking with the family, speak slowly in a quiet, calm voice and use simple terms, not medical terms. Pause every few seconds to ask if they understand what is being said. You may need to repeat information several times. Generally, you should make eye contact with the family members—except where cultural differences may exist. Enlist the assistance of a social worker, clergy, or grief support personnel as needed.

Conveying the News of a Death to Concerned Survivors

Healthcare professionals may not receive sufficient training regarding how the death of a loved one should be conveyed to survivors. In a survey of family members of patients who had died, the most important features of delivering bad news were determined to be:

- Attitude of the news-giver (ranked most important by 72%)
- Clarity of the message (70%)
- Privacy (65%)
- Knowledge/ability to answer questions (57%)

In this survey, the attire of the news-giver ranked as least important (3%). Sympathy, time for questions, and location of the conversation were ranked of intermediate importance. Touching was unwanted by 30% of the respondents, but encouraged or acceptable in 24%.[5]

If the resuscitation effort was unsuccessful, use the words "death," "dying," or "dead" instead of phrases such as "passed on," "no longer with us," "went to another place," or "we lost him" when speaking to the family. Allow time for the shock to be absorbed and as much time as necessary for questions and discussion. It is important to provide adequate information to the caregivers. This may require repeating answers or explanations to make sure they are understood.

Assume nothing as to how the news is going to be received. The family's reaction to the disclosure of bad news may be anger, shock, withdrawal, disbelief, extreme agitation, guilt, or sorrow. In some cases, there may be no observable response, or the response may seem inappropriate.

A statement such as "You have my (our) sincere sympathy" may be used to express your feelings. However, there are times that silence is appropriate. Silence respects the family's feelings and allows them to regain composure at their own pace.

Allow the family the opportunity to see their relative. In cases involving severe traumatic cardiac arrest, this may not be advisable. If equipment is still connected to the patient, prepare the family for what they will see. The patient should be gowned before the family views the body. Accompany them if necessary. Some caregivers may prefer not to view the body. If this is their preference, do not attempt to force them to do so.

Offer to contact the patient's attending or family physician and to be available if there are further questions. Arrange for follow-up and continued support during the grieving period.

Phase VI: Transfer

The resuscitation team's responsibility to the patient continues until patient care is transferred to a healthcare team with equal or greater expertise. When transferring care, provide information that is well organized, concise, and complete.

Phase VII: Critique

Regardless of the outcome of the resuscitation effort or its length, the team leader is responsible for making sure that the resuscitation effort is critiqued by the team. A critique of the resuscitation provides the following:

- An opportunity for education ("teachable moment")
- Feedback to hospital and prehospital personnel regarding the efforts of the team
- Review the events of the resuscitation effort including the following:
  - Relevant patient history and events preceding the arrest
  - Decisions made during the arrest and any variations from usual protocols
  - Discuss the elements of the resuscitation that went well, those areas that could be improved, and recommendations for future resuscitation efforts

Helping the Caregivers

An unsuccessful resuscitation effort is difficult for the family as well as the healthcare professionals involved in the resuscitation. Although each healthcare professional may deal with stress differently, reactions suggesting a need for assistance include persistent feelings of anger, self-doubt, sadness, depression, or a desire to withdraw from others. It is important to recognize the warning signs of stress in yourself and others and know how to deal with them. Strategies for dealing with stress may include exercise, practicing relaxation techniques, talking with family or friends, or meeting with a qualified mental health professional.

CARDIAC ARREST RHYTHMS

The initial rhythm recorded by emergency personnel is generally considered the electrical mechanism of a cardiac arrest.[6] This information is important because it impacts patient outcome. Patients who are in sustained VT at the time of initial contact have the best outcome. Those who present with a bradyarrhythmia or asystole at initial contact have the worst prognosis. If the initial rhythm recorded is VF, the patient's outcome is intermediate between the outcomes associated with sustained VT and bradyarrhythmia and asystole.[6]

Data from the 1970s and 1980s indicated that shockable rhythms (VT or VF) were the initial rhythms observed in 70% to 80% of cardiac arrests each year in the United States. PEA and asystole were the initial rhythms in 20% and 30% of victims.

Reviewing the ECG tracings of patients who died while wearing a Holter monitor helped researchers determine the electrical mechanisms of cardiac arrest.[7] In most cases, ventricular tachyarrhythmias were the most frequent cause of sudden death. VF was often preceded by VT. In some cases, VT leading to VF was preceded by sinus tachycardia or a new atrial tachyarrhythmia.

More recent data indicate that about 40% of victims are in VF at the time of initial contact.[8-10] PEA and asystole are being reported with increasing frequency as the initial rhythm in prehospital sudden cardiac deaths.[11] Based on studies of patients who died while their cardiac rhythm was being monitored, it is likely that prehospital cardiac arrest victims were in VT or VF, which deteriorated to PEA or asystole by the time the patient's initial cardiac rhythm was analyzed.

RHYTHMS: PULSELESS VENTRICULAR TACHYCARDIA/VENTRICULAR FIBRILLATION

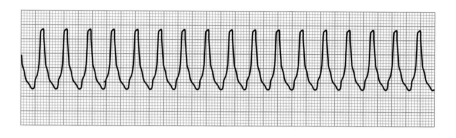

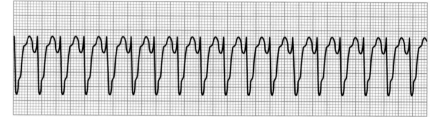

Figure 8-2 • Monomorphic VT.

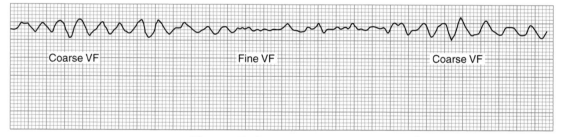

Figure 8-3 • Coarse and fine VF.

Monitor lead

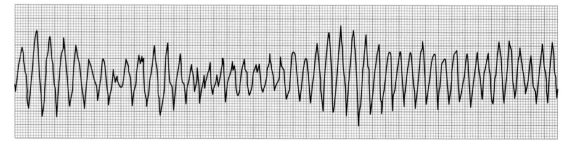

Figure 8-4 • Unstable, sustained polymorphic VT is treated as VF.

Medications

Medications used in pulseless VT/VF include epinephrine, vasopressin, amiodarone, lidocaine, and (in some cases) magnesium sulfate.

Vasopressors

Epinephrine and vasopressin are vasopressors. Epinephrine has many beneficial actions including bronchodilation, increased heart rate, and increased force of contraction. However, epinephrine is given in cardiac arrest primarily for its vasoconstricting (alpha-adrenergic) properties. Vasoconstriction helps increase coronary and cerebral perfusion pressures.

Epinephrine should be given IV or IO in cardiac arrest. The IV/IO dose of epinephrine is 1 mg of 1:10,000 solution. Although it can be given endotracheally, some studies suggest that endotracheal epinephrine can produce a transient *decrease* in BP (see Chapter 5). This effect is presumed to be due to beta$_2$-adrenergic receptor stimulation. This can cause hypotension and *lower* coronary artery perfusion pressure, which may lessen the potential for a return of spontaneous circulation. If epinephrine is given endotracheally, remember that the endotracheal (ET) dose is 2 to 2.5 times the IV/IO dose. Because the effects of epinephrine do not last long, epinephrine should be repeated every 3 to 5 minutes as long as the patient is in cardiac arrest.

 Epinephrine is available in different concentrations and in different medication containers such as a prefilled syringe, ampules, and multidose vials. Be sure you read the label carefully before giving epinephrine to ensure that you are giving the right dose and using the right concentration of the drug.

Vasopressin causes constriction of peripheral, coronary, and renal vessels. Vasopressin can be given IV/IO or endotracheally. When used, 40 U is given once in place of the first or second dose of epinephrine in cardiac arrest. Research has shown that endotracheal vasopressin produces an immediate increase in diastolic BP that lasts more than 1 hour (see Chapter 5). Elevated diastolic BP is important because it directly influences coronary perfusion pressure.

 During a cardiac arrest, drugs should be given at the time of the rhythm check. Remember to follow each IV/IO bolus dose of a drug used in cardiac arrest with a 20-mL IV fluid flush and elevate the extremity for 10 to 20 seconds to help speed delivery of the drug to the central circulation.

Antiarrhythmics

If pulseless VT/VF continues despite CPR, 2 or 3 shocks, and giving a vasopressor, consider giving an antiarrhythmic.

Amiodarone is an antiarrhythmic that blocks sodium channels, inhibits sympathetic stimulation, and blocks potassium channels as well as calcium channels. In cardiac arrest due to pulseless VT/VF, the initial IV/IO bolus of amiodarone is 300 mg. If the rhythm persists, consider a repeat IV/IO bolus dose of 150 mg in 5 minutes. If there is a return of spontaneous circulation after giving amiodarone, a continuous infusion of the drug may be considered.

 If there is a return of spontaneous circulation after giving an antiarrhythmic, it may be reasonable to begin a continuous infusion of the drug associated with a return of spontaneous circulation.[12]

Although amiodarone is the antiarrhythmic mentioned first in the pulseless VT/VF algorithm, lidocaine may be considered if amiodarone is unavailable. The initial dose of lidocaine is 1 to 1.5 mg/kg IV push. Repeat doses of 0.5 to 0.75 mg/kg IV push may be given at 5- to 10-minute intervals. The cumulative IV/IO bolus dose is 3 mg/kg. If there is a return of spontaneous circulation, consider a lidocaine infusion of 1 to 4 mg/min.

Magnesium sulfate is recommended for torsades de pointes (TdP) with or without cardiac arrest. In cardiac arrest, magnesium is given IV/IO at a dose of 1 to 2 g diluted in 10-mL D5W (5% dextrose in water).

It is important to consider possible reversible causes of a cardiac emergency. Possible reversible causes and interventions to consider are as follows:

PATCH-4-MD

Pulmonary embolism—anticoagulants? surgery?

Acidosis—ventilation, correct acid-base disturbances

Tension pneumothorax—needle decompression

Cardiac tamponade—pericardiocentesis

Hypovolemia—replace volume

Hypoxia—give O_2, ensure adequate ventilation

Heat/cold (hyperthermia/hypothermia)—cooling/warming methods

Hypokalemia/hyperkalemia (and other electrolytes)—correct electrolyte disturbances

Myocardial infarction—fibrinolytics?

Drug overdose/accidents—antidote/specific therapy

Pulseless Ventricular Tachycardia/Ventricular Fibrillation Algorithm

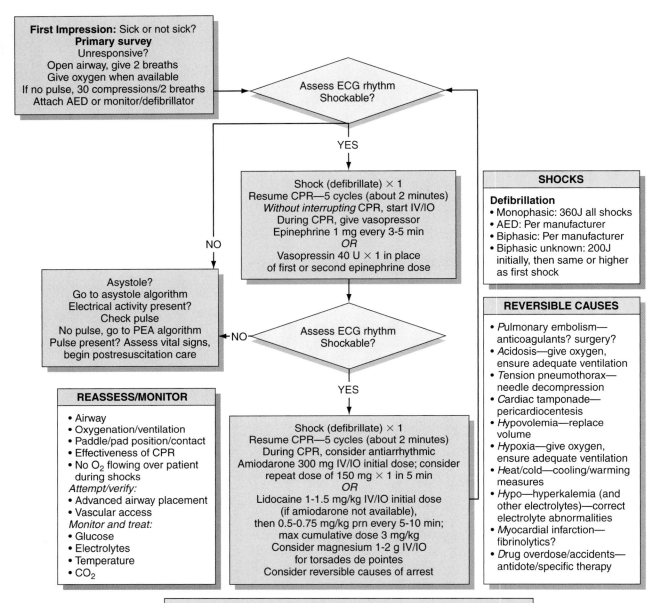

First Impression: Sick or not sick?
Primary survey
Unresponsive?
Open airway, give 2 breaths
Give oxygen when available
If no pulse, 30 compressions/2 breaths
Attach AED or monitor/defibrillator

Assess ECG rhythm
Shockable?

YES

Shock (defibrillate) × 1
Resume CPR—5 cycles (about 2 minutes)
Without interrupting CPR, start IV/IO
During CPR, give vasopressor
Epinephrine 1 mg every 3-5 min
OR
Vasopressin 40 U × 1 in place
of first or second epinephrine dose

NO

Asystole?
Go to asystole algorithm
Electrical activity present?
Check pulse
No pulse, go to PEA algorithm
Pulse present? Assess vital signs,
begin postresuscitation care

NO

Assess ECG rhythm
Shockable?

YES

REASSESS/MONITOR

- Airway
- Oxygenation/ventilation
- Paddle/pad position/contact
- Effectiveness of CPR
- No O_2 flowing over patient
  during shocks
Attempt/verify:
- Advanced airway placement
- Vascular access
Monitor and treat:
- Glucose
- Electrolytes
- Temperature
- CO_2

Shock (defibrillate) × 1
Resume CPR—5 cycles (about 2 minutes)
During CPR, consider antiarrhythmic
Amiodarone 300 mg IV/IO initial dose; consider
repeat dose of 150 mg × 1 in 5 min
OR
Lidocaine 1-1.5 mg/kg IV/IO initial dose
(if amiodarone not available),
then 0.5-0.75 mg/kg prn every 5-10 min;
max cumulative dose 3 mg/kg
Consider magnesium 1-2 g IV/IO
for torsades de pointes
Consider reversible causes of arrest

SHOCKS

Defibrillation
- Monophasic: 360J all shocks
- AED: Per manufacturer
- Biphasic: Per manufacturer
- Biphasic unknown: 200J
  initially, then same or higher
  as first shock

REVERSIBLE CAUSES

- *P*ulmonary embolism—
  anticoagulants? surgery?
- *A*cidosis—give oxygen,
  ensure adequate ventilation
- *T*ension pneumothorax—
  needle decompression
- *C*ardiac tamponade—
  pericardiocentesis
- *H*ypovolemia—replace
  volume
- *H*ypoxia—give oxygen,
  ensure adequate ventilation
- *H*eat/cold—cooling/warming
  measures
- *H*ypo—hyperkalemia (and
  other electrolytes)—correct
  electrolyte abnormalities
- *M*yocardial infarction—
  fibrinolytics?
- *D*rug overdose/accidents—
  antidote/specific therapy

Algorithm assumes scene safety has been assured, personal protective
equipment is used, no signs of obvious death or presence
of do not resuscitate order, and previous step was unsuccessful

Figure 8-5 • Pulseless VT/VF algorithm.

Putting It All Together

■ *Evaluator:*   Your patient is a 48-year-old man who was found unresponsive in bed by his wife. You have five other advanced life support personnel to assist you. Emergency equipment is immediately available.

■ *Team Leader:*   Is the scene safe to enter?

■ *Evaluator:*   The scene is safe.

Initial Assessment

First Impression

■ *Team Leader:*   I am putting on personal protective equipment. As I approach the patient and form a first impression, what do I see?

■ *Evaluator:*   The patient is supine in bed. His eyes are closed. You do not see any obvious chest rise and fall. The patient's skin is pale.

Primary Survey

■ *Team Leader:*   I will quickly approach the patient and assess his level of responsiveness.

■ *Evaluator:*   The patient is unresponsive.

■ *Team Leader:*   I will open the patient's airway using a head-tilt/chin-lift. Do I see anything in the patient's mouth such as blood, broken teeth or loose dentures, gastric contents, or a foreign object?

■ *Evaluator:*   The airway is clear. What should be done now?

■ *Team Leader:*   I will look, listen, and feel for breathing for up to 10 seconds.

■ *Evaluator:*   The patient is not breathing.

■ *Team Leader:*   I will ask the airway team member to size and insert an oral airway and begin positive-pressure ventilation with a bag-mask connected to 100% oxygen while I continue the primary survey. I want the airway team member to maintain proper head position and a good seal with the mask against the patient's face. I want a second team member to assume responsibility for compressing the bag with just enough force to produce gentle chest rise.

■ *Evaluator:*   An oral airway has been inserted. The patient is being ventilated with a bag-mask. You see gentle chest rise with bagging. At what rate should this patient be ventilated?

■ *Team Leader:*   The patient should be ventilated at a rate of 10 to 12 ventilations per minute (one ventilation every 5 to 6 seconds). Each ventilation should be given over 1 second. I will ask another assistant to assess baseline breath sounds while the patient is being ventilated. I want the defibrillation team member to attach self-adhesive combination pads to the patient's chest while I feel for a carotid pulse for up to 10 seconds. Do I feel a carotid pulse?

■ *Evaluator:*   Breath sounds are clear and equal with bagging. There is no pulse. What should be done now?

■ *Team Leader:*   I will ask for a defibrillator immediately. I want the CPR team member to begin chest compressions while I will begin the secondary survey. I want the CPR team member and airway team member to automatically rotate positions after every five cycles (about 2 minutes) of CPR so they don't become fatigued. I want the patient's ECG rhythm checked every 2 minutes as the team members change positions.

■ *Evaluator:*   Combination pads are in place on the patient's chest. A monophasic defibrillator is now present. You see this rhythm on the cardiac monitor (Figure 8-6). What is the rhythm on the monitor?

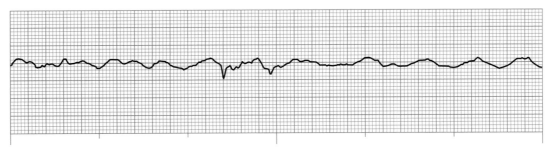

Figure 8-6

■ *Team Leader:*	The rhythm is ventricular fibrillation. I will ask the airway team member to temporarily shut off the oxygen as I prepare to shock the patient. I want the IV team member to prepare the initial drugs that will be used and start an IV after the first shock is delivered.
■ *Evaluator:*	What initial drugs do you want the IV team member to prepare?
■ *Team Leader:*	I want the IV team member to prepare epinephrine, vasopressin, and amiodarone for now.
■ *Evaluator:*	What energy setting will you use for your initial shock?
■ *Team Leader:*	When a monophasic defibrillator is used, all shocks are delivered using 360 J. As the machine charges, I want all team members, with the exception of the chest compressor, to immediately clear the patient. As the airway team member clears the patient, I will remind him to turn off the oxygen flow. I want the chest compressor to continue CPR while the machine is charging. Once the defibrillator is charged, I want the chest compressor to *immediately* clear the patient. I am ready to shock the patient. I will make sure the chest compressor is now clear of the patient and will deliver a shock with 360 J.
■ *Evaluator:*	Shock delivered. What would you like to do next?

Use the energy levels recommended by the manufacturer if a biphasic defibrillator is used. If you do not know what the recommended energy levels are, it is reasonable to use 200 J to start. Use 200 J or a higher dose for the second or subsequent shocks, depending on the capabilities of the defibrillator.

Secondary Survey/Focused History and Exam

■ *Team Leader:*	I want my team to resume CPR immediately, beginning with chest compressions. I will ask the airway team member to turn the oxygen on. After five cycles of CPR (about 2 minutes), I will recheck the patient's rhythm. Without interrupting CPR, I want the IV team member to start an IV of normal saline, give 40 units of vasopressin IV push, flush the dose with 20 mL of normal saline, and raise the arm. I am considering possible causes of the arrest. Is there someone available who may know what happened before the patient collapsed?
■ *Evaluator:*	(See Table 8-1 for SAMPLE history and Table 8-2 for physical exam findings.) An IV has been started with normal saline in the patient's left antecubital vein. Vasopressin has been given IV as ordered.
■ *Team Leader:*	I will recheck the patient's ECG rhythm.
■ *Evaluator:*	The monitor is unchanged. It has been about 2 minutes since your team resumed CPR.
■ *Team Leader:*	I will prepare to deliver another shock. I will clear all team members, except the chest compressor, from the patient. I will remind the airway team member to turn off the oxygen flow. I am ready to shock the patient. I will make sure the chest compressor is now clear of the patient and will deliver a shock with 360 J.
■ *Evaluator:*	Shock delivered. What would you like to do next?

TABLE 8-1. SAMPLE History

(History obtained from wife)

Signs/symptoms	Unwitnessed collapse
Allergies	None
Medications	Depakote
Past medical history	Seizures
Last oral intake	Unknown
Events prior	Unknown

TABLE 8-2. Physical Examination Findings

Head, ears, eyes, nose, and throat	No abnormalities noted
Neck	Trachea midline, no jugular venous distention
Chest	Breath sounds clear and equal with positive-pressure ventilation
Abdomen	No abnormalities noted
Pelvis	No abnormalities noted
Extremities	No abnormalities noted
Posterior body	No abnormalities noted

▪ *Team Leader:* I want my team to resume CPR immediately, starting with chest compressions. I will remind the airway team member to turn the oxygen on. I will recheck the patient's rhythm after five cycles of CPR. Without interrupting CPR, I want the IV team member to give 1 mg of 1:10,000 epinephrine IV push, flush the dose with 20 mL of normal saline, and raise the arm.

▪ *Evaluator:* CPR was resumed and epinephrine has been given as ordered. Two minutes have elapsed. The monitor is unchanged.

▪ *Team Leader:* I will prepare to deliver another shock. I will clear all team members, except the chest compressor, from the patient. I will remind the airway team member to turn off the oxygen flow. I am ready to shock the patient. I will make sure the chest compressor is now clear of the patient and will deliver a shock with 360 J.

▪ *Evaluator:* Shock delivered. What would you like to do next?

▪ *Team Leader:* I want my team to resume CPR immediately, starting with chest compressions. I will remind the airway team member to turn the oxygen on. I will recheck the patient's rhythm after five cycles of CPR. Without interrupting CPR, I want the IV team member to give 300 mg of amiodarone IV, flush the dose with 20 mL of IV fluid, and raise the arm.

▪ *Evaluator:* CPR was resumed and amiodarone has been given as ordered. Two minutes have elapsed.

▪ *Team Leader:* I will recheck the patient's ECG rhythm.

▪ *Evaluator:* The cardiac monitor shows the following rhythm (Figure 8-7). What is the rhythm?

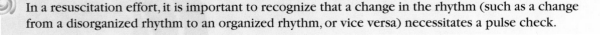

In a resuscitation effort, it is important to recognize that a change in the rhythm (such as a change from a disorganized rhythm to an organized rhythm, or vice versa) necessitates a pulse check.

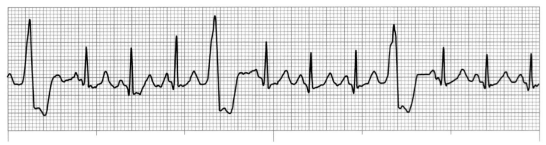

Figure 8-7

■ *Team Leader:* The rhythm is a sinus tachycardia with frequent uniform premature ventricular complexes (PVCs). I will ask the CPR team member to stop CPR and check for a pulse.

■ *Evaluator:* A strong carotid pulse is present. What should be done now?

Postresuscitation Support/Ongoing Assessment

■ *Team Leader:* I will ask an assistant to obtain a complete set of vital signs while I will repeat the primary survey. Is the patient responsive? Is he breathing?

■ *Evaluator:* The patient is moaning and breathing about 6 to 8 times per minute. A strong pulse is present at a rate of about 120 bpm. BP is 82/53. What should be done now?

■ *Team Leader:* I will recheck the patient's vital signs and ECG in about 5 minutes. I want the airway team member to assist the patient's breathing with a bag-mask connected to 100% oxygen and continue to monitor the patient's respiratory rate and effort. Because I gave an IV bolus dose of an antiarrhythmic during the arrest, I think it is reasonable to continue a maintenance infusion of that drug. The antiarrhythmic I used was amiodarone so I will ask the IV team member to hang an amiodarone drip. I want the drug infused at a rate of 1 mg/min for the next 6 hours.

■ *Evaluator:* An amiodarone drip is infusing as ordered. The patient is now awake but disoriented. He is breathing about 14 times per minute. His heart rate is about 100 bpm and the PVCs on the monitor have resolved. His BP is 117/65.

■ *Team Leader:* I will continue to closely monitor the patient's vital signs and ECG as I prepare to transfer the patient for further care.

What should you do if a shock terminates VF or pulseless VT and an accelerated idioventricular rhythm (AIVR) is now present on the monitor? A quick assessment reveals the patient has a pulse and is breathing on his own about 4 to 6 times/min. As you direct a team member to assist the patient's respirations, the patient's pulse and BP are assessed. The patient's BP is 94/53. The monitor shows AIVR at a rate of 100 bpm. Should anything be done about the patient's rhythm?

Confusion about what treatment should be instituted is common because the patient was previously pulseless and now has a pulse, although the rhythm on the monitor is ventricular in origin. AIVR can be mistaken for VT if the ventricular rate is not counted and the patient assessed. Keep in mind that most patients do not develop serious signs and symptoms related to a tachycardia until the rate exceeds 150 bpm. Although drugs are often used to suppress VT that causes serious signs and symptoms, they are not generally used to suppress AIVR. In our patient scenario, a patient who was pulseless now has a pulse and is attempting to breathe on his own. These are positive signs. In a case such as this, "watchful waiting" is a reasonable course of action. Remember, AIVR is usually a transient rhythm. Close monitoring of the patient's vital signs and cardiac rhythm is essential.

RHYTHMS: ASYSTOLE/PULSELESS ELECTRICAL ACTIVITY

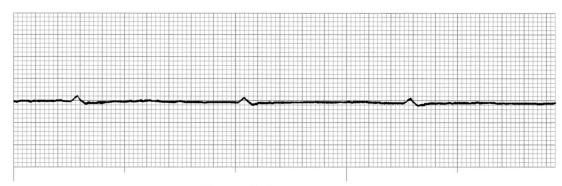

Figure 8-8 • P-wave asystole.

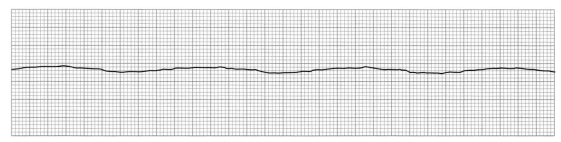

Figure 8-9 • Asystole.

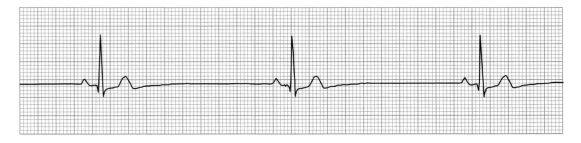

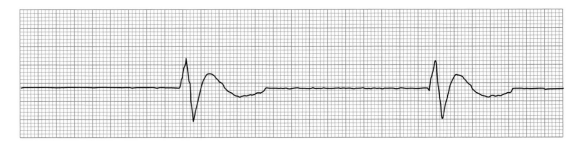

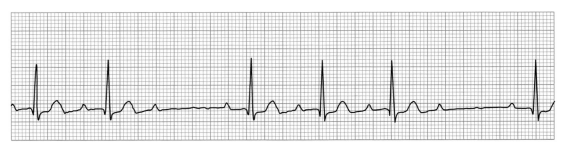

Figure 8-10 • PEA is an organized rhythm on the monitor, other than VT, that does not produce a palpable pulse.

Asystole is a total absence of ventricular electrical activity. There is no ventricular rate or rhythm, no pulse, and no cardiac output. Some atrial electrical activity may be evident. If atrial electrical activity is present, the rhythm is called "P-wave" asystole or ventricular standstill. "Bradyasystole refers to a cardiac rhythm that has a ventricular rate below 60 bpm in adults, periods of absent heart rhythm (asystole), or both. Bradyasystolic states are clinical situations during which bradyasystole is the dominant heart rhythm."[13]

Medications

Other than oxygen, the primary drugs used in the management of asystole and PEA are epinephrine or vasopressin, and atropine. Epinephrine was discussed earlier in this chapter. The 2005 resuscitation guidelines provide conflicting information about the use of vasopressin in cardiac arrest due to PEA: "If the rhythm check confirms asystole or PEA, resume CPR immediately. A vasopressor (epinephrine or vasopressin) may be administered at this time."[14] "Providers may consider vasopressin for treatment of asystole, but there is insufficient evidence to recommend for or against its use in PEA. Further studies are required."[15]

Atropine is a parasympathetic blocker. In cardiac arrest, it is possible that an absence of ventricular activity may be caused or worsened by excessive stimulation of the parasympathetic division of the autonomic nervous system. Because atropine blocks the effects of acetylcholine, it seems reasonable to give atropine in these situations. Although anecdotal reports of the return of sinus rhythm after atropine exist, definitive evidence of its usefulness is lacking. In cardiac arrest due to asystole or slow PEA, the recommended dose of atropine is 1 mg IV/IO bolus. This dose can be repeated every 3 to 5 minutes to a maximum total dose of 3 mg if the rhythm persists.

Note that atropine is given *after* epinephrine in cardiac arrest. In PEA, atropine is only given if the rate on the cardiac monitor is slow.

Defibrillating asystole is not recommended. Defibrillation is not indicated in PEA. According to the 2005 resuscitation guidelines, attempting transcutaneous pacing in asystole is also no longer recommended.

Asystole/Pulseless Electrical Activity Algorithm

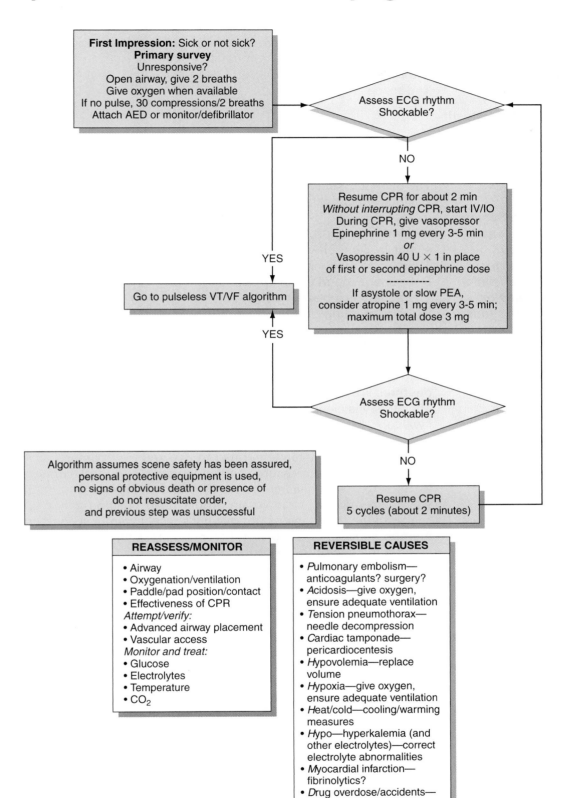

First Impression: Sick or not sick?
Primary survey
Unresponsive?
Open airway, give 2 breaths
Give oxygen when available
If no pulse, 30 compressions/2 breaths
Attach AED or monitor/defibrillator

Assess ECG rhythm
Shockable?

NO

Resume CPR for about 2 min
Without interrupting CPR, start IV/IO
During CPR, give vasopressor
Epinephrine 1 mg every 3-5 min
or
Vasopressin 40 U × 1 in place
of first or second epinephrine dose

If asystole or slow PEA,
consider atropine 1 mg every 3-5 min;
maximum total dose 3 mg

YES

Go to pulseless VT/VF algorithm

YES

Assess ECG rhythm
Shockable?

Algorithm assumes scene safety has been assured,
personal protective equipment is used,
no signs of obvious death or presence of
do not resuscitate order,
and previous step was unsuccessful

NO

Resume CPR
5 cycles (about 2 minutes)

REASSESS/MONITOR

- Airway
- Oxygenation/ventilation
- Paddle/pad position/contact
- Effectiveness of CPR
Attempt/verify:
- Advanced airway placement
- Vascular access
Monitor and treat:
- Glucose
- Electrolytes
- Temperature
- CO_2

REVERSIBLE CAUSES

- *P*ulmonary embolism—anticoagulants? surgery?
- *A*cidosis—give oxygen, ensure adequate ventilation
- *T*ension pneumothorax—needle decompression
- *C*ardiac tamponade—pericardiocentesis
- *H*ypovolemia—replace volume
- *H*ypoxia—give oxygen, ensure adequate ventilation
- *H*eat/cold—cooling/warming measures
- *H*ypo—hyperkalemia (and other electrolytes)—correct electrolyte abnormalities
- *M*yocardial infarction—fibrinolytics?
- *D*rug overdose/accidents—antidote/specific therapy

Figure 8-11 • Asystole/PEA algorithm.

Putting It All Together: Asystole

■ *Evaluator:*   Your patient is a 33-year-old woman who was found unresponsive by her boyfriend. You have four other ALS personnel to assist you. Emergency equipment is immediately available.

■ *Team Leader:*   Is the scene safe to enter?

■ *Evaluator:*   The scene is safe.

Initial Assessment

First Impression

■ *Team Leader:*   I am putting on personal protective equipment. As I approach the patient and form a first impression, what do I see?

■ *Evaluator:*   The patient is supine in bed. Her eyes are closed. You do not see any obvious chest rise and fall. The patient's skin is pale.

Primary Survey

■ *Team Leader:*   I will quickly approach the patient and assess her level of responsiveness. Does she respond when I call her name?

■ *Evaluator:*   There is no response.

■ *Team Leader:*   Does she respond when I pinch her hand?

■ *Evaluator:*   The patient is unresponsive.

■ *Team Leader:*   Is there anything on the scene or visible on the patient that would lead me to suspect possible trauma?

■ *Evaluator:*   No.

■ *Team Leader:*   I will open the patient's airway using a head-tilt/chin-lift. Do I see anything in the patient's mouth such as blood, broken teeth or loose dentures, gastric contents, or a foreign object?

■ *Evaluator:*   The airway is clear. What should be done now?

■ *Team Leader:*   I will look, listen, and feel for breathing for up to 10 seconds.

■ *Evaluator:*   The patient is not breathing.

■ *Team Leader:*   I will ask the airway team member to size and insert an oral airway and begin positive-pressure ventilation with a bag-mask connected to 100% oxygen while I continue the primary survey. I want the airway team member to maintain proper head position and a good seal with the mask against the patient's face. I want a second team member to assume responsibility for compressing the bag with just enough force to produce gentle chest rise.

■ *Evaluator:*   An oral airway has been inserted. The patient is being ventilated with a bag-mask. You see gentle chest rise with bagging. At what rate should this patient be ventilated?

■ *Team Leader:*   The patient should be ventilated at a rate of 10 to 12 ventilations/minute (one ventilation every 5 to 6 seconds). Each ventilation should be given over 1 second. I will ask another assistant to assess baseline breath sounds while the patient is being ventilated. I will ask the defibrillation team member to attach the ECG monitoring leads while I feel for a carotid pulse for up to 10 seconds. Do I feel a carotid pulse?

■ *Evaluator:*   Breath sounds are clear and equal with bagging. There is no pulse. What should be done now?

■ *Team Leader:*   I will request a defibrillator immediately, instruct the CPR team member to begin chest compressions, and I will begin the secondary survey. I want the CPR team member and airway team member to automatically rotate positions after every five cycles (about 2 minutes) of CPR so they don't become fatigued. I want the patient's ECG rhythm checked every 2 minutes as the team members change positions.

Secondary Survey/Focused History and Exam

■ *Evaluator:* The patient has been placed on the cardiac monitor (Figure 8-12). A defibrillator is now present. What is the rhythm on the monitor?

■ *Team Leader:* The rhythm is asystole. I want to confirm this rhythm in a second lead.

■ *Evaluator:* The rhythm is confirmed as asystole.

■ *Team Leader:* Is there someone available who may know what happened before the patient collapsed? I will ask the IV team member to start an IV of normal saline without interrupting CPR and then give 1 mg of 1:10,000 epinephrine IV push as soon as the IV is in. I want epinephrine given every 3 to 5 minutes as long as the patient has no pulse. Flush each dose with 20 mL of normal saline and raise the arm. I will perform a focused physical exam, looking for possible clues as to the cause of the arrest.

■ *Evaluator:* (See Table 8-3 for SAMPLE history and Table 8-4 for physical exam findings.) CPR is continuing as ordered. An IV has been established with normal saline. The first dose of epinephrine has been given as

TABLE 8-3. SAMPLE History

Signs/symptoms	Found unresponsive by boyfriend
Allergies	Unknown
Medications	Paxil
Past medical history	Depression
Last oral intake	Unknown
Events prior	Found unresponsive by boyfriend, last seen 40 minutes ago; according to the boyfriend, the patient lost her job two weeks ago

TABLE 8-4. Physical Examination Findings

Head, ears, eyes, nose, and throat	No abnormalities noted
Neck	Trachea midline, no jugular venous distention
Chest	Breath sounds clear and equal with positive-pressure ventilation
Abdomen	No abnormalities noted
Pelvis	No abnormalities noted
Extremities	No abnormalities noted
Posterior body	No abnormalities noted

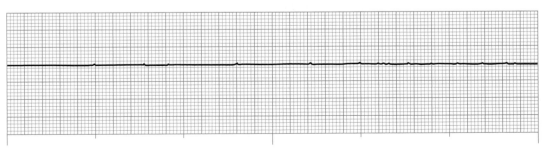

Figure 8-12

ordered. Other than asystole, what are possible causes of a flat line on the cardiac monitor?

■ *Team Leader:* Other than asystole, possible causes of a flat line on the cardiac monitor include no power, loose leads, no connection to the patient, and no connection to the defibrillator or monitor. I want the IV team member to give 1 mg of atropine IV push every 3 to 5 minutes until the maximum dose of 3 mg is reached. Flush each dose with 20 mL of normal saline and raise the arm.

■ *Evaluator:* Atropine order received.

■ *Team Leader:* After making sure that we have an esophageal detector device available, I want my most experienced assistant to intubate the patient. I want the defibrillation team member to assist by performing cricoid pressure during the procedure.

■ *Evaluator:* An endotracheal tube has been inserted and the cuff inflated. Cricoid pressure has been discontinued.

■ *Team Leader:* I will confirm placement of the ET tube starting with a five-point auscultation of the chest. I'm listening over the epigastrium. What do I hear?

■ *Evaluator:* There are no sounds heard over the epigastrium.

■ *Team Leader:* I am listening to the right and left sides of the chest in four areas. What do I hear?

■ *Evaluator:* Breath sounds with bag-mask ventilation are clear and equal bilaterally.

■ *Team Leader:* Does the esophageal detector device indicate that the ET tube is in the trachea?

■ *Evaluator:* The esophageal detector device confirms proper placement of the ET tube.

■ *Team Leader:* I will ask the airway team member to note the cm markings on the ET tube and then secure the tube in place. Has there been any change in the patient's ECG rhythm?

■ *Evaluator:* The ET tube has been secured. The monitor still shows asystole. What should be done now?

■ *Team Leader:* Because an advanced airway is now in place, I will instruct the airway team member to change the rate of positive-pressure ventilations from 10 to 12 per minute to 8 to 10 per minute. I will instruct the CPR team member to continue chest compressions without pausing for ventilations.

Postresuscitation Support/Ongoing Assessment

■ *Evaluator:* Forty-five minutes have now elapsed since resuscitation efforts began. CPR is continuing without interruption. Epinephrine has been given every 3 to 5 minutes with no response. A total of 3 mg of atropine has been given with no response. The patient's ECG rhythm has shown continuous asystole. What would you like to do now?

■ *Team Leader:* I will consult with the members of my team about termination of resuscitation efforts.

Putting It All Together: PEA

PEA (formerly called EMD [electromechanical dissociation]) is an organized rhythm on the monitor, other than VT, that does not produce a palpable pulse. The term was changed from EMD to PEA because research using ultrasonography and indwelling pressure catheters revealed that the electrical activity seen in some of these situations *is* associated with mechanical contractions—the contractions are simply too weak to produce a palpable pulse or measurable BP. The cause of many cases of sudden cardiac arrest from PEA is unknown.

■ Evaluator:	You are working on the medical/surgical floor of a local hospital. A laboratory technician can be heard calling for help down the hall. You arrive on the scene with four other members of the code team. When you arrive in the room, the technician is standing in the bathroom and informs you she found the patient unresponsive on the floor. Emergency equipment is immediately available.
■ Team Leader:	Is the scene safe to enter?
■ Evaluator:	The scene is safe.

Initial Assessment

First Impression

| ■ Team Leader: | I am putting on personal protective equipment. As I approach the patient and form a first impression, what do I see? |
| ■ Evaluator: | You see a 33-year-old man lying supine on the floor. His eyes are closed. You do not see any obvious chest rise and fall. The patient's skin is pale. |

Primary Survey

■ Team Leader:	I will quickly approach the patient and assess his level of responsiveness.
■ Evaluator:	The patient is unresponsive.
■ Team Leader:	Because the patient's collapse was not witnessed, I will assume there may be a possible cervical spine injury. I will open the patient's airway using a jaw thrust without head tilt. Do I see anything in the patient's mouth such as blood, broken teeth or loose dentures, gastric contents, or a foreign object?
■ Evaluator:	The airway is clear. What should be done now?
■ Team Leader:	I will look, listen, and feel for breathing for up to 10 seconds.
■ Evaluator:	The patient is not breathing.
■ Team Leader:	I will ask the airway team member to size and insert an oral airway and begin positive-pressure ventilation with a bag-mask connected to 100% oxygen while I continue the primary survey. I want the airway team member to maintain proper head position and a good seal with the mask against the patient's face. I want a second team member to assume responsibility for compressing the bag with just enough force to produce gentle chest rise. The patient should be ventilated at a rate of 10 to 12 ventilations per minute (one ventilation every 5 to 6 seconds). Each ventilation should be given over 1 second.
■ Evaluator:	An oral airway has been inserted. The patient is being ventilated with a bag-mask. You see gentle chest rise with bagging.
■ Team Leader:	I will ask another assistant to assess baseline breath sounds while the patient is being ventilated. I want the defibrillation team member to attach self-adhesive combination pads to the patient's chest while I feel for a carotid pulse for up to 10 seconds. Do I feel a carotid pulse?
■ Evaluator:	There is no pulse. What should be done now?
■ Team Leader:	I will request a defibrillator immediately and instruct the CPR team member to begin chest compressions. I will begin the secondary survey.

Secondary Survey/Focused History and Exam

| ■ Evaluator: | The cardiac monitor reveals the following rhythm (Figure 8-13). A defibrillator is now present. What is the rhythm on the monitor? |

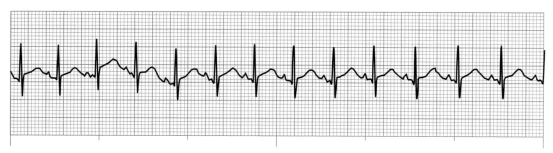

Figure 8-13

■ *Team Leader:*   The rhythm is a sinus tachycardia. Despite the presence of a sinus tachycardia on the monitor, the patient has no pulse. This clinical situation is called pulseless electrical activity. I want the CPR team member and airway team member to automatically rotate positions after every five cycles (about 2 minutes) of CPR so they don't become fatigued. I want the patient's ECG rhythm checked every 2 minutes as the team members change positions. I will perform a focused physical exam, looking for possible clues as to the cause of the arrest. Is there someone available who may know what happened before the patient collapsed?

■ *Evaluator:*   (See Table 8-5 for SAMPLE history and Table 8-6 for physical exam findings.)

■ *Team Leader:*   I will ask the IV team member to start an IV of normal saline without interrupting CPR.

■ *Evaluator:*   Where should the IV be started?

■ *Team Leader:*   During circulatory collapse or cardiac arrest, the preferred IV site is the largest, most accessible vein that does not require the interruption of resuscitation efforts. Because there is no IV in place, an IV

TABLE 8-5. SAMPLE History

Signs/symptoms	Found unresponsive by coworker
Allergies	Codeine
Medications	Tagamet
Past medical history	Unknown
Last oral intake	Unknown
Events prior	Admitted yesterday for abdominal pain; last seen 30 minutes ago. The lab technician recalls seeing a large amount of black-appearing stool in the bathroom toilet when she found the patient. Because of its odor, she flushed the toilet and did not think much of it.

TABLE 8-6. Physical Examination Findings

Head, ears, eyes, nose, and throat	No abnormalities noted
Neck	Trachea midline, no jugular venous distention
Chest	Breath sounds clear and equal with positive-pressure ventilation
Abdomen	No abnormalities noted
Pelvis	No abnormalities noted
Extremities	No abnormalities noted
Posterior body	No abnormalities noted

will be started using a peripheral vein—preferably the antecubital or external jugular vein.

■ *Evaluator:* An IV has been established with normal saline in the patient's right antecubital vein. Based on the information available thus far, what do you suspect is the most likely cause of this arrest?

■ *Team Leader:* Based on the patient's past medical history of ulcers, admission complaint of abdominal pain, and the lab technician's description of her findings in the bathroom at the time of the patient's collapse, hypovolemia is the most likely cause of the patient's situation. I want the IV team member to infuse 500 mL of normal saline and give 1 mg of 1:10,000 epinephrine IV push. I want epinephrine given every 3 to 5 minutes as long as the patient has no pulse. Flush each dose with 20 mL of normal saline and raise the arm.

■ *Evaluator:* CPR is continuing as ordered. Epinephrine is being given as ordered. Since the cardiac monitor shows a narrow-QRS rhythm with a rapid rate, why are you ordering epinephrine for this patient?

■ *Team Leader:* The primary beneficial effects of giving epinephrine in cardiac arrest are due to its alpha-adrenergic receptor stimulating action, resulting in peripheral vasoconstriction. Increased peripheral vasoconstriction improves cerebral and coronary blood flow.

■ *Evaluator:* If the rhythm on the cardiac monitor was slow (and the patient still had no pulse), another medication could be used. What is the name of this medication and its dosage?

■ *Team Leader:* Atropine could be given if the rate of the rhythm on the monitor was less than 60 per minute. The dose is 1 mg IV every 3 to 5 minutes to a maximum total dose of 3 mg.

■ *Evaluator:* What would you like to do now?

■ *Team Leader:* After making sure that we have an esophageal detector device available, I want my most experienced assistant to intubate the patient.

■ *Evaluator:* None of your team members are experienced in performing endotracheal intubation. They do know how to insert a laryngeal mask airway (LMA) and Combitube.

■ *Team Leader:* I would like the airway team member to insert an LMA. Has there been any change on the cardiac monitor or any change in the patient's pulse?

■ *Evaluator:* There has been no change in the rhythm on the monitor. The patient still has no pulse. The LMA has been inserted.

■ *Team Leader:* I will confirm placement of the LMA using a five-point auscultation of the chest and an esophageal detector device.

■ *Evaluator:* Proper placement of the LMA has been confirmed.

■ *Team Leader:* I will ask the airway team member to secure the tube in place. Has there been any change in the patient's ECG rhythm?

■ *Evaluator:* The ET tube has been secured. The cardiac monitor remains unchanged. What should be done now?

■ *Team Leader:* Because an advanced airway is now in place, I will ask the airway team member to change the rate of positive-pressure ventilations from 10 to 12 per minute to 8 to 10 per minute. I will ask the CPR team member to continue chest compressions without pausing for ventilations. I will ask the IV team member to infuse another 500 mL of normal saline.

Postresuscitation Support/Ongoing Assessment

■ *Evaluator:* After giving epinephrine and 1 L of normal saline, the patient has pulses consistent with the rhythm on the monitor. What should be done now?

■ *Team Leader:*   I will repeat the primary survey and ask the CPR team member to obtain a full set of vital signs.

■ *Evaluator:*   Strong carotid and radial pulses are present. The patient's breathing is shallow at about 4 breaths per minute. Breath sounds are clear and equal bilaterally. The patient's BP is 96/74, and oxygen saturation is 98%. The cardiac monitor still shows a sinus tachycardia, but the rate has decreased to about 110 per minute.

■ *Team Leader:*   I will ask the airway team member to assist ventilations with the bag-mask device and continue to monitor the patient's vital signs and ECG as I prepare to transfer the patient for further care.

POSTRESUSCITATION CARE

The **postresuscitation period** is the interval between restoration of spontaneous circulation and transfer to the intensive care unit. The immediate goals of postresuscitation care include the following:[16]

■ Provide cardiorespiratory support to optimize tissue perfusion—especially to the heart, brain, and lungs (the organs most affected by cardiac arrest).

■ Transport to the ED and then to an appropriately equipped critical care unit.

■ Attempt to identify the precipitating cause of the arrest and start specific treatment if necessary.

■ Take actions to prevent recurrence.

■ Take actions to improve long-term, neurologically intact survival.

Immediate Postresuscitation Care

Reassess the ABCDs:

■ Airway
- ❱ Reassess the effectiveness of initial airway maneuvers and interventions.
- ❱ If not already done, perform endotracheal intubation if needed.

■ Breathing
- ❱ Assess the adequacy ventilations.
- ❱ Confirm advanced airway placement.
- ❱ Provide positive-pressure ventilation with O_2.
- ❱ Assess the effectiveness of ventilations.
- ❱ Apply pulse oximeter and assess O_2 saturation.
- ❱ Rule out potential breathing complications from resuscitation (such as pneumothorax, rib fractures, sternal fractures, misplaced endotracheal tube).
- ❱ Mechanical ventilation may be necessary due to absent or inadequate spontaneous respirations.

■ Circulation
- ❱ Reassess vital signs, skin color, mental status.
- ❱ Establish IV access with NS or LR solution if not already done.
- ❱ Change IV lines that were placed without proper sterile technique.
- ❱ ECG monitoring (if not already done); order 12-lead ECG.
- ❱ If the arrest rhythm was VF or VT, it may be reasonable to continue an infusion of the antiarrhythmic that was associated with a return of spontaneous circulation.
- ❱ Use of beta-blockers in the postresuscitation setting seems practical if no contraindications.

■ Differential diagnosis
- ❱ Consider possible causes of the arrest.
  - • Myocardial infarction (MI)
  - • Primary dysrhythmias
  - • Electrolyte disturbances (such as tall T waves on the monitor)
  - • Aortic aneurysm (brachial pulses present, femoral pulses absent)

■ Additional actions
  ▶ Assess for complications that may have occurred during resuscitation (such as rib fracture, hemopneumothorax, pericardial tamponade, intra-abdominal trauma, misplaced endotracheal tube).
  ▶ Order cardiac biomarkers, serum electrolytes (including magnesium and calcium), complete blood count, renal profile, portable chest x-ray.
  ▶ Insert a nasogastric tube, urinary catheter—monitor intake and output.
  ▶ Evaluate IV infusions used during the resuscitation effort. Are the infusions currently running? Are they still needed?
  ▶ Arrange patient transfer to special care unit.
    • Transfer with O_2, ECG monitoring, resuscitation equipment.
    • Trained personnel should accompany patient.
  ▶ Ensure family has been updated regarding events.
  ▶ Finish documentation as needed.
  ▶ Acknowledge the efforts of the resuscitation team.
  ▶ Perform postresuscitation critique.

Temperature Regulation

■ Monitor the patient's body temperature closely.
■ Fever can impair brain recovery by creating an imbalance between O_2 supply and demand; avoid hyperthermia.
■ Do not actively rewarm stable patients who spontaneously develop mild hypothermia after resuscitation from cardiac arrest.[17]
  ▶ Mild hypothermia may be beneficial to neurological outcome.
  ▶ May be well tolerated without significant risk of complications.
■ After prehospital cardiac arrest, unresponsive adults who have a return of spontaneous circulation should be cooled to 89.6° F to 93.2° F (32° C to 34° C) for 12 to 24 hours when the initial rhythm was VF. Similar therapy may be beneficial for prehospital patients with cardiac arrest due to other rhythms or for in-hospital arrest.[17]

Glucose Control

■ Studies have documented poor neurologic outcomes in patients who have high blood glucose levels after resuscitation from cardiac arrest.
■ Signs of hypoglycemia are often not obvious in comatose patients.
■ Monitor serum glucose levels closely.

TOO SLOW RHYTHMS: SYMPTOMATIC BRADYCARDIAS

Remember that cardiac output = stroke volume × heart rate. Therefore, a decrease in either stroke volume or heart rate may result in a decrease in cardiac output. An **absolute bradycardia** is a heart rate of less than 60 bpm. When a patient has a **relative bradycardia,** his or her heart rate may be more than 60 bpm. This may occur when a hypotensive patient needs a tachycardia (as in hypovolemia) but is unable to increase his or her heart rate due to sinoatrial (SA) node disease, beta-blockers, or other medications. A patient with an unusually slow heart may complain of weakness and/or dizziness. Fainting (syncope) can occur. Decreasing cardiac output will eventually produce hemodynamic compromise.

Many patients tolerate a heart rate of 50 to 60 bpm but become symptomatic when the rate drops below 50.

If a patient presents with a bradycardia, assess how the patient is tolerating the rhythm. If the patient has no symptoms, no treatment is necessary; but the patient should be observed closely. Examples of serious signs and symptoms are shown in Box 8-1. The initial treatment of any patient with a symptomatic bradycardia should focus on support of airway and breathing. If serious signs and symptoms are present because of the slow rate, give O_2, start an IV, and then determine if the QRS is wide or narrow. If the QRS is wide, transcutaneous pacing should be started right away. If the QRS is narrow, atropine may be tried while making preparations for transcutaneous pacing.

If the cardiac monitor reveals an atrioventricular (AV) block, locating the probable site of the block plays a critical part in developing an effective treatment plan. Remember that the right coronary artery supplies the AV node in most of the population. Thus, blockage of the right coronary artery (as in an inferior wall MI) is often associated with AV blocks occurring in the AV node. A block in the AV node usually displays a narrow QRS complex. When AV block occurs in the setting of a blockage in the left coronary artery (septal and anterior infarctions), the block is usually located in the bundle branches (infranodal) and displays a wide QRS complex. This type of block is most likely due to serious tissue injury or tissue death. Infranodal AV blocks may quickly progress to a near-asystole state. Therefore, standby pacing is indicated when infranodal AV block complicates anterior wall MI. The rationale behind this strategy is this: If an AV block is known to be unstable and unlikely to respond to atropine, then applying the pacemaker on standby—even when the AV block is presently stable—is the best defense.[18]

BOX 8-1

Symptomatic Bradycardia: Serious Signs and Symptoms

Low BP
Pulmonary congestion
Acute altered mental status
Dizziness
Signs of shock
Ongoing chest pain
Congestive heart failure
Weakness or fatigue

RHYTHMS: NARROW-QRS BRADYCARDIAS

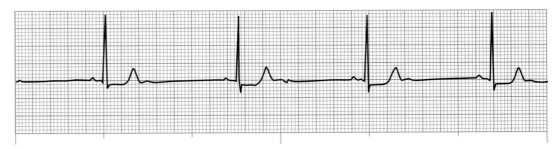

Figure 8-14 • Sinus bradycardia with ST-segment depression.

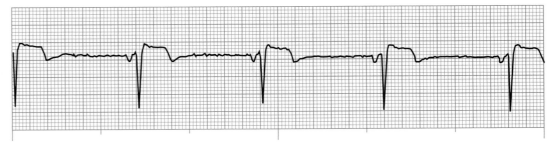

Figure 8-15 • Junctional escape rhythm with ST-segment elevation.

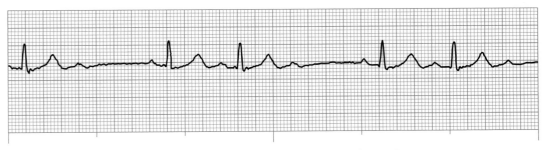

Figure 8-16 • Second-degree AV block, type I.

RHYTHMS: WIDE-QRS BRADYCARDIAS

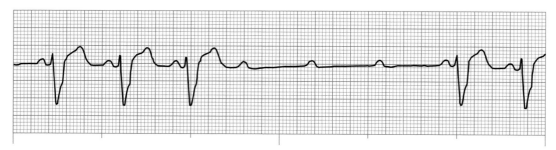

Figure 8-17 • Second-degree AV block, type II with ST-segment elevation.

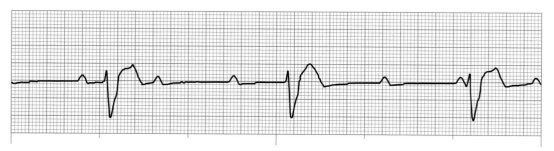

Figure 8-18 • Third-degree AV block with ST-segment elevation.

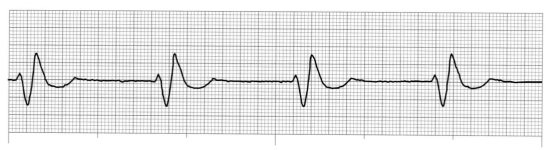

Figure 8-19 • Idioventricular (ventricular escape) rhythm.

MEDICATIONS

Atropine is a vagolytic drug that is used to increase heart rate (*vago* = vagus nerves [right and left], which are main nerves of the parasympathetic division of the autonomic nervous system [ANS]; *lytic* = "lyse," which means to interfere with). Atropine works by blocking acetylcholine at the endings of the vagus nerves. The vagus nerves innervate the heart at the SA and the AV nodes. Thus, atropine is most effective for narrow-QRS bradycardias. By blocking the effects of acetylcholine, atropine allows more activity from the sympathetic division of the ANS. As a result, the rate at which the SA node can fire is increased. Areas of the heart that are not innervated or are minimally innervated by the vagus nerves (such as the ventricles) will not respond to atropine. Thus, atropine is usually ineffective in the treatment of wide-QRS bradycardias. Atropine also increases the rate at which an impulse is conducted through the AV node. It has little or no effect on the force of contraction.

When given to a patient with a pulse, the IV dose of atropine is 0.5 mg. This dose can be repeated every 3 to 5 minutes as needed to a maximum total dose of 3 mg.

When a wide-QRS bradycardia is present, it is best to proceed immediately to transcutaneous pacing instead of using atropine.[19] Atropine can cause paradoxical slowing in patients with an AV block below the level of the AV node. This occurs because atropine will typically increase SA node activity and the speed of impulse conduction through the AV node. However, an ischemic or diseased AV junction can't handle the additional impulses that subsequently bombard it, resulting in worsening of the degree of AV block and further decreasing heart rate and BP.

According to the 2005 guidelines, atropine may be used with caution for patients who have a transplanted heart and symptomatic bradycardia. In situations such as this, it is unlikely that atropine will be effective because the transplanted heart lacks vagal innervation. If atropine is given, the patient must be monitored closely. Paradoxical slowing of the heart rate and high-degree AV block have been reported when atropine was given to patients after cardiac transplantation.[20]

If atropine is ineffective, or if pacing is delayed or ineffective, consider an IV infusion of dopamine or epinephrine. Dopamine is a dose-related drug. This means that the effects of the drug differ depending on the rate at which it is infused (see Chapter 5). In the management of a symptomatic bradycardia, the infusion is started at 2 mcg/kg/min and the patient's response assessed. The infusion is then titrated upward as needed to the desired response. The recommended dose range is 2 to 10 mcg/kg/min.

It is important to recognize the similarities and differences between dopamine and epinephrine administration when treating a symptomatic bradycardia. Although both drugs are given by continuous IV infusion, their dosing differs. Because the correct infusion rate for dopamine depends on the patient's weight, its dose range is 2 to 10 *mcg/kg/min*. An epinephrine infusion is *not* based on the patient's weight. Its dose range is 2 to 10 *mcg/min*.

Epinephrine can be used in the management of a symptomatic bradycardia. Remember that epinephrine increases heart rate, increases the force of contraction, and constricts blood vessels (increasing BP). In cardiac arrest, epinephrine is given IV bolus. However, in a symptomatic bradycardia, epinephrine is given as a *continuous IV infusion*—not as an IV bolus. The recommended dose range is 2 to 10 mcg/min. The infusion should be started at 1 to 2 mcg/min and the patient reassessed. The infusion is then titrated upward based on the patient's response.

SYMPTOMATIC BRADYCARDIA ALGORITHM

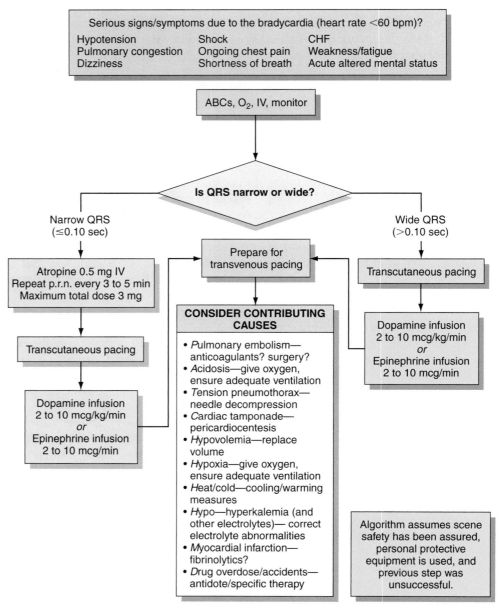

Serious signs/symptoms due to the bradycardia (heart rate <60 bpm)?

Hypotension	Shock	CHF
Pulmonary congestion	Ongoing chest pain	Weakness/fatigue
Dizziness	Shortness of breath	Acute altered mental status

ABCs, O₂, IV, monitor

Is QRS narrow or wide?

Narrow QRS (≤0.10 sec)

Wide QRS (>0.10 sec)

Atropine 0.5 mg IV
Repeat p.r.n. every 3 to 5 min
Maximum total dose 3 mg

Transcutaneous pacing

Dopamine infusion
2 to 10 mcg/kg/min
or
Epinephrine infusion
2 to 10 mcg/min

Prepare for transvenous pacing

Transcutaneous pacing

Dopamine infusion
2 to 10 mcg/kg/min
or
Epinephrine infusion
2 to 10 mcg/min

CONSIDER CONTRIBUTING CAUSES

- *P*ulmonary embolism—anticoagulants? surgery?
- *A*cidosis—give oxygen, ensure adequate ventilation
- *T*ension pneumothorax—needle decompression
- *C*ardiac tamponade—pericardiocentesis
- *H*ypovolemia—replace volume
- *H*ypoxia—give oxygen, ensure adequate ventilation
- *H*eat/cold—cooling/warming measures
- *H*ypo—hyperkalemia (and other electrolytes)— correct electrolyte abnormalities
- *M*yocardial infarction—fibrinolytics?
- *D*rug overdose/accidents—antidote/specific therapy

Algorithm assumes scene safety has been assured, personal protective equipment is used, and previous step was unsuccessful.

Figure 8-20 • Symptomatic bradycardia algorithm.

PUTTING IT ALL TOGETHER

■ *Evaluator:*   A 65-year-old man is complaining of severe dizziness. You have four advanced life support personnel to assist you. Emergency equipment is available.

■ *Team Leader:*   Is the scene safe to enter?

■ *Evaluator:*   The scene is safe.

Initial Assessment

First Impression

■ *Team Leader:*   I am putting on personal protective equipment. As I approach the patient and form a first impression, what do I see?

■ *Evaluator:*   You see an anxious-appearing man sitting in a chair. He is watching your approach. His breathing appears unlabored. You can see beads of sweat on his forehead. His skin looks pale.

Primary Survey

■ *Team Leader:*   I will approach the patient and begin a primary survey. Does the patient respond when I speak his name?

■ *Evaluator:*   The patient responds appropriately. He is alert and oriented to person, place, time, and event.

■ *Team Leader:*   How is his breathing? What is his pulse rate and quality?

■ *Evaluator:*   The patient's breathing is quiet and unlabored. You are unable to feel a radial pulse. The patient's carotid pulse is slow and weak.

■ *Team Leader:*   I will assist the patient to a supine position and make sure a defibrillator with pacemaker capability is within reach. I will ask the defibrillation team member to attach a pulse oximeter and place the patient on a cardiac monitor. I will ask the airway team member to place the patient on oxygen by nonrebreather mask. I want the CPR team member to obtain the patient's baseline vital signs while I begin the secondary survey.

Secondary Survey/Focused History and Exam

■ *Team Leader:*   What are the patient's vital signs?

■ *Evaluator:*   The patient's vital signs are as follows: BP 58/30, heart rate is about 40, and respirations 16. Breath sounds are clear and equal bilaterally. The patient's oxygen saturation (SpO_2) on room air was 92% and is now 98% on oxygen by nonrebreather mask. The patient is now supine and has been placed on the cardiac monitor (Figure 8-21). What is the rhythm on the monitor?

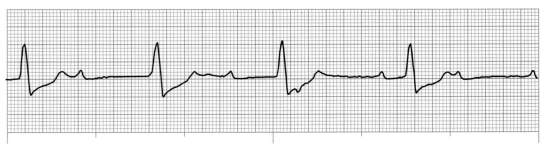

Figure 8-21

■ *Team Leader:* The rhythm is a third-degree AV block with a wide-QRS complex. I will obtain a SAMPLE history from the patient and perform a focused physical exam. I will ask the IV team member to start an IV of normal saline. I will ask the CPR team member to order a 12-lead ECG.

■ *Evaluator:* (See Table 8-7 for SAMPLE history and Table 8-8 for physical exam findings.) An IV has been started and the 12-lead has been ordered.

■ *Team Leader:* Based on the patient's history and physical findings, I am going to order transcutaneous pacing.

■ *Evaluator:* Where will you place the pacer pads?

■ *Team Leader:* I want the defibrillation team member to place the anterior pacer pad over the heart to the left of the sternum (Figure 8-22). I want the

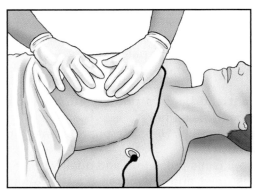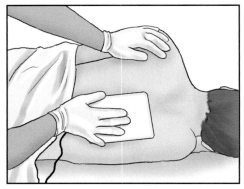

Figure 8-22

TABLE 8-7. **SAMPLE History**	
Signs/symptoms	Sudden onset of severe dizziness
Allergies	None
Medications	Cardizem
Past medical history	3-vessel coronary artery bypass graft 1 year ago
Last oral intake	Dinner
Events prior	Sudden onset of severe dizziness. Symptoms started about 15 minutes ago while at rest.

TABLE 8-8. **Physical Examination Findings**	
Head, ears, eyes, nose, and throat	No abnormalities noted
Neck	Trachea midline, no jugular venous distention
Chest	Breath sounds clear bilaterally, surgical scar noted over sternum
Abdomen	No abnormalities noted
Pelvis	No abnormalities noted
Extremities	No abnormalities noted
Posterior body	No abnormalities noted

posterior pad placed on the back of the patient's chest behind the heart (and the anterior pacer pad). I will make sure the pads do not overlap the sternum, spine, or scapula.

The recommended positioning of pacing pads varies depending on the transcutaneous pacemaker used. You must be familiar with the equipment you are using and the manufacturer's recommendations for pacer pad placement.

■ *Evaluator:*   If this patient was a female, would you position the pacemaker pads in the same way?

■ *Team Leader:*   In females, the anterior pacer pad should be positioned under (not on) the left breast.

■ *Evaluator:*   The pacemaker pads are in place. What should be done next?

■ *Team Leader:*   I will order the settings for the pacemaker's rate and output (milliamps, mA). The rate is usually set between 60 and 80 pulses per minute. I want the defibrillation team member to set the rate at 60. Because this patient has a pulse, I want the defibrillation team member to start with low energy (about 20 mA) and gradually increase the energy until capture is achieved.

■ *Evaluator:*   What do you mean by "capture?"

■ *Team Leader:*   I will watch the cardiac monitor closely for signs of *electrical* capture. This is usually evidenced by a wide QRS and a T wave that appears in a direction opposite the QRS. I will make sure there is *mechanical* capture by assessing the patient's pulse and BP.

■ *Evaluator:*   You see the following rhythm on the monitor (Figure 8-23). What is the rhythm?

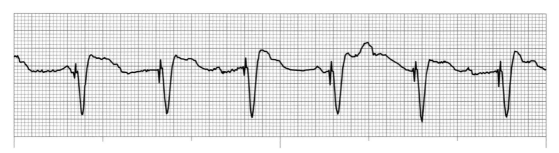

Figure 8-23

■ *Team Leader:*   I see a ventricular paced rhythm. Each pacemaker spike is followed by a wide-QRS complex. This represents 100% electrical capture. I will now assess a pulse to confirm mechanical capture.

■ *Evaluator:*   Does it make a difference where you choose to assess a pulse?

■ *Team Leader:*   Yes. I will check the patient's right arm or femoral pulses. It is important to avoid assessing pulses in the patient's neck or on the patient's left side. This helps minimize confusion between the presence of an actual pulse and skeletal muscle contractions caused by the pacemaker.

■ *Evaluator:*   You feel strong right brachial and femoral pulses. What would you like to do now?

■ *Team Leader:*   At what milliamp setting on the pacer did I obtain 100% capture?

■ *Evaluator:*   Capture was obtained at 70 mA.

■ *Team Leader:*   I will ask the defibrillation team member to adjust the output setting to continue pacing at 72 mA.

■ *Evaluator:*   The pacemaker settings have been adjusted as requested. What do you want to do next?

Postresuscitation Support/Ongoing Assessment

- **Team Leader:** I will repeat the primary survey and ask the CPR team member to obtain another set of vital signs. What is the patient's BP? Is he uncomfortable with pacing? Have his symptoms improved?

- **Evaluator:** The patient states that he is no longer dizzy, but he is very uncomfortable. His vital signs are BP 114/70, P 60 (paced), R 14, and SpO_2 is 98%.

- **Team Leader:** I will ask the IV team member to give the patient morphine for pain. I want this given in doses of 2 mg. It can be repeated as needed every 5 minutes until the patient is pain free. I want the patient's vital signs rechecked after each dose to watch his respiratory rate and make sure he does not become hypotensive. I will also arrange for a cardiology consult because this patient will most likely need a permanent pacemaker.

- **Evaluator:** If a transcutaneous pacemaker was not available, what other interventions would you have considered for this patient?

- **Team Leader:** I would have considered a dopamine or epinephrine IV infusion.

- **Evaluator:** If you had chosen a dopamine infusion, what would the correct infusion rate be?

- **Team Leader:** 2 to 10 mcg/kg/min

- **Evaluator:** What is the correct infusion rate for an epinephrine infusion?

- **Team Leader:** 2 to 10 mcg/min

- **Evaluator:** Explain why epinephrine may be useful in the management of a symptomatic bradycardia.

- **Team Leader:** Epinephrine 1) constricts peripheral blood vessels, increasing BP (vasopressor); 2) increases heart rate (chronotropic effect); and 3) increases the force of contraction (inotropic effect).

TOO FAST RHYTHMS: TACHYCARDIAS

Management of patients who present with a tachycardia is often complex. Consultation with a cardiologist is advised.

NARROW-QRS TACHYCARDIAS

"Treat the patient, not the monitor" is a caveat that has been used for many years in the delivery of ACLS. When a patient presents with signs and symptoms related to a tachycardia, ask yourself three questions:

1. Is the patient stable or unstable?
2. Is the QRS wide or narrow?
3. Is the ventricular rhythm regular or irregular?

The answers to these questions will help guide your treatment decisions. Most tachycardias do not cause serious signs and symptoms until the ventricular rate exceeds 150 bpm. Examples of serious signs and symptoms include low BP, pulmonary congestion, acute altered mental status, dizziness, signs of shock, ongoing chest pain, congestive heart failure, and weakness or fatigue. If the patient is symptomatic but does not have serious signs and symptoms because of the rapid rate, the patient is considered "stable." After assessing their ABCs, stable patients are given O_2, an IV is started, and drug therapy is begun. If the tachycardia produces serious signs and symptoms (typically with heart rates of 150 bpm or more), the patient is considered "unstable." Unstable patients who have serious signs and symptoms due to the tachycardia (and have a pulse) should receive immediate synchronized cardioversion.

With that said, it is important to recognize that not all patient situations are so simplistic. Patients often present with signs and symptoms that place them in a "gray area"—they are symptomatic, but not clearly stable or unstable. Consider the case of a 55-year-old woman complaining of palpitations that have been present for 40 minutes. She is awake and alert, but anxious. As the patient converses with you, you note that she pauses after every 5 or 6 words to take a breath, but she states she does not feel short of breath. Her vital signs are as follows: BP 114/78, P 180, R 20. She states her normal BP is around 130/80. Breath sounds reveal a few bibasilar rales. Her skin is pink, warm, and moist. Her calves and ankles appear swollen. The patient has no pertinent past medical history and takes no medications regularly. O_2 is being given and an IV has been started.

Remember the three important questions to ask yourself when treating a tachycardia. The first question is, Is the patient stable or unstable? The patient's BP is lower than normal for her (an important finding), but not yet in the clearly hypotensive range. Would you consider this patient stable or unstable? The patient's presentation is consistent with the "gray area" previously mentioned. She is symptomatic and signs of heart failure (pulmonary congestion, shortness of breath, and lower extremity swelling) are present. These are serious signs and symptoms. At the same time, she is awake, alert, and has a reasonable BP. The second question you must ask yourself is, Is the QRS wide or narrow? The cardiac monitor reveals a narrow-QRS tachycardia at a rate of 180. No P waves are visible. The third question to ask is, Is the ventricular rhythm regular or irregular? The ventricular rhythm is regular.

What should be done now? The decision regarding how to proceed will depend on your medical judgment, location and availability of resources, experience and, of course, the patient's condition. In this situation, a reasonable approach might include a combination of therapies. For example, because the patient is awake and alert and an IV is in place, make sure that emergency drugs and a defibrillator are within arm's reach. Then ask the patient to cough or bear down. If the rhythm does not convert, consider giving adenosine IV while preparing for synchronized cardioversion.

Rhythms: Narrow-QRS Tachycardias

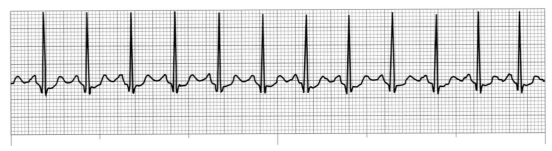

Figure 8-24 • Sinus tachycardia.

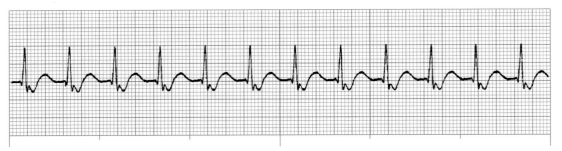

Figure 8-25 • Junctional tachycardia.

Normal sinus rhythm

Atrial tachycardia (AT)

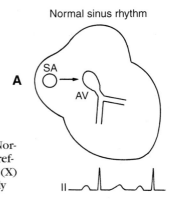

Figure 8-26 • Types of SVTs. **A,** Normal sinus rhythm is shown here as a reference. **B,** Atrial tachycardia—a focus (X) outside the SA node fires automatically at a rapid rate. **C,** AV nodal reentrant tachycardia—an impulse originates as a wave of excitation that spins around the area of the AV node. On the ECG, P waves may be buried in the QRS or appear just before or after the QRS complex because of the nearly simultaneous activation of the atria and ventricles. **D,** AV reentrant tachycardia—a similar type of reentrant (circus-movement) mechanism may occur with a bypass tract like that found in Wolff-Parkinson-White syndrome.

Atrioventricular nodal reentrant tachycardia (AVNRT)

Atrioventricular reentrant tachycardia (AVRT)

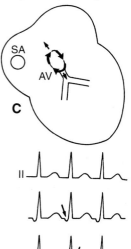

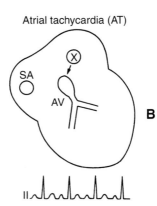

Medications

When vagal maneuvers fail to convert a narrow-QRS tachycardia, adenosine is the first drug that is used to try to terminate the rhythm. Adenosine is found naturally in all body cells and is rapidly metabolized in the blood vessels. Adenosine slows the rate of the SA node, slows conduction time through the AV node, can interrupt reentry pathways that involve the AV node, and can restore sinus rhythm in SVT. Reentry circuits are the underlying mechanism for many episodes of SVT. Adenosine acts at specific receptors to cause a temporary block in conduction through the AV node, interrupting these reentry circuits.

If a narrow-QRS tachycardia does not convert with adenosine (and the patient's condition remains stable), calcium channel blockers or beta-blockers may be used. Calcium channel blockers slow the movement of calcium ions across cell membranes in the heart and vascular smooth muscle. These actions result in a depressant effect on the heart's contractile function and slowed conduction through the AV node. By slowing conduction through the AV node, these drugs may terminate dysrhythmias that need the AV node in order to perpetuate the rhythm. Calcium channel blockers should be used with caution in patients with heart failure.

Beta-blockers may be used to slow the ventricular rate in narrow-QRS tachycardias that have not responded to vagal maneuvers or adenosine. Beta-blockers work by interfering with the ability of epinephrine and related chemicals to bind with beta-adrenergic receptors. Cardioselective beta-blockers (such as atenolol and metoprolol) work by blocking $beta_1$ receptors more than they block $beta_2$ receptors. Nonselective beta-blockers (such as propranolol, sotalol, and labetalol) block both $beta_1$ and $beta_2$ receptors. Stimulation of $beta_1$ receptor sites in the heart results in increased heart rate, contractility, and, ultimately, irritability of cardiac cells. By blocking $beta_1$ receptors, heart rate decreases, the force of contraction decreases, and dysrhythmias that depend on catecholamine stimulation can be controlled. Beta-blockers should not be used if the patient has signs of heart failure, evidence of a low output state, increased risk for cardiogenic shock (age greater than 70 years, systolic blood pressure less than 120 mm Hg, sinus tachycardia greater than 110 bpm or heart rate less than 60 bpm, and increased time since onset of symptoms of STEMI), or other relative contraindications to beta blockade (PR interval greater than 0.24 seconds, second- or third-degree AV block, active asthma, or reactive airway disease).

Narrow-QRS Tachycardia Algorithm

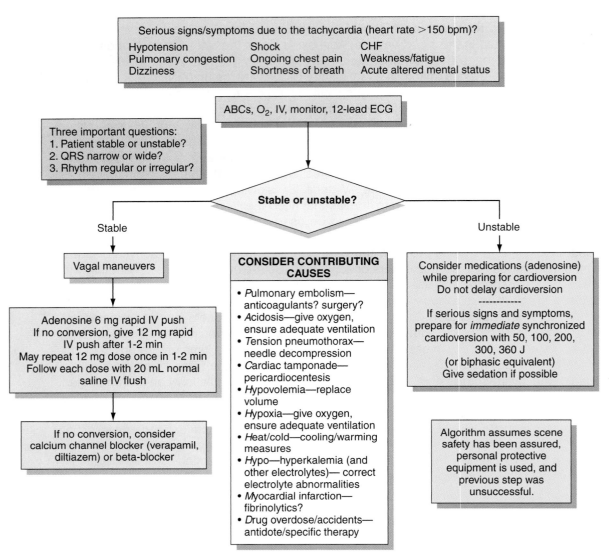

Serious signs/symptoms due to the tachycardia (heart rate >150 bpm)?

Hypotension	Shock	CHF
Pulmonary congestion	Ongoing chest pain	Weakness/fatigue
Dizziness	Shortness of breath	Acute altered mental status

ABCs, O₂, IV, monitor, 12-lead ECG

Three important questions:
1. Patient stable or unstable?
2. QRS narrow or wide?
3. Rhythm regular or irregular?

Stable or unstable?

Stable

Unstable

Vagal maneuvers

Adenosine 6 mg rapid IV push
If no conversion, give 12 mg rapid
IV push after 1-2 min
May repeat 12 mg dose once in 1-2 min
Follow each dose with 20 mL normal
saline IV flush

If no conversion, consider
calcium channel blocker (verapamil,
diltiazem) or beta-blocker

CONSIDER CONTRIBUTING CAUSES

- *P*ulmonary embolism—
  anticoagulants? surgery?
- *A*cidosis—give oxygen,
  ensure adequate ventilation
- *T*ension pneumothorax—
  needle decompression
- *C*ardiac tamponade—
  pericardiocentesis
- *H*ypovolemia—replace
  volume
- *H*ypoxia—give oxygen,
  ensure adequate ventilation
- *H*eat/cold—cooling/warming
  measures
- *H*ypo—hyperkalemia (and
  other electrolytes)— correct
  electrolyte abnormalities
- *M*yocardial infarction—
  fibrinolytics?
- *D*rug overdose/accidents—
  antidote/specific therapy

Consider medications (adenosine)
while preparing for cardioversion
Do not delay cardioversion

If serious signs and symptoms,
prepare for *immediate* synchronized
cardioversion with 50, 100, 200,
300, 360 J
(or biphasic equivalent)
Give sedation if possible

Algorithm assumes scene
safety has been assured,
personal protective
equipment is used, and
previous step was
unsuccessful.

Figure 8-27 • Narrow-QRS tachycardia algorithm (regular ventricular rhythm).

WIDE-QRS TACHYCARDIAS

Most wide-complex tachycardias are ventricular tachycardia. Some wide-complex tachycardias are actually SVT with aberrant conduction. It is best to consult a cardiologist when treating a patient who has a wide-complex tachycardia.

If the rhythm is most likely SVT with aberrant conduction and the patient is stable, adenosine is the first drug that is given to try to terminate the rhythm. If the rhythm is monomorphic VT (and the patient's symptoms are due to the tachycardia):

■ CPR and defibrillation are used if the patient is pulseless.

■ Stable but symptomatic patients are treated with O_2, IV access, and ventricular antiarrhythmics (such as amiodarone) to suppress the rhythm.

■ Unstable patients (usually a sustained heart rate of 150 bpm or more) are treated with O_2, IV access, and sedation (if awake and time permits) followed by synchronized cardioversion.

■ In all cases, an aggressive search must be made for the cause of the VT.

If the patient presents with serious signs and symptoms due to the tachycardia, specific diagnosis of the origin of the tachycardia is irrelevant—the patient needs *immediate* electrical therapy (synchronized cardioversion).

Rhythms: Wide-QRS Tachycardias

Monitor lead

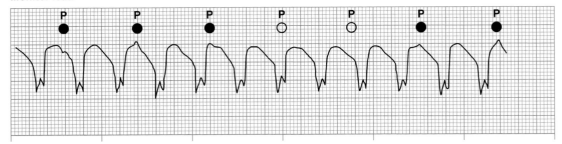

Figure 8-28 • Sustained monomorphic VT with AV dissociation. Visible sinus P waves are indicated by a dark circle. Hidden P waves are indicated by a clear circle.

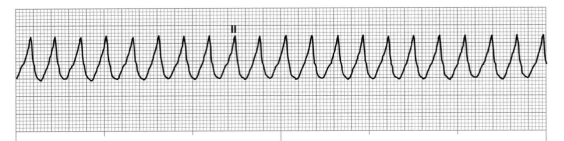

Figure 8-29 • Monomorphic VT.

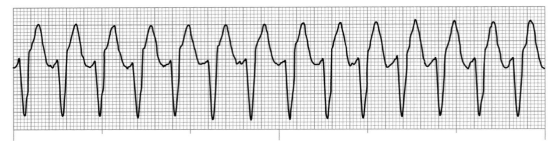

Figure 8-30 • Wide complex tachycardia of uncertain origin.

Medications

The medications recommended in the initial management of stable patients who present with a regular, wide-QRS tachycardia are adenosine or amiodarone. Adenosine is given if the rhythm on the cardiac monitor is likely to be SVT with aberrant conduction. If the tachycardia is most likely VT, amiodarone is the first drug that is recommended. Procainamide and sotalol are acceptable alternative choices. Amiodarone, procainamide, and sotalol are antiarrhythmics that have complex mechanisms of action. They are used for both atrial and ventricular dysrhythmias.

Because amiodarone, procainamide, and sotalol are antiarrhythmics that can cause prolongation of the QT interval, they are not used for dysrhythmias such as polymorphic VT associated with a long QT interval (TdP).

Wide-QRS Tachycardia Algorithm

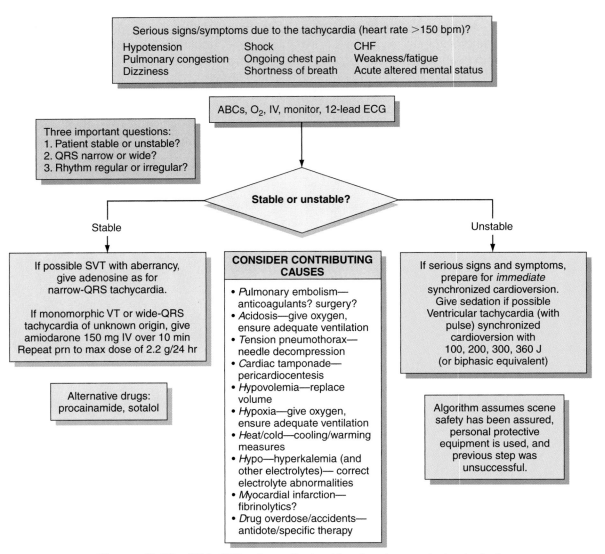

Serious signs/symptoms due to the tachycardia (heart rate >150 bpm)?

Hypotension	Shock	CHF
Pulmonary congestion	Ongoing chest pain	Weakness/fatigue
Dizziness	Shortness of breath	Acute altered mental status

ABCs, O₂, IV, monitor, 12-lead ECG

Three important questions:
1. Patient stable or unstable?
2. QRS narrow or wide?
3. Rhythm regular or irregular?

Stable or unstable?

Stable

Unstable

If possible SVT with aberrancy, give adenosine as for narrow-QRS tachycardia.

If monomorphic VT or wide-QRS tachycardia of unknown origin, give amiodarone 150 mg IV over 10 min Repeat prn to max dose of 2.2 g/24 hr

Alternative drugs: procainamide, sotalol

CONSIDER CONTRIBUTING CAUSES

- *P*ulmonary embolism—anticoagulants? surgery?
- *A*cidosis—give oxygen, ensure adequate ventilation
- *T*ension pneumothorax—needle decompression
- *C*ardiac tamponade—pericardiocentesis
- *H*ypovolemia—replace volume
- *H*ypoxia—give oxygen, ensure adequate ventilation
- *H*eat/cold—cooling/warming measures
- *H*ypo—hyperkalemia (and other electrolytes)— correct electrolyte abnormalities
- *M*yocardial infarction—fibrinolytics?
- *D*rug overdose/accidents—antidote/specific therapy

If serious signs and symptoms, prepare for *immediate* synchronized cardioversion. Give sedation if possible Ventricular tachycardia (with pulse) synchronized cardioversion with 100, 200, 300, 360 J (or biphasic equivalent)

Algorithm assumes scene safety has been assured, personal protective equipment is used, and previous step was unsuccessful.

Figure 8-31 • Wide-QRS tachycardia algorithm (regular ventricular rhythm).

IRREGULAR TACHYCARDIAS

The severity of signs and symptoms associated with an irregular tachycardia varies depending on the ventricular rate, how long the rhythm has been present, and the patient's cardiovascular status. The patient may be asymptomatic and not require treatment or may experience serious signs and symptoms. It is best to consult a cardiologist when treating a patient who has an irregular tachycardia.

Atrial Flutter and Atrial Fibrillation

When atrial flutter is present with 2:1 conduction, it may be difficult to tell the difference between atrial flutter and sinus tachycardia, atrial tachycardia, atrioventricular nodal reentrant tachycardia (AVNRT), atrioventricular reentrant tachycardia (AVRT), or paroxysmal supraventricular tachycardia (PSVT). Vagal maneuvers may help identify the rhythm by temporarily slowing AV conduction and revealing the underlying flutter waves. When vagal maneuvers are used in atrial flutter, the response is usually sudden slowing and then a return to the former rate. Vagal maneuvers will not usually convert atrial flutter because the reentry circuit is located in the atria, not the AV node.

The severity of signs and symptoms associated with atrial flutter or atrial fibrillation (AFib) varies, depending on the ventricular rate, how long the rhythm has been present, and the patient's cardiovascular status. The patient may be asymptomatic and not require treatment or may experience serious signs and symptoms.

Synchronized cardioversion should be considered for any patient in atrial flutter or AFib that has serious signs and symptoms because of the rapid ventricular rate (such as low BP, signs of shock, or heart failure). If synchronized cardioversion is performed, atrial flutter can be successfully converted to a sinus rhythm using low energy levels (starting with 50 J). Because the rhythm is more disorganized, AFib generally requires higher energy levels (starting with 100 J).

If atrial flutter or AFib is associated with a rapid ventricular rate and the patient is stable but symptomatic, treatment may be directed toward controlling the ventricular rate or converting the rhythm to a sinus rhythm. In the prehospital and ED setting, treatment is usually aimed at controlling the ventricular rate. If heart failure is not present, medications such as calcium channel blockers or beta-blockers are often used (if no contraindications exist).

If the decision is made to convert the rhythm, it is important to first consider how long the rhythm has been present. If the rhythm has been present for 48 hours or longer, anticoagulation is recommended before attempting to convert the rhythm with medications, synchronized cardioversion, or catheter ablation. A widely accepted practice is to begin prophylactic anticoagulation 2 to 3 weeks before and continue therapy for about 4 weeks after conversion.

Polymorphic Ventricular Tachycardia

If the rhythm is polymorphic VT, it is important to determine if the patient's QT interval just before the tachycardia is normal or prolonged (if this information is available). Remember that polymorphic VT that occurs in the presence of a long QT interval is called *TdP*. Polymorphic VT that occurs in the presence of a normal QT interval is simply referred to as *polymorphic VT* or *polymorphic VT resembling TdP.*

- If the QT interval is *normal* (that means the rhythm is polymorphic VT), the rhythm is sustained, and the patient is symptomatic due to the tachycardia:
  - ▶ Treat ischemia if present.
  - ▶ Correct electrolyte abnormalities.
  - ▶ If the patient is stable, amiodarone may be effective.
  - ▶ If the patient is unstable, proceed with defibrillation as for VF.
- If the QT interval is *prolonged* (that means the rhythm is TdP), the rhythm is sustained, and the patient is symptomatic due to the tachycardia:
  - ▶ Discontinue any medications that the patient may be taking that prolong the QT interval.
  - ▶ Correct electrolyte abnormalities.
  - ▶ If the patient is stable, give magnesium sulfate IV.
  - ▶ If the patient is unstable, proceed with defibrillation as for VF.

Rhythms: Irregular Tachycardias

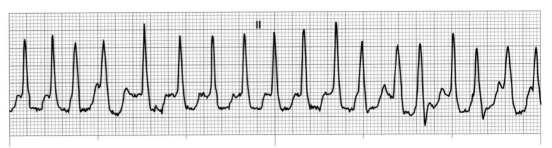

Figure 8-32 • AFib with a rapid ventricular response.

Lead I

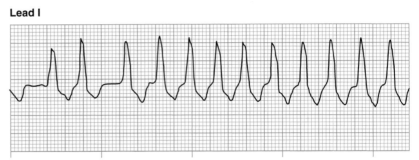

Figure 8-33 • AFib with a rapid ventricular response and left bundle branch block.

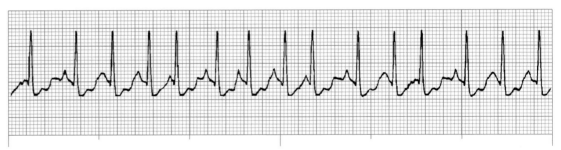

Figure 8-34 • Multifocal atrial tachycardia, also known as chaotic atrial tachycardia.

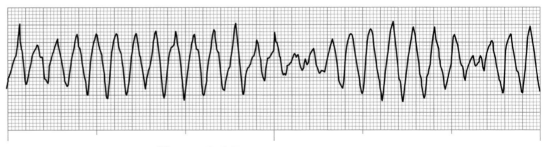

Figure 8-35 • Sustained polymorphic VT.

Medications

Calcium channel blockers are used to control the ventricular rate in many types of atrial dysrhythmias. Because of their depressant effect on the heart's contractile function, calcium channel blockers should be used with caution in patients with heart failure.

Beta-blockers may be used to slow the ventricular rate in AFib and atrial flutter in patients who have no signs or symptoms of heart failure (or other contraindications, such as pulmonary disease).

Amiodarone may be effective in the treatment of polymorphic VT with a normal QT interval. Magnesium sulfate is recommended for TdP (polymorphic VT with a prolonged QT interval with or without cardiac arrest. Some studies have shown that magnesium is also effective for AFib with a rapid ventricular response. If the patient has a pulse, magnesium sulfate is given IV in a dose of 1 to 2 g diluted in D5W over 5 to 60 minutes. If the patient is stable, infuse the drug slowly. If the patient is unstable, the drug can be given more rapidly.[21]

Irregular Tachycardia Algorithm

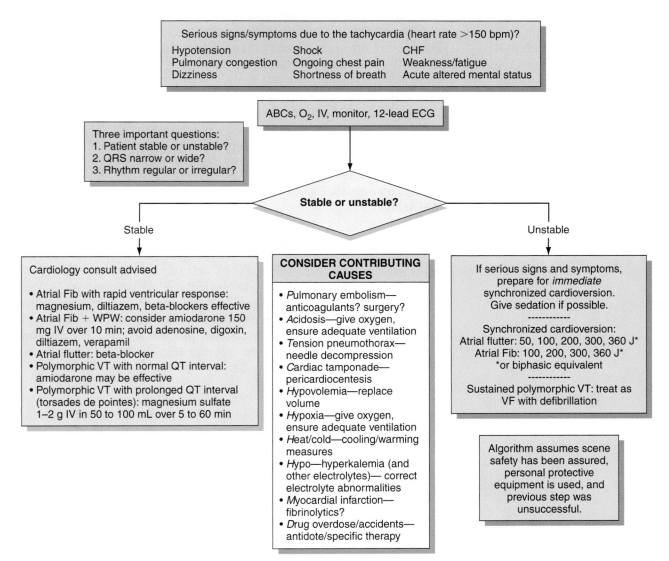

Figure 8-36 • Irregular tachycardia algorithm.

PUTTING IT ALL TOGETHER

■ *Evaluator:*   A 47-year-old man is complaining that he feels lightheaded and dizzy. You have four ALS personnel to assist you. Emergency equipment is available.

■ *Team Leader:*   Is the scene safe to enter?

■ *Evaluator:*   The scene is safe.

Initial Assessment

First Impression

■ *Team Leader:*   I am putting on personal protective equipment. As I approach the patient and form a first impression, what do I see?

■ *Evaluator:*   You see a man supine in bed. He is aware of your presence. His breathing appears adequate. His skin color looks normal.

Primary Survey

■ *Team Leader:*   I will approach the patient and begin a primary survey. Does the patient respond when I speak his name?

■ *Evaluator:*   The patient answers when you speak his name.

■ *Team Leader:*   How is his breathing? What is his pulse rate and quality?

■ *Evaluator:*   The patient's breathing is adequate. His radial and carotid pulses are strong but fast. You estimate the rate to be about 200 per minute.

■ *Team Leader:*   I will make sure a defibrillator is within reach. I want the defibrillation team member to attach a pulse oximeter and place the patient on a cardiac monitor. I will ask the airway team member to place the patient on oxygen by nonrebreather mask. I want the CPR team member to obtain the patient's baseline vital signs while I begin the secondary survey. I want the IV team member to start an IV of normal saline.

Secondary Survey/Focused History and Exam

■ *Team Leader:*   What are the patient's vital signs?

■ *Evaluator:*   The patient's vital signs are as follows: BP 161/98, heart rate is 214, and respirations 20. Breath sounds are clear and equal bilaterally. The patient's SpO_2 is 98% on oxygen by nonrebreather mask. An IV has been started in the patient's left antecubital vein. The patient has been placed on the cardiac monitor (Figure 8-37). What is the rhythm on the monitor?

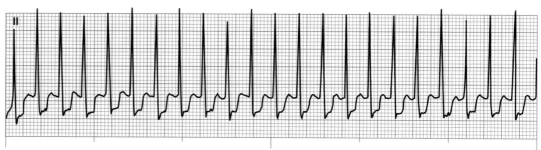

Figure 8-37

■ *Team Leader:*   The rhythm is a narrow-QRS tachycardia, probably AVNRT. I will obtain a SAMPLE history from the patient and perform a focused physical exam. I will order a 12-lead ECG.

■ *Evaluator:*   (See Table 8-9 for SAMPLE history and Table 8-10 for physical exam findings). A 12-lead has been ordered. What would you like to do now?

■ *Team Leader:*   Based on the patient's history and physical findings, the patient is stable at this time. I will ask the patient to cough forcefully or bear down in an attempt to convert the rhythm.

■ *Evaluator:*   The patient attempts the vagal maneuvers as requested, but the rhythm remains unchanged.

■ *Team Leader:*   Because the rhythm is AVNRT, I will ask the IV team member to give 6 mg of adenosine rapid IV push. I want the drug followed immediately with a 20-mL flush of normal saline and elevation of the patient's arm.

■ *Evaluator:*   What are some of the common side effects of adenosine?

■ *Team Leader:*   Flushing, dyspnea, and chest pain are common side effects of adenosine.

■ *Evaluator:*   As the IV team member is giving the adenosine you ordered, the patient's eyes roll back in his head. What do you want to do now?

■ *Team Leader:*   I will quickly repeat the primary survey and ask the CPR team member to obtain the patient's vital signs. What is my patient's level of responsiveness? Is his airway open? Is he breathing? Is a pulse present?

■ *Evaluator:*   The patient is unresponsive. His airway is open. He is breathing at a rate of about 6 per minute. You are unable to feel a radial pulse. A weak carotid pulse is present. The patient's BP is 63/40.

■ *Team Leader:*   What is the rhythm on the monitor?

TABLE 8-9. SAMPLE History

Signs/symptoms	Sudden onset of feeling lightheaded and dizzy
Allergies	None
Medications	None
Past medical history	None
Last oral intake	Lunch 4 hours ago
Events prior	Standing in line at the post office when he suddenly felt lightheaded and dizzy. No history of recent illness, denies chest pain, nausea, vomiting, and shortness of breath.

TABLE 8-10. Physical Examination Findings

Head, ears, eyes, nose, and throat	No abnormalities noted
Neck	Trachea midline, no jugular venous distention
Chest	Breath sounds clear bilaterally
Abdomen	No abnormalities noted
Pelvis	No abnormalities noted
Extremities	No abnormalities noted
Posterior body	No abnormalities noted

■ *Evaluator:* The patient's cardiac rhythm is unchanged. What should be done now?

■ *Team Leader:* The patient is now clearly unstable. I will ask the airway team member to begin positive-pressure ventilation with a bag-mask connected to 100% oxygen while preparations are made to shock the patient. Because the patient is unresponsive, I will not need to ask the IV team member to sedate the patient before the shock.

■ *Evaluator:* Are you going to perform synchronized cardioversion or will you defibrillate the patient?

■ *Team Leader:* Because the patient has a pulse and a narrow-QRS tachycardia is present on the monitor, I want the defibrillation team member to perform synchronized cardioversion.

■ *Evaluator:* A biphasic manual defibrillator is available to you. What initial energy setting will you use?

■ *Team Leader:* I will begin synchronized cardioversion using 50 J or the energy setting recommended by the manufacturer. I want the airway team member to temporarily shut off the oxygen flow while the defibrillation team member prepares to deliver the shock. When the defibrillation team member is ready, he will make sure all team members (including him) are clear of the patient and then deliver the shock.

■ *Evaluator:* The oxygen was shut off as ordered and a synchronized shock was delivered using 50 J as ordered. A team member calls your attention to the cardiac monitor (Figure 8-38). What do you see now?

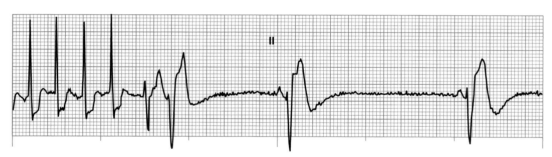

Figure 8-38

Postresuscitation Support/Ongoing Assessment

■ *Team Leader:* The monitor is showing conversion of the rhythm from AVNRT to a sinus bradycardia with ST-segment elevation. I will observe the ECG for a couple of minutes and see if the rate increases on its own. I will ask the CPR team member to check for a pulse and obtain a full set of vital signs while I repeat the primary survey. Is a pulse present? Is the patient responsive? Is he breathing?

■ *Evaluator:* The patient is awake. Strong carotid and radial pulses are present. The patient is breathing about 12 times per minute. Breath sounds are clear and equal bilaterally. The patient's BP is 130/88. His oxygen saturation is 98%.

■ *Team Leader:* What is the patient's heart rate? What do I see on the cardiac monitor?

■ *Evaluator:* The cardiac monitor shows a sinus rhythm at 78 bpm. The patient's carotid and radial pulses remain strong and consistent with the monitor.

■ *Team Leader:* I will continue to monitor the patient's vital signs and ECG and transfer the patient for continued observation.

ACUTE CORONARY SYNDROMES

Information pertaining to acute coronary syndromes was covered in depth in Chapter 6. Figure 8-39 shows the surfaces of the heart and the leads that view them. Table 8-11 shows the leads of the heart and the heart surface viewed to help localize ECG changes. The ischemic chest discomfort (Figure 8-40), acute pulmonary edema (Figure 8-41), and cardiogenic shock (Figure 8-42) algorithms appear on the following pages.

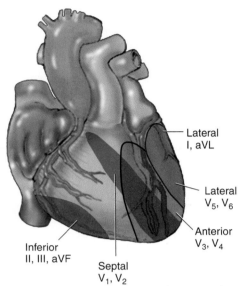

Lateral
I, aVL

Lateral
V_5, V_6

Anterior
V_3, V_4

Inferior
II, III, aVF

Septal
V_1, V_2

Figure 8-39 • The surfaces of the heart and the leads that view them. The posterior surface is not shown.

TABLE 8-11		Localizing ECG Changes						
I	Lateral	aVR	------------	V_1	Septum	V_4	Anterior	V_4R	Right Ventricle
II	Inferior	aVL	Lateral	V_2	Septum	V_5	Lateral	V_5R	Right Ventricle
III	Inferior	aVF	Inferior	V_3	Anterior	V_6	Lateral	V_6R	Right Ventricle

ISCHEMIC CHEST PAIN ALGORITHM

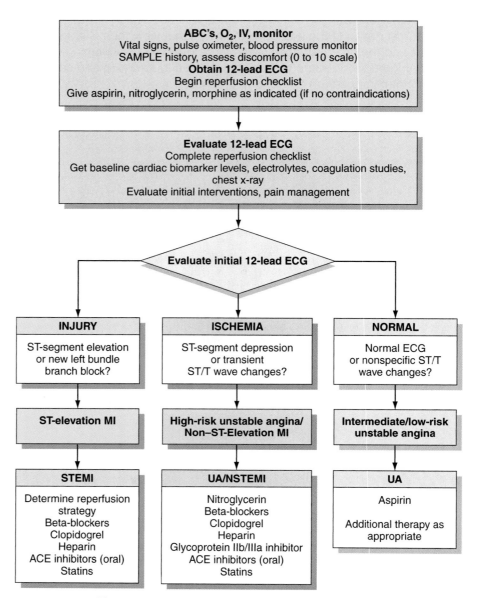

Figure 8-40 • Ischemic chest discomfort algorithm.

ACUTE PULMONARY EDEMA ALGORITHM

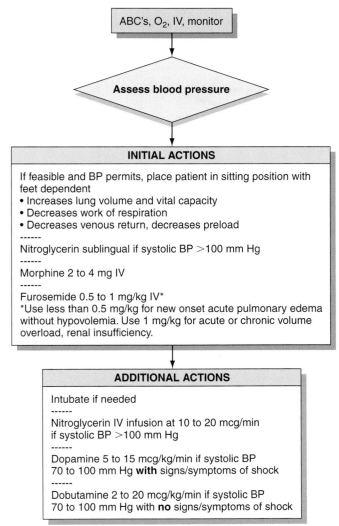

Figure 8-41 • Acute pulmonary edema.

CARDIOGENIC SHOCK ALGORITHM

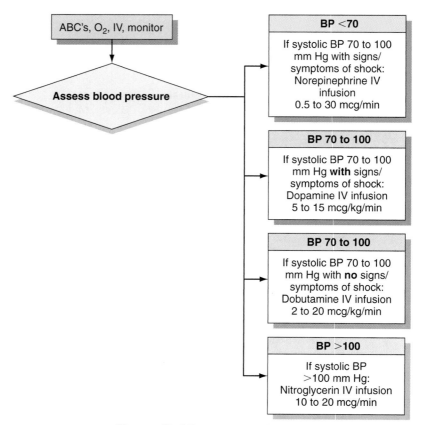

Figure 8-42 • Cardiogenic shock.

PUTTING IT ALL TOGETHER

■ *Evaluator:* Your patient is a 50-year-old man who presents with chest pain. You have four ALS personnel to assist you. Emergency equipment is immediately available.
■ *Team Leader:* Is the scene safe to enter?
■ *Evaluator:* The scene is safe.

Initial Assessment

First Impression

■ *Team Leader:* I am putting on personal protective equipment. As I approach the patient and form a first impression, what do I see?
■ *Evaluator:* You see the patient sitting in a chair clutching his chest. His breathing is unlabored. His skin looks pale.

Primary Survey

■ *Team Leader:* I will approach the patient and begin a primary survey. Does the patient respond when I speak his name?
■ *Evaluator:* Yes. The patient quickly introduces himself and asks that you do something about his pain.
■ *Team Leader:* How is his breathing? What is his pulse rate and quality?
■ *Evaluator:* The patient's breathing is adequate. His radial and carotid pulses are strong but slightly irregular. You estimate the rate to be about 100 per minute.
■ *Team Leader:* I will make sure a defibrillator is within reach, but it is not needed at this time. I will reassure the patient that I will do something about his pain very soon. I want the defibrillation team member to attach a pulse oximeter and place the patient on a cardiac monitor. I will ask the airway team member to place the patient on oxygen by nonrebreather mask. I want the CPR team member to obtain the patient's baseline vital signs while I begin the secondary survey. I want the IV team member to start an IV of normal saline. I want the defibrillation team member to order a 12-lead ECG.

Secondary Survey/Focused History and Exam

■ *Team Leader:* What are the patient's vital signs?
■ *Evaluator:* The patient's vital signs are as follows: BP 162/107, heart rate is about 110, and respirations 24. Breath sounds are clear and equal bilaterally. The patient's SpO_2 is 98% on oxygen by nonrebreather mask. An IV has been started. The 12-lead has been ordered. The patient has been placed on the cardiac monitor (Figure 8-43). What is the rhythm on the monitor?

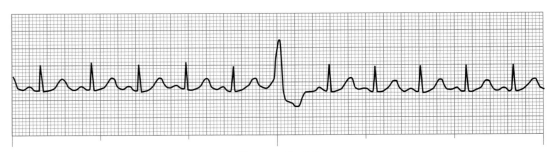

Figure 8-43

■ *Team Leader:*   The cardiac monitor shows a sinus tachycardia with a PVC. I will obtain a SAMPLE history from the patient and perform a focused physical exam.

■ *Evaluator:*   (See Table 8-12 for SAMPLE history and Table 8-13 for physical exam findings.) What would you like to do now?

■ *Team Leader:*   I want the IV team member to check to be sure there are no contraindications, and then give the patient 325 mg of baby aspirin and ask the patient to chew and swallow it. After making sure the patient has not used Viagra, Cialis, or a similar medication in the past 24 to 48 hours, I want the IV team member to give the patient sublingual nitroglycerin now and repeat every 5 minutes to a maximum of 3 doses. I want the patient's BP and pain reevaluated 5 minutes after each dose of nitroglycerin. I want the CPR team member to order cardiac biomarkers and other lab work, a portable chest x-ray, and begin a reperfusion therapy checklist right away. Is the patient's initial 12-lead available for review?

■ *Evaluator:*   The patient's 12-lead is available (Figure 8-44). Are there any significant findings on this 12-lead?

TABLE 8-12. **SAMPLE History**	
Signs/symptoms	Severe chest pain
OPQRST	"Squeezing" chest pain began 45 minutes ago; rates pain a "10" on 0 to 10 scale; points to center of chest and says pain radiates to left jaw and back; feels nauseated
Allergies	None
Medications	Metoprolol, Lotensin, BuSpar (states he has never used Viagra, Cialis, or similar medication)
Past medical history	Hypertension, anxiety, 2-vessel coronary artery bypass graft in 1999
Last oral intake	Breakfast 2 hours ago
Events prior	Awoke this morning feeling very tired; under additional stress lately (wife diagnosed yesterday with cancer); extensive family history of early coronary artery disease

TABLE 8-13. **Physical Examination Findings**	
Head, ears, eyes, nose, and throat	No abnormalities noted
Neck	Trachea midline, no jugular venous distention
Chest	Breath sounds clear bilaterally, well-healed surgical scar present over the sternum
Abdomen	No abnormalities noted
Pelvis	No abnormalities noted
Extremities	No abnormalities noted
Posterior body	No abnormalities noted

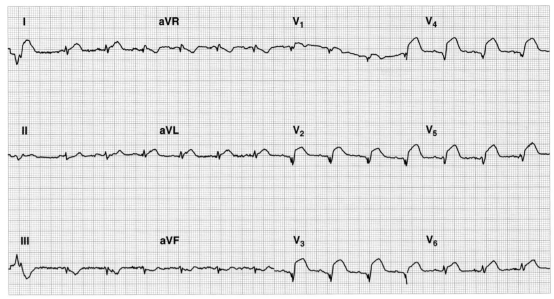

Figure 8-44

■ *Team Leader:*   The patient's heart rate is now about 80 bpm. There is ST-segment elevation in leads I, aVL, and V_1 to V_6.

■ *Evaluator:*   What would you like to do now?

■ *Team Leader:*   The patient's 12-lead ECG suggests an extensive anterior myocardial infarction. A physician needs to review the 12-lead right away and classify the patient as STEMI.

■ *Evaulator:*   What would you like to do next?

Postresuscitation Support/Ongoing Assessment

■ *Team Leader:*   I want to repeat the primary survey and obtain another set of vital signs. How is the patient's pain?

■ *Evaluator:*   The patient is resting more comfortably. His pain has steadily decreased from a "10" to "4" after a total of three nitroglycerin tablets. His heart rate is about 80 bpm, BP is 158/98, and respirations are 18.

■ *Team Leader:*   I would like the IV team member to give the patient 2 mg of morphine now. I want this repeated every 5 minutes as needed until the patient is pain free (assuming his vital signs remain stable). I want the patient's vital signs taken and recorded between doses. I want to make sure the reperfusion checklist is completed and schedule the patient for the cardiac catheterization laboratory.

STOP & REVIEW

Questions 1-26. Match each term or phrase below with its corresponding description.

a) Glucose level
b) Atropine
c) Ultrasound
d) Intropin
e) Two
f) Fibrinolytics
g) T waves
h) Normal
i) Three
j) Furosemide
k) Droop
l) Verapamil
m) Headache

n) Hypovolemia
o) Pericardiocentesis
p) Tachycardia
q) Cordarone
r) Pump
s) Bruits
t) Ventricular
u) Monomorphic
v) Muscle
w) Unstable angina
x) Aberrancy
y) Augmented
z) Eye opening

_____ 1. This drug is contraindicated in wide-QRS tachycardia of unknown origin

_____ 2. If a patient is hypotensive or has signs of shock, ask yourself, "Is there a rate problem, a __ problem, or a volume/vascular resistance problem?"

_____ 3. An acute coronary syndrome

_____ 4. Common cause of PEA

_____ 5. Drug of choice for symptomatic narrow-QRS bradycardia

_____ 6. In an acute coronary syndrome, time is __

_____ 7. The "A" in aVR, aVL, and aVF

_____ 8. Five cycles of CPR equal about __ minutes

_____ 9. One of the areas evaluated using the Glasgow Coma Scale

_____10. Most wide-QRS tachycardias are __ tachycardia

_____11. SVT with __ may appear on the ECG as a wide-QRS tachycardia

_____12. Assessment for a possible stroke includes looking for a facial __

_____13. Trade name for amiodarone

_____14. Trade name for dopamine

_____15. A severe __ is a common symptom of subarachnoid hemorrhage

_____16. "Clot-busters"

_____17. Definitive treatment for cardiac tamponade

_____18. A type of VT in which the QRS complexes are of similar shape and amplitude

____19. A(n) __ ECG does not rule out the diagnosis of an acute coronary syndrome

____20. Giving this drug too rapidly can cause tinnitus and transient deafness

____21. This increases myocardial oxygen demand and decreases time for coronary artery perfusion

____22. Listen for carotid __ before performing carotid sinus massage

____23. The maximum total dose of atropine for symptomatic bradycardia or asystole is __ mg

____24. Signs of hyperkalemia on the ECG are usually seen as tall __

____25. Do not use this type of gel for defibrillation

____26. This should be checked in all patients who present with an acute altered mental status

27. True or False. During a resuscitation effort, team members should frequently reassess the patient and keep the team leader informed of any changes in the patient's vital signs or ABCs.

28. A 47-year-old man is complaining of crushing chest pain, dizziness, and nausea. His BP is 74/40, pulse 48, respirations 16. The patient's breath sounds are clear. The cardiac monitor displays a second-degree AV block, type I. Recommended treatment for this patient includes which of the following?
   a. ABCs, O_2, IV, and adenosine rapid IV push
   b. ABCs, O_2, IV, sublingual nitroglycerin, and transcutaneous pacing
   c. ABCs, O_2, IV atropine IV, and/or transcutaneous pacing
   d. ABCs, O_2, IV, and morphine titrated to pain relief

29. In which of the following situations would an epinephrine IV bolus be indicated?
   a. Sinus bradycardia, junctional rhythm, and a ventricular escape rhythm
   b. Junctional rhythm, pulseless VT, and asystole
   c. PEA, pulseless VT, and asystole
   d. PEA, VF, and a ventricular escape rhythm

30. A 72-year-old man is anxious and complaining of palpitations. BP 110/64, P 190, and R 16. The patient denies chest pain. Breath sounds are clear. The cardiac monitor shows monomorphic VT. Recommended treatment in this situation includes which of the following?
   a. Begin CPR and defibrillate immediately
   b. ABCs, O_2, IV, sublingual nitroglycerin, and adenosine 6 mg rapid IV push
   c. ABCs, O_2, IV, and vasopressin 40 U rapid IV push
   d. ABCs, O_2, IV, and amiodarone 150 mg IV

31. A 57-year-old man is complaining of chest discomfort and difficulty breathing. He is disoriented and extremely anxious. Examination reveals bibasilar crackles, a weak carotid pulse, and a BP of 60/30. The cardiac monitor displays a regular narrow-QRS tachycardia at a rate of 210 bpm. The patient has been placed on oxygen and an IV has been established. Management of this patient should include:
   a. Giving sublingual nitroglycerin for pain relief
   b. Performing synchronized cardioversion with 50 J and reassessing the patient
   c. Giving 6 mg of adenosine rapid IV bolus and reassessing the patient
   d. Giving 2.5 mg of verapamil slow IV bolus and reassessing the patient

32. Morphine sulfate may be used in the management of acute pulmonary edema because it:
    a. Causes bronchodilation and increases cardiac output
    b. Increases myocardial contractility
    c. Is a potent, rapid-acting diuretic
    d. Causes vasodilation, reducing preload and afterload

33. A patient has experienced a cardiopulmonary arrest. The cardiac monitor displays a sinus tachycardia at 110 bpm. Appropriate treatment for this patient should include which of the following?
    a. CPR, IV access, epinephrine, and atropine
    b. CPR, transcutaneous pacing, and a search for the cause of the arrest
    c. CPR, IV access, epinephrine, and a search for the cause of the arrest
    d. CPR, defibrillation, IV access, epinephrine, and atropine

34. The initial treatment of any patient with a symptomatic bradycardia should focus on which of the following?
    a. Support of airway and breathing
    b. Preparations for transcutaneous pacing
    c. Preparations for synchronized cardioversion
    d. Assessing oxygen saturation and establishing IV access

35. When a "flat line" is observed on a cardiac monitor:
    a. Apply adhesive pads or hand-held paddles to the patient's chest and defibrillate immediately
    b. Check the lead/cable connections and make sure the correct lead is selected
    c. Prepare for immediate transcutaneous pacing
    d. Apply adhesive pads or hand-held paddles to the patient's chest and perform synchronized cardioversion

36. When atropine is used in the management of asystole, the correct IV dose is:
    a. 0.5 mg
    b. 1.0 mg
    c. 2 to 2.5 mg
    d. 5 mcg/kg

37. Examples of irregular tachycardias include:
    a. Idioventricular rhythm, AFib, and accelerated junctional rhythm
    b. Sinus tachycardia, accelerated junctional rhythm, and atrial flutter
    c. AFib, atrial flutter, and polymorphic VT
    d. Polymorphic VT, asystole, and sinus tachycardia

38. A 69-year-old woman presents with a sudden onset of palpitations, chest pain, and dizziness. The cardiac monitor reveals AFib with a rapid ventricular response ranging from 150 to 215 bpm. Her blood pressure is 77/30 and respirations are 16. The patient has been placed on oxygen and an IV has been started. Your best course of action will be to:
    a. Sedate the patient and perform synchronized cardioversion with 100 J
    b. Give dopamine by IV infusion to increase BP
    c. Begin transcutaneous pacing
    d. Give adenosine 6 mg IV slow IV push over 2 minutes

39. A 29-year-old man presents with acute altered mental status. His BP is 50 by palpation, respirations 14. The cardiac monitor reveals the following (Figure 8-45):

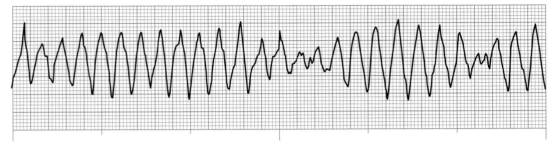

Figure 8-45

Your best course of action in this situation will be to:
a. Perform immediate synchronized cardioversion
b. Give adenosine rapid IV push
c. Consider sedation and defibrillate immediately
d. Give diltiazem IV push over 2 minutes

40. A 73-year-old woman is found unresponsive, not breathing, and without a pulse. She was last seen 15 minutes ago. CPR is in progress. The cardiac monitor reveals the following (Figure 8-46):

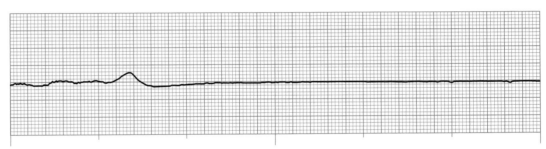

Figure 8-46

You should now:
a. Start an IV and give amiodarone
b. Start an IV and give epinephrine and atropine
c. Defibrillate with 360 J and reassess the patient
d. Give norepinephrine IV bolus

41. Which of the following correctly reflects the priorities of care during cardiac arrest?
a. CPR and establishing IV access
b. Defibrillation and drug administration
c. Establishing IV access and drug administration
d. CPR and defibrillation

42. Vasopressin:
a. Should be given every 3 to 5 minutes during cardiac arrest
b. May replace either the first or second dose of epinephrine in the treatment of cardiac arrest
c. Should be given as a continuous IV infusion at a rate of 40 U/hr in cardiac arrest
d. Can be used in cardiac arrest due to pulseless VT or VF, but not in cardiac arrest due to asystole or PEA

43. Which of the following statements is true about patients who present with a possible ACS?
    a. VF or pulseless VT is most likely to develop 48 hours after the onset of symptoms
    b. Prophylactic lidocaine should be given to all patients with a possible ACS to reduce the incidence of VF
    c. Patients who are most likely to benefit from reperfusion therapy are those who show ST-segment depression or nonspecific ST- or T-wave changes on their ECG
    d. A 12-lead ECG should be obtained with 10 minutes of patient contact (prehospital) or 10 minutes of patient arrival in the ED

44. Which of the following statements about lidocaine dosing in pulseless VT/VF is correct?
    a. The initial dose is 1 mg IV push, which may be repeated twice to a maximum dose of 3 mg
    b. Lidocaine is given as a continuous IV infusion of 2 to 10 mcg/min
    c. The initial dose is 1 to 1.5 mg/kg IV push; repeat doses of 0.5 to 0.75 mg/kg IV push may be given at 5- to 10-minute intervals, to a maximum IV bolus dose of 3 mg/kg
    d. Lidocaine is given as a continuous IV infusion of 10 to 20 mcg/kg/min

45. True or False. During cardiac arrest, rhythm checks should be brief, and pulse checks should generally be performed only if an organized rhythm is seen on the cardiac monitor.

46. Which of the following medications is recommended if the patient exhibits pump problems with a systolic pressure of 70 to 100 mm Hg and no signs of shock?
    a. Digoxin
    b. Diltiazem
    c. Dobutamine
    d. Dopamine

STOP & REVIEW ANSWERS

1. l

2. r

3. w

4. n

5. b

6. v

7. y

8. e

9. z

10. t

11. x

12. k

13. q

14. d

15. m

16. f

17. o

18. u

19. h

20. j

21. p

22. s

23. i

24. g

25. c

26. a

27. True. During a resuscitation effort, team members should frequently reassess the patient and inform the team leader of any changes in the patient's vital signs or ABCs. Patient reassessment and communication with the team leader should occur at least every 3 to 5 minutes through the resuscitation effort.

28. c. A second-degree AV block type I is usually associated with a narrow-QRS. Atropine is often effective in increasing the heart rate in symptomatic narrow-QRS bradycardias. Because atropine will likely result in an increase in heart rate, the resulting increased rate will also increase myocardial O_2 demand. This must be considered when giving atropine to a patient who may be experiencing an acute MI. Transcutaneous pacing is an appropriate treatment for any symptomatic bradycardia. Adenosine is used to slow the heart rate in symptomatic narrow-QRS tachycardias. Because this patient has a bradycardia, adenosine is not indicated. Sublingual nitroglycerin should not be given at this time because the patient's heart rate is less than 50 bpm and his BP is low. Although morphine is used to relieve pain, the patient's BP is very low. Because the patient's breath sounds are clear, consider a 250-mL IV fluid challenge of normal saline to try and increase the patient's BP. Give nitroglycerin and morphine as needed for pain relief if the patient's systolic blood pressure (SBP) rises above 90 to 100 mm Hg (check your local protocols) and the heart rate increases to more than 50 bpm (but less than 100).

29. c. An IV bolus of epinephrine is indicated in cardiac arrest. Cardiac arrest rhythms include PEA, asystole, pulseless VT, and VF. Epinephrine is not given IV bolus to treat a dysrhythmia in patients who have a pulse. Although epinephrine may be given to patients for symptomatic bradycardia, it is given as an IV infusion, not an IV bolus.

30. d. Based on the information presented, the patient appears to be stable. Because the patient has a pulse, CPR, defibrillation, and vasopressin are not indicated. The patient

denies chest pain, so nitroglycerin is not indicated. The drug of choice for a stable patient in monomorphic VT is amiodarone. Because the patient has a pulse, give amiodarone 150 mg IV over 10 minutes. Repeat as needed to a maximum dose of 2.2 g/24 hr. Alternative drugs include procainamide and sotalol.

31. b. This patient is unstable (chest discomfort, altered level of consciousness, hypotension, difficulty breathing). Consider sedation, perform synchronized cardioversion with 50 J, and reassess the patient. Nitroglycerin is contraindicated because of the patient's rapid heart rate and low BP. Adenosine and verapamil may be used for *stable* patients with a symptomatic narrow-QRS tachycardia.

32. d. Medications used in the management of a normotensive patient in acute pulmonary edema include nitroglycerin, furosemide, and morphine. Morphine reduces anxiety, increases venous capacitance (venous pooling) and decreases venous return (preload) (sometimes called "chemical phlebotomy"), decreases systemic vascular resistance (afterload), and decreases myocardial O_2 demand.

33. c. Despite the presence of an organized rhythm on the cardiac monitor, the patient is pulseless. The clinical situation is PEA. Start CPR, insert an IV, give epinephrine, and search for a reversible cause of the arrest. If the patient's rhythm was slow, the use of atropine would be appropriate. In this case, the patient's PEA is associated with a tachycardia, so atropine is not indicated.

34. a. The initial treatment of any patient with a symptomatic bradycardia should focus on support of airway and breathing.

35. b. When a "flat line" is observed on an ECG, make sure the power to the monitor is on, check the lead/cable connections, make sure the correct lead is selected, and turn up the gain (ECG size) on the monitor. Attempting transcutaneous pacing for asystole is no longer recommended.

36. b. When atropine is used to treat a symptomatic bradycardia, the correct dose is 0.5 mg IV every 3 to 5 minutes to a maximum dose of 3.0 mg. When atropine is used to treat asystole or slow PEA, the correct dose is 1.0 mg IV every 3 to 5 minutes to a maximum dose of 3.0 mg.

37. c. Examples of irregular tachycardias include AFib, atrial flutter, and polymorphic VT. Asystole, idioventricular rhythm, and accelerated junctional rhythm are not tachycardias.

38. a. This patient is unstable (hypotension, chest pain). The patient should be sedated and then synchronized cardioversion should be performed starting with 100 J or equivalent biphasic energy. Although dopamine will increase BP, it usually increases heart rate as well. A better course of action would be to treat the rate problem with synchronized cardioversion and then reassess the patient's BP. By correcting the rate problem, it is likely the patient's BP will improve. Transcutaneous pacing is used to increase heart rate. Because the patient is tachycardic, it is not indicated in this situation. Adenosine is used for narrow-QRS tachycardias that use the AV node to perpetuate the rhythm. Drugs that slow conduction through the AV node will not generally convert Afib (or atrial flutter) to a sinus rhythm because the reentry circuit is located in the atria (not the AV node) and is not affected. In AFib, the AV node does not play a part in the maintenance of the tachycardia. The AV node serves only to passively conduct the supraventricular rhythm into the ventricles.

39. c. The rhythm shown is polymorphic VT. The patient is unstable (acute altered mental status, hypotension). Consider sedation and defibrillate immediately. Although syn-

chronized cardioversion is an appropriate treatment for unstable patients with a tachycardia, it is used for tachycardias that have a relatively uniform amplitude. Because the amplitude of the waveforms in polymorphic VT varies, defibrillation should be used instead. Adenosine and diltiazem are not indicated.

40. b. The rhythm shown is asystole. Appropriate emergency care includes CPR, giving O_2, starting an IV, giving epinephrine and atropine, and considering possible reversible causes of the arrest. Vasopressin can be used in place of the first or second dose of epinephrine. Although amiodarone is used in the management of many atrial and ventricular dysrhythmias, it is not indicated in the treatment of asystole. Defibrillation is not indicated in the treatment of asystole. Norepinephrine is given by continuous IV infusion for severe hypotension (SBP < 70 mm Hg) that is not due to hypovolemia. It is not indicated in asystole.

41. d. Because no drugs used in cardiac arrest have been shown to improve survival to hospital discharge, the priorities of care in a cardiac arrest are CPR and defibrillation.

42. b. One dose of vasopressin 40 U IV/IO may replace either the first or second dose of epinephrine in the treatment of cardiac arrest.

43. d. A 12-lead ECG should be obtained with 10 minutes of patient contact (prehospital) or 10 minutes of patient arrival in the ED. Primary VF is VF that occurs during the acute phase of an MI. The incidence of VF is highest during the first 4 hours after onset of symptoms and remains an important contributing factor to death in the first 24 hours. For many years, PVCs observed in patients experiencing an acute MI were thought to be "warning" dysrhythmias of impending VF, particularly multiform PVCs, R-on-T PVCs, couplets, frequent (>6/min) PVCs. It is considered prudent clinical practice to observe these premature beats closely, consider the reason for their occurrence (such as hypoxemia, acid-base disturbance, electrolyte imbalance, or heart failure), and correct the underlying cause. Routine administration of lidocaine to prevent VF is no longer recommended. Reperfusion therapy is the mainstay of treatment for STEMI. Because STEMI is usually the result of a blocked coronary artery, the blockage may be removed by giving fibrinolytics (pharmacologic reperfusion) or primary percutaneous coronary intervention (PCI) (mechanical reperfusion).

44. c. Although amiodarone is the antiarrhythmic mentioned first in the pulseless VT/VF algorithm, lidocaine may be considered if amiodarone is not available. The initial dose of lidocaine is 1 to 1.5 mg/kg IV push. Repeat doses of 0.5 to 0.75 mg/kg IV push may be given at 5- to 10-minute intervals. The cumulative IV/IO bolus dose is 3 mg/kg. If there is a return of spontaneous circulation, consider a lidocaine infusion of 1 to 4 mg/min. This should be reduced after 24 hours (to 1 to 2 mg/min) or in the setting of altered metabolism (congestive heart failure, hepatic dysfunction, acute MI with hypotension or shock, patients >70 years, poor peripheral perfusion) and as guided by blood level monitoring.

45. True. During cardiac arrest, rhythm checks should be brief, and pulse checks should generally be performed only if an organized rhythm is seen on the cardiac monitor.

46. c. Dobutamine is used for the short-term management of patients with cardiac decompensation due to depressed contractility (e.g., congestive heart failure, pulmonary congestion) with a SBP of 70 to 100 mm Hg **and no signs of shock.** Hypovolemia must be corrected before treatment with dobutamine. Dobutamine is given as a continuous IV infusion at a rate of 2 to 20 mcg/kg/min.

REFERENCES

1. 2005 American Heart Association guidelines for cardiopulmonary resuscitation and emergency cardiovascular care, part 5: Electrical therapies. Automated external defibrillators, defibrillation, cardioversion, and pacing. *Circulation* 2005;112(suppl IV):IV-36.

2. Boyd R: Witnessed resuscitation by relatives. *Resuscitation* Feb 2000;43(3):171-176.

3. Meyers TA, Eichhorn DJ, Guzzetta CE: Do families want to be present during CPR? A retrospective survey. *J Emerg Nurs* 1998;24:400-405.

4. Doyle CJ, Post H, Burney RE, et al: Family participation during resuscitation: An option. *Ann Emerg Med* 1987;16:673-675.

5. Jurkovich GJ, Pierce B, Pananen L, et al: Giving bad news: The family perspective. *J Trauma* May 2000;48(5):865-870

6. Myerburg RJ, Castellanos A: Cardiac arrest and sudden cardiac death. In Zipes DP, Libby P, Bonow RO, Braunwald EB (Eds.), *Braunwald's heart disease: A textbook of cardiovascular medicine* (7th ed.). Philadelphia: Saunders, 2005, pp. 865-908.

7. Bayes de Luna A, Coumel P, Leclercq JF: Ambulatory sudden cardiac death: Mechanisms of production of fatal arrhythmia on the basis of data from 157 cases. *Am Heart J* Jan 1989;17(1): 151-159.

8. Cobb LA, Fahrenbruch CE, Olsufka M, Copass MK: Changing incidence of out-of-hospital ventricular fibrillation, 1980-2000. *JAMA* Dec 18, 2002;288(23):3008-3013.

9. Rea TD, Eisenberg MS, Sinibaldi G, White RD: Incidence of EMS-treated out-of-hospital cardiac arrest in the United States. *Resuscitation* Oct 2004;63(1):17-24.

10. Vaillancourt C, Stiell IG: Canadian cardiovascular outcomes research team. Cardiac arrest care and emergency medical services in Canada. *Can J Cardiol* Sep 2004;20(11):1081-1090. Review.

11. Niemann JT, Stratton SJ, Cruz B, Lewis RJ: Outcome of out-of-hospital postcountershock asystole and pulseless electrical activity versus primary asystole and pulseless electrical activity. *Crit Care Med* Dec 2001;29(12):2366-2370.

12. 2005 American Heart Association guidelines for cardiopulmonary resuscitation and emergency cardiovascular care, part 7.5: Postresuscitation support. *Circulation* 2005;112(suppl IV):IV-86.

13. Ornato JP, Peberdy MA: The mystery of bradyasystole during cardiac arrest. *Ann Emerg Med* May 1996;27:576-587.

14. 2005 American Heart Association guidelines for cardiopulmonary resuscitation and emergency cardiovascular care, part 7.2: Management of pulseless arrest. *Circulation* 2005;112(suppl IV): IV-61.

15. 2005 American Heart Association guidelines for cardiopulmonary resuscitation and emergency cardiovascular care, part 7.2: Management of pulseless arrest. *Circulation* 2005; 112(suppl IV): IV-62.

16. 2005 American Heart Association guidelines for cardiopulmonary resuscitation and emergency cardiovascular care, part 7.5: Postresuscitation support. *Circulation* 2005;112(suppl IV):IV-84.

17. 2005 American Heart Association guidelines for cardiopulmonary resuscitation and emergency cardiovascular care, part 7.5: Postresuscitation support. *Circulation* 2005;112(suppl IV):IV-85.

18. Phalen T, Aehlert B: *The 12-lead ECG in Acute Coronary Syndromes.* St. Louis: Mosby, 2006.

19. 2005 American Heart Association guidelines for cardiopulmonary resuscitation and emergency cardiovascular care, part 7.3: Management of symptomatic bradycardia and tachycardia. *Circulation* 2005;112(suppl IV):IV-67.

20. 2005 American Heart Association guidelines for cardiopulmonary resuscitation and emergency cardiovascular care, part 7.3: Management of symptomatic bradycardia and tachycardia. *Circulation* 2005;112(suppl IV):IV-69.

21. 2005 American Heart Association guidelines for cardiopulmonary resuscitation and emergency cardiovascular care, part 7.3: Management of symptomatic bradycardia and tachycardia. *Circulation* 2005;112(suppl IV):IV-75.

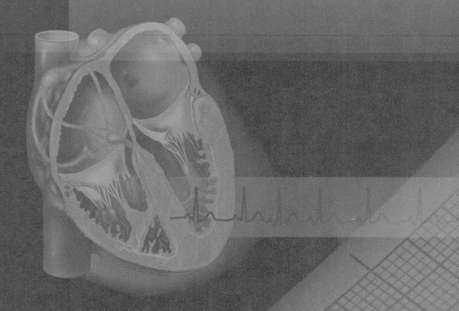

PART

II

CASE STUDIES

Case Studies

INTRODUCTION

The first section of this book provided the "why," "when," and "how" for the case studies that follow. It has been proved that in order to learn how to do something, you must actually *do* it. The opportunity to "do" the skills taught in an advanced cardiac life support (ACLS) course and make decisions regarding patient care is provided during 10 "core" case studies in the ACLS Provider course. The 10 "core" cases presented during an ACLS course include the following:

1. Respiratory arrest
2. Pulseless ventricular tachycardia (VT)/ventricular fibrillation (VF) treated with an automated external defibrillator (AED)
3. Pulseless VT/VF
4. Asystole
5. Pulseless electrical activity (PEA)
6. Acute coronary syndromes (ACSs)
7. Symptomatic bradycardia
8. Unstable tachycardia
9. Stable tachycardia
10. Acute ischemic stroke

During an ACLS course, discussion pertaining to each of the core ACLS cases may occur between the course instructor and the entire class, between several instructors and small groups of course participants, or between groups of students who alternate playing the role of the patient, rescuers, and coach with oversight by an instructor.

Each of the "core" ACLS cases is presented on the following pages. The case studies presented here are not intended to cover every possible dysrhythmia or patient condition that may be presented in an actual ACLS course. Rather, they are provided as examples to help you integrate the information presented in the preparatory section of this book.

Each ACLS case is presented using two styles. In the first, a scenario is presented and followed by a series of questions. The questions are intended to reinforce important points pertinent to the case that were presented in the preparatory section of this book. Read the scenario and answer each question that follows it. Compare your answers with the answers provided at the end of the case study. The questions are followed by a scenario sheet. A sample scenario sheet is shown below. Read the entire sheet, paying particular attention to the "Necessary Tasks" section, which reflects what you are expected to do.

After you have read the sheet, ask another person to assist you by assuming the role of "coach." Information that should be read aloud to you appears in italics. As you practice, assume you are the person responsible for directing the actions of a team providing emergency care for the patient. Assume that each team member will correctly carry out your instructions; however, they will not do anything without your direction. Perform a patient assessment as you would in an actual situation, including communicating with your patient. The coach should assume the role of the patient, family members, bystanders, or others as necessary. As you progress through the case study, state everything you are assessing. Ask the coach questions about the patient's vital signs, history, and response to the treatments performed as needed. If you have trouble deciding what to do, the coach can help you by reading what Emergency Action Step is next or by telling you what Necessary Tasks should be performed. The coach should acknowledge your interventions and ask you for additional information if clarification is needed. After completing each scenario, briefly review with the coach what went right and what needed improvement. Remember, practice makes perfect.

The case studies presented here simulate situations that you may encounter as an ACLS provider. Although case studies provide opportunities for problem solving and help "put it all together," they are imperfect simulations of reality. It is impossible to predict all possible actions for a given situation, or patient responses to a particular intervention. As you practice with each of the case studies presented here, please understand that there may be alternative actions that are perfectly acceptable, yet not presented in the case study.

SAMPLE SCENARIO SHEET:

EMERGENCY ACTION STEPS	NECESSARY TASKS
Scene Survey	Ensures scene safety. Takes or communicates standard/universal precautions.
	Coach: The scene is safe.

INITIAL ASSESSMENT

First Impression	Verbalizes general impression of patient (appearance, breathing, circulation)
	Coach: The patient is not moving. There is no obvious movement of his chest. His skin looks pale.

PRIMARY SURVEY

Responsiveness/Airway	Assesses airway . . .
	Coach:
Breathing	Assesses breathing . . .
	Coach:
Circulation	Assesses pulses, skin (color, temperature, and moisture), estimates heart rate
	Coach:
Defibrillation	Based on information obtained, determines need for an AED or monitor/defibrillator
	Coach:

SECONDARY SURVEY/FOCUSED HISTORY & EXAM

Vital Signs/History	Obtains baseline vital signs, history *Coach:*
Airway, Breathing, Circulation	Assesses need for advanced airway, gives O_2, starts IV, . . . *Coach:*
Differential Diagnosis, Evaluates Interventions	Determines treatment plan, begins appropriate care, evaluates patient response, facilitates family presence when applicable *Coach:*

POSTRESUSCITATION SUPPORT/ONGOING ASSESSMENT

Begins Postresuscitation Support/Performs Ongoing Assessment	Repeats initial assessment *Coach:* Repeats vital signs *Coach:* Evaluates response to care *Coach:*

CASE 1: RESPIRATORY ARREST

Objective	Given a patient situation, describe and demonstrate the initial emergency care for a patient who has experienced a respiratory arrest.
Skills to Master	◆ Primary and secondary surveys ◆ Recognition of a patient with respiratory compromise/arrest. ◆ Head-tilt/chin-lift, jaw thrust without head tilt ◆ Insertion of an oral or nasal airway ◆ Pocket mask or bag-mask ventilation (1- and 2-rescuer technique) ◆ Suctioning ◆ Attachment and use of electrocardiogram (ECG) monitoring leads ◆ Advanced airway insertion (laryngeal mask airway, Combitube, endotracheal [ET] intubation) ◆ Use of a pulse oximeter, end-tidal carbon dioxide ($ETCO_2$) detector, esophageal detector device ◆ IV access
Rhythms to Master	◆ Sinus bradycardia ◆ Sinus rhythm
Medications to Master	O_2
Related Text Chapters	Chapter 1: The ABCDs of Emergency Cardiovascular Care Chapter 2: Airway Management: Oxygenation and Ventilation Chapter 3: Vascular Access

CASE 1: QUESTIONS

SCENARIO: Your patient is a 78-year-old woman who is complaining of difficulty breathing. You have four other advanced life support (ALS) personnel to assist you. Emergency equipment is immediately available. The scene is safe.

1. You are putting on personal protective equipment as you approach the patient. What are the first impression ABCs?

   A:

   B:

   C:

2. You see an elderly woman sitting up in bed with 3 or 4 pillows behind her back. Her breathing appears faster than normal and labored. Her skin looks pale. As you reach the patient's side, the patient slumps backward into the pillows. What memory aid can you use to evaluate the patient's level of responsiveness?

3. The patient is unresponsive. What should be done next?

4. At your direction, your assistants remove the pillows from the bed and quickly position the patient on her back. How will you open the patient's airway?

5. You see a significant amount of mucus in the patient's mouth. What should be done now?

6. What is the maximum length of time for a suctioning attempt?

7. The patient's airway is clear. What should be done now?

8. The patient is not breathing. How should you proceed?

9. How will you determine the proper size oral airway for this patient?

10. Name two possible complications of oral airway insertion.

11. Describe two methods for insertion of an oral airway in the adult patient.

12. An oral airway has been inserted. The patient is still not breathing. Should a nasal cannula be considered at this point?

13. When use of a nasal cannula is indicated, what is the liter flow recommended for use with this device? What is the approximate O_2 concentration that can be delivered with this device?

14. Should a simple face mask be considered at this point?

15. When use of a simple face mask is indicated, what is the liter flow recommended for use with this device? What is the approximate O_2 concentration that can be delivered with this device?

16. What percentage of O_2 can be delivered with a bag-mask device?

17. Name three advantages of ventilation with a bag-mask device.
    1.
    2.
    3.

18. What is the most common problem associated with the use of the bag-mask device?

19. An oral airway has been inserted and the patient is being ventilated with a bag-mask device. There are no spontaneous respirations, but you do see gentle chest rise with bagging. At what rate should this patient be ventilated?

20. The patient is being ventilated as instructed. What should be done now?

21. A carotid pulse is present. The rate is slow, weak, and regular. What should be done now?

22. The patient remains unresponsive and apneic. Breath sounds with bag-mask ventilation reveal clear upper lobes and diminished sounds in the lower lobes bilaterally. The patient's heart rate is 37 bpm. Her BP is 108/74. The patient has been placed on the cardiac monitor (see Case 1 Rhythm 1 and Case 1 SAMPLE history and physical examination tables). What is the rhythm on the monitor? What should be done now?

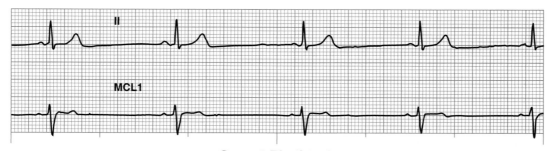

Case 1 Rhythm 1.

CASE 1

SAMPLE History

Signs/symptoms	Increasing shortness of breath since yesterday
Allergies	Sulfa
Medications	Protonix, Prevacid, magnesium oxide
Past medical history	Chronic obstructive pulmonary disease, smoker since age 17
Last oral intake	Yesterday
Events prior	Before she collapsed, the patient mentioned a constant, localized pain under her right breast since yesterday that "kept getting worse." She was watching television when it started. Nothing made it better or worse.

CASE 1

Physical Examination Findings

Head, ears, eyes, nose, and throat	Mucus initially present in mouth (cleared with suctioning)
Neck	Trachea midline, no jugular venous distention
Chest	Breath sounds are clear in upper lobes/diminished in lower lobes
Abdomen	No abnormalities noted
Pelvis	No abnormalities noted
Extremities	Bilateral pedal edema
Posterior body	Unremarkable

23. After making sure that an $ETCO_2$ monitor is available, you have asked your most experienced assistant to intubate the patient. You have asked another team member to assist by performing cricoid pressure during the procedure. What is the purpose of cricoid pressure? At what point should cricoid pressure be released?

24. Name three indications for ET intubation:
    1.
    2.
    3.

25. What is the maximum length of time ventilation should be interrupted for an intubation attempt? At what point does this time interval begin and end?

26. What is the average ET tube size for an adult male? An adult female?

27. Name five possible complications of ET intubation.
    1.
    2.
    3.
    4.
    5.

28. An IV has been established with normal saline. An ET tube has been inserted and the cuff inflated. Cricoid pressure has been discontinued. How will you confirm placement of the ET tube?

29. After placement of the tube, there are no sounds heard over the epigastrium. Breath sounds are diminished in the upper and lower lobes on the left side of the chest. They are clearly heard in the right upper lobe and diminished in the right lower lobe. What do you suspect?

30. After repositioning the ET tube, breath sounds with bag-mask ventilation reveal clear upper lobes and diminished sounds in the lower lobes bilaterally. An ETCO$_2$ monitor confirms the presence of CO$_2$ and the ET tube has been secured in place. What should be done now?

31. The patient is making no attempt to breathe spontaneously. Her vital signs now: BP 112/74, P 72, strong and regular; R 12/min via bag-mask device; SpO$_2$ 97%. What is the rhythm on the cardiac monitor (Case 1 Rhythm 2)? What should be done now?

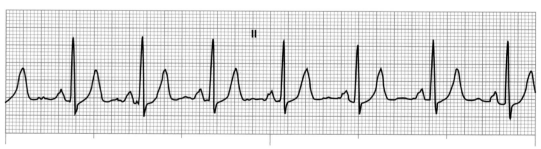

Case 1 Rhythm 2.

CASE 1: ANSWERS

1. The first impression ABCs are appearance, (work of) breathing, and circulation.

2. The memory aid used to assess responsiveness is AVPU. A = alert, V = responds to a verbal stimulus, P = responds to a painful stimulus, U = unresponsive.

3. Perform a primary survey starting with assessment of the patient's airway. Primary survey: A = Airway, B = Breathing, C = Circulation, D = Defibrillation, if necessary.

4. Because you have seen nothing to suspect trauma, open the patient's airway using a head-tilt/chin-lift. If there were anything that suggested trauma in this situation, you would open the airway with a jaw thrust without head tilt. Look in the mouth for blood, broken teeth or loose dentures, gastric contents, and foreign objects.

5. Ask an assistant to clear the patient's airway with suctioning.

6. In an adult, suction should not be applied for more than 10 to 15 seconds.

7. Look, listen, and feel for breathing for up to 10 seconds.

8. Ask the airway team member to size and insert an oral airway and begin positive-pressure ventilation with a bag-mask device connected to 100% O_2 while you continue the primary survey. Be sure that the airway team member maintains proper head position and a good seal with the mask against the patient's face. Ask a second team member to assume responsibility for compressing the bag with just enough force to produce gentle chest rise.

9. Proper airway size is determined by holding the device against the side of the patient's face and selecting an airway that extends from the corner of the mouth to the tip of the earlobe or the angle of the jaw.

10. Trauma/bleeding of oropharynx, bradycardia because of stimulation of gag reflex. Insertion in responsive or semiresponsive patient may stimulate vomiting or laryngospasm. If the oral airway is improperly positioned, the tongue may be pushed back into the posterior pharynx, causing an airway obstruction. If the airway is too long, it may press the epiglottis against the entrance of the larynx, resulting in a complete airway obstruction. If the airway is too short, it will not displace the tongue and may advance out of the mouth.

11. *Method #1:* The oral airway is inserted with the tip pointing toward the roof of the patient's mouth. It is advanced along the roof of the mouth and rotated 180 degrees when the distal end reaches the back of the throat so that it is positioned over the tongue. *Method #2:* Requires the use of a tongue blade to depress the tongue. If this method is used, the oral airway is inserted with the tip of the oral airway facing the floor of the patient's mouth (curved side down). Using the tongue blade to depress the tongue, the oral airway is gently advanced into place over the tongue.

12. No. A nasal cannula is used only in spontaneously breathing patients with adequate ventilation.

13. 1 to 6 L/min, 25% to 45% (actual amount of inspired O_2 depends on respiratory rate and depth)

14. No. A simple face mask is used only in spontaneously breathing patients with adequate ventilation.

15. At 6 to 10 L/min, the simple face mask can provide an inspired O_2 concentration of approximately 40% to 60%; the recommended flow rate is 8 to 10 L/min. The patient's actual inspired O_2 concentration will vary because the amount of air that mixes with supplemental O_2 is dependent on the patient's inspiratory flow rate.

16. Without supplemental O_2: 21% (room air); 12 to 15 L/min supplemental O_2 but no reservoir: 40% to 60%; 12 to 15 L/min supplemental O_2 and reservoir: 90% to 100%

17. Provides a means for delivery of an O_2-enriched mixture to the patient; conveys a sense of compliance of the patient's lungs to the bag-mask operator; provides a means for immediate ventilatory support; can be used with the spontaneously breathing patient as well as the nonbreathing patient.

18. The most frequent problem with the bag-mask device is the inability to provide an adequate ventilatory volume. This is due to the difficulty in providing a leak-proof seal to the face while maintaining an open airway at the same time.

19. The patient should be ventilated at a rate of 10 to 12 ventilations/min (one ventilation every 5 to 6 seconds). Each ventilation should be given over 1 second. Ask an assistant to assess baseline breath sounds while the patient is being ventilated and then prepare the intubation equipment.

20. Ask a team member to attach a pulse oximeter and the ECG monitoring leads while you feel for a carotid pulse for up to 10 seconds. While you are feeling for a pulse, assess the patient's skin temperature, color, and moisture.

21. Assess the need for a defibrillator. Because the patient has a pulse and the heart rate is slow, defibrillation is not necessary right now. Ask a team member to obtain the patient's baseline vital signs while you begin the secondary survey. If not already done, find out if there is someone available who may know what happened before the patient collapsed.

22. The rhythm is a sinus bradycardia. Instruct the airway team member to prepare to intubate the patient. Ask the IV team member to start an IV with normal saline. Order a 12-lead ECG and portable chest x-ray and perform a focused physical exam. Resist the temptation to treat the patient's initial bradycardia with atropine. The most likely cause of the patient's bradycardia is hypoxia. Make sure the patient is adequately oxygenated and ventilated before considering other possible causes of the patient's situation or the use of atropine.

23. Remember: Cricoid pressure is not intended to aid visualization of the vocal cords during intubation. Cricoid pressure (the Sellick maneuver) compresses the esophagus between the cricoid cartilage and the fifth and sixth cervical vertebrae. This minimizes gastric distention and aspiration during positive-pressure ventilation. Pressure is maintained until the cuff of the ET tube is inflated. If the patient vomits while cricoid pressure is being applied, pressure is released to avoid rupture of the stomach or esophagus.

24. Inability of the patient to protect his or her own airway due to the absence of protective reflexes (such as coma, respiratory and/or cardiac arrest); inability of the rescuer to ventilate the unresponsive patient with less invasive methods; present or impending airway obstruction/respiratory failure (e.g., inhalation injury, severe asthma, exacerbation of chronic obstructive pulmonary disease, severe pulmonary edema, severe flail chest or pulmonary contusion); when prolonged ventilatory support is required

25. 30 seconds. The 30-second interval begins when ventilation of the patient ceases to allow insertion of the laryngoscope blade into the patient's mouth and ends when the patient is ventilated again upon placement of the ET tube.

26. Adult male: 8.0 to 8.5; adult female: 7.0 to 8.0; emergency rule: 7.5 will fit

27. Bleeding, laryngospasm, vocal cord damage, mucosal necrosis, barotrauma, aspiration, cuff leak, esophageal intubation, right mainstem intubation, occlusion caused by patient biting tube or secretions, laryngeal or tracheal edema, tube occlusion, inability to talk, hypoxia due to prolonged or unsuccessful intubation, dysrhythmias; trauma to lips, teeth, tongue, or soft tissues of the oropharynx; increased intracranial pressure

28. Attach a ventilation device to the ET tube and ventilate the patient. Confirm proper placement of the tube by first auscultating over the epigastrium (should be silent) and then in the midaxillary and anterior chest line on the right and left sides of the patient's chest. Observe the patient's chest for adequate chest rise with ventilation. It is important to note that auscultation for breath sounds over the lungs and abdomen and observing chest rise are not always indicative of correct ET tube placement. After visualizing the ET tube passing through the vocal cords and confirming placement of the tube by auscultation, be sure to verify tube placement using an exhaled carbon dioxide detector and/or an esophageal detector device. Once placement is confirmed, note and record the depth (cm marking) of the tube at the patient's teeth. When an ET tube has been properly placed, the cm markings on the side of the tube should be observed and recorded. This value is typically between the 19- and 23-cm marks on the tube at the front teeth. Average tube depth in men is 23 cm at the lips, 22 cm at the teeth; average tube depth in women is 22 cm at the lips, 21 cm at the teeth.

29. If breath sounds are diminished or absent on the left after intubation but present on the right, assume right mainstem bronchus intubation. Deflate the ET cuff, pull back the ET tube slightly, reinflate the cuff, and reassess breath sounds.

30. Repeat the primary survey and obtain another set of vital signs. Is the patient attempting to breathe spontaneously? What is the rate and quality of the patient's pulse? What is the patient's BP?
31. The monitor shows a sinus rhythm with tall T waves. Order laboratory studies, evaluate the patient's 12-lead ECG and chest x-ray, and attempt to determine possible causes of the patient's respiratory arrest. Arrange for continued mechanical ventilation and transfer the patient for definitive care.

CASE 1: SCENARIO SHEET

SCENARIO: Your patient is a 78-year-old woman who is complaining of difficulty breathing. You have four other ALS personnel to assist you. Emergency equipment is immediately available.

EMERGENCY ACTION STEPS	NECESSARY TASKS
Scene Survey	I am putting on personal protective equipment. Is the scene safe to enter? *Coach: The scene is safe.*

INITIAL ASSESSMENT

First Impression	As I approach the patient and form a first impression (assessing the patient's appearance, work of breathing, and circulation), what do I see? *Coach: You see an elderly woman sitting up in bed with 3 or 4 pillows behind her back. Her breathing appears faster than normal and labored. Her skin looks pale. As you reach the patient's side, the patient slumps backward into the pillows.*

PRIMARY SURVEY

Responsiveness/Airway	I will quickly approach the patient and assess her level of responsiveness. Does she respond when I call her name? *Coach: There is no response.* Does she respond when I pinch her hand? *Coach: The patient is unresponsive.* I will ask my assistants to remove the pillows from the bed and quickly help me position the patient on her back so that I can assess her airway. *Coach: The pillows have been removed and the patient is now supine.* Since I have seen nothing to suspect trauma, I will open the patient's airway using a head-tilt/chin-lift. Do I see anything in the patient's mouth such as blood, broken teeth or loose dentures, gastric contents, or a foreign object? *Coach: You see a significant amount of mucus in the patient's mouth.* I will ask an assistant to clear the patient's airway with suctioning. *Coach: The airway is now clear. What should be done now?*
Breathing	I will look, listen, and feel for breathing for up to 10 seconds. *Coach: The patient is not breathing.* I will ask the airway team member to size and insert an oral airway and begin positive-pressure ventilation with a bag-mask device connected to 100% O$_2$ while I continue the primary survey. I want the airway team member to maintain proper head position and a good seal with the mask against the patient's face. I want a sec-

ond team member to assume responsibility for compressing the bag with just enough force to produce gentle chest rise.

Coach: An oral airway has been inserted. The patient is being ventilated with a bag-mask device. There are no spontaneous respirations, although you do see gentle chest rise with bagging. At what rate should this patient be ventilated?

The patient should be ventilated at a rate of 10 to 12 ventilations/min (one ventilation every 5 to 6 seconds). Each ventilation should be given over 1 second. I will ask another assistant to assess baseline breath sounds while the patient is being ventilated and then prepare the intubation equipment.

Circulation	I will ask the defibrillation team member to attach a pulse oximeter and the ECG monitoring leads while I feel for a carotid pulse for up to 10 seconds. Do I feel a pulse? While I am feeling the patient's pulse, I will assess her skin condition. What is her skin temperature, color, and condition? *Coach: A slow, weak carotid pulse is present. You estimate the rate to be about 40. Her skin is warm, pale, and dry. What should be done now?*
Defibrillation	I will assess the need for a defibrillator. Since the patient has a slow pulse, defibrillation is not necessary right now. I will ask the IV team member to obtain the patient's baseline vital signs while I begin the secondary survey.

SECONDARY SURVEY/FOCUSED HISTORY & EXAM

Vital Signs/History	What are the patient's vital signs? *Coach: The patient remains unresponsive and apneic. Breath sounds with bag-mask ventilation reveal clear upper lobes and diminished sounds in the lower lobes bilaterally. The patient's heart rate is 37 bpm. Her BP is 108/74. The patient has been placed on the cardiac monitor. What is the rhythm on the monitor? (See Case 1 Rhythm 1.)* The rhythm is a sinus bradycardia. Is there someone available who may know what happened before the patient collapsed? *Coach: (See Case 1 SAMPLE history table.)*
Airway, Breathing, Circulation	After making sure that we have an ETCO$_2$ monitor available, I want my most experienced assistant to intubate the patient now. I want the defibrillation team member to assist by performing cricoid pressure during the procedure. I want the IV team member to start an IV with normal saline. I would also like to order a 12-lead ECG and portable chest x-ray while I perform a focused physical exam. *Coach: (See Case 1 physical exam findings table.) An ET tube has been inserted and the cuff inflated. Cricoid pressure has been discontinued. An IV has been established with normal saline.* I will confirm placement of the ET tube starting with a 5-point auscultation of the chest. I'm listening over the epigastrium. I am listening to the right and left sides of the chest in four areas. What do I hear? *Coach: There are no sounds heard over the epigastrium. Breath sounds are diminished in the upper and lower lobes on the left side of the chest. They are clearly heard in the right upper lobe and diminished in the right lower lobe.* Based on these findings, I suspect a right mainstem intubation. I will ask the airway team member to deflate the cuff, pull back slightly on the ET tube, reinflate the cuff, and reassess breath sounds.

Differential Diagnosis, Evaluates Interventions

Coach: Breath sounds with bag-mask ventilation reveal clear upper lobes and diminished sounds in the lower lobes bilaterally.

If the ETCO$_2$ monitor confirms the presence of CO$_2$, I will ask the airway team member to note the cm markings on the ET tube and then secure the tube in place.

Coach: The ETCO$_2$ monitor confirms the presence of CO$_2$. The ET tube has been secured. What should be done now?

POSTRESUSCITATION SUPPORT/ONGOING ASSESSMENT

Begins Postresuscitation Support/Performs Ongoing Assessment

I would like to repeat the primary survey and obtain another set of vital signs. Is the patient attempting to breathe spontaneously? What is the rate and quality of the patient's pulse? What is the patient's BP?

Coach: The patient is making no attempt to breathe spontaneously. Her vital signs now: BP 112/74; P 72, strong and regular; R 12/min via bag-mask; SpO$_2$ 97%. What is the rhythm on the cardiac monitor? (See Case 1 Rhythm 1.)

The monitor shows a sinus rhythm with tall T waves. I will order laboratory studies, evaluate the patient's 12-lead ECG and chest x-ray, and attempt to determine possible causes of the patient's respiratory arrest. I will also arrange for continued mechanical ventilation and transfer the patient for definitive care.

CASE 1: ESSENTIAL ACTIONS

Essential Actions

Ensure scene safety, use personal protective equipment
Perform a primary survey
- ◆ Assess level of responsiveness, call for help
- ◆ Open airway and assess breathing
- ◆ If patient is not breathing, insert an oral airway and begin rescue breathing with bag-mask device
- ◆ Assess pulse; if present, continue ventilations and continue survey

Perform secondary survey
- ◆ Reassess effectiveness of initial airway maneuvers and emergency care
- ◆ Insert an advanced airway, confirm tube placement (visualization, rise and fall of chest, presence of bilateral breath sounds, use of ETCO$_2$ detector, esophageal detector device)
- ◆ Establish IV access, connect ECG monitor, give medications if appropriate
- ◆ Consider possible causes of the event

Transfer patient for definitive care

Unacceptable Actions

Failure to use personal protective equipment
Failure to recognize signs of deterioration to respiratory failure or arrest and the need for more aggressive intervention
Giving O$_2$ by a means other than positive-pressure ventilation
Failure to ventilate patient at appropriate rate
Failure to preoxygenate patient before advanced airway placement
Failure to confirm advanced airway placement
Failure to properly secure an advanced airway
Failure to recognize right mainstem intubation or esophageal intubation

Interruption of ventilations for more than 30 seconds at any time

Failure to oxygenate the patient between intubation attempts

◆ Failure to monitor the cardiac rhythm in any patient who displays abnormal respiratory rate or effort, abnormal heart rate, perfusion, blood pressure (BP), or acute altered mental status

CASE 2: PULSELESS VT/VF WITH AN AED

Objective	Given a patient situation, describe and demonstrate the initial emergency care for a patient in cardiac arrest due to pulseless VT/VF and with an AED immediately available.
Skills to Master	Primary and secondary surveys
	Recognition of a patient in cardiac arrest
	Head-tilt/chin-lift, jaw thrust without head tilt
	Insertion of an oral or nasal airway
	Cardiopulmonary resuscitation (CPR)
	Pocket mask or bag-mask ventilation (1- and 2-rescuer technique)
	Suctioning
	Operation of an AED
	Advanced airway insertion (laryngeal mask airway, Combitube, ET intubation)
	Use of an ETCO$_2$ detector, esophageal detector device
	IV/intraosseous (IO) access
	IV/IO drug administration
Rhythms to Master	None (rhythm analysis performed by AED)
Medications to Master	O$_2$
	Epinephrine
	Vasopressin
	Amiodarone
	Lidocaine
Related Text Chapters	Chapter 1: The ABCDs of Emergency Cardiac Care
	Chapter 2: Airway Management: Oxygenation and Ventilation
	Chapter 3: Rhythm Recognition
	Chapter 4: Electrical Therapy
	Chapter 5: Vascular Access and Medications
	Chapter 8: Putting It All Together

CASE 2: QUESTIONS

SCENARIO: You are a nurse at an outpatient surgery center. The receptionist rushes to tell you that a patient has collapsed in the front lobby. Another nurse has arrived to assist you. She has brought an AED and emergency O$_2$ kit with her. The scene is safe.

1. You are putting on personal protective equipment as you approach the patient. You see an elderly man supine on the lobby floor. You recognize him as a patient scheduled for cataract surgery this morning. His eyes are closed. You do not see any signs of breathing. His skin is pale. How should you proceed?

2. The patient is unresponsive. What should be done now? (See Case 2 SAMPLE history and physical examination tables.)

CASE 2	
SAMPLE History	
Signs/symptoms	Witnessed collapse in lobby
Allergies	No known allergies
Medications	Lopressor
Past medical history	Hypertension
Last oral intake	Unknown
Events prior	Per a bystander in lobby, patient suddenly clutched his chest and collapsed to the floor

*History obtained from prescreening done via phone yesterday afternoon.

CASE 2	
Physical Examination Findings	
Head, ears, eyes, nose, and throat	No abnormalities noted
Neck	Trachea midline, no jugular venous distention
Chest	Breath sounds are clear and equal with positive-pressure ventilation
Abdomen	No abnormalities noted
Pelvis	No abnormalities noted
Extremities	No abnormalities noted
Posterior body	No abnormalities noted

3. The patient's airway is open and clear. What should be done now?

4. The patient is not breathing. How would you like to proceed?

5. Two additional nurses have arrived to assist you. An oral airway has been inserted. The patient is being ventilated with a bag-mask device. You see gentle chest rise with bagging. What should be done now?

6. The patient is pulseless. How would you like to proceed?

7. What is the purpose of defibrillation?

8. What is the difference between manual defibrillation and automated external defibrillation?

9. You have applied the AED to the patient and pressed the analyze button. While waiting for the machine to analyze the patient's rhythm, should you ask your assistants to insert an advanced airway and/or start an IV? Why or why not?

10. The AED advises a shock. How would you like to proceed?

11. You confirmed that everyone is clear of the patient and the O_2 is off before pressing the shock button. As the shock is delivered, you see the fire department pull up in front of the lobby doors. What should be done now?

12. The AED states, "No shock advised." Paramedics are now at your side. How would you like to proceed?

13. A strong carotid pulse is present. What should be done now?

14. The patient is waking up and breathing on his own about 12 times/min. The patient's heart rate is strong and regular at a rate of 80 bpm. BP is 98/60. What should be done now?

CASE 2: ANSWERS

1. Call for additional help. Ask the receptionist to call 9-1-1. Quickly approach the patient and begin the primary survey by assessing his level of responsiveness.
2. Open the patient's airway using a jaw thrust without head-tilt maneuver. Look in the patient's mouth for blood, broken teeth or loose dentures, gastric contents, or a foreign object.
3. Look, listen, and feel for breathing for up to 10 seconds.
4. While you continue the primary survey, ask the other nurse to size and insert an oral airway and begin positive-pressure ventilation with a bag-mask device connected to 100% O_2. Make sure the patient is ventilated at a rate of 10 to 12 ventilations/min (one ventilation every 5 to 6 seconds). Each ventilation should be given over 1 second.
5. Feel for a carotid pulse for up to 10 seconds.
6. Ask one of the nurses to begin chest compressions while you prepare the AED. Without interrupting CPR, expose the patient's chest and apply the AED pads. Then turn the power on to the machine.
7. Defibrillation is delivery of an electrical current across the heart muscle over a very brief period to terminate an abnormal heart rhythm. Defibrillation is also called unsynchronized countershock or asynchronous countershock because the delivery of current has no relationship to the cardiac cycle.
8. Manual defibrillation refers to the placement of paddles or pads on a patient's chest, interpretation of the patient's cardiac rhythm by a trained healthcare professional, and the healthcare professional's decision to deliver a shock (if indicated). AED refers to the placement of paddles or pads on a patient's chest and interpretation of the patient's cardiac rhythm by the defibrillator's computerized analysis system.
9. No. Do not delay defibrillation to insert an advanced airway, establish an IV, or give drugs.
10. All team members, with the exception of the chest compressor, should immediately clear the patient. As the nurse managing the patient's airway clears the patient, ask her to turn off the O_2 flow. The chest compressor should continue CPR until you are ready to press

the shock button. This will minimize the time chest compressions are interrupted. As soon as you indicate that you are ready to deliver the shock, the chest compressor should *immediately* clear the patient.

11. Ask your assistants to resume CPR immediately, beginning with chest compressions. Ask the airway team member to turn the O_2 on. After five cycles of CPR (about 2 minutes), reanalyze the patient's rhythm.
12. Ask an assistant to check for a pulse.
13. Repeat the primary survey and ask an assistant to obtain a complete set of vital signs.
14. Transfer patient care to the paramedics on the scene with a verbal report of what has occurred.

CASE 2: SCENARIO SHEET

SCENARIO: You are a nurse at outpatient surgery center. The receptionist rushes to tell you that a patient has collapsed in the front lobby. Another nurse has arrived to assist you. She has brought an AED and emergency O_2 kit with her.

EMERGENCY ACTION STEPS	NECESSARY TASKS
Scene Survey	I am putting on personal protective equipment. Is the scene safe to enter? *Coach: The scene is safe.*

INITIAL ASSESSMENT

First Impression	As I approach the patient and form a first impression (assessing the patient's appearance, work of breathing, and circulation), what do I see? *Coach: You see an elderly man supine on the lobby floor. You recognize him as a patient scheduled for cataract surgery this morning. His eyes are closed. You do not see any signs of breathing. His skin is pale.*

PRIMARY SURVEY

Responsiveness/Airway	I will quickly approach the patient and assess his level of responsiveness. Does he respond when I call his name? *Coach: The patient is unresponsive. (See Case 2 SAMPLE history and physical exam findings tables.)* I will ask the receptionist to call 9-1-1 right away. I will open the patient's airway using a jaw thrust without head tilt. Do I see anything in the patient's mouth such as blood, broken teeth or loose dentures, gastric contents, or a foreign object? *Coach: The patient's airway is open and clear. What should be done now?*
Breathing	I will look, listen, and feel for breathing for up to 10 seconds. *Coach: The patient is not breathing. How would you like to proceed?* I will ask the other nurse to size and insert an oral airway and begin positive-pressure ventilation with a bag-mask connected to 100% O_2 while I continue the primary survey. I want the patient ventilated at a rate of 10 to 12 ventilations/min (one ventilation every 5 to 6 seconds). Each ventilation should be given over 1 second. *Coach: Two additional nurses have arrived to assist you. An oral airway has been inserted. The patient is being ventilated with a bag-mask device. You see gentle chest rise with bagging.*

Circulation	I will feel for a carotid pulse for up to 10 seconds. Do I feel a carotid pulse? While I am feeling the patient's pulse, I will assess his skin temperature, color, and moisture.
	Coach: There is no pulse. His skin is cool, pale, and dry. What should be done now?
Defibrillation	I will ask one of the nurses to begin chest compressions while I prepare the AED. Without interrupting CPR, I will expose the patient's chest and apply the AED pads. I will then turn the power on to the machine.
	Coach: The AED pads are in place. The power is on.
	I will ask everyone (including myself) to clear the patient and press the analyze button on the AED.
	Coach: The AED advises a shock.
	I want all team members, with the exception of the chest compressor, to remain clear of the patient. As the nurse managing the patient's airway clears the patient, I will ask her to turn off the O$_2$ flow. I want the chest compressor to continue CPR until I am ready to press the shock button. This will minimize the time chest compressions are interrupted. As soon as I indicate that I am ready to shock, I want the chest compressor to immediately clear the patient. I am now ready to shock the patient.
	Coach: Everyone is clear of the patient. The oxygen is off. As you press the shock button, you see the fire department pull up in front of the lobby doors.
	I want my assistants to resume CPR immediately, beginning with chest compressions. I will ask the airway nurse to turn the oxygen on. After 5 cycles of CPR (about 2 minutes), I will reanalyze the patient's rhythm.
	Coach: The AED states, "No shock advised." Paramedics are now at your side.
	I will ask an assistant to check for a pulse.
	Coach: A strong carotid pulse is present. What should be done now?
	I will repeat the primary survey. Is the patient responsive? Is he breathing?
	Coach: The patient is waking up and breathing on his own about 12 times/min.

SECONDARY SURVEY/FOCUSED HISTORY & EXAM

Vital Signs/History	I will ask an assistant to obtain a complete set of vital signs.
	Coach: The patient's heart rate is strong and regular at a rate of 80 bpm. Respirations are 12/min. BP is 98/60. What should be done now?

POSTRESUSCITATION SUPPORT/ONGOING ASSESSMENT

Begins Postresuscitation Support/Performs Ongoing Assessment	I will transfer patient care to the paramedics on the scene with a verbal report of what has occurred.

CASE 2: ESSENTIAL ACTIONS

Essential Actions	Ensure scene safety, use personal protective equipment
	Perform primary and secondary surveys
	Begin CPR

Give O_2 using positive-pressure ventilation as soon as it is available
Start an IV/IO
Know the actions, indications, dosages, side effects, and contraindications for the drugs used in the treatment of pulseless VT/VF
Follow each drug given in a cardiac arrest with a 20-mL IV fluid flush and elevation of the extremity
Consider possible reversible causes of the arrest
Facilitate family presence during resuscitative efforts according to agency/institution protocol

Unacceptable Actions
Failure to use personal protective equipment
Failure to begin CPR
Performs CPR incorrectly (incorrect hand position, depth of compressions, compression rate, ventilation rate)
Unsafe operation of AED (failure to clear self or others before shocking)
Failure to start an IV
Failure to give O_2 and/or other drugs appropriate for the dysrhythmia
Gives O_2 by a means other than positive-pressure ventilation
Failure to consider the possible reversible causes of the arrest
Medication errors

CASE 3: PULSELESS VT/VF

Objective
Given a patient situation, describe and demonstrate the initial emergency care for a patient in cardiac arrest due to pulseless VT/VF.

Skills to Master
Primary and secondary surveys
Recognition of a patient in cardiac arrest
Head-tilt/chin-lift, jaw thrust without head tilt
Insertion of an oral or nasal airway
CPR
Pocket mask or bag-mask ventilation (1- and 2-rescuer technique)
Suctioning
Operation of a defibrillator
Advanced airway insertion (laryngeal mask airway, Combitube, ET intubation)
Use of an $ETCO_2$ detector, esophageal detector device
IV/IO access
IV/IO drug administration

Rhythms to Master
VT
VF

Medications to Master
O_2
Epinephrine
Vasopressin
Amiodarone
Lidocaine
Magnesium sulfate (if torsades de pointes)

Related Text Chapters
Chapter 1: The ABCDs of Emergency Cardiac Care
Chapter 2: Airway Management: Oxygenation and Ventilation
Chapter 3: Rhythm Recognition
Chapter 4: Electrical Therapy
Chapter 5: Vascular Access and Medications
Chapter 8: Putting It All Together

CASE 3: QUESTIONS

SCENARIO: You are a paramedic called to a local restaurant for a "possible code." Anxious bystanders tell you that the patient, a 58-year-old man, collapsed while having lunch. His coworkers state they were in the middle of a high-stress meeting when the patient "started sweating and collapsed." Coworkers helped him to the floor and immediately called 9-1-1. It has been 5 minutes since the patient collapsed. You have five other ALS personnel to assist you. Emergency equipment, including a biphasic manual defibrillator, is immediately available. The scene is safe.

1. As you approach the patient and put on personal protective equipment, your first impression reveals that the patient's eyes are closed. He does not appear to be breathing. His skin looks very pale. What should be done now?

2. The patient is unresponsive. How would you like to proceed?

3. The airway is clear. What should be done now?

4. The patient is not breathing. How would you like to proceed?

5. An oral airway has been inserted. The patient is being ventilated with a bag-mask device. You see gentle chest rise with bagging. What should be done now?

6. There is no pulse. What should be done now?

7. Combination pads are in place on the patient's chest. A biphasic defibrillator is within arm's reach. You see this rhythm on the cardiac monitor (Case 3 Rhythm 1). What is the rhythm? How do you want to proceed?

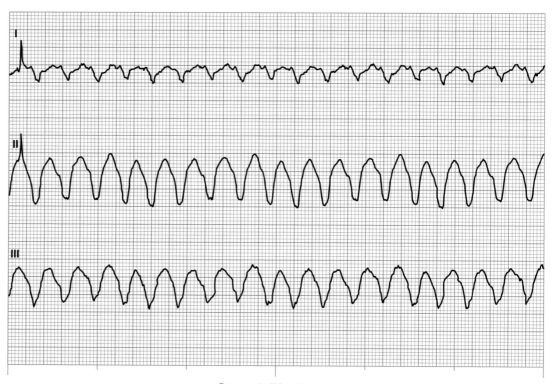

Case 3 Rhythm 1.

8. What initial drugs do you want the IV team member to prepare to give?

9. What energy setting will you use for your initial shock?

10. Shock delivered. What would you like to do next?

11. An IV has been started with normal saline in the patient's left antecubital vein. Epinephrine has been given IV. What should be done now? (See Case 3 SAMPLE history and physical examination tables.)

CASE 3

SAMPLE History

Signs/symptoms	Witnessed collapse
Allergies	None
Medications	"Little round white pills"
Past medical history	3-vessel coronary artery bypass graft 1 year ago
Last oral intake	Soft drink with Italian food for lunch
Events prior	Sudden collapse

*History obtained from coworkers.

CASE 3

Physical Examination Findings

Head, ears, eyes, nose, and throat	No abnormalities noted
Neck	Trachea midline, no jugular venous distention
Chest	Breath sounds are clear and equal with positive-pressure ventilation
Abdomen	No abnormalities noted
Pelvis	No abnormalities noted
Extremities	No abnormalities noted
Posterior body	No abnormalities noted

12. It has been 2 minutes since you gave epinephrine. A team member calls your attention to a rhythm change on the cardiac monitor. What is the rhythm on the monitor (Case 3 Rhythm 2)? What would you like to do next?

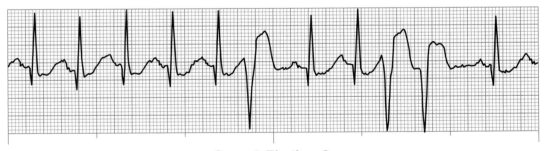

Case 3 Rhythm 2.

13. A strong carotid pulse is present. What should be done now?

14. The patient is unresponsive but is breathing about 12 times/min. A strong pulse is present at a rate of about 115 bpm. BP is 94/50. His color is improving. What should be done now?

CASE 3: ANSWERS

1. Quickly approach the patient and assess his level of responsiveness.
2. Open the patient's airway using a jaw thrust without head tilt. Look in the patient's mouth for blood, broken teeth or loose dentures, gastric contents, or a foreign object that may cause an airway obstruction.
3. Look, listen, and feel for breathing for up to 10 seconds.
4. Ask the airway team member to size and insert an oral airway and begin positive-pressure ventilation with a bag-mask device connected to 100% O_2 while continuing the primary survey. The airway team member must maintain proper head position and a good seal with the mask against the patient's face. Ask a second team member to assume responsibility for compressing the bag with just enough force to produce gentle chest rise. The patient should be ventilated at a rate of 10 to 12 ventilations/min (one ventilation every 5 to 6 seconds). Each ventilation should be given over 1 second.
5. Ask another assistant to assess baseline breath sounds while the patient is being ventilated. Ask the defibrillation team member to attach self-adhesive combination pads to the patient's chest while you feel for a carotid pulse for up to 10 seconds.
6. Ask for a defibrillator immediately. Ask the CPR team member to begin chest compressions while you will begin the secondary survey. The CPR team member and airway team member should rotate positions after every five cycles (about 2 minutes) of CPR so they don't become fatigued. Check the patient's ECG rhythm every 2 minutes as the team members change positions.
7. The rhythm is monomorphic VT. Ask the airway team member to temporarily shut off the O_2 as you prepare to shock the patient. Ask the IV team member to prepare the initial drugs that will be used and start an IV after the first shock is delivered.
8. Although your personal preference may differ, for this scenario we will ask the IV team member to prepare epinephrine, vasopressin, and amiodarone.
9. The manufacturer of the biphasic defibrillator you are using recommends 200 J for the initial shock. As the machine charges, ask all team members, with the exception of the chest compressor, to immediately clear the patient. As the airway team member clears the patient, remind him or her to turn off the O_2 flow. Ask the chest compressor to continue CPR while the machine is charging. Once the defibrillator is charged, ask the chest compressor to *immediately* clear the patient. After making sure the chest compressor is clear, deliver a shock with 200 J.
10. Resume CPR immediately, beginning with chest compressions. Ask the airway team member to turn the O_2 on. After five cycles of CPR (about 2 minutes), recheck the patient's rhythm. Without interrupting CPR, ask the IV team member to start an IV of normal saline and then give 1 mg of epinephrine using 1:10,000 solution IV push. Flush all drugs given IV push during the arrest with 20 mL of normal saline and then raise the arm for about 20 seconds.
11. Consider possible causes of the arrest. Try to find out if there is someone available who may know what happened before the patient collapsed and may know something of the patient's medical history.
12. The monitor shows a sinus tachycardia with a premature ventricular complex (PVC) and a ventricular couplet. Ask the CPR team member to stop CPR and check for a pulse.
13. Ask an assistant to obtain a complete set of vital signs while you repeat the primary survey.
14. Recheck the patient's vital signs and ECG every 5 minutes. Ask the airway team member to assess the quality of the patient's respiratory effort and assist the patient's breathing with a bag-mask device connected to 100% O_2 as needed. Continue to closely monitor the patient's vital signs and ECG and prepare to transport the patient for further care.

CASE 3: SCENARIO SHEET

SCENARIO: You are a paramedic called to a local restaurant for a "possible code." Anxious bystanders tell you that the patient, a 58-year-old man, collapsed while having lunch. His coworkers state they were in the middle of a high-stress meeting when the patient "started sweating and collapsed." Coworkers helped him to the floor and immediately called 9-1-1. It has been 5 minutes since the patient collapsed. You have five other ALS personnel to assist you. Emergency equipment, including a biphasic manual defibrillator, is immediately available.

EMERGENCY ACTION STEPS	NECESSARY TASKS
Scene Survey	I am putting on personal protective equipment. Is the scene safe to enter? *Coach: The scene is safe.*

INITIAL ASSESSMENT

First Impression	As I approach the patient and form a first impression, what do I see? *Coach: You can see that the patient's eyes are closed. He does not appear to be breathing. His skin looks very pale.*

PRIMARY SURVEY

Responsiveness/Airway	I will quickly approach the patient and assess his level of responsiveness. *Coach: The patient is unresponsive.* I will open the patient's airway using a jaw thrust without head tilt. Do I see anything in the patient's mouth such as blood, broken teeth or loose dentures, gastric contents, or a foreign object? *Coach: The patient's airway is clear. What should be done now?*
Breathing	I will look, listen, and feel for breathing for up to 10 seconds. *Coach: The patient is not breathing. How would you like to proceed?* I will ask the airway team member to size and insert an oral airway and begin positive-pressure ventilation with a bag-mask connected to 100% O_2 while I continue the primary survey. I want the airway team member to maintain proper head position and a good seal with the mask against the patient's face. I want a second team member to assume responsibility for compressing the bag with just enough force to produce gentle chest rise. The patient should be ventilated at a rate of 10 to 12 ventilations/min (one ventilation every 5 to 6 seconds). Each ventilation should be given over 1 second. *Coach: An oral airway has been inserted. The patient is being ventilated with a bag-mask device. You see gentle chest rise with bagging. What should be done now?*
Circulation	I will ask another assistant to assess baseline breath sounds while the patient is being ventilated. I want the defibrillation team member to attach self-adhesive combination pads to the patient's chest while I feel for a carotid pulse for up to 10 seconds. Do I feel a carotid pulse? *Coach: There is no pulse. What should be done now?*
Defibrillation	I will ask for the defibrillator immediately. I want the CPR team member to begin chest compressions while I will begin the secondary survey. I want the CPR team member and airway team member to automatically rotate positions after every 5 cycles

(about 2 minutes) of CPR so they don't become fatigued. I want the patient's ECG rhythm checked every 2 minutes as the team members change positions.

Coach: Combination pads are in place on the patient's chest. A biphasic defibrillator is within arm's reach. You see this rhythm on the cardiac monitor (See Case 3 Rhythm 1.) What is the rhythm on the monitor? How do you want to proceed?

The rhythm is monomorphic VT. I will ask the airway team member to temporarily shut off the O_2 as I prepare to shock the patient. I want the IV team member to prepare the initial drugs that will be used and start an IV after the first shock is delivered.

Coach: What initial drugs do you want the IV team member to prepare?

I want the IV team member to prepare epinephrine, vasopressin, and amiodarone for now.

Coach: What energy setting will you use for your initial shock?

I am using a biphasic defibrillator. The manufacturer of the machine I am using recommends 200 J for the initial shock. As the machine charges, I want all team members, with the exception of the chest compressor, to immediately clear the patient. As the airway team member clears the patient, I will remind him to turn off the O_2 flow. I want the chest compressor to continue CPR while the machine is charging. Once the defibrillator is charged, I want the chest compressor to immediately clear the patient. I am ready to shock the patient. I will make sure the chest compressor is now clear of the patient and will deliver a shock with 200 J.

Coach: Shock delivered. What would you like to do next?

SECONDARY SURVEY/FOCUSED HISTORY & EXAM

Vital Signs/History	I want my team to resume CPR immediately, beginning with chest compressions. I will ask the airway team member to turn the O_2 on. After 5 cycles of CPR (about 2 minutes), I will recheck the patient's rhythm.
Airway, Breathing, Circulation	Without interrupting CPR, I want the IV team member to start an IV of normal saline and then give 1 mg of epinephrine using 1:10,000 solution IV push. I want the drug flushed with 20 mL of normal saline and then raise the arm for about 20 seconds. *Coach: An IV has been started with normal saline in the patient's left antecubital vein. Epinephrine has been given IV as ordered.*
Differential Diagnosis, Evaluates Interventions	I am considering possible causes of the arrest. Is there someone available who may know what happened before the patient collapsed? *Coach: (See Case 3 SAMPLE history and physical exam findings tables.) It has been 2 minutes since you gave epinephrine. A team member calls your attention to a rhythm change on the cardiac monitor (See Case 3 Rhythm 2.) What is the rhythm on the monitor?* The monitor shows a sinus tachycardia with a PVC and a ventricular couplet. *Coach: What would you like to do next?* I will ask the CPR team member to stop CPR and check for a pulse. *Coach: A strong carotid pulse is present. What should be done now?*

POSTRESUSCITATION SUPPORT/ONGOING ASSESSMENT

Begins Postresuscitation Support/Performs Ongoing Assessment	I will ask an assistant to obtain a complete set of vital signs while I repeat the primary survey. Is the patient responsive? Is he breathing? *Coach: The patient is unresponsive but is breathing about 12 times/ min. A strong pulse is present at a rate of about 115 bpm. BP is 94/50. His color is improving. What should be done now?* I will recheck the patient's vital signs and ECG every 5 minutes. I want the airway team member to assess the quality of the patient's respiratory effort and assist the patient's breathing with a bag-mask device connected to 100% O_2 as needed. I will continue to closely monitor the patient's vital signs and ECG as I prepare to transport the patient for further care.

CASE 3: ESSENTIAL ACTIONS

Essential Actions	Ensure scene safety, use personal protective equipment. Perform primary and secondary surveys. Begin CPR. Give O_2 using positive-pressure ventilation as soon as it is available. Start an IV/IO. Know the actions, indications, dosages, side effects, and contraindications for the drugs used in the treatment of pulseless VT/VF. Follow each drug given in a cardiac arrest with a 20-mL IV fluid flush and elevation of the extremity for 10 to 20 seconds. Consider possible reversible causes of the arrest. Recognize that the presence of an organized rhythm on the monitor necessitates a pulse check. If a pulse is present, assess BP and respirations. Facilitate family presence during resuscitative efforts according to agency/institution protocol.
Unacceptable Actions	Failure to use personal protective equipment Failure to begin CPR Performs CPR incorrectly (incorrect hand position, depth of compressions, compression rate, ventilation rate) Unsafe operation of defibrillator (failure to clear self or others before shocking) Failure to start an IV Failure to give O_2 and/or other drugs appropriate for the dysrhythmia Gives O_2 by a means other than positive-pressure ventilation Failure to consider the possible reversible causes of the arrest Medication errors

CASE 4: ASYSTOLE

Objective	Given a patient situation, describe and demonstrate the initial emergency care for a patient in asystole.
Skills to Master	Primary and secondary surveys
	Recognition of a patient in cardiac arrest
	Head-tilt/chin-lift, jaw thrust without head tilt
	Insertion of an oral or nasal airway
	CPR
	Pocket mask or bag-mask ventilation (1- and 2-rescuer technique)
	Suctioning
	Attachment and use of ECG monitoring leads
	Advanced airway insertion (laryngeal mask airway, Combitube, ET intubation)
	Use of an $ETCO_2$ detector, esophageal detector device
	IV/IO access
	IV/IO drug administration
Rhythms to Master	Asystole
Medications to Master	O_2
	Epinephrine
	Atropine
Related Text Chapters	Chapter 1: The ABCDs of Emergency Cardiac Care
	Chapter 2: Airway Management: Oxygenation and Ventilation
	Chapter 3: Rhythm Recognition
	Chapter 5: Vascular Access and Medications
	Chapter 8: Putting It All Together

CASE 4: QUESTIONS

SCENARIO: Your patient is an 80-year-old man who was found unresponsive by his wife. She says he was fine about 15 minutes ago. You have four other ALS personnel to assist you. Emergency equipment is immediately available. The scene is safe.

1. As you put on personal protective equipment and form a first impression, you see an elderly man slumped over in a chair. He is not aware of your approach. There is no obvious rise and fall of his chest. His skin is pale. After determining that he is unresponsive, your assistants help you move the patient to the floor. What should be done now?

2. The airway is clear. What should be done now?

3. The patient is not breathing. How should you proceed?

4. The patient does not have a do not resuscitate (DNR) order. An oral airway has been inserted. The patient is being ventilated with a bag-mask device. You see gentle chest rise with bagging. At what rate should this patient be ventilated?

5. The patient has no pulse. His skin is cool, pale, and dry. What should be done now? (See Case 4 SAMPLE history and physical examination tables.)

CASE 4

SAMPLE History

Signs/symptoms	Found unresponsive by wife
Allergies	Penicillin
Medications	Synthroid, aspirin, vitamins, calcium
Past medical history	Hypothyroidism, acid reflux, pacemaker insertion 4 years ago
Last oral intake	Dinner 4 hours ago
Events prior	Found unresponsive by wife, last seen 15 minutes ago

CASE 4

Physical Examination Findings

Head, ears, eyes, nose, and throat	No abnormalities noted
Neck	Trachea midline, no jugular venous distention
Chest	Breath sounds are clear and equal with positive-pressure ventilation; bulge present in upper right chest consistent with permanent pacemaker
Abdomen	No abnormalities noted
Pelvis	No abnormalities noted
Extremities	No abnormalities noted
Posterior body	No abnormalities noted

6. Combination pads are in place on the patient's chest. A biphasic defibrillator is within arm's reach. You see the rhythm on the cardiac monitor (Case 4 Rhythm 1). What is the rhythm on the monitor?

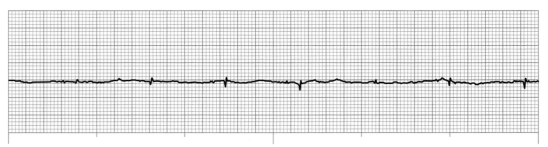

Case 4 Rhythm 1.

7. The rhythm is confirmed as asystole. The airway team member states that the ET tube is in place. The IV team member has not yet been successful starting an IV. What should be done now?

8. There are no sounds heard over the epigastrium. Breath sounds are present and equal bilaterally with positive pressure ventilation. An esophageal detector device confirms proper placement of the ET tube. The IV team member has successfully started an IV of normal saline in the right antecubital vein. What should be done next?

9. The monitor still shows asystole. The ET tube has been secured. Now that an advanced airway in place, what changes should be made in the rate of positive pressure ventilation?

10. Epinephrine has been given IV. What is the dose of atropine that should be given in this situation?

11. Forty minutes have now elapsed since resuscitation efforts began. CPR is continuing without interruption. Epinephrine has been given every 3 to 5 minutes with no response. A total of 3 mg of atropine has been given with no response. The patient's ECG rhythm has shown continuous asystole. What would you like to do now?

CASE 4: ANSWERS

1. Open the patient's airway using a head-tilt/chin-lift. Look in the patient's mouth for blood, broken teeth or loose dentures, gastric contents, a foreign object, or other possible airway obstructions.
2. Look, listen, and feel for breathing for up to 10 seconds.
3. Ask the airway team member to size and insert an oral airway and begin positive-pressure ventilation with a bag-mask device connected to 100% O_2 while you continue the primary survey. Make sure the airway team member maintains proper head position and a good seal with the mask against the patient's face. Ask a second team member to assume responsibility for compressing the bag with just enough force to produce gentle chest rise. It is important and appropriate to ask the patient's wife if the patient has a DNR order.
4. The patient should be ventilated at a rate of 10 to 12 ventilations/min (one ventilation every 5 to 6 seconds). Each ventilation should be given over 1 second. Ask another assistant to assess baseline breath sounds while the patient is being ventilated and then prepare the intubation equipment.
5. Ask for the defibrillator immediately. Ask the CPR team member to begin chest compressions. Ask the defibrillation team member to apply combination pads to the patient's bare chest. Ask the CPR team member and airway team member to automatically rotate positions after every five cycles (about 2 minutes) of CPR so they don't become fatigued. Recheck the patient's ECG rhythm every 2 minutes as the team members change positions. Perform a focused physical exam, looking for possible clues as to the cause of the arrest. Talk to the patient's wife to find out what happened before the patient collapsed and learn about his medical history.

6. The rhythm is asystole. The electrical activity shown is caused by pacemaker spikes from the patient's permanent pacemaker (no capture). Confirm asystole in a second lead. Ask the airway team member to intubate the patient. Ask the IV team member to prepare epinephrine and atropine and start an IV of normal saline.

7. Confirm placement of the ET tube starting with a five-point auscultation of the chest. Begin by listening over the epigastrium. Then listen to the right and left sides of the chest in four areas.

8. Ask the airway team member to note the cm markings on the ET tube and then secure the tube in place. Ask the IV team member to give 1 mg of 1:10,000 epinephrine IV push now and repeat the same dose every 3 to 5 minutes as long as the patient has no pulse. Flush each dose with 20 mL of normal saline and raise the arm. Perform a focused physical exam, looking for possible clues as to the cause of the arrest.

9. Because an advanced airway is now in place, instruct the airway team member to change the rate of positive-pressure ventilations from 10 to 12/min to 8 to 10/min. Instruct the CPR team member to continue chest compressions without pausing for ventilations.

10. Atropine can be given in cardiac arrest due to asystole and slow PEA. In these situations, the IV/IO dose of atropine is 1 mg every 3 to 5 minutes to a maximum total dose of 3 mg. Remember to flush each dose with 20 mL of normal saline and raise the arm.

11. Consult with the members of your team about termination of resuscitation efforts.

CASE 4: SCENARIO SHEET

SCENARIO: Your patient is an 80-year-old man who was found unresponsive by his wife. She says he was fine about 15 minutes ago. You have four other ALS personnel to assist you. Emergency equipment is immediately available.

EMERGENCY ACTION STEPS	NECESSARY TASKS
Scene Survey	I am putting on personal protective equipment. Is the scene safe to enter? *Coach: The scene is safe.*

INITIAL ASSESSMENT

First Impression	As I approach the patient and form a first impression (assessing the patient's appearance, work of breathing, and circulation), what do I see? *Coach: You see an elderly man slumped over in a chair. He is not aware of your approach. There is no obvious rise and fall of his chest. His skin is pale.*

PRIMARY SURVEY

Responsiveness/Airway	I will quickly approach the patient and assess his level of responsiveness. Does he respond when I call his name? *Coach: The patient is unresponsive.* I will ask my assistants to help me move the patient to the floor so I can assess his airway. *Coach: The patient is now supine on the floor.* Since I have seen nothing to suspect trauma, I will open the patient's airway using a head-tilt/chin-lift. Do I see anything in the patient's mouth such as blood, broken teeth or loose dentures, gastric contents, or a foreign object? *Coach: The airway is clear. What should be done now?*
Breathing	I will look, listen, and feel for breathing for up to 10 seconds. *Coach: The patient is not breathing.*

I will ask the airway team member to size and insert an oral airway and begin positive-pressure ventilation with a bag-mask connected to 100% O_2 while I continue the primary survey. I want the airway team member to maintain proper head position and a good seal with the mask against the patient's face. I want a second team member to assume responsibility for compressing the bag with just enough force to produce gentle chest rise. Does the patient's wife know if the patient has a DNR order?

Coach: The patient does not have a DNR order. An oral airway has been inserted. The patient is being ventilated with a bag-mask device. You see gentle chest rise with bagging. At what rate should this patient be ventilated?

The patient should be ventilated at a rate of 10 to 12 ventilations/min (one ventilation every 5 to 6 seconds). Each ventilation should be given over 1 second. I will ask another assistant to assess baseline breath sounds while the patient is being ventilated and then prepare the intubation equipment.

Circulation	I will ask the defibrillation team member to attach combination pads to the patient's chest while I feel for a carotid pulse for up to 10 seconds. Do I feel a pulse? While I am feeling the patient's pulse, I will assess his skin condition. What is his skin temperature, color, and condition? *Coach: There is no pulse. The patient's skin is cool, pale, and dry. What should be done now?*
Defibrillation	I will ask for the defibrillator immediately. I want the CPR team member to begin chest compressions while I will begin the secondary survey. I want the defibrillation team member to apply combination pads to the patient's bare chest. I want the CPR team member and airway team member to automatically rotate positions after every 5 cycles (about 2 minutes) of CPR so they don't become fatigued. I want the patient's ECG rhythm checked every 2 minutes as the team members change positions.

SECONDARY SURVEY/FOCUSED HISTORY & EXAM

Vital Signs/History	I will perform a focused physical exam, looking for possible clues as to the cause of the arrest. Is the patient's wife available to tell us what happened before the patient collapsed? What can she tell me about his medical history? *Coach: (See Case 4 SAMPLE history and physical exam findings tables.) Combination pads are in place on the patient's chest. A biphasic defibrillator is within arm's reach. You see this rhythm on the cardiac monitor. (See Case 4 Rhythm 1.) What is the rhythm? What do you want to do next?*
Airway, Breathing, Circulation	The rhythm is asystole. It appears the patient has an internal pacemaker. I want to confirm this rhythm in a second lead. I will ask the airway team member to intubate the patient. I want the IV team member to prepare epinephrine and atropine and start an IV of normal saline. *Coach: The rhythm is confirmed as asystole. The airway team member states that the ET tube is in place. The IV team member has not yet been successful starting the IV.* I will confirm placement of the ET tube starting with a 5-point auscultation of the chest. I'm listening over the epigastrium. I am

listening to the right and left sides of the chest in four areas. What do I hear?

Coach: There are no sounds heard over the epigastrium. Breath sounds are present, and equal bilaterally with positive pressure ventilation.

Does the esophageal detector device indicate that the ET tube is in the trachea?

Coach: The esophageal detector device confirms proper placement of the ET tube. The IV team member has successfully placed an IV in the right antecubital vein.

I will ask the airway team member to note the cm markings on the ET tube and then secure the tube in place.

Coach: The ET tube has been secured. The monitor still shows asystole. What should be done now?

Since an advanced airway is now in place, I will instruct the airway team member to change the rate of positive-pressure ventilations from 10 to 12/min to 8 to 10/min. I will instruct the CPR team member to continue chest compressions without pausing for ventilations. I want the IV team member to give 1 mg of 1:10,000 epinephrine IV push now and every 3 to 5 minutes as long as the patient has no pulse. Flush each dose with 20 mL of normal saline and raise the arm.

Coach: What is the dose of atropine that should be given in this situation?

Differential Diagnosis, Evaluates Interventions

In cardiac arrest, the IV/IO dose of atropine is 1 mg every 3 to 5 minutes to a maximum total dose of 3 mg.

Coach: 40 minutes have now elapsed since resuscitation efforts began. CPR is continuing without interruption. Epinephrine has been given every 3 to 5 minutes with no response. A total of 3 mg of atropine has been given with no response. The patient's ECG rhythm has shown continuous asystole. What would you like to do now?

I would like to consult with the members of my team about termination of resuscitation efforts.

CASE 4: ESSENTIAL ACTIONS

Essential Actions

Ensure scene safety, use personal protective equipment.
Perform primary and secondary surveys.
Recognize asystole.
Check for signs of obvious death, do not attempt resuscitation order.
Begin CPR.
Give O_2 using positive-pressure ventilation as soon as it is available.
Start an IV/IO.
Know the actions, indications, dosages, side effects, and contraindications for the drugs used in the treatment of asystole.
Follow each drug given in a cardiac arrest with a 20-mL IV fluid flush and elevation of the extremity for 10 to 20 seconds.
Consider possible reversible causes of the arrest.
Recognize that the presence of an organized rhythm on the monitor necessitates a pulse check. If a pulse is present, assess BP and respirations.
Facilitate family presence during resuscitative efforts according to agency/institution protocol.

Unacceptable Actions	Failure to use personal protective equipment
	Performs CPR incorrectly (incorrect hand position, depth of compressions, compression rate, ventilation rate)
	Failure to correctly identify the ECG rhythm
	Failure to start an IV
	Failure to give O_2 and/or other drugs appropriate for the dysrhythmia
	Defibrillating asystole
	Failure to begin CPR
	Gives O_2 by a means other than positive-pressure ventilation
	Failure to consider the possible reversible causes of PEA
	Failure to recognize rhythm change
	Medication errors
	Performs any technique resulting in potential harm to the patient

CASE 5: PEA

Objective	Given a patient situation, describe and demonstrate the initial emergency care for a patient in cardiac arrest due to PEA.
Skills to Master	Primary and secondary surveys
	Recognition of a patient in cardiac arrest
	Head-tilt/chin-lift, jaw thrust without head tilt
	Insertion of an oral or nasal airway
	CPR
	Pocket mask or bag-mask ventilation (1- and 2-rescuer technique)
	Suctioning
	Attachment and use of ECG monitoring leads
	Advanced airway insertion (laryngeal mask airway, Combitube, ET intubation)
	Use of an $ETCO_2$ detector, esophageal detector device
	IV/IO access
	IV/IO drug administration
	Needle decompression (needle thoracostomy)
Rhythms to Master	Junctional escape rhythm
	Accelerated junctional rhythm
	Idioventricular (ventricular escape) rhythm
	Sinus tachycardia
	Sinus bradycardia
	Atrial fibrillation
	Polymorphic VT
Medications to Master	O_2
	Epinephrine
	Atropine
Related Text Chapters	Chapter 1: The ABCDs of Emergency Cardiac Care
	Chapter 2: Airway Management: Oxygenation and Ventilation
	Chapter 3: Rhythm Recognition
	Chapter 5: Vascular Access and Medications
	Chapter 8: Putting It All Together

CASE 5: QUESTIONS

SCENARIO: Your patient is a 15-year-old boy who was "dropped off" in front of the emergency department (ED) doors by gang members. You have five other ALS personnel to assist you. Emergency equipment is immediately available. The scene is safe.

1. As you put on personal protective equipment and form a first impression, you see a 15-year-old boy lying supine on the ground in front of the ED doors. You estimate the patient weighs about 70 kg. His eyes are closed. You do not see any obvious chest rise and fall. The patient's skin is pale. You ask one of your assistants to maintain manual in-line stabilization of the patient's cervical spine while the remainder of your assistants help you place the patient on a backboard and then onto a stretcher. The stretcher has been wheeled into the trauma room. What should be done now?

2. The airway is clear. What should be done now?

3. The patient is not breathing. How should you proceed?

4. An oral airway has been inserted. The patient is being ventilated with a bag-mask device. You see gentle chest rise with bagging. As you watch the patient's chest rise, you notice a small amount of blood on the patient's left upper abdomen. At what rate should this patient be ventilated?

5. The patient has no pulse. His skin is cool, pale, and moist. What should be done now? (See Case 5 SAMPLE history and physical examination tables.)

CASE 5	
SAMPLE History	
Signs/symptoms	Unresponsive, apneic, pulseless
Allergies	Unknown
Medications	Unknown
Past medical history	Unknown
Last oral intake	Unknown
Events prior	Dropped off at the ED doors by gang members

CASE 5

Physical Examination Findings

Head, ears, eyes, nose, and throat	No abnormalities noted
Neck	Trachea midline, jugular veins flat
Chest	Breath sounds are clear and equal with positive-pressure ventilation
Abdomen	Stab wound to left upper abdomen; firm, distended
Pelvis	No abnormalities noted
Extremities	No abnormalities noted
Posterior body	No abnormalities noted

6. Combination pads are in place on the patient's chest. A biphasic defibrillator is within arm's reach. You see this rhythm on the cardiac monitor (Case 5 Rhythm 1). What is the rhythm on the monitor?

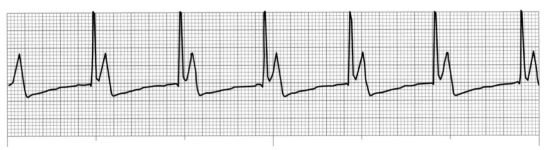

Case 5 Rhythm 1.

7. The airway team member states that the ET tube is in place. The IV team member has successfully started an IV of normal saline in the left antecubital vein. ECG leads have been applied to the patient's chest. A team member calls your attention to a change on the cardiac monitor (Case 5 Rhythm 2). What is the rhythm?

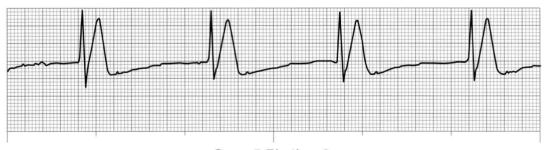

Case 5 Rhythm 2.

8. An IV of normal saline is being infused. There are loud sounds heard over the epigastrium. No breath sounds are heard with positive pressure ventilation. The patient still has no pulse. What should be done next?

9. The ET tube has been removed. 1 mg of 1:10,000 epinephrine has been given IV. There is another change in the cardiac monitor (Case 5 Rhythm 3). What is the rhythm? What should be done now?

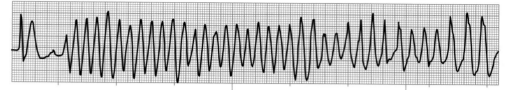

Case 5 Rhythm 3.

10. There is no pulse. How should you proceed?

11. Will you defibrillate the patient or perform synchronized cardioversion? What energy setting will you use for your initial shock?

12. After the shock is delivered, the cardiac monitor shows a change in rhythm (Case 5 Rhythm 4). What is the rhythm on the monitor?

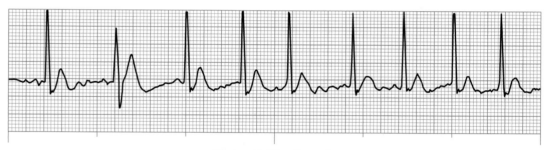

Case 5 Rhythm 4.

13. A pulse is present. What should be done now?

14. The patient is unresponsive but breathing spontaneously about 4 times/min. His BP is 90/50. His heart rate is irregular at a rate of about 90. His color is improving. What should be done next?

CASE 5: ANSWERS

1. Open the patient's airway using a jaw thrust without head tilt. Look in the patient's mouth for blood, broken teeth, gastric contents, a foreign object, or other possible airway obstructions.
2. Look, listen, and feel for breathing for up to 10 seconds.
3. Ask the airway team member to size and insert an oral airway and begin positive-pressure ventilation with a bag-mask device connected to 100% O_2 while you continue the primary survey. Make sure the airway team member maintains proper head position and a good seal with the mask against the patient's face. Ask a second team member to assume responsibility for compressing the bag with just enough force to produce gentle chest rise.
4. The patient should be ventilated at a rate of 10 to 12 ventilations/min (one ventilation every 5 to 6 seconds). Each ventilation should be given over 1 second. Ask another assistant to assess baseline breath sounds while the patient is being ventilated and then prepare the intubation equipment.
5. Ask for the defibrillator immediately. Ask the CPR team member to begin chest compressions. Ask the defibrillation team member to apply combination pads to the patient's bare chest. Ask the CPR team member and airway team member to automatically rotate positions after every five cycles (about 2 minutes) of CPR so they don't become fatigued. Recheck the patient's ECG rhythm checked every 2 minutes as the team members change positions. Perform a focused physical exam, looking for possible clues as to the cause of the arrest.
6. The monitor shows an accelerated junctional rhythm. Although an organized rhythm is present on the monitor, the patient has no pulse, which means this cardiac arrest is due to PEA. Ask the airway team member to intubate the patient. Ask the IV team member to prepare epinephrine and start an IV of normal saline. Ask a member of the team to contact the operating room (OR) and determine the availability of an OR.
7. The monitor shows a junctional rhythm. It is important to note that although an organized rhythm is present on the monitor and there is still no pulse, the heart rate on the monitor is decreasing. Consider possible causes of the arrest (firm, distended abdomen suggests internal bleeding due to abdominal stab wound) and this change in heart rate (such as hypoxia). Confirm placement of the ET tube starting with a five-point auscultation of the chest. Begin by listening over the epigastrium. Then listen to the right and left sides of the chest in four areas. Ask the IV team member to give a fluid challenge of normal saline. The amount given often varies depending on agency policy/local protocol. For the purposes of this scenario, we will give a 20 mL/kg fluid challenge of normal saline to start with. Because this patient weighs 70 kg, our initial fluid challenge will be 1400 mL.
8. Ask the airway team member to deflate the cuff on the ET tube and remove it. Make sure the patient is adequately oxygenated and then try again to intubate. Ask the IV team member to give 1 mg of 1:10,000 epinephrine IV push now and repeat the same dose every 3 to 5 minutes as long as the patient has no pulse. Flush each dose with 20 mL of normal saline and raise the arm.
9. The monitor shows polymorphic VT. Because there is a rhythm change on the monitor, it is reasonable to check a pulse.
10. Although the patient has had no pulse despite the organized electrical activity seen on the monitor throughout this arrest (PEA), the rhythm on the monitor now is sustained polymorphic VT. This is a shockable rhythm. The presence of a shockable rhythm changes the algorithm from PEA to pulseless VT/VF. Prepare to shock the patient immediately.
11. Because of the changing amplitude of the waveforms in polymorphic VT, synchronizing to a QRS complex is unreliable. (Even if the rhythm was monomorphic VT, defibrillation is used when the patient has no pulse, not synchronized cardioversion.) This patient should be defibrillated using the energy recommended by the defibrillator manufacturer. For the purpose of this scenario, we will assume that the recommended initial energy is 200 J.
12. The monitor shows atrial fibrillation. Ask the CPR team member to stop compressions. The presence of an organized rhythm on the monitor warrants a pulse check.

13. If a pulse is present, check the patient's other vital signs and repeat the primary survey.
14. Recheck the patient's vital signs and ECG every 5 minutes. Ask the airway team member to continue to assist the patient's breathing with a bag-mask device connected to 100% O_2. Continue to monitor the patient's vital signs and ECG as you prepare to transport the patient to the OR. Weigh the decision to place an advanced airway and to give additional IV fluids now (delaying definitive care) versus transporting the patient to the OR and having these interventions performed by the anesthesiologist. Consultation with the anesthesiologist is advised.

CASE 5: SCENARIO SHEET

SCENARIO: Your patient is a 15-year-old boy who was "dropped off" in front of the ED doors by gang members. You have five other ALS personnel to assist you. Emergency equipment is immediately available.

EMERGENCY ACTION STEPS	NECESSARY TASKS
Scene Survey	I am putting on personal protective equipment. Is the scene safe to enter? *Coach: The scene is safe.*

INITIAL ASSESSMENT

First Impression	As I approach the patient and form a first impression (assessing the patient's appearance, work of breathing, and circulation), what do I see? *Coach: You see a 15-year-old boy lying supine on the ground in front of the emergency department doors. You estimate the patient weighs about 70 kg. His eyes are closed. You do not see any obvious chest rise and fall. The patient's skin is pale.*

PRIMARY SURVEY

Responsiveness/Airway	I will quickly approach the patient and assess his level of responsiveness. Does he respond when I call his name? *Coach: The patient is unresponsive.* I will ask one of my assistants to maintain manual in-line stabilization of the patient's cervical spine while the remainder of my assistants help me place the patient on a backboard and then onto a stretcher so that I can begin my assessment. *Coach: The patient is now on a backboard, which was placed on a stretcher and wheeled into the trauma room.* I will open the patient's airway using a jaw thrust without head tilt. Do I see anything in the patient's mouth such as blood, broken teeth, gastric contents, or a foreign object? *Coach: The airway is clear. What should be done now?*
Breathing	I will look, listen, and feel for breathing for up to 10 seconds. *Coach: The patient is not breathing.* I will ask the airway team member to size and insert an oral airway and begin positive-pressure ventilation with a bag-mask device connected to 100% O_2 while I continue the primary survey. I want the airway team member to maintain proper head position and a good seal with the mask against the patient's face. I want a second team member to assume responsibility for compressing the bag with just enough force to produce gentle chest rise. *Coach: An oral airway has been inserted. The patient is being ventilated with a bag-mask device. You see gentle chest rise with bag-*

ging. As you watch the patient's chest rise, you notice a small amount of blood on his left upper abdomen. At what rate should this patient be ventilated?

The patient should be ventilated at a rate of 10 to 12 ventilations/min (one ventilation every 5 to 6 seconds). Each ventilation should be given over 1 second. I will ask another assistant to assess baseline breath sounds while the patient is being ventilated and then prepare the intubation equipment.

Circulation

I will ask the defibrillation team member to attach combination pads to the patient's bare chest while I feel for a carotid pulse for up to 10 seconds. Do I feel a pulse? While I am feeling the patient's pulse, I will assess his skin condition. What is his skin temperature, color, and condition?

Coach: There is no pulse. The patient's skin is cool, pale, and moist. Combination pads have been placed on the patient's chest. What should be done now?

Defibrillation

I will ask for the defibrillator immediately. I want the CPR team member to begin chest compressions while I begin the secondary survey. I want the CPR team member and airway team member to automatically rotate positions after every 5 cycles (about 2 minutes) of CPR so they don't become fatigued. I want the patient's ECG rhythm checked every 2 minutes as the team members change positions.

SECONDARY SURVEY/FOCUSED HISTORY & EXAM

Vital Signs/History

I will perform a focused physical exam, looking for possible clues as to the cause of the arrest.

Coach: (See Case 5 SAMPLE history and physical exam findings tables.) A biphasic defibrillator is within arm's reach. You see this rhythm on the cardiac monitor. (See Case 5 Rhythm 1.) What is the rhythm? What do you want to do next?

Airway, Breathing, Circulation

The monitor shows an accelerated junctional rhythm. Although an organized rhythm is present on the monitor, the patient has no pulse, which means this cardiac arrest is due to PEA. I will ask the airway team member to intubate the patient. I want the IV team member to prepare epinephrine and then start an IV of normal saline without interrupting CPR.

Coach: The airway team member states that the ET tube is in place. The IV team member has successfully placed an IV in the left antecubital vein. ECG leads have been applied to the patient's chest. A team member calls your attention to a change on the cardiac monitor. (See Case 5 Rhythm 2.) What is the rhythm?

Differential Diagnosis, Evaluates Interventions

The monitor shows a junctional rhythm. The heart rate on the monitor is decreasing. I suspect a cause of the patient's PEA is hypovolemia due to the abdominal stab wound. I want to give a 20-mL/kg IV fluid challenge of normal saline. I want to confirm placement of the ET tube starting with a 5-point auscultation of the chest. I'm listening over the epigastrium. I am listening to the right and left sides of the chest in four areas. What do I hear?

Coach: The fluid challenge is being given as ordered. You hear loud sounds over the epigastrium. No breath sounds are heard with bag-mask ventilation. The patient still has no pulse.

I will ask the airway team member to deflate the cuff on the ET tube and remove it. I want the patient adequately oxygenated before attempting another intubation. I want the IV team member to give 1 mg of 1:10,000 epinephrine IV push now and every 3 to 5 minutes as long as the patient has no pulse. I want each dose flushed with 20 mL of normal saline and the arm raised.

Coach: The ET tube has been removed, and 1 mg of epinephrine has been given IV. There is another change on the cardiac monitor. (See Case 5 Rhythm 3.) What is the rhythm? What should be done now?

The rhythm on the monitor is polymorphic VT. Does the patient have a pulse with this rhythm?

Coach: There is no pulse. How should you proceed?

Sustained polymorphic VT is a shockable rhythm. I will prepare to shock the patient immediately.

Coach: Will you defibrillate the patient or perform synchronized cardioversion? What energy setting will you use for your initial shock?

I will defibrillate the patient. I am using a biphasic defibrillator. The manufacturer of the machine I am using recommends 200 J for the initial shock. As the machine charges, I want all team members, with the exception of the chest compressor, to immediately clear the patient. As the airway team member clears the patient, I will remind him to turn off the O_2 flow. I want the chest compressor to continue CPR while the machine is charging. Once the defibrillator is charged, I want the chest compressor to immediately clear the patient. I am ready to shock the patient. I will make sure the chest compressor is now clear of the patient and will deliver a shock with 200 J.

Coach: Shock delivered. The cardiac monitor shows a change in rhythm. (See Case 5 Rhythm 4.) What is the rhythm on the monitor?

The monitor shows atrial fibrillation. I will ask the CPR team member to stop CPR and check for a pulse. Does the patient have a pulse?

Coach: A strong carotid pulse is present. What should be done now?

POSTRESUSCITATION SUPPORT/ONGOING ASSESSMENT

Begins Postresuscitation Support/Performs Ongoing Assessment

I will ask an assistant to obtain a complete set of vital signs while I repeat the primary survey. Is the patient responsive? Is he breathing?

Coach: The patient is unresponsive but breathing spontaneously about 4 times/min. His BP is 90/50. His heart rate is irregular at a rate of about 90. His color is improving. What should be done next?

I will recheck the patient's vital signs and ECG every 5 minutes. I want the airway team member to continue to assist the patient's breathing with a bag-mask device connected to 100% O_2. I will continue to monitor the patient's vital signs and ECG as we prepare to transport the patient to the operating room.

CASE 5: ESSENTIAL ACTIONS

Essential Actions	Ensure scene safety, use personal protective equipment.
	Perform primary and secondary surveys.
	Check for signs of obvious death, do not attempt resuscitation order.
	Begin CPR.
	Give O_2 using positive-pressure ventilation as soon as it is available.
	Start an IV/IO.
	Know the actions, indications, dosages, side effects, and contraindications for the drugs used in the treatment of PEA.
	Follow each drug given in a cardiac arrest with a 20-mL IV fluid flush and elevation of the extremity.
	Consider possible reversible causes of the arrest.
	Recognize that a change in the rhythm necessitates a pulse check.
	If a pulse is present, assess BP and respirations.
	Facilitate family presence during resuscitative efforts according to agency/institution protocol.
Unacceptable Actions	Failure to use personal protective equipment
	Performs CPR incorrectly (incorrect hand position, depth of compressions, compression rate, ventilation rate)
	Failure to correctly identify the ECG rhythm
	Failure to start an IV
	Defibrillating PEA
	Failure to give O_2 and/or other drugs appropriate for the dysrhythmia
	Failure to begin CPR
	Gives O_2 by a means other than positive-pressure ventilation
	Failure to consider the possible reversible causes of PEA
	Failure to recognize rhythm change
	Medication errors

CASE 6: ACS

Objective	Given a patient situation, describe and demonstrate the initial emergency care for a patient experiencing an ACS.
Skills to Master	Primary and secondary surveys
	Supplemental O_2 delivery devices
	Attachment and use of ECG monitoring leads
	IV access
	IV drug administration
	Know the ECG criteria for myocardial ischemia, injury, and infarction
	Recognize clinical signs and symptoms of right and left ventricular failure
Rhythms to Master	Sinus rhythm, sinus bradycardia, sinus tachycardia
	Atrial fibrillation, atrial flutter
	Atrioventricular (AV) blocks: first-degree, second-degree type I, second-degree type II, third-degree AV block
	Premature atrial complexes
	Premature ventricular complexes
	VF, VT

Medications to Master
O_2
Nitroglycerin (NTG)
Morphine sulfate
Aspirin
Fibrinolytics
Beta-blockers
Heparin
Glycoprotein IIb/IIIa Inhibitors
Angiotensin-converting enzyme (ACE) inhibitors
Furosemide
Dopamine
Dobutamine
Norepinephrine

Related Text Chapters
Chapter 1: The ABCDs of Emergency Cardiac Care
Chapter 2: Airway Management: Oxygenation and Ventilation
Chapter 3: Rhythm Recognition
Chapter 5: Vascular Access and Medications
Chapter 6: Acute Coronary Syndromes
Chapter 8: Putting It All Together

CASE 6: QUESTIONS

SCENARIO: Your patient is a 50-year-old woman who is complaining of nausea, light-headedness, and "pain between my shoulder blades." You have five other ALS personnel to assist you. Emergency equipment is immediately available. The scene is safe.

1. As you put on personal protective equipment and form a first impression, you see a 50-year-old woman sitting in a chair. She looks anxious. She appears to be breathing rapidly, but her breathing does not appear labored. Her skin is pink. You see beads of sweat on her upper lip and forehead. How would you like to proceed?

2. The patient tells you she thinks she may be having a heart attack. She is breathing 32 times/min. Her breathing is not labored. Radial and carotid pulses are strong and regular. You estimate the rate to be about 60/min. Her skin is warm, pink, and moist. What should be done now?

3. The patient's vital signs are as follows: BP 178/104, heart rate is about 60, and respirations are now 24. Breath sounds are clear and equal bilaterally. The patient's SpO_2 was 96% on room air. Since placing the patient on O_2 by nonrebreather mask, it is now 98%. (See Case 6 SAMPLE history and physical examination tables.) The patient has been placed on the cardiac monitor. How would you like to proceed?

CASE 6

SAMPLE History

Signs/symptoms	Nausea, lightheadedness, and "pain between my shoulder blades"
OPQRST	Pain between her shoulder blades has steadily increased in intensity; rates her discomfort 9/10; symptoms have been present for about 2 hours
Allergies	None
Medications	Zestril
Past medical history	Hypertension; patient's mother died at age 72 of breast cancer; her father, age 74, is living and had a coronary artery bypass graft at age 62; patient is 5'5" and weighs 190 pounds
Last oral intake	Breakfast 3 hours ago
Events prior	The patient, an accountant, states that she was working at her desk when her symptoms began; denies any recent unusual physical activity or illness that may have precipitated her symptoms

CASE 6

Physical Examination Findings

Head, ears, eyes, nose, and throat	No abnormalities noted
Neck	Trachea midline, no jugular venous distention
Chest	Breath sounds are clear bilaterally
Abdomen	No abnormalities noted
Pelvis	No abnormalities noted
Extremities	No abnormalities noted
Posterior body	No abnormalities noted

4. An IV has been started. Aspirin has been given. A 12-lead ECG has been obtained as ordered (Case 6 Rhythm 1). Are there any significant findings on this 12-lead ECG?

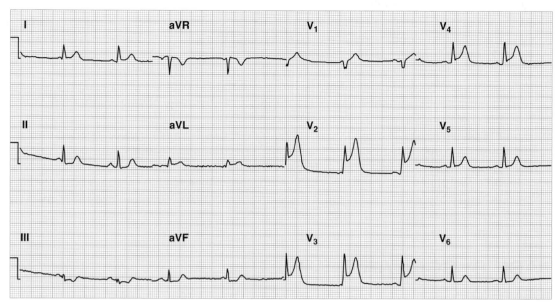

Case 6 Rhythm 1.

I	Lateral	aVR	------------	V₁	Septum	V₄	Anterior	V₄R	Right Ventricle
II	Inferior	aVL	Lateral	V₂	Septum	V₅	Lateral	V₅R	Right Ventricle
III	Inferior	aVF	Inferior	V₃	Anterior	V₆	Lateral	V₆R	Right Ventricle

5. What do these 12-lead ECG findings suggest? How would you like to proceed?

6. The patient's BP is now 164/90, her heart rate is 66, and respirations are 24. After two doses of sublingual NTG, she rates her discomfort 7/10. What should be done now?

CASE 6: ANSWERS

1. Approach the patient and begin a primary survey.
2. Ask a team member to attach a pulse oximeter and place the patient on a cardiac monitor. Ask your team members to place the patient on O_2 by nonrebreather mask and obtain the patient's baseline vital signs while you obtain a SAMPLE history and perform a focused physical examination.
3. After making sure there are no contraindications, ask the IV team member to give the patient 325 mg of aspirin to chew and swallow, and then start an IV of normal saline. After the IV is in place, reassess the patient's chest discomfort and order a 12-lead ECG.
4. The 12-lead ECG shows a sinus bradycardia at 57 bpm. There is ST-segment elevation in leads V_2 to V_4.

5. The patient's 12-lead ECG shows evidence of an anterior infarction. This area is normally supplied by the diagonal branch of the left anterior descending (LAD) artery. Because the LAD artery supplies about 40% of the heart's blood and a critical section of the left ventricle, a blockage in this area can lead to complications such as left ventricular dysfunction, including congestive heart failure and cardiogenic shock. Dysrhythmias including PVCs, atrial flutter, or atrial fibrillation are common with this type of myocardial infarction (MI). Because the bundle branches travel through this area, bundle branch blocks may result from injury in this area. A physician needs to review the 12-lead right away and classify the patient as an ST-elevation MI. Give sublingual NTG (if no contraindications). Order cardiac biomarkers and other lab work, order a portable chest x-ray, and begin a reperfusion therapy checklist right away. Repeat the primary survey, obtain another set of vital signs, and reassess the patient's discomfort.

6. Give the patient 2 mg of morphine now and repeat it every 5 minutes as needed until the patient is pain free (assuming her vital signs remain stable). Assess and record the patient's vital signs between doses. Make sure the reperfusion checklist is completed. Schedule the patient for the cardiac catheterization laboratory (or prepare fibrinolytics if ordered and no contraindications). If there are no contraindications, give other medications (such as beta-blockers) as ordered.

CASE 6: SCENARIO SHEET

SCENARIO: Your patient is a 50-year-old woman who is complaining of nausea, lightheadedness, and "pain between my shoulder blades." You have five other ALS personnel to assist you. Emergency equipment is immediately available.

EMERGENCY ACTION STEPS	NECESSARY TASKS
Scene Survey	I am putting on personal protective equipment. Is the scene safe to enter? *Coach: The scene is safe.*

INITIAL ASSESSMENT

First Impression	As I approach the patient and form a first impression (assessing the patient's appearance, work of breathing, and circulation), what do I see? *Coach: You see a 50-year-old woman sitting in a chair. She looks anxious. She appears to be breathing rapidly, but her breathing does not appear labored. Her skin is pink. You see beads of sweat on her upper lip and forehead. How would you like to proceed?*

PRIMARY SURVEY

Responsiveness/Airway	I will approach the patient and begin a primary survey. Is the patient aware of my approach? Does she respond when I speak her name? *Coach: Yes. The patient quickly tells you that she thinks she may be having a heart attack.*
Breathing	What is the rate and quality of the patient's breathing? *Coach: The patient's respiratory rate is 32 and unlabored.*
Circulation	What is her pulse rate and quality? What is her skin condition? *Coach: Radial and carotid pulses are strong and regular. You estimate the rate to be about 60/min. Her skin is warm, pink, and moist.*
Defibrillation	I will make sure a defibrillator is within reach, although it is not needed at this time. *Coach: A biphasic defibrillator is available to you.*

SECONDARY SURVEY/FOCUSED HISTORY & EXAM

Vital Signs/History | I want the defibrillation team member to attach a pulse oximeter and place the patient on a cardiac monitor. I will ask the airway team member to place the patient on O_2 by nonrebreather mask. I want a team member to obtain the patient's baseline vital signs while I obtain a SAMPLE history from the patient and perform a focused physical exam. What are the patient's vital signs?
Coach: The patient's vital signs are as follows: BP 178/104, heart rate is about 60, and respirations are now 24. Breath sounds are clear and equal bilaterally. The patient's SpO_2 was 96% on room air. Since placing the patient on O_2 by nonrebreather mask, it is now 98%. The patient has been placed on the cardiac monitor. (See Case 6 SAMPLE history and physical exam findings.) How would you like to proceed?

Airway, Breathing, Circulation | I want the IV team member to check to be sure there are no contraindications, and then give the patient 325 mg of baby aspirin and ask the patient to chew and swallow it. I want the IV team member to start an IV of normal saline, and I want to order a 12-lead ECG. I want to reassess the patient's discomfort. How does the patient rate her discomfort now?
Coach: An IV has been started. Aspirin has been given. The patient rates her discomfort 9/10. A 12-lead ECG has been obtained as ordered. (See Case 6 Rhythm 1.) Are there any significant findings on this 12-lead ECG?

Differential Diagnosis, Evaluates Interventions | The 12-lead ECG shows a sinus bradycardia at 57 bpm. There is ST-segment elevation in leads $V_2 - V_4$. I want a team member to order cardiac biomarkers and other lab work and a portable chest x-ray, and to begin a reperfusion therapy checklist right away.
Coach: How would you like to proceed?
The patient's 12-lead ECG suggests an anterior myocardial infarction. A physician needs to review the 12-lead ECG right away and classify the patient as an ST-elevation MI. I want the IV team member to give the patient sublingual NTG now and repeat every 5 minutes as needed to a maximum of three doses. I want the patient's BP and pain reevaluated 5 minutes after each dose of NTG.
Coach: What would you like to do next?

POSTRESUSCITATION SUPPORT/ONGOING ASSESSMENT

Begins Postresuscitation Support/Performs Ongoing Assessment | I want to repeat the primary survey and obtain another set of vital signs. How is the patient's discomfort?
Coach: The patient's BP is now 164/90, her heart rate is 66, and respirations are 24. After two doses of sublingual NTG, she rates her discomfort 7/10. What should be done now?
I would like the IV team member to give the patient 2 mg of morphine now. I want this repeated every 5 minutes as needed until the patient is pain free (assuming her vital signs remain stable). I want the patient's vital signs taken and recorded between doses. I want to make sure the reperfusion checklist is completed and schedule the patient for the cardiac catheterization laboratory.

CASE 6: ESSENTIAL ACTIONS

Essential Actions	Ensure scene safety, use personal protective equipment
	Perform primary and secondary surveys
	Give O_2, start an IV, obtain vital signs, attach a pulse oximeter and cardiac monitor, obtain a 12-lead ECG, order laboratory studies
	Review the patient's initial 12-lead ECG for evidence of myocardial ischemia, injury, or infarction
	Know the actions, indications, dosages, side effects, and contraindications for the drugs used in the treatment of acute coronary syndromes
	Use a reperfusion checklist to evaluate the patient's candidacy for reperfusion therapy
Unacceptable Actions	Failure to use personal protective equipment
	Failure to start an IV
	Failure to correctly identify the ECG rhythm
	Failure to give O_2 and/or other drugs appropriate for patients with ischemic chest discomfort
	Failure to attempt to control a patient's chest discomfort
	Medication errors
	Failure to monitor the cardiac rhythm in any patient who displays an abnormal respiratory rate or effort, abnormal heart rate, perfusion, BP, or acute altered mental status

CASE 7: SYMPTOMATIC BRADYCARDIA

Objective	Given a patient situation, describe and demonstrate the initial emergency care for a patient with a symptomatic bradycardia.
Skills to Master	Primary and secondary surveys
	Supplemental O_2 delivery devices
	Attachment and use of ECG monitoring leads
	IV access
	IV drug administration
	Operation of a transcutaneous pacemaker
Rhythms to Master	Sinus rhythm
	Sinus bradycardia
	Junctional rhythm
	Idioventricular (ventricular escape) rhythm
	AV blocks: first-degree, second-degree type I, second-degree type II, third-degree AV block
Medications to Master	O_2
	Atropine
	Dopamine
	Epinephrine
Related Text Chapters	Chapter 1: The ABCDs of Emergency Cardiac Care
	Chapter 2: Airway Management: Oxygenation and Ventilation
	Chapter 3: Rhythm Recognition
	Chapter 4: Electrical Therapy
	Chapter 5: Vascular Access and Medications
	Chapter 6: Acute Coronary Syndromes
	Chapter 8: Putting It All Together

CASE 7: QUESTIONS

SCENARIO: Your patient is a 37-year-old man who is complaining of dizziness. You have five other ALS personnel to assist you. Emergency equipment is immediately available. The scene is safe.

1. As you put on personal protective equipment and form a first impression, you see an ill-appearing man lying in bed. His eyes are closed. You can see equal rise and fall of his chest. His skin is pale. How would you like to proceed?

2. The patient tells you he feels very dizzy. He is breathing 18 times/min. His breathing is not labored. The patient's carotid pulse is weak but regular. You estimate the rate to be about 40/min. His skin is cool, pale, and moist. What should be done now?

3. The patient's vital signs are as follows: BP 58/32, heart rate is about 45, and respirations are18. Breath sounds are clear and equal bilaterally. The patient's SpO_2 is 97% on room air. The patient has been placed on the cardiac monitor (see Case 7 Rhythm 1 and Case 7 SAMPLE history and physical examination tables). What is the rhythm on the monitor? How would you like to proceed?

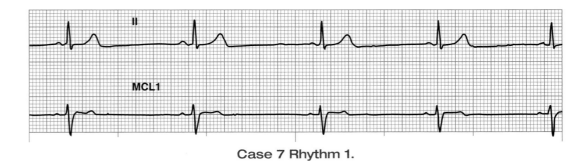

Case 7 Rhythm 1.

CASE 7	
SAMPLE History	
Signs/symptoms	Sudden onset of severe dizziness
Allergies	Codeine
Medications	None
Past medical history	Asthma as a child
Last oral intake	Lunch 2 hours ago
Events prior	Sudden onset of dizziness. Symptoms started about 30 minutes ago while at rest.

CASE 7	
Physical Examination Findings	
Head, ears, eyes, nose, and throat	No abnormalities noted
Neck	Trachea midline, no jugular venous distention
Chest	Breath sounds are clear bilaterally
Abdomen	No abnormalities noted
Pelvis	No abnormalities noted
Extremities	No abnormalities noted
Posterior body	No abnormalities noted

4. An IV has been started. A 12-lead ECG has been ordered. The defibrillator available to you has transcutaneous pacing capability. How would you like to proceed?

5. Atropine has been given as ordered. Lab work and a chest x-ray have been ordered. A reperfusion checklist has been started. What would you like to do next?

6. The patient's BP is now 112/70, his heart rate is 88, and respirations are 16. His skin is now warm, pink, and dry. The patient states that he feels much better. What should be done now?

CASE 7: ANSWERS

1. Approach the patient and begin a primary survey.
2. Ask a team member to attach a pulse oximeter and place the patient on a cardiac monitor. Ask your team members to place the patient on O_2 by nonrebreather mask and obtain the patient's baseline vital signs while you obtain a SAMPLE history and perform a focused physical examination.
3. The monitor shows a sinus bradycardia. Ask the airway team member to place the patient on O_2 by nonrebreather mask. Ask the IV team member to start an IV of normal saline. Order a 12-lead ECG. Make sure that your defibrillator has transcutaneous pacing capability.
4. Because the rhythm on the monitor is a narrow-QRS bradycardia, it is reasonable to try atropine to increase the patient's heart rate. In a patient with a pulse, atropine is given in doses of 0.5 mg IV every 3 to 5 minutes as needed to a maximum total dose of 3 mg. You should also order cardiac biomarkers and other lab work and begin a reperfusion therapy checklist in case the patient's bradycardia is the result of an acute coronary syndrome.
5. After giving atropine, be sure to repeat the primary survey and obtain another set of vital signs to assess the patient's response to your treatment.
6. Continue to monitor the patient's ECG and vital signs closely. Review the results of the patient's 12-lead ECG and lab work to try to determine the cause of the patient's bradycardia.

CASE 7: SCENARIO SHEET

SCENARIO: Your patient is a 37-year-old man who is complaining of dizziness. You have five other ALS personnel to assist you. Emergency equipment is immediately available.

EMERGENCY ACTION STEPS	NECESSARY TASKS
Scene Survey	I am putting on personal protective equipment. Is the scene safe to enter? *Coach: The scene is safe.*

INITIAL ASSESSMENT

First Impression	As I approach the patient and form a first impression (assessing the patient's appearance, work of breathing, and circulation), what do I see? *Coach: You see an ill-appearing man lying in bed. His eyes are closed. You can see equal rise and fall of his chest. His skin is pale. How would you like to proceed?*

PRIMARY SURVEY

Responsiveness/Airway	I will approach the patient and begin a primary survey. Is the patient aware of my approach? Does he respond when I speak his name? *Coach: Yes. The patient tells you that he is very dizzy.*
Breathing	What is the rate and quality of the patient's breathing? *Coach: The patient's respiratory rate is 18 and unlabored.*
Circulation	What is his pulse rate and quality? What is his skin condition? *Coach: The patient's carotid pulse is weak but regular. You estimate the rate to be about 40/min. His skin is cool, pale, and moist.*
Defibrillation	I will make sure a defibrillator is within reach, although it is not needed at this time. *Coach: A biphasic defibrillator is available to you.*

SECONDARY SURVEY/FOCUSED HISTORY & EXAM

Vital Signs/History	I want a team member to attach a pulse oximeter and place the patient on a cardiac monitor. I want a team member to obtain the patient's baseline vital signs while I obtain a SAMPLE history from the patient and perform a focused physical exam. What are the patient's vital signs? *Coach: The patient's vital signs are as follows: BP 58/32, heart rate is about 45, and respirations are 18. Breath sounds are clear and equal bilaterally. The patient's SpO$_2$ is 97% on room air. The patient has been placed on the cardiac monitor. (See Case 7 SAMPLE history and physical exam findings tables and Case 7 Rhythm 1.) What is the rhythm on the monitor? How would you like to proceed?*
Airway, Breathing, Circulation	The monitor shows a sinus bradycardia. I will ask the airway team member to place the patient on O$_2$ by nonrebreather mask. I want the IV team member to start an IV of normal saline and I want to order a 12-lead ECG. I also want to make sure that my defibrillator has transcutaneous pacing capability. *Coach: An IV has been started. A 12-lead ECG has been ordered. The defibrillator available to you does have transcutaneous pacing capability.*

Differential Diagnosis, Evaluates Interventions	I want to give the patient 0.5 mg of atropine IV now. I also want to order cardiac biomarkers, other lab work, and a portable chest x-ray. I also want to begin a reperfusion therapy checklist. *Coach: Atropine has been given as ordered. Lab work and a chest x-ray have been ordered. A reperfusion checklist has been started. What would you like to do next?*

POSTRESUSCITATION SUPPORT/ONGOING ASSESSMENT

Begins Postresuscitation Support/Performs Ongoing Assessment	I want to repeat the primary survey and obtain another set of vital signs. Has there been any improvement in the patient's symptoms? *Coach: The patient's BP is now 112/70, his heart rate is 88, and respirations are 16. His skin is now warm, pink, and dry. The patient states that he feels much better. What should be done now?* I will continue to monitor the patient's ECG and vital signs closely. I will review the results of the patient's 12-lead ECG and lab work to try to determine the cause of the patient's bradycardia.

CASE 7: ESSENTIAL ACTIONS

Essential Actions	Ensure scene safety, use personal protective equipment Perform primary and secondary surveys Give O_2, start an IV, obtain vital signs, attach a pulse oximeter and cardiac monitor, obtain a 12-lead ECG Recognize first-degree, second-degree type I, second-degree type II, and third-degree AV blocks Obtain a history and perform a physical exam, recognizing a symptomatic bradycardia Give drugs as indicated Perform transcutaneous pacing as indicated Consider reperfusion therapy if the patient's signs and symptoms are consistent with an acute coronary syndrome and there are no contraindications
Unacceptable Actions	Failure to use personal protective equipment Failure to start an IV Failure to correctly identify the ECG rhythm Failure to prepare the transcutaneous pacemaker while trying atropine (if atropine is indicated) Giving lidocaine for ventricular escape rhythms Treating an asymptomatic bradycardia with drugs or pacing Medication errors Failure to monitor the cardiac rhythm in any patient who displays abnormal respiratory rate or effort, abnormal heart rate, perfusion, BP, or acute altered mental status

CASE 8: UNSTABLE TACHYCARDIA

Objective	Given a patient situation, describe and demonstrate the initial emergency care for an unstable patient with a narrow- or wide-QRS tachycardia.

Skills to Master	Primary and secondary surveys
	Supplemental O_2 delivery devices
	Attachment and use of ECG monitoring leads
	IV access
	IV drug administration
	Synchronized cardioversion
Rhythms to Master	AV nodal reentrant tachycardia (AVNRT)
	AV reentrant tachycardia (AVRT)
	Atrial tachycardia (AT)
	Junctional tachycardia
	Monomorphic VT
	Polymorphic VT
	Wide-complex tachycardia of unknown origin
Medications to Master	O_2
	Adenosine
	Amiodarone
	Magnesium sulfate
	Procainamide
	Sotalol
Related Text Chapters	Chapter 1: The ABCDs of Emergency Cardiac Care
	Chapter 2: Airway Management: Oxygenation and Ventilation
	Chapter 3: Rhythm Recognition
	Chapter 4: Electrical Therapy
	Chapter 5: Vascular Access and Medications
	Chapter 8: Putting It All Together

CASE 8: QUESTIONS

SCENARIO: Your patient is a 72-year-old man who was found unresponsive by his wife. He was last seen about 10 minutes ago. The patient's wife says he had complained to her a few minutes ago that his heart was beating "too fast." She left the room to find his doctor's phone number and found him unresponsive when she returned. You have five other ALS personnel to assist you. Emergency equipment is immediately available. The scene is safe.

1. As you put on personal protective equipment and form a first impression, you see a man lying supine on the bed. His eyes are closed. His skin looks very pale. You can see rise and fall of his chest. How would you like to proceed?

2. The patient is unresponsive. He is breathing shallowly at a rate of 4 to 6/min. You are unable to feel a radial pulse. A weak carotid pulse is present. You estimate the rate to be about 150. The patient's skin is cool, pale, and moist. How would you like to proceed?

3. A biphasic defibrillator is available to you. The patient's vital signs are as follows: BP 50/24, heart rate is 150, and respirations 20. Breath sounds are clear and equal bilaterally with bagging. The patient's SpO_2 is 97%. The patient has been placed on the cardiac monitor. (See Case 8 Rhythm 1 and Case 8 SAMPLE history and physical examination tables). What is the rhythm on the monitor? How would you like to proceed?

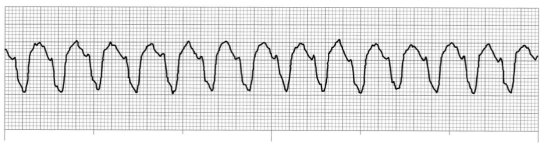

Case 8 Rhythm 1.

CASE 8	
SAMPLE History*	
Signs/symptoms	Sudden onset of palpitations
Allergies	Darvon, codeine
Medications	Albuterol, diazepam prn
Past medical history	Asthma, hypertension, anxiety
Last oral intake	Lunch 20 minutes ago
Events prior	Reading the newspaper when his heart "started beating too fast"

*History was obtained from wife.

CASE 8	
Physical Examination Findings	
Head, ears, eyes, nose, and throat	No abnormalities noted
Neck	Trachea midline, no jugular venous distention
Chest	Breath sounds are clear bilaterally
Abdomen	No abnormalities noted
Pelvis	No abnormalities noted
Extremities	No abnormalities noted
Posterior body	No abnormalities noted

4. An IV has been started. A 12-lead ECG has been ordered. Are you going to perform synchronized cardioversion or will you defibrillate the patient?

5. A biphasic manual defibrillator is available to you. What initial energy setting will you use?

6. The O_2 was shut off and a synchronized shock was delivered as ordered. You see the following rhythm on the monitor. (See Case 8 Rhythm 2 and Case 8 SAMPLE history and physical examination tables). What is the rhythm? What would you like to do next?

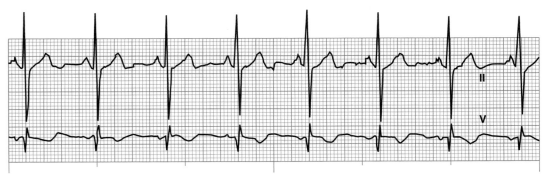

Case 8 Rhythm 2.

7. Strong carotid and radial pulses are present. The patient is awake. He is breathing about 14 times/min. Breath sounds are clear and equal bilaterally. The patient's BP is 133/80. His O_2 saturation is 98%. The cardiologist is here. What would you like done now?

CASE 8: ANSWERS

1. Approach the patient and begin a primary survey.
2. Based on the information available to you so far, you know that you have an unresponsive patient who has a tachycardia. You need to work quickly and find out what the rhythm is on the monitor. Once you know what the rhythm is, you can begin forming a more definitive treatment plan. For now, make sure a defibrillator is within reach. Ask a team member to attach a pulse oximeter and place the patient on a cardiac monitor. Ask your airway team member to assist the patient's breathing with a bag-mask device connected to 100% O_2. Ask a team member to obtain the patient's baseline vital signs while you obtain a SAMPLE history from the patient's wife and perform a focused physical exam.
3. The monitor shows monomorphic VT. The patient is clearly unstable (unresponsive, severe hypotension). Because the rhythm is a wide-QRS tachycardia, it is a good idea to order a cardiology consult as soon as possible. Ask the defibrillation team member to apply combination pads to the patient's bare chest and prepare to shock the patient. If it won't delay delivery of a shock, ask the IV team member to start an IV of normal saline. Order a 12-lead ECG. Because the patient is unresponsive, it will not be necessary to sedate the patient before the shock.
4. Because the patient has a pulse and the rhythm is monomorphic VT, you will perform synchronized cardioversion. If the patient had *no pulse* with this rhythm, you would defibrillate.
5. Begin synchronized cardioversion using 100 J or the energy setting recommended by the manufacturer. (In the management of the hemodynamically unstable patient in monomor-

phic VT with a pulse, synchronized shocks are delivered with 100 J and, if unsuccessful, 200 J, 300 J, and 360 J [or equivalent biphasic energy] as needed.) Make sure the airway team member temporarily shuts off the O_2 flow while the defibrillation team member prepares to deliver the shock. When the defibrillation team member is ready, he must make sure all team members (including him) are clear of the patient and then deliver the shock.

6. The monitor shows a sinus rhythm. Make sure the patient still has a pulse (a pulse is present). Repeat the primary survey and obtain another set of vital signs.

7. Ask the airway team member to remove the bag-mask device and replace it with a non-rebreather mask. Ask that the patient's vital signs be monitored every 5 minutes for the next 30 minutes and transfer patient care to the cardiologist.

CASE 8: SCENARIO SHEET

SCENARIO: Your patient is a 72-year-old man who was found unresponsive by his wife. He was last seen about 10 minutes ago. The patient's wife says he had complained to her a few minutes ago that his heart was beating "too fast." She left the room to find his doctor's phone number and found him unresponsive when she returned. You have five other ALS personnel to assist you. Emergency equipment is immediately available.

EMERGENCY ACTION STEPS	NECESSARY TASKS
Scene Survey	I am putting on personal protective equipment. Is the scene safe to enter? *Coach: The scene is safe.*

INITIAL ASSESSMENT

First Impression	As I approach the patient and form a first impression (assessing the patient's appearance, work of breathing, and circulation), what do I see? *Coach: You see a man lying supine on the bed. His eyes are closed. His skin looks very pale. You can see rise and fall of his chest. How would you like to proceed?*

PRIMARY SURVEY

Responsiveness/Airway	I will approach the patient and begin a primary survey. Is the patient aware of my approach? Does he respond when I speak his name? *Coach: The patient is unresponsive.*
Breathing	What is the rate and quality of the patient's breathing? *Coach: The patient is breathing shallowly at a rate of 4 to 6/min.*
Circulation	I will ask the airway team member to assist the patient's breathing with a bag-mask device connected to 100% O_2. What is his pulse rate and quality? What is his skin condition? *Coach: You are unable to feel a radial pulse. A weak carotid pulse is present. You estimate the rate to be about 150. The patient's skin is cool, pale, and moist.*
Defibrillation	I want to make sure that a defibrillator is within reach. *Coach: A biphasic defibrillator is available to you.*

SECONDARY SURVEY/FOCUSED HISTORY & EXAM

Vital Signs/History	I want a team member to attach a pulse oximeter and place the patient on a cardiac monitor. I want a team member to obtain the patient's baseline vital signs while I obtain a SAMPLE history from the patient's wife and perform a focused physical exam. What are the patient's vital signs?

	Coach: The patient's vital signs are as follows: BP 50/24, heart rate is 150, and respirations 20. Breath sounds are clear and equal bilaterally with bagging. The patient's SpO$_2$ is 97%. The patient has been placed on the cardiac monitor. (See Case 8 SAMPLE history and physical exam findings tables and Case 8 Rhythm 1.) What is the rhythm on the monitor? How would you like to proceed?
Airway, Breathing, Circulation	The monitor shows monomorphic VT. The patient is clearly unstable. I would like to order a cardiology consult as soon as possible. I will ask the defibrillation team member to apply combination pads to the patient's chest and prepare to shock the patient. While we are preparing to shock the patient, I want the IV team member to start an IV of normal saline and I want to order a 12-lead ECG. Because the patient is unresponsive, I will not need to ask the IV team member to sedate the patient before the shock.
	Coach: An IV has been started. A 12-lead ECG has been ordered. Are you going to perform synchronized cardioversion or will you defibrillate the patient?
	Since the patient has a pulse and the rhythm is monomorphic VT, I want the defibrillation team member to perform synchronized cardioversion.
	Coach: A biphasic manual defibrillator is available to you. What initial energy setting will you use?
Differential Diagnosis, Evaluates Interventions	I will begin synchronized cardioversion using 100 J or the energy setting recommended by the manufacturer. I want the airway team member to temporarily shut off the O$_2$ flow while the defibrillation team member prepares to deliver the shock. When the defibrillation team member is ready, he will make sure all team members (including him) are clear of the patient and then deliver the shock.
	Coach: The O$_2$ was shut off as ordered and a synchronized shock was delivered using 100 J. What is the rhythm on the monitor? (See Case 8 Rhythm 2.)
	The monitor shows a sinus rhythm.
	Coach: What would you like to do next?

POSTRESUSCITATION SUPPORT/ONGOING ASSESSMENT

Begins Postresuscitation Support/Performs Ongoing Assessment	I want to repeat the primary survey and obtain another set of vital signs.
	Coach: Strong carotid and radial pulses are present. The patient is awake. He is breathing about 14 times/min. Breath sounds are clear and equal bilaterally. The patient's BP is 133/80. His O$_2$ saturation is 98%. The cardiologist is here.
	I want the airway team member to remove the bag-mask device and replace it with a nonrebreather mask. I want the patient's vital signs monitored every 5 minutes for the next 30 minutes and will now transfer patient care to the cardiologist.

CASE 8: ESSENTIAL ACTIONS

Essential Actions	Ensure scene safety, use personal protective equipment
	Perform primary and secondary surveys
	Quickly recognize if the patient is stable or unstable
	Quickly identify the ECG rhythm, determining if the QRS is narrow or wide, regular or irregular

Recognize sinus tachycardia, AVNRT, AVRT, AT, junctional tachycardia, monomorphic VT, polymorphic VT, and wide-complex tachycardia of unknown origin

Give O_2, start an IV, obtain vital signs, attach a pulse oximeter and cardiac monitor, obtain a 12-lead ECG

Obtain a history and perform a physical exam, recognizing a symptomatic tachycardia

Know the actions, indications, dosages, side effects, and contraindications for the drugs used in the treatment of a narrow-QRS or wide-QRS tachycardia

Deliver the correct type of energy (synchronized cardioversion versus defibrillation) and the correct energy level for the tachycardia if electrical therapy is indicated

Demonstrate safe operation of the defibrillator, including turning off the O_2 flow during each shock if electrical therapy is indicated

Perform synchronized cardioversion as indicated

Recognize the need to change from synchronized cardioversion to defibrillation if the patient goes into pulseless VT or VF

Unacceptable Actions   Failure to use personal protective equipment

Failure to start an IV

Failure to correctly identify the ECG rhythm

Inability to quickly determine if the patient is stable or unstable

Failure to press the sync control after delivery of an initial synchronized shock to deliver additional synchronized shocks (if necessary)

Medication errors

Failure to monitor the cardiac rhythm in any patient who displays an abnormal respiratory rate or effort, abnormal heart rate, perfusion, BP, or acute altered mental status

CASE 9: STABLE TACHYCARDIA

Objective	Given a patient situation, describe and demonstrate the initial emergency care for a stable but symptomatic patient with a narrow- or wide-QRS tachycardia.
Skills to Master	Primary and secondary surveys
	Supplemental O_2 delivery devices
	Attachment and use of ECG monitoring leads
	IV access
	IV drug administration
Rhythms to Master	Sinus tachycardia
	AVNRT
	AVRT
	AT
	Junctional tachycardia
	Monomorphic VT
	Polymorphic VT
	Wide-complex tachycardia of unknown origin
Medications to Master	O_2
	Adenosine
	Amiodarone
	Beta-blockers
	Diltiazem
	Magnesium sulfate

Procainamide
Sotalol
Verapamil
Related Text Chapters   Chapter 1: The ABCDs of Emergency Cardiac Care
Chapter 2: Airway Management: Oxygenation and Ventilation
Chapter 3: Rhythm Recognition
Chapter 4: Electrical Therapy
Chapter 5: Vascular Access and Medications
Chapter 8: Putting It All Together

CASE 9: QUESTIONS

SCENARIO: A 67-year-old man presents with a complaint of a "racing heart." You have four ALS personnel to assist you. Emergency equipment is available. The scene is safe.

1. As you put on personal protective equipment and form a first impression, you see an anxious-appearing man sitting in a chair. His breathing is unlabored. His skin appears pink. How would you like to proceed?

2. As you approach, the patient immediately begins speaking to you. He tells you that his heart is racing and he is worried that he is going to die. The patient's respiratory rate is 18 and unlabored. His radial and carotid pulses are strong but too fast to count accurately. You estimate the rate to be about 200/min. His skin is cool, pink, and moist. What should be done now?

3. The patient's vital signs are as follows: BP 156/90, heart rate is 214, and respirations 20. Breath sounds are clear and equal bilaterally. The patient's SpO_2 on room air was 95% and is now 98% on O_2 by nonrebreather mask. The patient has been placed on the cardiac monitor. (See Case 9 Rhythm 1 and Case 9 SAMPLE history and physical examination tables.) What is the rhythm on the monitor? How would you like to proceed?

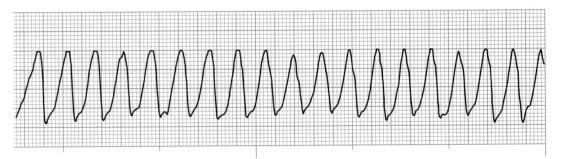

Case 9 Rhythm 1.

CASE 9

SAMPLE History

Signs/symptoms	"Racing heart"
Allergies	Bactrim
Medications	Glyburide, Prevacid
Past medical history	Diabetes, hypertension
Last oral intake	Sugar-free 2 hours ago
Events prior	Sudden onset of "racing heart"; symptoms started 40 minutes ago

CASE 9

Physical Examination Findings

Head, ears, eyes, nose, and throat	No abnormalities noted
Neck	Trachea midline, no jugular venous distention
Chest	Breath sounds are clear bilaterally
Abdomen	No abnormalities noted
Pelvis	No abnormalities noted
Extremities	No abnormalities noted
Posterior body	No abnormalities noted

4. An IV has been started. A 12-lead ECG has been ordered. How would you like to proceed?

5. A cardiology consult has been requested. The cardiologist is en route and is expected to arrive in about 20 minutes. What would you like to do next?

6. The IV/meds team member is preparing to give amiodarone as requested. How much amiodarone should the patient receive at this time?

7. Amiodarone has been ordered. What would you like to do next?

8. The monitor now shows the following rhythm (Case 9 Rhythm 2). The patient's BP is 134/70, his heart rate is 94, and his respirations are 16. His skin is now warm, pink, and dry. The patient states that he "feels great." What should be done now?

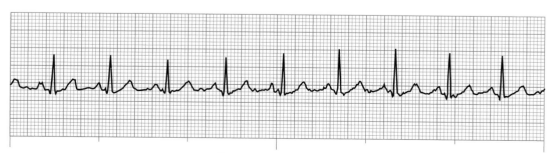

Case 9 Rhythm 2.

CASE 9: ANSWERS

1. Approach the patient and begin a primary survey.
2. Ask a team member to attach a pulse oximeter and place the patient on a cardiac monitor. Ask your team members to place the patient on O_2 by nonrebreather mask and obtain the patient's baseline vital signs while you obtain a SAMPLE history and perform a focused physical examination.
3. The monitor shows monomorphic VT. Ask the airway team member to place the patient on O_2 by nonrebreather mask. Ask the IV team member to start an IV of normal saline. Order a 12-lead ECG.
4. It is best to consult a cardiologist when treating a patient who has a wide-QRS tachycardia.
5. A stable but symptomatic patient in monomorphic VT is treated with oxygen, IV access, and ventricular antiarrhythmics (such as amiodarone) to suppress the rhythm.
6. Give 150 mg of amiodarone IV over 10 minutes.
7. Repeat the primary survey, obtain another set of vital signs, and check the cardiac monitor to assess the patient's response to your treatment.
8. The monitor now shows a sinus rhythm. Continue to monitor the patient's ECG and vital signs closely. Since amiodarone converted the rhythm from VT to a sinus rhythm, consult with the cardiologist about starting a continuous IV infusion of amiodarone.

CASE 9: SCENARIO SHEET

SCENARIO: A 67-year-old man presents with a complaint of a "racing heart." You have four ALS personnel to assist you. Emergency equipment is available.

EMERGENCY ACTION STEPS	NECESSARY TASKS
Scene Survey	I am putting on personal protective equipment. Is the scene safe to enter? *Coach: The scene is safe.*

INITIAL ASSESSMENT

First Impression	As I approach the patient and form a first impression (assessing the patient's appearance, work of breathing, and circulation), what do I see? *Coach: You see an anxious appearing man sitting in a chair. His breathing is unlabored. His skin appears pink. How would you like to proceed?*

PRIMARY SURVEY

Responsiveness/Airway	I will approach the patient and begin a primary survey. Is the patient aware of my approach? Does he respond when I speak his name? *Coach: As you approach, the patient immediately begins speaking to you. He tells you that his heart is racing and he is worried that he is going to die.*
Breathing	What is the rate and quality of the patient's breathing? *Coach: The patient's respiratory rate is 18 and unlabored.*
Circulation	What is his pulse rate and quality? What is his skin condition? *Coach: His radial and carotid pulses are strong but too fast to count accurately. You estimate the rate to be about 200/min. His skin is cool, pink, and moist.*
Defibrillation	I will assist the patient to a supine position and make sure a defibrillator is within reach. *Coach: A biphasic defibrillator is available to you.*

SECONDARY SURVEY/FOCUSED HISTORY & EXAM

Vital Signs/History	I want a team member to attach a pulse oximeter and place the patient on a cardiac monitor. I will ask the airway team member to place the patient on O_2 by nonrebreather mask. I want a team member to obtain the patient's baseline vital signs while I obtain a SAMPLE history from the patient and perform a focused physical exam. What are the patient's vital signs?
	Coach: The patient's vital signs are as follows: BP 156/90, heart rate is 214, and respirations 20. Breath sounds are clear and equal bilaterally. The patient's SpO2 on room air was 95% and is now 98% on O_2 by nonrebreather mask. The patient has been placed on the cardiac monitor. (See Case 9 SAMPLE history and physical exam findings tables and Case 9 Rhythm 1.) What is the rhythm on the monitor? How would you like to proceed?
Airway, Breathing, Circulation	The monitor shows monomorphic VT. I want the IV team member to start an IV of normal saline and I want to order a 12-lead ECG.
	Coach: An IV has been started. A 12-lead ECG has been ordered.
Differential Diagnosis, Evaluates Interventions	Based on the patient's history and physical findings, I believe the patient is stable at this time. Since the rhythm is monomorphic VT, I will ask the IV team member to give 150 mg of amiodarone IV over 10 minutes.
	Coach: Amiodarone has been given as ordered. What would you like to do next?

POSTRESUSCITATION SUPPORT/ONGOING ASSESSMENT

Begins Postresuscitation Support/Performs Ongoing Assessment	I would like to order a cardiology consult as soon as possible. I want to repeat the primary survey and obtain another set of vital signs. Has there been any change in the patient's rhythm or in the patient's condition?
	Coach: A cardiology consult has been requested. The cardiologist is en route and is expected to arrive in about 20 minutes. The monitor now shows the following rhythm. (See Case 9 Rhythm 2.) The patient's BP is 134/70, his heart rate is 94, and respirations are 16. His skin is now warm, pink, and dry. The patient states that he "feels great." What should be done now?
	I will continue to monitor the patient's ECG and vital signs closely. I will consult with the cardiologist about starting a continuous IV infusion of amiodarone.

CASE 9: ESSENTIAL ACTIONS

Essential Actions	Ensure scene safety, use personal protective equipment
	Perform primary and secondary surveys
	Quickly recognize if the patient is stable or unstable
	Quickly identify the ECG rhythm, determining if the QRS is narrow or wide, regular or irregular
	Give O_2, start an IV, obtain vital signs, attach a pulse oximeter and cardiac monitor, obtain a 12-lead ECG
	Recognize sinus tachycardia, AVNRT, AVRT, AT, junctional tachycardia, monomorphic VT, polymorphic VT, and wide-complex tachycardia of unknown origin
	Know what a vagal maneuver is, types, and when they are performed

	Know the actions, indications, dosages, side effects, and contra-indications for the drugs used in the treatment of a narrow-QRS or wide-QRS tachycardia
Unacceptable Actions	Failure to use personal protective equipment
	Failure to start an IV
	Failure to correctly identify the ECG rhythm
	Inability to quickly determine if the patient is stable or unstable
	Failure to give O_2 and/or other drugs appropriate for the dysrhythmia
	Medication errors
	Failure to monitor the cardiac rhythm in any patient who displays an abnormal respiratory rate or effort, abnormal heart rate, perfusion, BP, or acute altered mental status

CASE 10: ACUTE ISCHEMIC STROKE

Objective	Given a patient situation, describe and demonstrate the initial emergency care for a patient experiencing an acute ischemic stroke.
Skills to Master	Primary and secondary surveys
	Supplemental O_2 delivery devices
	Attachment and use of ECG monitoring leads
	Suctioning
	Serum glucose determination
	IV access
	IV drug administration
Rhythms to Master	Atrial fibrillation
	Sinus rhythm
Medications to Master	O_2
	Fibrinolytics
	Dextrose (if documented hypoglycemia)
	Thiamine (if malnourished or alcoholic individual)
Related Text Chapters	Chapter 1: The ABCDs of Emergency Cardiac Care
	Chapter 2: Airway Management: Oxygenation and Ventilation
	Chapter 3: Rhythm Recognition
	Chapter 5: Vascular Access and Medications
	Chapter 7: Stroke and Special Resuscitation Situations

CASE 10: QUESTIONS

SCENARIO: A 76-year-old man presents with a sudden onset of difficulty speaking. The patient's anxious wife is present. You have four ALS personnel to assist you. Emergency equipment is available. The scene is safe.

1. As you put on personal protective equipment and form a first impression, you see a patient supine in bed. He is awake and aware of your presence. You see equal rise and fall of his chest. His skin is pink and appears dry. How would you like to proceed?

2. The patient is aware of your approach and attempts to answer you, but his speech is garbled and unintelligible. His breathing is quiet and unlabored at a rate of 16 to 18/min. The patient's radial and carotid pulses are strong but irregular. The patient's skin is warm, pink, and dry. What should be done now?

3. A biphasic defibrillator is available to you. The patient's vital signs are as follows: BP 204/102 (left arm) 198/100 (right arm), heart rate is strong but irregular, and respirations 16. Breath sounds are clear and equal bilaterally. The patient's SpO$_2$ was 94% on room air and is now 97% on O$_2$ by nasal cannula. The patient has been placed on the cardiac monitor (see Case 10 Rhythm 1 and Case 10 SAMPLE history and physical examination tables). What is the rhythm on the monitor? How would you like to proceed?

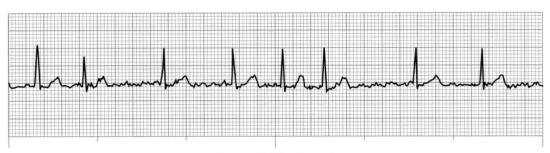

Case 10 Rhythm 1.

CASE 10

SAMPLE History

Signs/symptoms	Sudden onset of difficulty speaking; it is apparent that the patient can understand you, although you cannot understand him
Allergies	Demerol
Medications	Plavix, Wellbutrin, Coumadin, K-Dur
Past medical history	Transient ischemic attack 1 year ago, depression
Last oral intake	Lunch
Events prior	The patient's symptoms started about 1/2 hour ago. He has lost consciousness four times for about 2 minutes each time per his wife. No recent illness or injury. They had just finished lunch when his symptoms began.

CASE 10

Physical Examination Findings

Head, ears, eyes, nose, and throat	Pupils equal and reactive, but sluggish
Neck	Trachea midline, no jugular venous distention
Chest	Breath sounds are clear bilaterally
Abdomen	No abnormalities noted
Pelvis	No abnormalities noted
Extremities	Unable to grip with right hand, unable to move right leg
Posterior body	No abnormalities noted

4. An IV has been started. The patient's serum glucose is 140 mg/dL. Why is it important to determine the serum glucose level of a patient with a suspected stroke?

5. In addition to the SAMPLE history, list three questions you should ask a patient who presents with signs and symptoms of an acute stroke.
   1.
   2.
   3.

6. What would you like to do now?

7. What areas are assessed using the Cincinnati Prehospital Stroke Scale?

8. The patient is able to smile, but is unable to repeat a phrase clearly. He is also unable to move his right arm. What would you like to do now?

9. What is the time target for a possible stroke patient evaluation by a physician? What are the time targets to obtain and read a computed tomography (CT) scan?

10. The patient's airway remains clear and his breathing is adequate. BP is 190/104, respirations are 18, SpO_2 is 97%, and there is no change in the patient's heart rate. The patient's skin is warm and dry. What would you like to do now?

CASE 10: ANSWERS

1. Approach the patient and begin a primary survey.
2. Make sure that a defibrillator is within reach, but it is not needed at this time. Ask a team member to attach a pulse oximeter and place the patient on a cardiac monitor. Ask your team members to place the patient on O_2 by nasal cannula and obtain the patient's baseline vital signs while you obtain a SAMPLE history from the patient's wife and perform a focused physical examination. Ask your team to assess the patient's BP in both arms.
3. The rhythm is atrial fibrillation. Ask the IV team member to start an IV of normal saline and check the patient's serum glucose level.
4. A serum glucose level helps differentiate a possible stroke from other common causes of stroke symptoms such as hypoglycemia.
5. When was the last time the patient was known to be without symptoms? What was the patient doing when the symptoms began? Did the patient complain of a headache? Did he have a seizure? Has there been a change in his level of responsiveness? Is there a history of any recent trauma?
6. Based on the patient's history and physical findings, alert the stroke team right away and order a 12-lead ECG, lab tests, and portable chest x-ray. Ask the IV team member to infuse the IV at a keep-open rate (30 mL/hr). Perform an initial neurologic evaluation using the Cincinnati Prehospital Stroke Scale.
7. The Cincinnati Prehospital Stroke Scale assesses facial droop/weakness, arm drift, and speech.
8. Begin completing a fibrinolytic therapy checklist to determine if the patient is a candidate for therapy and order a noncontrast CT scan.

9. A patient who presents with a possible stroke should be seen by a physician within 10 minutes of arrival in the ED. A CT scan should be completed within 25 minutes of patient arrival and read by a physician within 45 minutes.

10. Repeat the primary survey; obtain another set of vital signs. Transfer patient care to the stroke team.

CASE 10: SCENARIO SHEET

SCENARIO: A 76-year-old man presents with a sudden onset of difficulty speaking. The patient's anxious wife is present. You have four ALS personnel to assist you. Emergency equipment is available. The scene is safe.

EMERGENCY ACTION STEPS	NECESSARY TASKS
Scene Survey	I am putting on personal protective equipment. Is the scene safe to enter? *Coach: The scene is safe.*

INITIAL ASSESSMENT

First Impression	As I approach the patient and form a first impression (assessing the patient's appearance, work of breathing, and circulation), what do I see? *Coach: You find the patient supine in bed. He is awake and aware of your presence. You see equal rise and fall of his chest. His skin is pink and appears dry.*

PRIMARY SURVEY

Responsiveness/Airway	I will approach the patient and begin a primary survey. Is the patient aware of my approach? Does he respond when I speak his name? *Coach: The patient is aware of your approach and attempts to answer you, but his speech is garbled and unintelligible.* I will look in the patient's mouth to make sure there is nothing present that may cause an airway obstruction or may explain the reason for the patient's garbled speech. *Coach: The patient's airway is clear.*
Breathing	What is the rate and quality of the patient's breathing? *Coach: His breathing is quiet and unlabored at a rate of 16 to 18/min.*
Circulation	What is his pulse rate and quality? What is his skin condition? *Coach: The patient's radial and carotid pulses are strong but irregular. The patient's skin is warm, pink, and dry.*
Defibrillation	I want to make sure that a defibrillator is within reach, although it is not needed at this time. *Coach: A biphasic defibrillator is available to you.*

SECONDARY SURVEY/FOCUSED HISTORY & EXAM

Vital Signs/History	I want a team member to attach a pulse oximeter and place the patient on a cardiac monitor. I will ask the airway team member to place the patient on O_2 by nasal cannula. I want the CPR team member to obtain the patient's baseline vital signs while I obtain a SAMPLE history from the patient's wife and perform a focused physical exam. I would like the patient's BP assessed in both arms. *Coach: The patient's vital signs are as follows: BP 204/102 (left arm) and 198/100 (right arm), heart rate is strong, but irregular, and*

respirations 16. Breath sounds are clear and equal bilaterally. The patient's SpO$_2$ was 94% on room air and is now 97% on O$_2$ by nasal cannula. The patient has been placed on the cardiac monitor (See Case 10 SAMPLE history and physical exam findings tables and Case 10 Rhythm 1.) What is the rhythm on the monitor? How would you like to proceed?

Airway, Breathing, Circulation

The rhythm is atrial fibrillation. I will ask the IV team member to start an IV of normal saline and check the patient's serum glucose level. I want to order a 12-lead ECG.

Coach: An IV has been started. A 12-lead ECG has been ordered. The patient's serum glucose is 140 mg/dL. Why is it important to determine the serum glucose level of a patient with a suspected stroke?

Differential Diagnosis, Evaluates Interventions

A serum glucose level helps differentiate a possible stroke from other common causes of stroke symptoms such as hypoglycemia.

Coach: In addition to the SAMPLE history, what questions should you ask a patient who presents with signs and symptoms of an acute stroke?

When was the last time the patient was known to be without symptoms? What was the patient doing when the symptoms began? Did the patient complain of a headache? Did he have a seizure? Has there been a change in his level of responsiveness? Is there a history of any recent trauma?

Coach: What would you like to do now?

Based on the patient's history and physical findings, I will alert the stroke team right away and order a 12-lead ECG, lab tests, and portable chest x-ray. I will ask the IV team member to infuse the IV at a keep-open rate (30 mL/hr). I will perform an initial neurologic evaluation using the Cincinnati Prehospital Stroke Scale.

Coach: What areas are assessed using this scale?

The Cincinnati Prehospital Stroke Scale assesses facial droop/weakness, arm drift, and speech.

Coach: The patient is able to smile, but is unable to repeat a phrase clearly. He is also unable to move his right arm.

I will begin completing a fibrinolytic therapy checklist to determine if the patient is a candidate for therapy and order a noncontrast CT scan.

Coach: What is the time target for a possible stroke patient evaluation by a physician?

A patient who presents with a possible stroke should be seen by a physician within 10 minutes of arrival in the ED.

Coach: What are the time targets to obtain and read a CT scan?

A CT scan should be completed within 25 minutes of patient arrival and read by a physician within 45 minutes.

Coach: What would you like to do now?

POSTRESUSCITATION SUPPORT/ONGOING ASSESSMENT

Begins Postresuscitation Support/Performs Ongoing Assessment

I want to repeat the primary survey, obtain another set of vital signs, and transfer patient care to the stroke team.

Coach: The patient's airway remains clear and his breathing is adequate. BP is 190/104, respirations are 18, SpO$_2$ is 97%, and there is no change in the patient's heart rate. The patient's skin is warm and dry.

CASE 10: ESSENTIAL ACTIONS

Essential Actions	Ensure scene safety, use personal protective equipment
	Perform primary and secondary surveys
	Give O$_2$, start an IV, obtain vital signs, attach a pulse oximeter and cardiac monitor, check serum glucose, obtain 12-lead ECG, laboratory studies
	Give dextrose if documented hypoglycemia present
	Obtain a focused history and perform a physical examination including vital signs, recognizing signs and symptoms of possible stroke
	Determine time of symptom onset
	Perform a general neurological screening assessment
	Order an urgent noncontrast CT scan
	Consider fibrinolytics if the patient's presentation is consistent with acute ischemic stroke verified by CT scan and there are no contraindications
	Use a reperfusion checklist to determine the patient's eligibility for therapy
Unacceptable Actions	Failure to use personal protective equipment
	Failure to establish IV access
	Failure to give O$_2$ and/or other drugs appropriate for patients with acute ischemic stroke
	Medication errors
	Failure to monitor the cardiac rhythm in any patient who displays abnormal respiratory rate or effort, abnormal heart rate, perfusion, BP, or acute altered mental status

Posttest

1. Which of the following situations does not require a reduction in the initial dose of IV adenosine?
   a. A patient who has a transplanted heart
   b. A patient who is taking carbamazepine (Tegretol)
   c. Giving adenosine through a central IV line
   d. A patient who is taking theophylline

2. A 62-year-old man is complaining of palpitations that came on suddenly after walking up a short flight of stairs. His symptoms have been present for about 20 minutes. He denies chest pain and is not short of breath. His skin is warm and dry; breath sounds are clear. His BP is 144/88, P 186, R 18. The cardiac monitor reveals sustained monomorphic VT. The patient has been placed on O_2, and an IV has been established. Which of the following medications is most appropriate in this situation?
   a. Amiodarone
   b. Dopamine
   c. NTG
   d. Furosemide

3. Which of the following statements is correct about the use of amiodarone in cardiac arrest?
   a. Amiodarone should be given as soon as possible after an IV is established in cardiac arrest
   b. Amiodarone can be considered if pulseless VT/VF continues despite 2 to 3 shocks, CPR, and administration of a vasopressor
   c. Amiodarone is the drug of choice for cardiac arrest due to asystole
   d. Amiodarone should be given immediately before the first shock if pulseless VT/VF is present

4. A 50-year-old woman is complaining of substernal chest discomfort and nausea. On a 0 to 10 scale, she rates her discomfort an 8. Her symptoms began about 3 hours ago. Her BP is 162/94, P 122, R 16. Breath sounds are clear. The cardiac monitor shows a sinus tachycardia with ST-segment depression in lead II. An IV has been started, and a 12-lead ECG has been ordered. Which of the following reflects the most appropriate treatment for this patient?
   a. O_2, atropine 1-mg IV, sublingual NTG, and morphine 2- to 4-mg IV
   b. O_2, aspirin 160 to 325 mg (chewed), sublingual nitroglycerin, and morphine 2- to 4-mg IV
   c. O_2, sublingual nitroglycerin, adenosine 6-mg IV, and a 250-mL IV fluid challenge
   d. O_2, aspirin 160 to 325 mg (chewed), vasopressin 20-U IV, and lidocaine 1.5-mg/kg IV

Questions 5 through 11 pertain to the following scenario:

A 55-year-old man is complaining of severe chest discomfort. He describes his discomfort as a "heavy pressure" in the middle of his chest that has been present for about 1 hour. On a 0-to-10 scale, he rates his discomfort a 9. His BP is 126/72 and respirations are 14. The cardiac monitor shows a sinus tachycardia.

5. Immediate management of this patient should include:
   a. ABCs, O_2, IV, and aspirin
   b. ABCs, O_2, IV, and adenosine
   c. ABCs, O_2, IV, and amiodarone
   d. ABCs, O_2, IV, and atropine

6. A 12-lead ECG has been obtained.

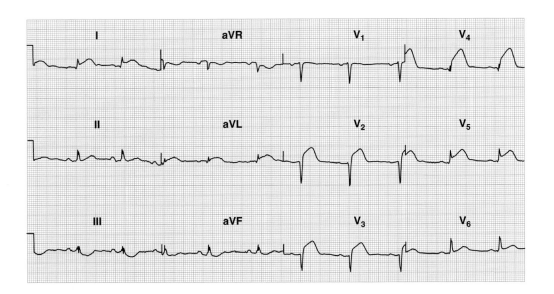

The patient's 12-lead ECG shows:
   a. ST-segment elevation in leads II, III, and aVF
   b. ST-segment depression in leads I, II, III, and aVL
   c. ST-segment elevation in leads I, aVL, V_2, V_3, V_4, and V_5
   d. ST-segment depression in leads V_1, V_4, V_5, and V_6

7. In the following table, indicate the area of the heart viewed by each lead.

I _____	aVR None	V_1 _____	V_4 _____
II _____	aVL _____	V_2 _____	V_5 _____
III _____	aVF _____	V_3 _____	V_6 _____

8. Label the following surfaces of the heart on the drawing below: anterior, inferior, septum, lateral. Some words may be used more than once.

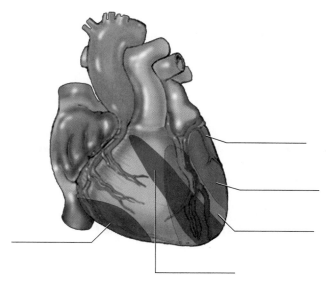

9. In order to be considered significant, ECG findings (such as ST-segment elevation or depression) need to be viewed in two or more contiguous leads. Which of the following are contiguous leads?
   a. I, II, III, and aVL
   b. III, aVL, and aVF
   c. V_1, V_4, and V_5
   d. V_2, V_3, and V_4

10. The patient's 12-lead ECG findings suggest:
   a. An inferior wall MI
   b. An anterolateral MI
   c. An inferolateral MI
   d. An NSTEMI

11. O_2 is being administered, and an IV has been established. The patient's BP is 130/70, pulse is now 98, and respirations are 14. Assuming there are no contraindications to any of the following medications, which would be appropriate for this patient at this time?
   a. NTG, morphine, and a beta-blocker
   b. NTG, a calcium channel blocker, and lidocaine
   c. A beta-blocker, morphine, and magnesium
   d. Lidocaine, magnesium, and a calcium channel blocker

12. The correct dose of epinephrine, when given by means of an ET tube during cardiac arrest, is:
   a. 0.5 mg
   b. 1 mg
   c. 2 to 2.5 mg
   d. 1 to 1.5 mg/kg

13. A 60-year-old woman has suffered a cardiac arrest. A healthcare professional trained in ET intubation has intubated the patient. Which of the following findings would indicate inadvertent esophageal intubation?
   a. Subcutaneous emphysema
   b. Gurgling sounds heard over the epigastrium
   c. Jugular vein distention
   d. Breath sounds heard on only the right side of the chest

14. Atypical symptoms or unusual presentations of acute coronary syndromes are more common in:
    a. Men, patients who have a history of coronary artery disease, and patients who have a history of hypertension
    b. Older adults, women, and diabetic individuals
    c. Men, older adults, and individuals who have liver disease
    d. Women, diabetic individuals, and individuals who have liver disease

15. A 56-year-old man has a permanent pacemaker in place. Should it be necessary to defibrillate this patient, adhesive pads or hand-held defibrillator paddles should be placed:
    a. At least one inch from the pacemaker generator
    b. It makes no difference where the paddles or pads are placed
    c. Directly over the pacemaker generator
    d. 6 to 8 inches from the pacemaker generator

16. A 53-year-old woman is unresponsive with BP 50/P and RR 10. The cardiac monitor initially showed a narrow-QRS tachycardia at 220 beats per minute. O$_2$ therapy was initiated and an IV established before the patient's collapse. You promptly delivered a synchronized shock. Reassessment reveals the patient is not breathing and has no pulse. The cardiac monitor now reveals VF. What course of action should you take at this time?
    a. Place an advanced airway and then begin transcutaneous pacing
    b. Defibrillate immediately
    c. Press the "sync" control and deliver another synchronized shock
    d. Perform CPR for 5 minutes and then prepare to defibrillate

Questions 17 through 20 pertain to the following scenario:

A 65-year-old man is complaining of a sudden onset of chest pain. He is awake, alert, and diaphoretic. Questions asked of the patient thus far reveal a possible acute coronary syndrome.

17. The patient states that his symptoms began 45 minutes ago while cleaning his garage. He denies nausea and has not vomited. The patient states that his discomfort is located in the center of his chest and radiates to his jaw. He rates the discomfort a 10 on a 0-to-10 scale. His BP is 130/50, R 24. The cardiac monitor reveals the following rhythm (lead II).

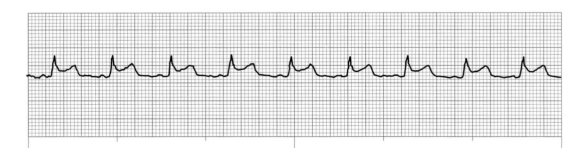

This rhythm is:
    a. Second-degree AV block type I
    b. Junctional rhythm with ST-segment elevation
    c. Sinus rhythm with ST-segment elevation
    d. Wide-QRS tachycardia

18. ST-segment elevation is considered significant if it is:
    a. More than 1/2 mm in at least two leads
    b. More than 1 mm in at least two contiguous leads
    c. More than 2 mm in at least two leads
    d. More than 5 mm in at least two contiguous leads

19. When the patient's 12-lead ECG is reviewed, the results should be used to classify the patient into one of three groups. Which of the following correctly reflects these categories?
    a. ST-segment depression, normal ECG, inconclusive ECG
    b. ST-segment elevation, normal ECG, Q waves
    c. Q waves, ST-segment depression, inconclusive ECG
    d. ST-segment elevation, ST-segment depression, normal/nondiagnostic ECG

20. O_2 has been applied, and an IV is in place. The patient's 12-lead ECG reveals ST-segment elevation in leads II, III, and aVF. Which of the following statements is correct?
    a. Leads II, III, and aVF view the anterior wall of the left ventricle. Since this patient is at extreme risk for congestive heart failure and cardiogenic shock, furosemide should be given without delay
    b. Leads II, III, and aVF view the inferior wall of the left ventricle. Since an inferior MI is suspected, right chest leads should be quickly used to rule out right ventricular infarction before giving medications for pain relief
    c. The patient's 12-lead results are inconclusive. Additional testing is needed before treatment is begun
    d. Since relief of pain is a priority in acute coronary syndrome patients, NTG and morphine should be given without further delay

21. Transcutaneous pacing is no longer recommended for which of the following rhythms?
    a. Junctional rhythm
    b. Asystole
    c. Second-degree AV block type II
    d. Third-degree AV block

Questions 22 and 23 pertain to the following scenario:

A 70-year-old man presents with acute altered mental status and dizziness.

22. O_2 has been applied, and the cardiac monitor reveals the following rhythm:

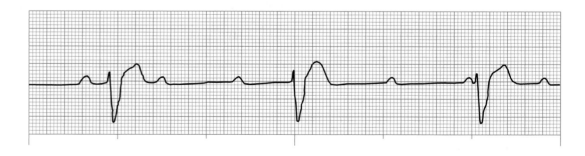

This rhythm is:
    a. Junctional rhythm
    b. Second-degree AV block type I
    c. Second-degree AV block type II
    d. Third-degree AV block

23. Based on the patient's signs and symptoms associated with this rhythm, your best course of action will be to:
    a. Observe the patient and monitor for signs of deterioration
    b. Give atropine 1-mg IV every 3 to 5 minutes
    c. Give epinephrine 1-mg IV bolus and reassess
    d. Prepare for immediate transcutaneous pacing

24. Furosemide is:
    a. A venodilator and potent diuretic
    b. Given as an initial bolus of 5-mg/kg slow IV push over 1 to 2 minutes
    c. A beta-adrenergic stimulator
    d. Indicated in the management of acute pulmonary embolism

25. Which of the following statements is true about giving antiarrhythmics during cardiac arrest?
    a. Antiarrhythmics are indicated only if an organized rhythm is seen on the cardiac monitor
    b. An antiarrhythmic should be the first drug given in every cardiac arrest
    c. An antiarrhythmic can be considered, but there is no evidence that any antiarrhythmic drug given routinely during human cardiac arrest increases survival to hospital discharge
    d. An antiarrhythmic is recommended for cardiac arrests involving nonshockable rhythms because studies clearly show that this action increases survival to hospital discharge

26. True or False. When pulseless VT/VF is present, the rescuer providing chest compressions should be prepared to resume CPR, beginning with chest compressions, as soon as a shock is delivered.

27. True or False. Complications associated with an inferior wall MI often include bradydysrhythmias.

28. A 62-year-old man is presenting with signs and symptoms suggesting a stroke. Realizing that the benefits of IV or intraarterial fibrinolytics are time-dependent, which of the following is the most important question that you should ask this patient, family, and/or bystanders?
    a. "Do you have a history of hypertension?"
    b. "When did you last see a physician?"
    c. "When did your symptoms begin?"
    d. "What were you doing when your symptoms began?"

29. Which of the following statements is correct about NTG administration?
    a. Common side effects include tinnitus, seizures, and hypertension
    b. Before giving NTG, make sure the patient's systolic BP is >90 mm Hg and heart rate is >50 and <100 bpm
    c. NTG is a potent vasoconstrictor
    d. NTG's onset of action is typically delayed 15 to 20 minutes after administration

30. When magnesium sulfate is administered during a cardiac arrest, the recommended dose is:
    a. 1- to 2-g IV push diluted in 10 mL
    b. 1.5-mg/kg IV push repeated in 3 to 5 minutes with the same dose
    c. 2.5- to 5-mg slow IV push
    d. 5-mg/kg continuous IV infusion

31. Which of the following dysrhythmias is most easily confused with multifocal atrial tachycardia?
    a. Junctional rhythm
    b. Sinus tachycardia
    c. Atrial fibrillation
    d. VT

32. Select the correct statement regarding airway management.
    a. The laryngeal mask airway protects the lower airway from aspiration
    b. The purpose of cricoid pressure is to aid visualization of the vocal cords during intubation
    c. An ET tube cuff is inflated to isolate the lungs from the upper airway and reduce the risk of aspiration
    d. Use of a Combitube requires visualization of the vocal cords for proper placement

33. True or False. Some AEDs can detect the patient's transthoracic resistance through the adhesive pads applied to the patient's chest. The AED automatically adjusts the voltage and length of the shock, thus customizing how the energy is delivered to that patient.

34. An oral airway:
    a. Is of no value once an ET tube is inserted
    b. Eliminates the possibility of aspiration
    c. Eliminates the need for proper head positioning of an unresponsive patient
    d. May stimulate vomiting or laryngospasm in a semiresponsive patient

35. Synchronized cardioversion:
    a. Delivers a shock a few milliseconds after the highest or deepest part of the QRS complex
    b. Is used only for atrial dysrhythmias
    c. Delivers a shock between the peak and end of the T wave
    d. Is used only for rhythms with a ventricular rate of less than 60 per minute

36. Which of the following statements is **incorrect** regarding safety precautions during defibrillation or synchronized cardioversion?
    a. Remove supplemental O_2 sources from the area of the patient's bed before defibrillation and cardioversion attempts, placing them at least 3 1/2 to 4 feet away from the patient's chest
    b. Use adult defibrillator paddles/pads for all patients
    c. When using hand-held paddles, use gels or pastes that are specifically made for defibrillation
    d. When applying combination pads to a patient's bare chest, press from one edge of the pad across the entire surface to remove all air

37. Under optimal conditions, a nasal cannula will deliver approximately __ O_2 at a flow rate of 4 L/min.
    a. 25%
    b. 29%
    c. 37%
    d. 45%

38. If atropine is given endotracheally during a cardiac arrest, the correct dose is:
    a. 0.5 to 1 mg
    b. 2 to 2.5 mg
    c. 3 to 4 mg
    d. 4 to 5 mg

39. Which of the following statements is true about the administration of epinephrine during cardiac arrest?
    a. 1 mg of epinephrine 1:10,000 solution should be given rapid IV push every 3 to 5 minutes
    b. 1 mg of epinephrine 1:1000 solution should be given slow IV push over 3 to 5 minutes
    c. 2 to 2.5 mg of epinephrine 1:10,000 solution should be given rapid IV push every 3 to 5 minutes
    d. 2 to 2.5 mg of epinephrine 1:1000 solution should be given slow IV push over 3 to 5 minutes

40. CPR is in progress for a 44-year-old woman in cardiac arrest. The arrest was not witnessed. The cardiac monitor reveals the rhythm below.

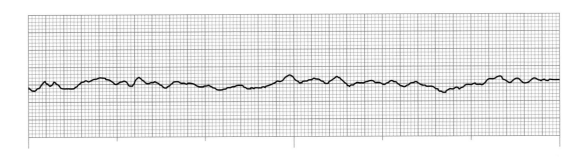

    Your next intervention should be to:
    a. Perform CPR for 2 minutes and then defibrillate
    b. Start an IV, give epinephrine, and then circulate the drug with CPR for 2 minutes
    c. Confirm the rhythm in a second lead, intubate, and then attempt transcutaneous pacing
    d. Insert an advanced airway, start an IV, give vasopressin, and then circulate the drug with CPR for 2 minutes

41. After witnessing the sudden cardiac arrest of a 48-year-old man, you delivered a shock that resulted in a sinus tachycardia on the cardiac monitor. A strong pulse is present. An IV is in place. No medications have been given. Which of the following statements is correct?
    a. Give amiodarone 300-mg IV bolus and then begin a maintenance infusion of the drug
    b. There is insufficient evidence to recommend for or against prophylactic administration of antiarrhythmic drugs to patients who have survived cardiac arrest from any cause
    c. There is clear evidence that giving antiarrhythmics after cardiac arrest is detrimental
    d. Give lidocaine 1.5-mg/kg IV over 10 minutes and then begin a maintenance infusion of the drug

42. The three major physical findings evaluated with the Cincinnati Prehospital Stroke Scale are:
    a. Eye movement, pupil reaction, and arm drift
    b. Best verbal response, facial droop, and eye opening
    c. Facial droop, arm drift, and speech abnormalities
    d. Best motor response, pupil reaction, and speech abnormalities

43. An 89-year-old man is complaining of chest discomfort and a "racing heart." He rates his discomfort a 4 on a 0-to-10 scale. He states his symptoms began while playing a card game with friends. He had an MI 15 years ago and a coronary artery bypass graft 5 years ago. His BP is 140/90, R 16. Breath sounds are clear. You have placed the patient on O_2 and started an IV. The cardiac monitor reveals the following rhythm:

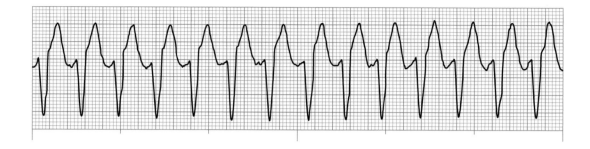

You should:
   a. Sedate the patient and then defibrillate with 360 joules
   b. Give a 2.5- to 5-mg IV bolus of verapamil over 3 minutes
   c. Give adenosine if you believe the rhythm is SVT, or amiodarone if you think it is more likely VT
   d. Give magnesium sulfate 1- to 2-g IV over 10 minutes

44. In the management of a symptomatic narrow-QRS bradycardia, if the maximum dose of atropine had been given and a pacemaker was not immediately available, your next course of action would include:
   a. Dopamine infusion, 2 to 10 mcg/kg/min
   b. Epinephrine 1-mg IV bolus followed by a 20-mL saline flush
   c. Amiodarone 150-mg IV over 10 minutes
   d. Lidocaine 1- to 1.5-mg/kg IV bolus followed by a 10-mL saline flush

45. Patients who experience a(n) __ MI have a greater incidence of CHF and cardiogenic shock than those who have MIs affecting other areas of the left ventricle.
   a. Inferior wall
   b. Anterior wall
   c. Lateral wall
   d. Posterior wall

Questions 46 through 49 pertain to the following scenario:

Paramedics arrive in the ED with a 23-year-old man who was shot in the chest.

46. The patient is unresponsive, not breathing, and has no pulse. CPR is in progress. An IV was established en route to the hospital. The patient is being ventilated with a bag-mask device connected to 100% O_2. A rhythm check reveals the following:

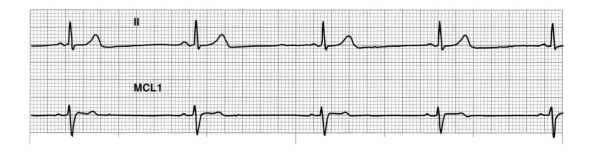

Which of the following ACLS treatment guidelines should be used in the initial treatment of this patient?
a. Symptomatic bradycardia
b. Asystole
c. Narrow-QRS tachycardia
d. PEA

47. While CPR is performed, positive-pressure ventilations should be delivered at a rate of:
a. 4 to 6 ventilations/min
b. 8 to 10 ventilations/min
c. 10 to 12 ventilations/min
d. 20 to 24 ventilations/min

48. You observe an entrance wound on the patient's left anterior chest. The team member who is ventilating the patient tells you that the patient is becoming more difficult to ventilate. You are able to hear breath sounds with positive-pressure ventilation on the right chest, but no sounds on the left. Based on these findings and the patient's mechanism of injury, you suspect:
a. Cardiac tamponade
b. Hypovolemia
c. Tension pneumothorax
d. Massive pulmonary embolism

49. Appropriate treatment at this time should include:
a. Needle decompression of the left chest
b. Immediate defibrillation
c. Preparations for transcutaneous pacing
d. Pericardiocentesis

50. Atypical chest discomfort is a phrase used to describe:
a. The absence of chest pain or discomfort
b. Chest pain or discomfort that is localized to the chest area but has musculoskeletal, positional, or pleuritic features
c. A patient who presents with dyspnea, palpitations, or syncope but no chest pain or discomfort
d. Chest pain or discomfort described as a pressure or tightness that may radiate to the left arm or neck

POSTTEST ANSWERS

1. d. The dose of adenosine should be decreased in patients on dipyridamole (Persantine), carbamazepine (Tegretol), those with transplanted hearts, or if given via a central IV line. Consider increasing the dose in patients on theophylline, caffeine, or theobromine.

2. a. From the information provided, the patient appears to be clinically stable despite the presence of monomorphic VT on the cardiac monitor. Amiodarone would be appropriate to consider in this situation. Dopamine increases the force of myocardial contraction, heart rate, and BP. Since this patient is not hypotensive and he has a rapid heart rate, dopamine is not indicated. NTG is a vasodilator. The patient has no complaint of chest pain and shows no signs of heart failure, so NTG is not indicated. Furosemide (Lasix) is also not indicated since there are no signs of pulmonary congestion.

3. b. No drugs used in cardiac arrest have been shown to improve survival to hospital discharge. In cardiac arrest due to pulseless VT/VF, a vasopressor (such as epinephrine or

vasopressin) should be given if the rhythm persists after delivery of 1 or 2 shocks and CPR. An antiarrhythmic can be considered if the rhythm persists after 2 to 3 shocks, CPR, and administration of a vasopressor. Amiodarone is not indicated in all cardiac arrests. For example, it may be used in cardiac arrest due to pulseless VT or VF but it is not indicated in cardiac arrest due to asystole or PEA.

4. b. From the information presented, it appears this patient is probably experiencing an acute coronary syndrome. Appropriate interventions in the management of this patient would include O_2, aspirin (if no contraindications), IV access, sublingual NTG, and morphine. The memory aid "MONA" (morphine, O_2, NTG, aspirin) is used to help recall the immediate general treatment measures that should be considered for a patient experiencing an acute coronary syndrome.

5. a. Immediate management of a patient who is experiencing a possible acute coronary syndrome includes ABCs, O_2, starting an IV, and giving aspirin as soon as possible (if there are no contraindications). The cardiac monitor shows a sinus tachycardia, which is most likely due to the patient's chest comfort and anxiety. Since atropine is used to increase heart rate, it is not indicated in this situation. Adenosine is used for symptomatic narrow-QRS tachycardias such as AVNRT and AVRT. It is not used for sinus tachycardia. Amiodarone may be used to treat many atrial and ventricular dysrhythmias, but it is not used for sinus tachycardia. The treatment of a sinus tachycardia is correction of the underlying cause.

6. c. The patient's 12-lead ECG shows ST-segment elevation in leads I, aVL, V_2, V_3, V_4, and V_5.

7.

I	Lateral	aVR	------------	V_1	Septum	V_4	Anterior	V_4R	Right Ventricle
II	Inferior	aVL	Lateral	V_2	Septum	V_5	Lateral	V_5R	Right Ventricle
III	Inferior	aVF	Inferior	V_3	Anterior	V_6	Lateral	V_6R	Right Ventricle

8.

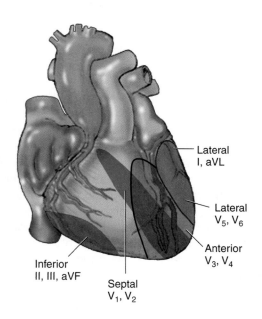

Lateral
I, aVL

Lateral
V_5, V_6

Anterior
V_3, V_4

Inferior
II, III, aVF

Septal
V_1, V_2

9. d. Two leads are contiguous if they look at the same area of the heart or if they are numerically consecutive chest leads. V_2, V_3, and V_4 are numerically consecutive chest leads.

10. b. The patient's 12-lead ECG shows ST-segment elevation in lead I, aVL, and V_2 through V_5. Because these leads view the lateral and anterior surfaces of the left ventricle, an anterolateral infarction is suspected.

11. a. NTG relaxes vascular smooth muscle, including dilation of the coronary arteries (particularly in the area of plaque disruption). It also decreases myocardial O_2 consumption. Morphine decreases anxiety, pain, and myocardial O_2 requirements. Beta-blockers have been shown to decrease the incidence of VF and decrease the incidence of sudden death associated with acute MI when given to patients without contraindications. Calcium channel blockers have not been shown to reduce mortality after acute MI and may be harmful in some patients with cardiovascular disease. They can be added as an alternative or additional therapy if beta-blockers are contraindicated or if the maximum dose has been given. Prophylactic administration of lidocaine to prevent VT or VF is not recommended. Routine administration of magnesium to patients with acute MI is not recommended.

12. c. The recommended dose of epinephrine, when administered via an ET tube, is 2 to 2.5 times the IV dose. Since the recommended IV dose is 1 mg, the ET dose would be 2 to 2.5 mg.

13. b. Absence of chest wall expansion and gurgling heard over the epigastrium indicate misplacement of the ET tube into the esophagus. If breath sounds were present bilaterally with bag-mask ventilation before placement of an ET tube, the presence of breath sounds on only the right side of the chest after placement of the tube suggests right mainstem bronchus intubation.

14. b. Atypical symptoms or unusual presentations of acute coronary syndromes are more common in older adults, women, and diabetic individuals.

15. a. When defibrillating (or cardioverting) a patient with a permanent (implanted) pacemaker or implantable cardioverter-defibrillator (ICD), be careful not to place the defibrillator paddles or combination pads directly over the device. Place defibrillator paddles or combination pads at least 1 inch (2.5 cm) from the pulse generator (bulge under the patient's skin). If the device is located in the patient's left pectoral area, standard sternum-apex paddle/pad placement for defibrillation is acceptable. If the device is located in the right pectoral area, anterior-posterior paddle/pad placement can be used. Because some of the defibrillation current flows down the pacemaker leads, a patient who has a permanent pacemaker or ICD should have the device checked to ensure proper function after defibrillation.

16. b. Appropriate care at this time includes immediate defibrillation.

17. c. The rhythm shown is a sinus rhythm with ST-segment elevation.

18. b. ST-segment elevation is considered significant when it is >1 mm in two or more contiguous leads. Some cardiologists use a more stringent requirement for ST-segment elevation. In this alternate means of infarct recognition, at least 2 mm of ST-segment elevation is required in the chest leads before infarction is suspected. Each method has its advantage: The 1-mm threshold for ST-segment elevation favors sensitivity, and the 2-mm criteria favors specificity. Sensitivity refers to a test's ability to identify true disease. Specificity refers to a test that is correctly negative in the absence of disease. A test with high specificity has few false-positives.

19. d. The patient's initial 12-lead ECG should be reviewed and the patient classified into one of three categories: ST-segment elevation, ST-segment depression, or normal/nondiagnostic ECG.

20. b. Leads II, III, and aVF view the inferior wall of the left ventricle. About 50% of patients with inferior infarction have some involvement of the right ventricle. Since an inferior MI is suspected, right chest leads should be quickly used to rule out RVI before giving medications for pain relief. Morphine and NTG are vasodilators, and thus they reduce preload. This reduction in preload, while usually beneficial, can be undesirable in the setting of RVI and may cause profound hypotension. Therefore, caution must be exercised when giving NTG and morphine to patients experiencing RVI.

21. b. Transcutaneous pacing is an appropriate treatment option for any symptomatic bradycardia. It is no longer recommended for asystolic cardiac arrest.

22. d. The rhythm shown is a third-degree AV block with ST-segment elevation.

23. d. Atropine is usually ineffective for wide-QRS bradycardias. Your best course of action will be to prepare for immediate transcutaneous pacing. Although epinephrine can be used in the management of a symptomatic bradycardia, it is given as a continuous IV infusion, <u>not</u> as an IV bolus.

24. a. Furosemide is a venodilator and potent diuretic used in the management of acute pulmonary edema. The usual dose is 0.5 to 1 mg/kg. Use less than 0.5 mg/kg for new onset acute pulmonary edema without hypovolemia. Use 1 mg/kg for acute or chronic volume overload or renal insufficiency.

25. c. An antiarrhythmic can be considered during cardiac arrest, but there is no evidence that any antiarrhythmic drug given routinely during human cardiac arrest increases survival to hospital discharge.

26. True. When pulseless VT/VF is present, defibrillation is indicated. When the team leader indicates it is time to deliver a shock, all team members with the exception of the person performing chest compressions should immediately clear the patient. The airway team member must make sure that O_2 is not flowing near the patient's chest. Once the defibrillator is charged, the chest compressor should clear the patient and a shock should be delivered immediately to the patient. In this way, chest compressions are interrupted for the least amount of time possible during the resuscitation effort. After the shock is delivered, immediately resume CPR, starting with chest compressions. Perform five cycles of CPR (about 2 minutes), and then recheck the patient's rhythm.

27. True. Bradydysrhythmias, including second-degree AV block type I (Wenckebach), are common complications of an inferior wall MI.

28. c. Currently, the window of opportunity to use IV recombinant tissue-type plasminogen activator (rtPA) to treat ischemic stroke patients is 3 hours. The window for intra-arterial fibrinolytics is about 6 hours. The time from onset of stroke symptoms until treatment is a key factor for success of any therapy. The earlier the treatment for stroke, the more favorable the results are likely to be. Blood flow needs to be restored to the affected area as quickly as possible.

29. b. NTG relaxes vascular smooth muscle, including dilation of the coronary arteries (particularly in the area of plaque disruption). It also decreases myocardial O_2 consumption. Before giving NTG, make sure an IV is in place, the patient's systolic BP is >90 mm Hg, the patient's heart rate is >50 and <100 bpm, there are no signs of RVI, and the patient has not used Viagra, Cialis, or similar medication in the previous 24 to 48 hours. The onset of action of sublingual NTG is typically within 1 to 3 minutes; IV NTG within about 1.5 minutes.

30. a. In cardiac arrest due to torsades de pointes, magnesium sulfate is given via an IV/IO push. The dosage is 1 to 2 g (2 to 4 mL of 50% solution) diluted in 10 mL.

31. c. Multifocal AT may be confused with atrial fibrillation since both rhythms are irregular; however, P waves (although varying in size, shape, and direction) are clearly visible in multifocal AT.

32. c. An ET cuff is inflated to isolate the lungs from the upper airway and reduce the risk of aspiration. ET intubation *reduces*, but does not eliminate, the risk of aspiration. The laryngeal mask airway may be used as an alternative to either an ET tube or a face mask with either spontaneous or positive-pressure ventilation; however, the laryngeal mask airway does **not** provide protection against aspiration. Cricoid pressure (Sellick maneuver) compresses and occludes the esophagus between the cricoid cartilage and the fifth and sixth cervical vertebrae, minimizing gastric distention and aspiration during positive-pressure ventilation. Cricoid pressure is <u>not</u> intended to facilitate visualization of the vocal cords during intubation. The esophageal-tracheal Combitube allows ventilation of the lungs and reduces the risk of aspiration of gastric contents. It does not require visualization of the vocal cords (blind insertion) to ventilate the trachea.

33. True. Some AEDs can detect the patient's transthoracic resistance through the adhesive pads applied to the patient's chest. The AED automatically adjusts the voltage and length of the shock, thus customizing how the energy is delivered to that patient.

34. d. An oral airway is used to help maintain an open airway in an unresponsive patient who is not intubated, help maintain an open airway in an unresponsive patient with no gag reflex who is being ventilated with a bag-mask or other positive-pressure device, and may be used as a bite block after insertion of an ET tube or orogastric tube. It does not protect the lower airway from aspiration and may produce vomiting if used in a responsive or semiresponsive patient with a gag reflex. Use of the device does not eliminate the need for maintaining proper head position.

35. a. Synchronized cardioversion is the timed delivery of a shock during the QRS complex. It is indicated in the management of a patient who is exhibiting serious signs and symptoms related to a tachycardia. It is used to treat rhythms that have a clearly identifiable QRS complex and a rapid ventricular rate (such as some narrow-QRS tachycardias and VT).

36. b. To prevent fires during defibrillation attempts, remove supplemental O_2 sources from the area of the patient's bed before defibrillation and cardioversion attempts and place them at least 3 1/2 to 4 feet away from the patient's chest. Be sure to use defibrillator paddles/pads of the appropriate size. Adult paddles/pads should be used for patients >10 kg. Use pediatric paddles/pads for patients <10 kg. When applying combination pads to a patient's bare chest, press from one edge of the pad across the entire surface to remove all air. Do not use gels or pastes that are not specifically made for defibrillation (such as ultrasound gel). Use of improper pastes, creams, gels, or pads can cause burns or sparks and pose a risk of fire in an O_2-enriched environment.

37. c. Although the actual inspired O_2 concentration depends on the patient's respiratory rate and depth, a nasal cannula can deliver O_2 concentrations of about 25% to 45% at 1 to 6 L/min flow. Using the formula (4 × the O_2 flow rate in L/min) + 21% (room air) = (4 × 4) + 21 = 37%.

38. b. Although the optimal ET dose of most drugs is unknown, the resuscitation guidelines recommend 2 to 2.5 times the IV dose for some ET drugs. Since the cardiac arrest dose of atropine is 1 mg, the ET dose is 2 to 2.5 mg.

39. a. When giving IV epinephrine in cardiac arrest, use the 1:10,000 solution. Give the drug as quickly as possible, follow it with a 20-mL flush of IV solution, and raise the extremity to help speed the delivery of the drug to the central circulation.

40. a. During a cardiac arrest, your two most important priorities are CPR and, if a shockable rhythm is present, defibrillation. Vascular access, giving drugs, and inserting an advanced airway are of secondary importance. In this situation, the cardiac monitor shows VF. After five cycles of CPR (about 2 minutes), attempt defibrillation.

41. b. There is insufficient evidence to recommend for or against prophylactic administration of antiarrhythmic drugs to patients who have survived cardiac arrest from any cause.

42. c. The three major physical findings evaluated with the Cincinnati Prehospital Stroke Scale are facial droop, arm drift, and speech abnormalities. If any one of these signs is abnormal, the stroke probability = 72%.

43. c. The rhythm shown is a wide-QRS tachycardia with a regular ventricular rhythm. Based on a single rhythm strip, it is difficult to tell if the rhythm is monomorphic VT or SVT with aberrant conduction. A 12-lead ECG should be obtained to help determine the origin of the rhythm. Give adenosine if you believe the rhythm is SVT, or amiodarone if you think it is more likely VT. Verapamil is contraindicated in the treatment of a wide-QRS tachycardia unless it is **known with certainty** to be supraventricular in origin. Magnesium sulfate is used in the treatment of torsades de pointes and for rhythm control of atrial fibrillation ≤48 hours duration. It is not indicated in this situation.

44. a. Your next course of action would include a dopamine infusion at 2 to 10 mcg/kg/min. Epinephrine is given by continuous IV infusion (not IV bolus) in the treatment of a symptomatic bradycardia. Amiodarone and lidocaine are not indicated in the treatment of a symptomatic bradycardia.

45. b. Patients who experience an **anterior** MI have a greater incidence of congestive heart failure and cardiogenic shock than those who have MIs affecting other areas of the left ventricle.

46. d. Despite the presence of an organized rhythm on the monitor, the patient has no pulse. This situation is PEA.

47. c. Positive-pressure ventilations should be delivered at a rate of 10 to 12 ventilations per minute (1 ventilation every 5 to 6 seconds). If an advanced airway is inserted, the rate of ventilations should be decreased to 8 to 10 per minute with no pauses for ventilations during chest compressions.

48. c. Based on the patient's mechanism of injury, the absence of breath sounds with positive-pressure ventilation on the left chest, and the increasing difficulty in ventilating the patient, you should suspect a tension pneumothorax.

49. a. Since a tension pneumothorax is suspected, definitive treatment includes needle decompression (also called needle thoracostomy). Needle decompression is the insertion of an over-the-needle catheter into the chest (second intercostal space, midclavicular line on the affected side, which is the left side in this case) to relieve a tension pneumothorax. The procedure converts a tension pneumothorax to a simple open pneumothorax. In the hospital, this procedure is typically followed by insertion of a chest tube.

50. b. Atypical chest discomfort is localized to the chest area but has musculoskeletal, positional, or pleuritic features.

Glossary

absolute refractory period   Corresponds with the onset of the QRS complex to approximately the peak of the T wave; cardiac cells cannot be stimulated to conduct an electrical impulse, no matter how strong the stimulus.

accelerated idioventricular rhythm (AIVR)   Dysrhythmia originating in the ventricles with a rate between 41 and 100 bpm.

accessory pathway   Extra muscle bundle consisting of working myocardial tissue that forms a connection between the atria and ventricles outside the normal conduction system.

acute coronary syndromes (ACS)   A term used to refer to patients presenting with ischemic chest discomfort. Acute coronary syndromes consist of three major syndromes: unstable angina, non–ST-segment elevation MI, and ST-segment elevation MI.

advance directive   A written document recording an individual's decisions concerning medical treatment that is applied (or not applied) in the event of physical or mental inability to communicate these wishes.

afterload   The pressure or resistance against which the ventricles must pump to eject blood.

angina   Chest discomfort of sudden onset that may occur because the increased oxygen demand of the heart temporarily exceeds the blood supply.

anginal equivalents   Symptoms of myocardial ischemia other than chest pain or discomfort.

arteriosclerosis   A chronic disease of the arterial system characterized by abnormal thickening and hardening of the vessel walls.

asthma   A reversible obstructive airway disease characterized by chronic airway inflammation, episodes of bronchoconstriction, and mucus plugging.

atherosclerosis   Athero = gruel or paste; sclerosis = hardness. A form of arteriosclerosis in which the thickening and hardening of the vessel walls are caused by a buildup of fat-like deposits in the inner lining of large and middle-sized muscular arteries. As the fatty deposits build up, the opening of the artery slowly narrows and blood flow to the muscle decreases.

automated external defibrillation   The placement of paddles or pads on a patient's chest and interpretation of the patient's cardiac rhythm by the defibrillator's computerized analysis system. Depending on the type of automated external defibrillator (AED) used, the machine will deliver a shock (if a shockable rhythm is detected) or instruct the operator to deliver a shock.

automated external defibrillator (AED)   A machine with a sophisticated computer system that analyzes a patient's heart rhythm using an algorithm to distinguish shockable rhythms from nonshockable rhythms. If a shockable rhythm is detected, it directs the rescuer to deliver an electrical shock.

automaticity   The ability of cardiac pacemaker cells to spontaneously initiate an electrical impulse without being stimulated from another source (such as a nerve).

AV junction   Atrioventricular node and the bundle of His.

biphasic   A waveform that is partly positive and partly negative.

bipolar limb lead   ECG lead consisting of a positive and negative electrode.

bypass tract   Term used when one end of an accessory pathway is attached to normal conductive tissue.

capacitor   A device for storing an electrical charge.

capnograph   A device that provides a numerical reading of exhaled CO_2 concentrations and a waveform (tracing).

capnography   The continuous analysis and recording of CO_2 concentrations in respiratory gases.

capnometer   A device that measures the concentration of CO_2 at the end of exhalation.

capnometry   A numerical reading of exhaled CO_2 concentrations without a continuous written record or waveform.

cardiac output   The amount of blood pumped into the aorta each minute by the heart. It is defined as the stroke volume (amount of blood ejected from a ventricle with each heartbeat) times the heart rate.

cardiopulmonary arrest   The absence of cardiac mechanical activity, confirmed by the absence of a detectable pulse, unresponsiveness, and apnea or agonal, gasping respiration; also called cardiac arrest.

cardiovascular disorders   A collection of diseases and conditions that involve the heart (cardio) and blood vessels (vascular).

carina   The point where the trachea divides into the right and left mainstem bronchi.

cellulitis   A diffuse inflammation and infection of cellular and subcutaneous connective tissue that can lead to abscess formation and ulceration of deeper tissues.

cerebral resuscitation   A term used to emphasize the need to preserve the viability of the cardiac arrest victim's brain.

Chain of Survival   Four interrelated steps that represent the ideal series of events that should take place immediately following the recognition of onset of sudden illness.

compliance   The resistance of the patient's lung tissue to ventilation.

conductivity   Ability of a cardiac cell to receive an electrical stimulus and conduct that impulse to the next cardiac cell.

contractility   Ability of cardiac cells to shorten, causing cardiac muscle contraction in response to an electrical stimulus.

coronary artery disease   Disease that affects the arteries that supply the heart muscle with blood.

coronary heart disease   Disease of the coronary arteries and their resulting complications, such as angina pectoris or acute myocardial infarction.

coronary perfusion pressure (CPP)   The difference between the aortic relaxation (diastolic) pressure and the right atrial relaxation (diastolic) blood pressure during CPR.

cough version Forceful and repetitive coughing every 1 to 3 seconds; also called "cough CPR."

countershock The delivery of an electrical current through the myocardium over a very brief period to terminate a cardiac dysrhythmia. There are two types of countershock: defibrillation and cardioversion.

C-reactive protein (CRP) A protein produced by the liver and released into the bloodstream when there is active inflammation in the body.

cricothyroid membrane A fibrous membrane located between the cricoid and thyroid cartilages.

defibrillation Delivery of an unsynchronized electrical current across the heart muscle over a very brief period to terminate an abnormal heart rhythm.

defibrillation threshold The least amount of energy in joules or volts delivered to the heart that reproducibly reverts VF to a normal rhythm.

defibrillator A device used to administer an electrical shock at a preset energy level to terminate a cardiac dysrhythmia.

delta wave Slurring of the beginning portion of the QRS complex, caused by preexcitation.

depolarization Movement of ions across a cell membrane, causing the inside of the cell to become more positive; an electrical event expected to result in contraction.

drowning A process resulting in primary respiratory impairment from submersion/immersion in a liquid medium.

durable power of attorney for healthcare A type of advance directive that identifies a legal guardian to make healthcare decisions for a patient when the patient can no longer make such decisions for him- or herself; also called a "healthcare proxy" or "appointment of a healthcare agent."

ejection fraction The percentage of total ventricular volume ejected during each myocardial contraction; used as a measure of ventricular function; normal is about 65%.

electrocardiogram (ECG) A recording of the heart's electrical activity that appears on ECG paper as specific waveforms and complexes.

electrode A paper, plastic, or metal device that contains conductive gel and is applied to the patient's skin.

endocardium Innermost layer of the heart that lines the inside of the myocardium and covers the heart valves.

endotracheal (ET) intubation An advanced airway procedure in which a tube is placed directly into the trachea.

epicardium Also known as the visceral pericardium; the external layer of the heart wall that covers the heart muscle.

epiglottis A small, leaf-shaped cartilage located at the top of the larynx that prevents food from entering the respiratory tract during swallowing.

excitability Ability of cardiac muscle cells to respond to an external stimulus, such as that from a chemical, mechanical, or electrical source; also known as irritability.

exhaled CO_2 detector A capnometer that provides a noninvasive estimate of alveolar ventilation, the concentration of exhaled carbon dioxide (CO_2) from the lungs, and arterial CO_2 content; also called an end-tidal CO_2 detector.

extravasation The actual (unintentional) escape or leakage of an agent that is irritating and causes blistering (a vesicant) from a vessel into the surrounding tissue.

failure to capture The inability of a pacemaker stimulus to depolarize the myocardium.

failure to pace A pacemaker malfunction that occurs when the pacemaker fails to deliver an electrical stimulus or when it fails to deliver the correct number of electrical stimulations per minute.

fibrinogen A protein produced by the liver and necessary for normal blood clotting.

fibrinolysis Dissolving of a blood clot; occurs naturally by plasmin or by a class of medications called fibrinolytics.

glottis The true vocal cords and the space between them.

hard palate Bony portion of the roof of the mouth that forms the floor of the nasal cavity.

heart disease A broad term that refers to conditions affecting the heart.

impedance Resistance to the flow of current. Transthoracic impedance (resistance) refers to the resistance of the chest wall to current.

infiltration The intentional or unintentional process in which a substance enters or infuses into another substance or a surrounding area.

insulin resistance A condition in which the normal amount of insulin secreted by the pancreas is not enough to cause an effect in body cells.

intraosseous infusion The infusion of fluids, medications, or blood directly into the bone marrow cavity.

intravenous cannulation The placement of a catheter into a vein to gain access to the body's venous circulation.

irritability Ability of cardiac muscle cells to respond to an external stimulus, such as that from a chemical, mechanical, or electrical source; also known as excitability.

ischemia A decreased supply of oxygenated blood to a body part or organ.

isoelectric A waveform that rests on the baseline.

J-point The point where the QRS complex and ST-segment meet.

joule The basic unit of energy; equivalent to watt-seconds.

living will A type of advance directive in which the patient puts in writing his or her wishes about medical treatment should he or she become terminally ill and incapable of making decisions regarding his or her medical care.

Lown-Ganong-Levine (LGL) syndrome A type of preexcitation syndrome in which part or all of the AV conduction system is bypassed by an abnormal AV connection from the atrial muscle to the bundle of His; characterized by a short PR interval (PRI; usually less than 0.12 sec) and a normal QRS duration.

manual defibrillation The placement of paddles or pads on a patient's chest, interpretation of the patient's cardiac rhythm by a trained healthcare professional, and the healthcare professional's decision to deliver a shock (if indicated).

medical emergency team (MET) In the hospital setting, a team typically consisting of a physician and nurse with critical care training who are available at all times to respond when summoned by other hospital staff.

minute volume The amount of air moved in and out of the lungs in 1 minute.

monomorphic Having the same shape.

myocardial infarction (MI) Death of some mass of the heart muscle due to an inadequate blood supply.

nasal cannula A piece of plastic tubing with two soft prongs that project from the tubing; used to delivery supplemental oxygen to a spontaneously breathing patient.

neurotransmitter A chemical responsible for transmission of an impulse across a synapse.

ohm The basic unit of measurement of resistance.

pacemaker Artificial pulse generator that delivers an electrical current to the heart to stimulate depolarization.

pacemaker spike   A vertical line on the ECG that indicates the pacemaker has discharged.

paroxysmal supraventricular tachycardia (PSVT)   A regular, narrow-QRS tachycardia that starts or ends suddenly.

periarrest period   The interval preceding a cardiac arrest and the immediate postresuscitation interval; 1 hour before and 1 hour after a cardiac arrest.

pocket mask   A clear semirigid mask designed for mouth-to-mask ventilation of a nonbreathing adult, child, or infant.

poison   A substance that, on ingestion, inhalation, absorption, application, injection, or development within the body in relatively small amounts, may cause structural damage or functional disturbance.

polarization   The resting state during which no electrical activity occurs in the heart.

polymorphic   Varying in shape.

positive-pressure ventilation   Forcing air into the lungs.

prearrest period   The interval preceding a cardiac arrest.

precordial thump   A forceful blow delivered to the lower half of the sternum to terminate VT or VF.

preexcitation   A term used to describe rhythms that originate from above the ventricles but in which the impulse travels via a pathway other than the AV node and bundle of His.

preload   The force exerted by the blood on the walls of the ventricles at the end of diastole.

proarrhythmia   A new or worsened rhythm disturbance paradoxically precipitated by treatment with antiarrhythmic medications.

public access defibrillation   Defibrillation performed by citizens at the scene of a cardiac arrest.

pulse oximetry   A noninvasive method of measuring the percentage of oxygen saturated in the blood (SpO_2).

pulseless electrical activity (PEA)   Organized electrical activity observed on a cardiac monitor (other than VT) without the patient having a palpable pulse.

refractoriness   The extent to which a cell is able to respond to a stimulus.

relative refractory period   Corresponds with the downslope of the T wave; cardiac cells can be stimulated to depolarize if the stimulus is strong enough.

repolarization   Movement of ions across a cell membrane in which the inside of the cell is restored to its negative charge.

reversible ischemic neurologic deficit (RIND)   A neurological deficit that last more than 24 hours but leaves little or no neurologic deficit.

risk factors   Traits and lifestyle habits that may increase a person's chance of developing a disease.

Sedentary Death Syndrome (SeDS)   A term used by researchers to represent the growing number of health conditions caused or worsened by a lack of adequate physical activity.

Sellick maneuver   Technique used to compress the cricoid cartilage against the cervical vertebrae, causing occlusion of the esophagus, thereby reducing the risk of aspiration; cricoid pressure.

shock   Inadequate tissue perfusion that results from the failure of the cardiovascular system to deliver enough oxygen and nutrients to sustain vital organ function.

simple face mask   An oxygen delivery device that consists of a plastic reservoir that fits over a patient's nose and mouth and a small diameter tube connected to the base of the mask through which oxygen is delivered.

sinoatrial node   Primary pacemaker of the heart that normally discharges at a rhythmic rate of 60 to 100 bpm.

soft palate   The back part of the roof of the mouth that is made up of mucous membrane, muscular fibers, and mucous glands.

speed shock   A systemic reaction to the rapid or excessive infusion of medication or solution into the circulation.

stroke   A sudden change in neurologic function caused by a change in cerebral blood flow.

stylet   A flexible plastic-coated wire that is inserted into an endotracheal tube to mold and maintain the shape of the tube.

sudden cardiac death   An unexpected death due to a cardiac cause that occurs either immediately or within 1 hour of the onset of symptoms.

supernormal period   Time during repolarization in which a weaker than normal stimulus can cause depolarization of cardiac cells.

supraventricular   Originating from a site above the bifurcation of the bundle of His, such as the sinoatrial node, atria, or AV junction.

supraventricular arrhythmias (SVA)   Rhythms that begin in the SA node, atrial tissue, or the AV junction.

synapse   The junction between two neurons.

synchronized cardioversion   The timed delivery of a shock during the QRS complex.

tidal volume   The volume of air moved into or out of the lungs during a normal breath.

transient ischemic attack (TIA)   A brief episode of neurologic dysfunction caused by focal brain or retinal ischemia, with clinical symptoms typically lasting less than 1 hour, and without evidence of acute infarction.

transthoracic impedance (resistance)   The resistance of the chest wall to current.

uvula   Fleshy tissue resembling a grape that hangs down from the soft palate.

vallecula   The space or "pocket" between the base of the tongue and the epiglottis.

vital capacity   The maximum volume of air that can be exhaled at the normal rate of exhalation after a maximum inhalation; the sum of the inspiratory reserve volume, tidal volume, and expiratory reserve volume; normally about 4600 mL.

voltage   The electrical pressure that drives current through a defibrillator circuit (such as the chest). The process of active medical resuscitation in the presence of family members.

Wolff-Parkinson-White (WPW) syndrome   Type of preexcitation syndrome, characterized by a slurred upstroke of the QRS complex (delta wave) and wide QRS.

Illustration Credits

Pretest

All illustrations from Aehlert B: ECGs Made Easy Study Cards, St. Louis, 2004, Mosby.

Chapter 1

1-1 Zipes D: Braunwald's Heart Disease: A Textbook of Cardiovascular Medicine, ed 7, Philadelphia, 2005, Saunders.

1-3, 1-4 Chapleau W: Emergency First Responder: Making the Difference, St. Louis, 2004, Mosby.

1-5 Zipes D: Braunwald's Heart Disease: A Textbook of Cardiovascular Medicine, ed 7, Philadelphia, 2005, Saunders.

1-8, 1-9, 1-10, 1-11, 1-12, 1-13 Chapleau W: Emergency First Responder: Making the Difference, St. Louis, 2004, Mosby.

1-16 Cummins R: ACLS Scenarios: Core Concepts for Case-Based Learning. St. Louis, 1996, Mosby Year-Book.

Chapter 2

2-1, 2-2, 2-3, 2-4, 2-5 Thibodeau G, Patton K: Anatomy & Physiology, ed 5, St. Louis, 2003, Mosby.

2-6, 2-7 Herlihy B, Maebius N: The Human Body in Health and Illness, ed 2, St. Louis, 2003, Saunders.

2-8, 2-9 Shade B, Rothenberg M, Wertz E, Jones S, Collins T: Mosby's EMT-Intermediate Textbook, ed 2, St. Louis, 2002, Mosby.

2-10 Sanders M: Mosby's Paramedic Textbook, ed 3, St. Louis, 2005, Mosby.

2-11 Henry M, Stapleton E: EMT Prehospital Care, ed 3, St. Louis, 2004, Mosby.

2-12 Stoy W: Mosby's EMT-Basic Textbook, St. Louis, 1996, Mosby.

2-13a: Henry M, Stapleton E: EMT Prehospital Care, ed 3, St. Louis, 2004, Mosby.

2-13b: Adapted from Kersten LD: Comprehensive Respiratory Nursing: A Decision-Making Approach. Philadelphia, WB Saunders, 1989.

2-14 Stoy W, Platt T, Lejeune D: Mosby's EMT-Basic Textbook, ed 2, St. Louis, 2005, Mosby.

2-15 Sanders M: Mosby's Paramedic Textbook, ed 3, St. Louis, 2005, Mosby.

2-16 Cummins R: ACLS Scenarios: Core Concepts for Case-Based Learning. St. Louis, 1996, Mosby Year-Book.

2-17, 2-18 Sanders M: Mosby's Paramedic Textbook, ed 3, St. Louis, 2005, Mosby.

2-19 Stoy W, Platt T, Lejeune D: Mosby's EMT-Basic Textbook, ed 2, St. Louis, 2005, Mosby.

2-20, 2-21, 2-22, 2-23 Shade B, Rothenberg M, Wertz E, Jones S, Collins T: Mosby's EMT-Intermediate Textbook, ed 2, St. Louis, 2002, Mosby.

2-24 Stoy W, Platt T, Lejeune D: Mosby's EMT-Basic Textbook, ed 2, St. Louis, 2005, Mosby.

2-25, 2-26 McSwain N, Paturas J: The Basic EMT, ed 2, St. Louis, 2003, Mosby.

2-27 Stoy W, Platt T, Lejeune D: Mosby's EMT-Basic Textbook, ed 2, St. Louis, 2005, Mosby.

2-28 Sanders M: Mosby's Paramedic Textbook, ed 3, St. Louis, 2005, Mosby.

2-29 McSwain N, Paturas J: The Basic EMT, ed 2, St. Louis, 2003, Mosby.

2-30 Sanders M: Mosby's Paramedic Textbook, ed 3, St. Louis, 2005, Mosby.

2-31 Stoy W, Platt T, Lejeune D: Mosby's EMT-Basic Textbook, ed 2, St. Louis, 2005, Mosby.

2-32 Henry M, Stapleton E: EMT Prehospital Care, ed 3, St. Louis, 2004, Mosby.

2-33 Stoy W, Platt T, Lejeune D: Mosby's EMT-Basic Textbook, ed 2, St. Louis, 2005, Mosby.

2-34 Sanders M: Mosby's Paramedic Textbook, ed 3, St. Louis, 2005, Mosby.

2-35, 2-36, 2-37, 2-38 Shade B, Rothenberg M, Wertz E, Jones S, Collins T: Mosby's EMT-Intermediate Textbook, ed 2, St. Louis, 2002, Mosby.

2-39, 2-40, 2-41, 2-42 Cummins R: ACLS Scenarios: Core Concepts for Case-Based Learning. St. Louis, 1996, Mosby Year-Book.

2-43a Courtesy Allied Healthcare Products, Inc.

2-43b Courtesy O Two Medical Technologies, Inc.

2-44 Sanders M: Mosby's Paramedic Textbook, ed 3, St. Louis, 2005, Mosby.

2-45, 2-46 Shade B, Rothenberg M, Wertz E, Jones S, Collins T: Mosby's EMT-Intermediate Textbook, ed 2, St. Louis, 2002, Mosby.

2-47 Basket PJF, Brain AIJ: The use of the LMA. In Basket PJF, Brain AIJ (eds): Cardiopulmonary Resuscitation Handbook. London, Intavent Research, 1994.

2-48 Shade B, Rothenberg M, Wertz E, Jones S, Collins T: Mosby's EMT-Intermediate Textbook, ed 2, St. Louis, 2002, Mosby.

2-49 Sanders M: Mosby's Paramedic Textbook, ed 3, St. Louis, 2005, Mosby.

2-50 Shade B, Rothenberg M, Wertz E, Jones S, Collins T: Mosby's EMT-Intermediate Textbook, ed 2, St. Louis, 2002, Mosby.

2-51 Sanders M: Mosby's Paramedic Textbook, ed 3, St. Louis, 2005, Mosby.

2-52 Shade B, Rothenberg M, Wertz E, Jones S, Collins T: Mosby's EMT-Intermediate Textbook, ed 2, St. Louis, 2002, Mosby.

2-53 Shade B, Rothenberg M, Wertz E, Jones S, Collins T: Mosby's EMT-Intermediate Textbook, ed 2, St. Louis, 2002, Mosby.

2-54 Sanders M: Mosby's Paramedic Textbook, ed 3, St. Louis, 2005, Mosby.

2-55 Roberts J, Hedges J: Clinical Procedures in Emergency Medicine, ed 4, Philadelphia, 2004, Saunders.

2-56 Sanders M: Mosby's Paramedic Textbook, ed 3, St. Louis, 2005, Mosby.

2-57, 2-58 Shade B, Rothenberg M, Wertz E, Jones S, Collins T: Mosby's EMT-Intermediate Textbook, ed 2, St. Louis, 2002, Mosby.

2-59 Sanders M: Mosby's Paramedic Textbook, ed 3, St. Louis, 2005, Mosby.

2-60 Shade B, Rothenberg M, Wertz E, Jones S, Collins T: Mosby's EMT-Intermediate Textbook, ed 2, St. Louis, 2002, Mosby.

2-61, 2-62 Sanders M: Mosby's Paramedic Textbook, ed 3, St. Louis, 2005, Mosby.

2-63, 2-64 Shade B, Rothenberg M, Wertz E, Jones S, Collins T: Mosby's EMT-Intermediate Textbook, ed 2, St. Louis, 2002, Mosby.

2-65 Sanders M: Mosby's Paramedic Textbook, ed 3, St. Louis, 2005, Mosby.

2-66 Shade B, Rothenberg M, Wertz E, Jones S, Collins T: Mosby's EMT-Intermediate Textbook, ed 2, St. Louis, 2002, Mosby.

2-15 Roberts J, Hedges J: Clinical Procedures in Emergency Medicine, ed 4, Philadelphia, 2004, Saunders.

Chapter 3

3-1 Herlihy B, Maebius N: The Human Body in Health and Illness, ed 2, St. Louis, 2003, Saunders.

3-2 Thibodeau G, Patton K: Anatomy & Physiology, ed 5, St. Louis, 2003, Mosby.

3-3 Huszar R: Basic Dysrhythmias: Interpretation & Management, ed 3, St. Louis, 2002, Mosby.

3-4, 3-5, 3-6, 3-7 Herlihy B, Maebius N: The Human Body in Health and Illness, ed 2, St. Louis, 2003, Saunders.

3-8 Aehlert B: ECGs Made Easy, ed 3, St. Louis, 2006, Mosby.

3-9 Courtesy Medtronic Emergency Response Systems.

3-10 Phalen T, Aehlert B: The 12-Lead ECG in Acute Coronary Syndromes, ed 2, St. Louis, 2006, Mosby.

3-11 Urden L, Stacy K, Lough M: Thelan's Critical Care Nursing: Diagnosis and Management, ed 5, St. Louis, 2006, Mosby.

3-12 Phalen T, Aehlert B: The 12-Lead ECG in Acute Coronary Syndromes, ed 2, St. Louis, 2006, Mosby.

3-13 Urden L, Stacy K, Lough M: Thelan's Critical Care Nursing: Diagnosis and Management, ed 5, St. Louis, 2006, Mosby.

3-14 Lounsbury P, Frye S: Cardiac Rhythm Disorders, A Nursing Approach, ed 2, St. Louis, 1992, Mosby.

3-15 Urden L, Stacy K, Lough M: Thelan's Critical Care Nursing: Diagnosis and Management, ed 5, St. Louis, 2006, Mosby.

3-16 Aehlert B: ECGs Made Easy, ed 3, St. Louis, 2006, Mosby.

3-17, 3-18 Thibodeau G, Patton K: Anatomy & Physiology, ed 5, St. Louis, 2003, Mosby.

3-19 Urden L, Stacy K, Lough M: Thelan's Critical Care Nursing: Diagnosis and Management, ed 5, St. Louis, 2006, Mosby.

3-20 Grauer K: A Practical Guide to ECG Interpretation, ed 2, St. Louis, 1998, Mosby.

3-21 Goldberger A: Clinical Electrocardiography: A Simplified Approach, ed 6, St. Louis, 1999, Mosby.

3-22 Aehlert B: ECGs Made Easy, ed 3, St. Louis, 2006, Mosby.

3-23 Crawford MV, Spence MI: Commonsense Approach to Coronary Care, rev ed 6, St. Louis, 1994, Mosby.

3-24 Urden L, Stacy K, Lough M: Thelan's Critical Care Nursing: Diagnosis and Management, ed 5, St. Louis, 2006, Mosby.

3-25 Crawford MV, Spence MI: Commonsense Approach to Coronary Care, rev ed 6, St. Louis, 1994, Mosby.

3-26, 3-27 Aehlert B: ECGs Made Easy Study Cards, St. Louis, 2004, Mosby.

3-28A Shade B, Rothenberg M, Wertz E, Jones S, Collins T: Mosby's EMT-Intermediate Textbook, ed 2, St. Louis, 2002, Mosby.

3-28B Aehlert B: ECGs Made Easy Study Cards, St. Louis, 2004, Mosby.

3-29 Goldberger A: Clinical Electrocardiography: A Simplified Approach, ed 6, St. Louis, 1999, Mosby.

3-30 Phalen T, Aehlert B: The 12-Lead ECG in Acute Coronary Syndromes, ed 2, St. Louis, 2006, Mosby.

3-31 Goldman L, Braunwald E: Primary Cardiology, Philadelphia, 1998, Saunders.

3-32 Aehlert B: ECGs Made Easy, ed 2, St. Louis, 2002, Mosby.

3-33 Urden L, Stacy K, Lough M: Thelan's Critical Care Nursing: Diagnosis and Management, ed 4, St. Louis, 2006, Mosby.

3-34 Crawford MV, Spence MI: Commonsense Approach to Coronary Care, rev ed 6, St. Louis, 1994, Mosby.

3-35 Surawicz B, Knilans TK: Chou's Electrocardiography in Clinical Practice: Adult and Pediatric, ed 5, Philadelphia, 1996, Saunders.

3-36, 3-37 Aehlert B: ECGs Made Easy, ed 3, St. Louis, 2006, Mosby.

3-38, 3-39 Phalen T, Aehlert B: The 12-Lead ECG in Acute Coronary Syndromes, ed 2, St. Louis, 2006, Mosby.

3-40 Aehlert B: ECGs Made Easy, ed 3, St. Louis, 2006, Mosby.

3-41 Crawford MV, Spence MI: Commonsense Approach to Coronary Care, rev ed 6, St. Louis, 1994, Mosby.

3-42 Aehlert B: ECGs Made Easy Study Cards, St. Louis, 2004, Mosby.

3-43 Goldberger A: Clinical Electrocardiography: A Simplified Approach, ed 6, St. Louis, 1999, Mosby.

3-44 Aehlert B: ECGs Made Easy, ed 3, St. Louis, 2006, Mosby.

3-45 Shade B, Rothenberg M, Wertz E, Jones S, and Collins T: Mosby's EMT-Intermediate Textbook, ed 2, St. Louis, 2002, Mosby.

3-46 Grauer K: A Practical Guide to ECG Interpretation, ed 2, St. Louis, 1998, Mosby.

3-47 Shade B, Rothenberg M, Wertz E, Jones S, Collins T: Mosby's EMT-Intermediate Textbook, ed 2, St. Louis, 2002, Mosby.

3-48, 3-49 Aehlert B: ECGs Made Easy Study Cards, St. Louis, 2004, Mosby.

3-50 Aehlert B: ECGs Made Easy, ed 3, St. Louis, 2006, Mosby.

3-51 Shade B, Rothenberg M, Wertz E, Jones S, Collins T: Mosby's EMT-Intermediate Textbook, ed 2, St. Louis, 2002, Mosby.

3-52, 3-53, 3-54 Aehlert B: ECGs Made Easy, ed 3, St. Louis, 2006, Mosby.

3-55 Shade B, Rothenberg M, Wertz E, Jones S, Collins T: Mosby's EMT-Intermediate Textbook, ed 2, St. Louis, 2002, Mosby.

3-56 Aehlert B: ECGs Made Easy, ed 3, St. Louis, 2006, Mosby.

3-57 Shade B, Rothenberg M, Wertz E, Jones S, Collins T: Mosby's EMT-Intermediate Textbook, ed 2, St. Louis, 2002, Mosby.

3-58 Aehlert B: ECGs Made Easy Study Cards, St. Louis, 2004, Mosby.

3-59, 3-60, 3-61: Aehlert B: ECGs Made Easy, ed 3, St. Louis, 2006, Mosby.

3-62 Grauer K: A Practical Guide to ECG Interpretation, ed 2, St. Louis, 1998, Mosby.

3-63 Shade B, Rothenberg M, Wertz E, Jones S, Collins T: Mosby's EMT-Intermediate Textbook, ed 2, St. Louis, 2002, Mosby.

3-64 Aehlert B: ECGs Made Easy Study Cards, St. Louis, 2004, Mosby.

3-65, 3-66, 3-67 Aehlert B: ECGs Made Easy, ed 3, St. Louis, 2006, Mosby.

3-68 Aehlert B: ECGs Made Easy Study Cards, St. Louis, 2004, Mosby.

3-69 Aehlert B: ECGs Made Easy, ed 3, St. Louis, 2006, Mosby.

3-70 Aehlert B: ECGs Made Easy Study Cards, St. Louis, 2004, Mosby.

3-71, 3-72 Aehlert B: ECGs Made Easy, ed 3, St. Louis, 2006, Mosby.

3-73 Aehlert B: ECGs Made Easy Study Cards, St. Louis, 2004, Mosby.

3-74, 3-75, 3-76, 3-77: Aehlert B: ECGs Made Easy, ed 3, St. Louis, 2006, Mosby.

3-78 Grauer K: A Practical Guide to ECG Interpretation, ed 2, St. Louis, 1998, Mosby.

3-79, 3-80, 3-81 Aehlert B: ECGs Made Easy, ed 3, St. Louis, 2006, Mosby.

3-82 Grauer K: A Practical Guide to ECG Interpretation, ed 2, St. Louis, 1998, Mosby.

3-83, 3-84, 3-85, 3-86, 3-87 Aehlert B: ECGs Made Easy Study Cards, St. Louis, 2004, Mosby.

3-88 Grauer K: A Practical Guide to ECG Interpretation, ed 2, St. Louis, 1998, Mosby.

3-89, 3-90, 3-91 Aehlert B: ECGs Made Easy Study Cards, St. Louis, 2004, Mosby.

Chapter 4

4-1 Flynn J: Introduction to Critical Care Skills, St. Louis, 1993, Mosby.

4-2 Courtesy Medtronic Emergency Response Systems.

4-3A EMSC Slide Set (CD-ROM). 1996. Courtesy the Emergency Medical Services for Children Program, administered by the U.S. Department of Health and Human Service's Health Resources and Services Administration, Maternal and Child Health Bureau.

4-3B Courtesy Medtronic Emergency Response Systems.

4-5, 4-6 Flynn J: Introduction to Critical Care Skills, St. Louis, 1993, Mosby.

4-12 Shade B, Rothenberg M, Wertz E, Jones S, Collins T: Mosby's EMT-Intermediate Textbook, ed 2, St. Louis, 2002, Mosby.

4-13 Courtesy Philips Medical Systems.

4-14 Chapleau W: Emergency First Responder: Making the Difference, St. Louis, 2004, Mosby.

4-15 Sanders M: Mosby's Paramedic Textbook, ed 3, St. Louis, 2005, Mosby.

4-16 Aehlert B: Mosby's Comprehensive Pediatric Emergency Care, St. Louis, 2005, Mosby.

4-17, 4-18 Aehlert B: ECGs Made Easy, ed 3, St. Louis, 2006, Mosby.

Chapter 5

5-1, 5-2 Shade B, Rothenberg M, Wertz E, Jones S, Collins T: Mosby's EMT-Intermediate Textbook, ed 2, St. Louis, 2002, Mosby.

5-3 Drake R, Vogl W, Mitchell A: Gray's Anatomy for Students, Philadelphia, 2005, Churchill Livingstone.

5-4 Sanders M: Mosby's Paramedic Textbook, ed 3, St. Louis, 2005, Mosby.

5-5, 5-6, 5-7 Drake R, Vogl W, Mitchell A: Gray's Anatomy for Students, Philadelphia, 2005, Churchill Livingstone.

5-8, 5-9, 5-10, 5-11 Reprinted with permission from Ethicon, Inc.

5-12A Courtesy Pyng Corporation.

5-12B Courtesy Vidacare Corporation.

5-13, 5-14 Sanders M: Mosby's Paramedic Textbook, ed 3, St. Louis, 2005, Mosby.

5-15 Weiderhold R: Electrocardiography: The Monitoring & Diagnostic Leads, ed 2, Philadelphia, 1999, Saunders.

5-16 Sanders M: Mosby's Paramedic Textbook, ed 3, St. Louis, 2005, Mosby.

5-17 Weiderhold R: Electrocardiography: The Monitoring & Diagnostic Leads, ed 2, Philadelphia, 1999, Saunders.

Chapter 6

6-1 Herlihy B, Maebius N: The Human Body in Health and Illness, ed 2, St. Louis, 2003, Saunders.

6-2 Modified and redrawn from Schoen FJ: Interventional and Surgical Cardiovascular Pathology: Clinical Correlations and Basic Principles. Philadelphia, 1989, Saunders.

6-3 Goldman L, Braunwald E: Primary Cardiology, Philadelphia, 1998, Saunders.

6-4 Falk, Anderson: Pathology of Atherosclerotic Plaque: Stable, Unstable, and Infarctional. In Roubin G, Califf R, O'Neill W (editors): Interventional Cardiovascular Medicine: Principles and Practice, New York, 1994, Churchill Livingstone. pp. 57-88.

6-5 Phalen T, Aehlert B: The 12-Lead ECG in Acute Coronary Syndromes, ed 2, St. Louis, 2006, Mosby.

6-6 Herlihy B, Maebius N: The Human Body in Health and Illness, ed 2, St. Louis, 2003, Saunders.

6-7, 6-8, 6-9, 6-10 Urden L, Stacy K, Lough M: Thelan's Critical Care Nursing: Diagnosis and Management, ed 4, St. Louis, 2006, Mosby.

6-11 Aehlert B: ECGs Made Easy, ed 3, St. Louis, 2006, Mosby.

6-12 Butler HA, Caplin M, McCaully E, et al (editors): Managing Major Diseases: Cardiac Disorders vol 2, St. Louis, 1999, Mosby

6-13 Sanders M: Mosby's Paramedic Textbook, ed 3, St. Louis, 2005, Mosby.

6-14 Grauer K: A Practical Guide to ECG Interpretation, ed 2, St. Louis, 1998, Mosby.

6-15, 6-16, 6-17, 6-18, 6-19, 6-20, 6-21 Phalen T, Aehlert B: The 12-Lead ECG in Acute Coronary Syndromes, ed 2, St. Louis, 2006, Mosby.

6-22 Surawicz B, Knilans TK: Chou's electrocardiography in clinical practice: adult and pediatric, ed 5, Philadelphia, 1996, Saunders.

6-23, 6-24, 6-25 Phalen T, Aehlert B: The 12-Lead ECG in Acute Coronary Syndromes, ed 2, St. Louis, 2006, Mosby.

6-26 Grauer K: A Practical Guide to ECG Interpretation, ed 2, St. Louis, 1998, Mosby.

6-27, 6-28 Phalen T, Aehlert B: The 12-Lead ECG in Acute Coronary Syndromes, ed 2, St. Louis, 2006, Mosby.

6-29 2005 American Heart Association Guidelines for Cardiopulmonary Resuscitation and Emergency Cardiovascular Care, Part 8: Stabilization of the Patient With Acute Coronary Syndromes. *Circulation* 2005;112(suppl IV):IV-90.

6-30 Shade B, Rothenberg M, Wertz E, Jones S, Collins T: Mosby's EMT-Intermediate Textbook, ed 2, St. Louis, 2002, Mosby.

6-31 Urden L, Stacy K, Lough M: Thelan's Critical Care Nursing: Diagnosis and Management, ed 5, St. Louis, 2006, Mosby.

6-32 Henry M, Stapleton E: EMT Prehospital Care, ed 3, St. Louis, 2004, Mosby.

Chapter 7

7-1 Thibodeau G, Patton K: Anatomy & Physiology, ed 5, St. Louis, 2003, Mosby.

7-2 Huether S, McCance K: Understanding Pathophysiology, ed 3, St. Louis, 2004, Mosby.

7-3 Thibodeau G, Patton K: Anatomy & Physiology, ed 5, St. Louis, 2003, Mosby.

7-6: Shade B, Rothenberg M, Wertz E, Jones S, Collins T: Mosby's EMT-Intermediate Textbook, ed 2, St. Louis, 2002, Mosby.

7-7 Courtesy National Institute of Neurological Disorders and Stroke: National Institutes of Health.

7-8, 7-9 Grauer K: A Practical Guide to ECG Interpretation, ed 2, St. Louis, 1998, Mosby.

7-13 Huether S, McCance K: Understanding Pathophysiology, ed 3, St. Louis, 2004, Mosby.

7-14, 7-15 Gould B: Pathophysiology for the Health Professions, ed 2, Philadelphia, 2002, Saunders.

7-16: Pre-Hospital Trauma Life Support Committee of the National Association of Emergency Medical Technicians in Cooperation with the Committee on Trauma of the American College of Surgeons: Pre-Hospital Trauma Life Support, ed 5, St. Louis, 2003, Mosby.

7-17 Gould B: Pathophysiology for the Health Professions, ed 2, Philadelphia, 2002, Saunders.

7-18 Sanders M: Mosby's Paramedic Textbook, ed 3, St. Louis, 2005, Mosby.

7-19 Gould B: Pathophysiology for the Health Professions, ed 2, Philadelphia, 2002, Saunders.

Chapter 8

8-1, 8-2: Cummins R: ACLS Scenarios: Core Concepts for Case-Based Learning, St. Louis, 1996, Mosby Year-Book.

8-3, 8-4 Goldberger A: Clinical Electrocardiography: A Simplified Approach, ed 6, St. Louis, 1999, Mosby.

8-5 2005 American Heart Association Guidelines for Cardiopulmonary Resuscitation and Emergency Cardiovascular Care, Part 7.2: Management of Cardiac Arrest. *Circulation* 2005:112(suppl IV):IV-58.

8-6, 8-7 Aehlert B: ECGs Made Easy Study Cards, St. Louis, 2004, Mosby.

8-8, 8-9: Cummins R: ACLS Scenarios: Core Concepts for Case-Based Learning. St. Louis, 1996. Mosby Year-Book.

8-10 Sanders M: Mosby's Paramedic Textbook, ed 3, St. Louis, 2005, Mosby.

8-11 2005 American Heart Association Guidelines for Cardiopulmonary Resuscitation and Emergency Cardiovascular Care, Part 7.2: Management of Cardiac Arrest. *Circulation* 2005:112(suppl IV):IV-58.

8-12, 8-13, 8-14, 8-15, 8-16, 8-17, 8-18, 8-19 Aehlert B: ECGs Made Easy Study Cards, St. Louis, 2004, Mosby.

8-20 2005 American Heart Association Guidelines for Cardiopulmonary Resuscitation and Emergency Cardiovascular Care, Part 7.3: Management of Symptomatic Bradycardia and Tachycardia. *Circulation* 2005:112(suppl IV):IV-68.

8-21 Aehlert B: ECGs Made Easy Study Cards, St. Louis, 2004, Mosby.

8-22 Cummins R: ACLS Scenarios: Core Concepts for Case-Based Learning, St. Louis, 1996, Mosby Year-Book.

8-23, 8-24 Aehlert B: ECGs Made Easy Study Cards, St. Louis, 2004, Mosby.

8-25 Aehlert B: ECGs Made Easy, ed 3, St. Louis, 2006, Mosby.

8-26 Goldberger A: Clinical Electrocardiography: A Simplified Approach, ed 6, St. Louis, 1999, Mosby.

8-27 2005 American Heart Association Guidelines for Cardiopulmonary Resuscitation and Emergency Cardiovascular Care, Part 7.3: Management of Symptomatic Bradycardia and Tachycardia. *Circulation* 2005:112(suppl IV):IV-70.

8-28 Goldberger A: Clinical Electrocardiography: A Simplified Approach, ed 6, St. Louis, 1999, Mosby.

8-29, 8-30 Aehlert B: ECGs Made Easy Study Cards, St. Louis, 2004, Mosby.

8-31 2005 American Heart Association Guidelines for Cardiopulmonary Resuscitation and Emergency Cardiovascular Care, Part 7.3: Management of Symptomatic Bradycardia and Tachycardia. *Circulation* 2005:112(suppl IV):IV-70.

8-32 Aehlert B: ECGs Made Easy Study Cards, St. Louis, 2004, Mosby.

8-33 Goldberger A: Clinical Electrocardiography: A Simplified Approach, ed 6, St. Louis, 1999, Mosby.

8-34 Aehlert B: ECGs Made Easy, ed 2, St. Louis, 2002, Mosby.

8-35 Aehlert B: ECGs Made Easy Study Cards, St. Louis, 2004, Mosby.

8-36 2005 American Heart Association Guidelines for Cardiopulmonary Resuscitation and Emergency Cardiovascular Care, Part 7.3: Management of Symptomatic Bradycardia and Tachycardia. *Circulation* 2005:112(suppl IV):IV-70.

8-37, 8-38 Aehlert B: ECGs Made Easy Study Cards, St. Louis, 2004, Mosby.

8-39 Sanders M: Mosby's Paramedic Textbook, ed 3, St. Louis, 2005, Mosby.

8-40 2005 American Heart Association Guidelines for Cardiopulmonary Resuscitation and Emergency Cardiovascular Care, Part 8: Stabilization of the Patient With Acute Coronary Syndromes. *Circulation* 2005;112(suppl IV):IV-90.

8-41, 8-42 Antman EM, Armstrong DT, Armstrong PW, et al: ACC/AHA Guidelines for the Management of Patients with ST-Elevation Myocardial Infarction: A Report of the American College of Cardiology/American Heart Association Task Force on Practice Guidelines (Committee to Revise the 1999 Guidelines for the Management of Patients with Acute Myocardial Infarction). 2004. Available at www.acc.org/clinical/guidelines/stemi/index.pdf. Accessed 01/23/06

8-43 Aehlert B: ECGs Made Easy Study Cards, St. Louis, 2004, Mosby.

8-44 Phalen T, Aehlert B: The 12-Lead ECG in Acute Coronary Syndromes, ed 2, St. Louis, 2006, Mosby.

8-45, 8-46 Aehlert B: ECGs Made Easy Study Cards, St. Louis, 2004, Mosby.

Chapter 9

All illustrations from Aehlert B: ECGs Made Easy Study Cards, St. Louis, 2004, Mosby, with the exception of Case 6 Rhythm 1 from Phalen T, Aehlert B: The 12-Lead ECG in Acute Coronary Syndromes, ed 2, St. Louis, 2006, Mosby.

Posttest

(unnumbered figures in order of appearance)

1 Phalen T, Aehlert B: The 12-Lead ECG in Acute Coronary Syndromes, ed 2, St. Louis, 2006, Mosby.

2 Sanders M: Mosby's Paramedic Textbook, ed 3, St. Louis, 2005, Mosby.

3 through 7 Aehlert B: ECGs Made Easy Study Cards, St. Louis, 2004, Mosby.

Index*

*Note: Page numbers followed by *f* indicate figures; those followed
by *t* indicate tables; those followed by *b* indicated boxed material.